AF327287

MR
and imaging
of the
FEMALE PELVIS

MR
and imaging
of the
FEMALE PELVIS

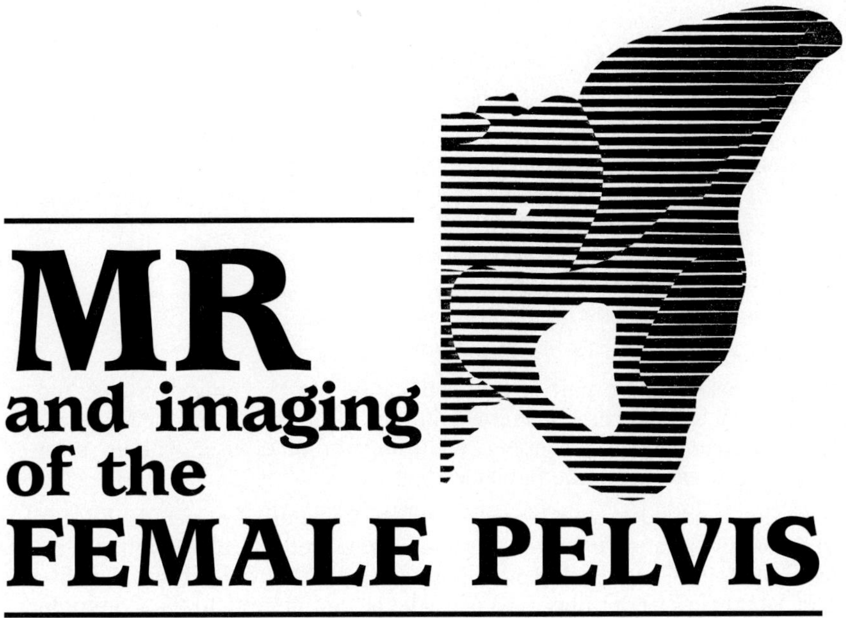

Clare M.C. Tempany, M.D.

Assistant Professor of Diagnostic Radiology
Harvard Medical School
Director of Body MRI, Department of Radiology
Brigham and Women's Hospital
Boston, Massachusetts

Mosby

St. Louis Baltimore Berlin Boston Carlsbad Chicago London Madrid
Naples New York Philadelphia Sydney Tokyo Toronto

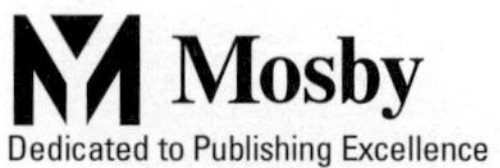

Mosby
Dedicated to Publishing Excellence

Executive Editor: Susan M. Gay
Developmental Editor: Sandra Clark Brown
Project Manager: Linda Clarke
Project Supervisor: Victoria Hoenigke
Manufacturing Supervisor: Karen Lewis
Book Designer: Sheilah Barrett

Printed in the United States of America
Composition by Graphic World
Printing/binding by Maple Vail

Mosby–Year Book, Inc.
11830 Westline Industrial Drive
St. Louis, MO 63146

Library of Congress Cataloging-in-Publication Data

MR and imaging of the female pelvis / [edited by] Clare M.C. Tempany.
     p.   cm.
   Includes bibliographical references and index.
   ISBN 1-55664-387-X
    1. Generative organs, Female—Magnetic resonance imaging.
  2. Genitourinary organs—Magnetic resonance imaging. I. Tempany, Clare M. C.
    [DNLM: 1. Genitalia, Female—anatomy & histology. 2. Magnetic Resonance Imaging—methods. 3. Genital Diseases, Female—diagnosis. 4. Pelvis—anatomy & histology.   WP 101 M939 1995]
   RG107.5.M34M7 1995
   618.1′07548—dc20
   DNLM/DLC
   for Library of Congress   94-32427
                                 CIP

95 96 97 98 / 9 8 7 6 5 4 3 2 1

Contributors

Stephen J. Blackband, Ph.D.
Senior Lecturer
MRI Center
Hull Royal Infirmary
England

Douglas L. Brown, M.D.
Assistant Professor of Radiology
Department of Radiology
Brigham and Women's Hospital
Harvard Medical School
Boston, Massachusetts

Richard A. Cooper, M.D.
Associate Professor of Radiology and Anatomy
Department of Diagnostic Radiology
Loyola Strich School of Medicine
Loyola University Medical Center
Maywood, Illinois

Julia Rose Fielding, M.D.
Instructor
Department of Radiology
Harvard Medical School
Radiologist
Brigham and Women's Hospital
Boston, Massachusetts

Karen Margaret Horton, M.D.
Resident
Department of Radiology
The Johns Hopkins University School of
    Medicine
Baltimore, Maryland

Ronald A. Morton, Jr., M.D.
Instructor
Department of Urology
The Johns Hopkins University School of
    Medicine
Baltimore, Maryland

Mary C. Olson, M.D.
Associate Professor
Department of Radiology
Loyola University Medical Center
Stritch School of Medicine
Maywood, Illinois

Harold Victor Posniak, M.D.
Associate Professor
Department of Radiology
Loyola University Medical Center
Stritch School of Medicine
Maywood, Illinois

Mitchell D. Schnall, M.D., Ph.D.
Associate Professor
Department of Radiology
The Hospital of the University of Pennsylvania
Philadelphia, Pennsylvania

Stuart George Silverman, M.D.
Assistant Professor
Harvard Medical School
Head, Uroradiology
Brigham and Women's Hospital
Boston, Massachusetts

Clare M.C. Tempany, M.D.
Assistant Professor of Diagnostic Radiology
Harvard Medical School
Director of Body MRI, Department of Radiology
Brigham and Women's Hospital
Boston, Massachusetts

Naveed Yousuf, M.D.
Clinical Fellow of Radiology
Harvard Medical School
Brigham and Women's Hospital
Boston, Massachusetts

This work is dedicated
*to my husband **Nezam***
and daughter
Sophie.

MR of the female pelvis now plays a major role in imaging patients with gynecologic diseases. Because of its high resolution, multiplanar capabilities, and relatively noninvasive nature, MRI has replaced or become complementary to other imaging modalities and surgical diagnostic procedures, such as diagnostic laparoscopy. There have been major advances in MR technology, with improvements in magnet hardware and more particularly, in surface coil technology with multicoil array systems (phased array coils), which have led to these increases in clinical applications. These have been further expanded by the introduction of intravenous, and now, oral contrast agents. These rapid developments in the technology have slowed more recently, allowing for stability and a more critical assessment of the appropriate applications of MRI. In the future, the applications of MR in the female pelvis appear to be in the field of image-guided, minimally invasive therapy.

This book is intended to provide the reader with a comprehensive review of the applications of MR imaging in gynecology. This is done with reference to other imaging modalities where indicated, following the natural divisions of the organs of the female genital tract. While it is primarily intended for radiologists both in training and in daily practice, it is also intended to be of value to obstetricians and gynecologists. This book has been written by each author according to their own "how I do it" approaches. It is not intended to be encyclopedic, nor to replace many of the excellent texts which cover the other imaging modalities, such as ultrasound or computed tomography, in greater detail. The intent is to provide the reader with the current, up-to-date approaches in clinical practice and even some that are still being researched in a "preclinical" phase (specifically, the applications of intracavitary coils for imaging the cervix). Both body coil and multicoil (phased array) images and, where possible, the pathology correlations, are presented throughout the book.

The initial chapters provide the reader with a comprehensive overview of the physical principles behind NMR and MRI. The same chapter also focuses on the methods available to maximize image quality. There is a review of the normal MR anatomy of the pelvis and a chapter describing the different imaging techniques (e.g. pulse sequences, coils, contrast agents). It also provides actual clinical imaging protocols that can be utilized. These are reviewed in general in this chapter and in more detail in the chapters on the organ under discussion. Throughout the book, the predominant emphasis is on MRI, but other applicable imaging studies are included as indicated. Specifically, a review of transabdominal and transvaginal ultrasound with color flow Doppler application is included in the chapter on imaging of the adnexa and the ovaries. Applications and correlations with hysterosalpingography are included for evaluation of benign diseases and conditions of infertility. With the kind permission of Springer-Verlag, I have included an appendix, which contains exerts from their "TNM Atlas." These illustrate the staging systems for gynecologic malignancies according to both the TNM and the International Federation of Gynecology and Obstetrics (FIGO).

All of the co-authors have provided excellent contributions, representing their broad experiences and the current clinical applications in their own practices. Without these contributions, this book would not have been possible, and a very sincere debt of gratitude is due to all of them.

Sincere thanks are due to my teachers and mentors for their superb teaching and guidance and especially for passing on their great enthusiasm for radiology in general and MRI in particular. These include Dr. Leon Love (Loyola University of Chicago), Dr. R.N. Bryan, and Dr. S.J. Zinreich (Johns Hopkins Medical Institutions). In particular, sincere gratitude is due to Dr. Elias Zerhouni, who was my first and foremost teacher and mentor in this exciting area of imaging. His persistence led to my understanding of the clinical and diagnostic demands of MR, which in turn have led to a most rewarding relationship with the obstetrician/gynecologists, to whom I am also indebted, both at John Hopkins Medical Institutes and the Brigham and Women's Hospital. They have provided excellent clinical correlation, continued interest, and support in this project. I am also grateful for the secretarial assistance provided by Nola Miller (Johns Hopkins Medical Institutions) and Sue McLaughlin (Brigham and Women's Hospital).

A particular acknowledgement is due to my many colleagues over the years who have very kindly shared their insight and their cases with me. Specific thanks are due to Drs. Alex Chaco, Ron Lee, Lawrence Schwartz, and Oliver Pomeroy for their great help and many contributions. I also acknowledge the original support and encouragement of Dana Dreibelbis (previously of BC Decker) and the editorial staff of Mosby-Year Book.

I would also like to thank Don Sucher, Children's Hospital, Boston, for his skillful photographing of many of the illustrations.

Clare M.C. Tempany

Contents

MR
and imaging
of the
FEMALE PELVIS

1 Introduction to the Physical Principles of NMR and MRI

Stephen J. Blackband

Many texts are now available that discuss nuclear magnetic resonance (NMR)[1-6] and magnetic resonance imaging (MRI)[7-12] techniques and applications in detail. There are also numerous clinical texts with a brief introductory chapter describing the basic principles of MRI. Rather than producing yet another similar introductory chapter, I propose, after a cursory review of the basic principles of MRI, to look in more detail at two aspects: phase encoding and the factors controlling the signal-to-noise ratio (SNR) in the MR images. In my experience, these aspects are the sources of greatest confusion and misunderstanding among clinicians. In particular, while frequency encoding is often easily grasped since it is analogous to projections used in computed tomography (CT) x-ray

scanning, phase encoding often remains something of a mystery. It is hoped that this chapter will give a physical feel for what phase encoding is and how it works.

Key words and phrases have been italicized. References are minimal and constrained to published texts rather than papers (except one). The author recommends an examination of these texts before the reader plunges into the voluminous journal publications.

NUCLEAR MAGNETIC RESONANCE

MRI methods are based on NMR spectroscopic principles, needing only the introduction of gradients in order to spatially encode the NMR signal so that an image may be produced. Before NMR imaging techniques are described, it is therefore essential to understand the basics of the NMR phenomenon. The following sections discuss NMR in a basic but, it is hoped, illuminating fashion, and with the exception of a couple of fundamental relationships, no mathematics is introduced.

NMR signal

The following sections offer a classic representation of NMR, albeit one often used and simplistic. It is worth noting, however, that this is only a model and it cannot be used to understand or describe all features of NMR. A proper understanding of the phenomenon of NMR requires a quantum mechanical description that for the uninitiated is mathematically intense and difficult. Fortunately, the classic model is adequate for an appreciation of most aspects of NMR imaging, and is used exclusively in this chapter.

Nuclei, spins, and magnets. As a starting point, I will introduce several basic physical concepts arising from classic electromagnetism.[13] It is known that although static charges do not generate magnetic fields, moving charges have magnetic fields associated with them. A current moving down a wire produces a magnetic field—a property that is used to make electric motors work. The protons in the nuclei of atoms are charged particles, i.e., they have intrinsic electric fields associated with them. These protons also have an intrinsic property known as angular momentum. These protons are spinning (the angular momentum) and charged with an electric field, and thus are in themselves little moving charges. Consequently, they have their own associated magnetic field called the *magnetic moment* of the protons. The sum of the proton magnetic moments within the nucleus may then be regarded as a single entity called the nuclear magnetic moment. This nuclear magnetic moment is extremely small and has associated with it a direction corresponding to the north and south polarities familiar to us in simple bar magnets. In most materials, these nuclear magnetic moments or nuclear bar magnets are randomly oriented. On average, then, their fields cancel each other out (each north pole is balanced by an opposing south pole), and the material has no net magnetic moment. Some special materials, such as iron, have an internal structure that automatically aligns the nuclear magnetic moments, producing a net magnetic moment. These materials are called ferromagnetic and are used to make the permanent magnets we are familiar with. In general, however, this is not the case; certainly water, for example, has no net magnetic moment.

If, however, we place a normally nonmagnetic material inside a very strong magnetic field, the small magnetic moments in the material will align parallel or antiparallel to that field. Slightly more nuclei align parallel to the field (around one in 1 million), resulting in a small net excess of spins pointing along the field. This excess is small but nevertheless results in the material being "magnetized," or having a net magnetic moment that we label M_0. The stronger the applied field, the larger this excess of spins will be. Consequently, we generally use a strong magnetic field for NMR experiments with respect to practical compromises (discussed later). The magnetic field strength is given in units of tesla (T), and a typical clinical magnet today has a field strength of 0.5 to 2T. (The earth's field is about 2×10^{-5}T, so these magnets are around 100,000 times stronger than the earth's magnetic field that is seen influencing a compass needle.) We label this applied *static magnetic field* with the symbol B_0.

As described so far, the net magnetic moment produced in the material is parallel with the applied magnetic field. Since this moment is over 1 million times smaller than that main field, we cannot detect it on top of that extremely large applied field. So how do we measure this net magnetic moment? Detection of the moments may be achieved by tipping the spins away from the B_0 axis, as I shall now describe.

Precession. Now suppose that our spins are not

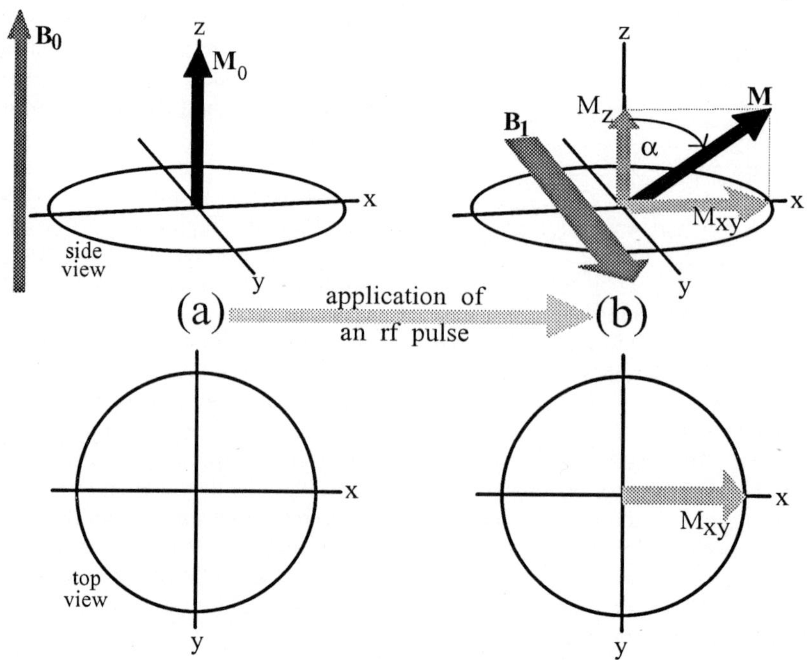

Fig. 1-1 (a), Magnetization (M), initially at equilibrium and aligned along B_0, can be tipped **(b)** into the transverse plane by application of a perpendicular B_1 field. M moves perpendicular to both B_0 and B_1.

aligned with B_0 but are tipped somehow away from B_0, as shown in Fig. 1-1. Remember that our nuclei are not actually bar magnets but small spinning entities with an associated charge. When tipped away from the direction of the applied field, the nuclei rotate around the axis of the applied field. This is equivalent to the motion observed with a child's spinning top if it is tipped off its axis a little. The top also rotates in a circular fashion around the vertical or central axis, and in this case the applied field is gravity. This rotational motion of a spinning object around a static applied field is called *precession*. The stronger the magnetic field the nuclei are placed in, the faster they will precess around it. (Similarly, if gravity were stronger, the child's spinning top would precess faster. Would a child's top precess in space where there is no gravity?) Further, the faster the nuclei are spinning around their own axis, the faster they will precess around B_0. (Similarly, the faster you get the child's top to spin, the faster it will precess. Would the top precess if it were not spinning?)

The above paragraph can be reiterated in NMR terminology. The frequency at which the spins precess, i.e., the number of times per second that the spins travel full circle around the B_0 field, is directly proportional to the strength of the magnetic field, B_0, in which the spins are placed:

$$2\pi f = \omega = \gamma B_0 \qquad \text{(Eq.1)}$$

where f is the frequency in hertz (rotations per unit time), which when multiplied by 2π gives the frequency in radians (2π radians is equivalent to 360 degrees). γ (gamma) is the gyromagnetic ratio and is a measure of how fast a particular nuclear type spins; e.g., the ^1H nucleus has a different γ to the ^{31}P, ^{23}Na, and ^{13}C nuclei. Roughly, the smaller the nucleus, the higher the gyromagnetic ratio will be (in effect, smaller nuclei can spin faster). ^1H has one of the highest gyromagnetic ratios and thus resonates at one of the highest frequencies in a given magnetic field.

Resonance condition. Suppose that the magnetic moments were aligned not with B_0 but at an angle to it, as described above. The spins would precess around B_0. Suppose we then place a copper wire near the spins. The magnetic field produced by the spins in the region of the wire is continuously increasing and decreasing as the precessional motion of the spins moves them closer to, and then farther away from, the wire. Classic electromagnetism tells us that a changing magnetic field induces a current in a wire (note that this is the reverse of the situation in which a moving electric field generates a magnetic field to work a motor). By measuring the current produced in the

wire, we would be able to detect the spins. The more spins there were, or the bigger their magnetic moments, the more electric current we would measure. How then can we knock or tip the spins so that they are no longer aligned along B_0 but precess around it so that we can detect them?

In order to tip the spins so as to detect the induced current, a second magnetic field is applied perpendicular to the main field, the effect of which is to push or tip the net magnetic moment away from the main field. This is illustrated in Fig. 1-1, and this perpendicular magnetic field is labeled as B_1. Note that in a similar fashion to that in which the spins precess *around* B_0, the spins rotate *around* B_1 and are thus tipped in the direction perpendicular to both B_0 and B_1. In three-dimensional space (x, y, and z coordinates) the z direction is parallel to the main field B_0 by convention. Spins pointing along B_0 are tipped away from the z axis and are thus tipped into the x-y plane, referred to as the *transverse plane*. The component of **M** that is in the transverse plane (i.e., the projection of M onto the transverse plane) is then referred to as the *transverse magnetization,* M_{xy}. Similarly the projection of **M** onto the z axis, M_z, is referred to as the *longitudinal magnetization.* After being tipped, the magnetic moment will precess around the main field, i.e., around the z axis. However, it is not sufficient to simply apply a second *static* perpendicular magnetic field to the spins because the energy transfer will be very inefficient.

To appreciate why the energy transfer would be inefficient, we may use the analogy of pushing young Molly around on a roundabout. Suppose Molly wants to go faster. This means that somehow you have to transfer energy into the roundabout to make it go faster. Suppose also that you are tired and don't want to run around pushing, but you do have a rather large wind machine that can blow air over a large area. To make the roundabout spin, Molly could hold a small sail to catch the wind and push the roundabout around. However, it would only push Molly around a little away from the wind machine, and after half a rotation Molly would then be facing into the wind and would be pushed back again. The wind would therefore simply rotate the roundabout until Molly was at the farthest point from the machine. Instead, we must place the wind machine on a track that circles the roundabout so that it moves around the roundabout at the same rate at which Molly is spinning. In that way the wind always faces into the sail, and Molly is continuously pushed. Note also that it is inefficient to have the wind machine move around at a faster or slower rate than Molly is rotating, because it will not face into the sail all the time. Thus, the wind machine must move around at the same rate or frequency at which the roundabout is rotating to ensure the most effective coupling with the roundabout to transfer energy to it.

So imagine that Molly is our spinning nucleus and that its rotation on the roundabout represents the precessional motion of the spin. The sail Molly is holding represents the magnetic moment that you need to "push." In order to efficiently transfer energy to the spin, the magnetic field that you use to push the spin must rotate at the same rate as the spin precesses. The applied perpendicular magnetic field must thus oscillate at the same frequency as the spin is precessing, i.e., at the resonant frequency of the spins. When this condition is satisfied, the applied magnetic field is termed to be *on resonance*. B_0 is then the applied static magnetic field, and B_1 is the applied and perpendicular *radiofrequency (rf)* magnetic field (i.e., rotating at the resonant frequency of the spins, which is in the megahertz range or radiofrequency range). Incidentally, we can also see from the Molly analogy why the applied rf field must be perpendicular to B_0: it would do us no good to blow wind into the ground or sky; it must blow perpendicular to the sky-ground axis.

Rotating frame of reference. Note that Fig. 1-1 has been drawn with the magnetic moments represented as static vectors, even though we know that they are precessing around B_0. This procedure is adopted to simplify the diagrams and also to simplify the mathematics. To appreciate the usefulness of this approach, imagine several children on a roundabout. If you were standing in the park watching the children, they would be rotating rapidly relative to your position, and describing where the children were would be difficult: you would have to use a time-dependent description of their position, the time dependence being related to the speed or frequency at which the roundabout turns (this is called the *laboratory frame of reference*). If the children then moved around on the roundabout, describing their positions would be very difficult. To make the children's positions simpler to describe, you could get on the roundabout yourself. The children would thus initially appear stationary relative to your position, and it would be easier to describe where they were. In effect, you have removed the necessity of including the time dependence due the roundabout's motion in your description (this is called the *rotating frame of reference*). If the children then move around on the roundabout, you need only describe their motion relative to your position. This "trick" also greatly simplifies the mathematics for the NMR, in that it is easier to describe the relative positions of the spin vectors in the rotating frame than to describe the laboratory frame of reference. We shall see later that we are concerned only with the rel-

ative positions (or phases) of the spin vectors for our description of imaging. We can then at any time transform from one frame to the other if required.

As we have seen, the rf pulse used to excite the spins must oscillate at the same frequency as the spins precess. Therefore, in the rotating frame of reference in which the magnetization vector appears static, the B_1 vector will also appear static, again simplifying the graphic representation (and the mathematics) of this process. The rotating reference frame will be used in the remainder of this chapter, and thus all spins resonating at ω_0 appear static on the vector diagrams.

Rf pulses and tip angles. How much energy can we put into the spins by this method and how much do we actually need? As we apply the B_1 field on resonance, the spins absorb energy and are tipped over into the x-y plane, creating the transverse magnetization. We may tip them through greater angles to the z axis by applying more energy, i.e., applying the rf pulse for a longer time. However, we are then going to try to detect the magnetic field produced by the spins that is perpendicular to the z axis, i.e., M_{xy} (note that we cannot detect signal that is parallel to the z axis and B_0). Consequently, the largest signal will be detected when the spins are at 90 degrees to the main field, B_0 (i.e., when $\mathbf{M} = M_{xy}$). We therefore apply a short burst of the B_1 field, referred to as an *rf pulse,* that is sufficient to tip the spins by 90 degrees. This is then referred to as a 90-degree rf pulse, and it excites maximal signal from the spins. Similarly, we may arrange to tip the spins by any amount, e.g., to the negative z direction using a 180-degree pulse (where there is thus no transverse magnetization and hence no signal) or the opposite direction in the x-y plane via a 270-degree pulse (maximal signal again), or indeed anything in between. The angle, α, through which the spins are tipped is known as the *tip angle* (Fig. 1-1).

Exciting and detecting the NMR signal. The rf pulse is applied by placing a coil of wire, the *rf transmitter coil,* around the sample, down which a radiofrequency alternating current is passed. The spins can now generate a signal, or have been *excited.* After the rf pulse is turned off, the spins freely precess in the static magnetic field, B_0, producing an oscillating magnetic field of their own. This spin-generated field is very small and may be detected by a second rf coil, the *rf receiver coil,* which is placed around the sample. It is often convenient to use the same physical coil for both transmission and reception, which we can thus term the rf transmitter/receiver coil. The current induced by the excited spins in the rf coil constitutes the NMR signal we detect and that we use to produce NMR spectra or images. Since the signal is small (microamperes or milliamperes at best), it is first amplified and then digitized for use by a computer in subsequent processing. The signal itself, if displayed on an oscilloscope, will appear as a small voltage oscillating in a sinusoidal fashion. The frequency of the sine wave will be equal to the resonant frequency of the spins. Thus, by measuring the frequency of the signal, we can tell which nucleus is in the magnet (since γ determines the frequency at which each nuclear type will precess). We see then that already our NMR machine is potentially useful: if an unknown material were placed in the magnet, we could tell what nuclear species (e.g., ^{1}H, ^{31}P, ^{13}C, ^{23}Na) it is made of. The size or amplitude of the signal we detect will tell us how much of that nuclear type is in the magnet, since a larger number of nuclei will induce a proportionately larger current in the receiver coil.

Summary. Spins inside a strong static magnetic field, B_0, can be excited from equilibrium by the application of a second perpendicular magnetic field, B_1, oscillating at the resonance frequency. The spins then precess and induce a voltage in a receiver coil. The spin system is easier to visualize in the rotating reference frame. Maximal signal is obtained after a 90 degree rf pulse.

T1 and T2 relaxation

Free induction decay. The excited magnetization precesses in the x-y plane after a 90-degree rf pulse, as briefly described, producing an oscillating voltage in a receiver coil. This precession (and hence the detected signal) does not continue indefinitely but decays away under *relaxation* processes. This relaxation occurs because of the interaction of the precessing nuclei with their environment, and is in effect a sort of "NMR friction." Although this may initially appear undesirable, it is this interaction with the environment that is responsible for the unique power of NMR, because differing environments cause differing amounts of signal decay. Thus, by measuring the signal decay, we can learn something about the environment the nuclei are in. These relaxation mechanisms also allow us to control the contrast in NMR images and distinguish differing pathologies in tissues. This oscillating voltage, which is varying in time, is called the *free induction decay (FID),* (Fig. 1-2), since it is induced in the NMR receiver by the freely precessing spins (B_1 is off) and decays over time under relaxation processes.

Spin-lattice relaxation, T1. The signal decay occurs via two independent relaxation processes. The first occurs because of an exchange of energy between the precessing spins and the molecular lattice in which they exist. This is called the *spin-lattice relaxation time,* or *T1.* The T1 relaxation represents the realignment of the spins with the

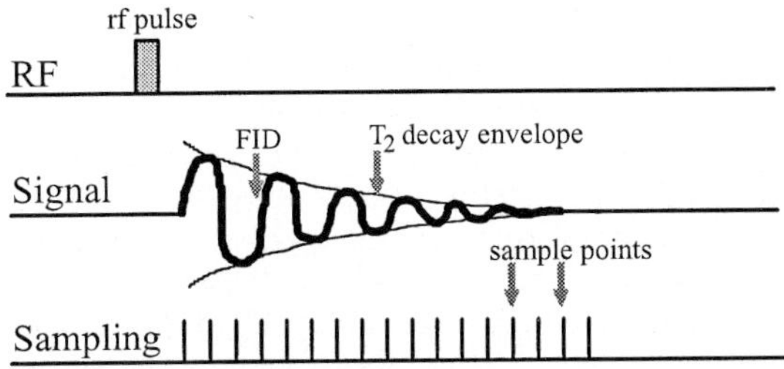

Fig. 1-2 Diagrammatic representation (pulse sequence) showing an rf excitation pulse generating a free induction decay (FID) that decays under T2 relaxation. This FID is digitized by discrete sample points for subsequent processing by computer.

magnetic field B_0 (i.e., the regrowth of M_z). This return of the magnetization along the z axis is exponential in nature, and the T1 time characterizes this exponential growth. T1 is in fact a time constant for the exponential curve and is the time it takes for 63% of the signal to return to equilibrium. (The time constant, T1, is equivalent to the half-life in radioactive decay, which is also exponential.) Nearly all the signal (99%) will have returned to equilibrium after approximately 5 times the T1 relaxation time.

Spin-spin relaxation, T2. The second relaxation mechanism occurs because of interactions between the precessing spins themselves and is called the *spin-spin relaxation time,* or *T2.* This relaxation can occur only when the spins are in the transverse (x-y) plane, i.e., when they have been tipped away from the z axis by an rf pulse. This is because while a particular spin precesses in the transverse plane, it is generating a changing magnetic field that influences nearby spins. Consequently, each spin experiences a small fluctuating magnetic field, causing them to precess at slightly different frequencies. This results in a gradual dephasing of the spins in the transverse plane, and the signal decays away. While the spins are aligned along the B_0 field, they do not generate a changing net transverse magnetic field, and consequently do not interact with each other, i.e., no T2 decay occurs. This signal loss is irreversible and exponential in nature, and T2 is the time constant that characterizes it (i.e., the time after which 63% of the signal has decayed away). On our rotating frame diagram (see Fig. 1-1), T2 decay would be represented by a shortening of the M_{xy} vector.

Clinical relaxation times. When T1 relaxation is complete, all the magnetization is realigned along B_0, and thus there can be no T2 decay (since there is no transverse magnetization). T2 must thus always be less than or equal to T1. In biologic tissues, T1 values are typically several times longer than T2 values. Typically, T1 varies from 0.3 to 1 second in biologic tissues at 1.5T, while T2 values are in the range of 20 to 100 msec. As a very rough rule of thumb, the more solid the material, the shorter is the T2. In liquids the molecules are generally relatively unbound and tumbling around. This reduces the spin-spin interaction, and thus T2 values are quite long. In solid materials the molecules are more tightly bound in a rigid lattice, and the spins interact much more strongly. In bone, for example, the T2 values are of the order of a few tens of microseconds. It is thus very difficult to image solid materials because the signal dies away so rapidly. Consequently, solid imaging is not clinically feasible and is unlikely to be so in the foreseeable future. (Note here that some success has been achieved imaging solids on very-small-diameter high-field magnets[14], and solid imaging is becoming a useful tool for materials research. However, tremendous gradient strengths and rf power requirements were necessitated. Currently, these requirements cannot technically or safely be met on larger clinical magnets.)

Since the T2 is always the faster relaxation mechanism for the spins and represents the loss of transverse magnetization, i.e., the loss of the oscillating magnetic field that produces our signal, we can see directly the T2 effect on the signal. Our signal without relaxation processes, as described above, is an oscillating sine wave as seen as a voltage induced in the receiver coil. Since the signal loss under T2 is exponential in nature, this sine wave signal will be damped out by an exponential envelope. The FID thus appears as an oscillating signal that decays away in amplitude, as illustrated in Fig. 1-2. This is exactly what you would see if the NMR receiver coil were hooked directly up to an oscilloscope.

Summary. Magnetization peturbed by an rf excitation pulse will decay back to equilibrium via spin-lattice (T_1) and spin-spin (T_2) interactions in an exponential manner. These relaxation times are characteristic of the nuclear environment.

NMR spectrum

So far I have described what happens if a particular nuclear type, e.g., the hydrogen nucleus ^{1}H, is placed in a magnetic field and excited. It will precess in the transverse plane at a frequency defined by γ and B_0. The precessing nucleus generates a magnetic field that induces a current in the NMR receiver (a coil of wire) placed around the sample. What we have thus detected is a signal at a defined frequency. If we then plot the frequency versus the amplitude of this signal, i.e., the frequency *spectrum,* it will consist of a single peak at that frequency, as shown in Fig. 1-3, *A.* The height or amplitude of this peak indicates the amount of sig-

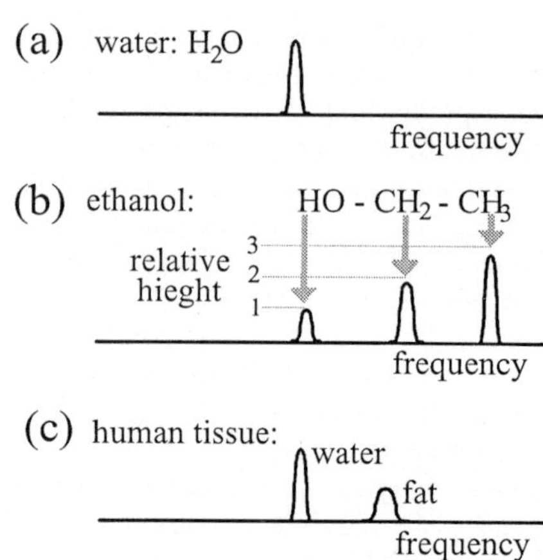

Fig. 1-3 (a), The protons in the hydrogen nucleus of water give rise to a frequency spectrum consisting of a single peak. **(b),** Ethanol contains three distinct hydrogen groups, producing a three-peak spectrum. The height of each peak indicates the relative numbers of hydrogen nuclei in each hydrogen group. **(c),** Most human tissues contain two ^{1}H resonances arising from the hydrogen nuclei in water and lipids.

nal, i.e., the number of ^{1}H nuclei that produced this signal. It is this signal that we will later encode in order to produce our image.

However, before I get to imaging, I will briefly describe what is called NMR spectroscopy, which involves the examination of these frequency spectra obtained from a sample. As just described, our spectrum isn't particularly useful. The frequency of the resonance peak tells us that ^{1}H is in the magnet, and the height of the peak tells us how much is there. Fortunately, however, things are far more interesting. It turns out that the environment of the ^{1}H nuclei can affect the frequency at which the nuclear spins resonate. The nucleus of an atom is surrounded by a cloud of electrons. This electron cloud acts as a small shield for the nucleus, so that the nucleus does not experience the full effect of the applied B_0 but experiences a slightly smaller field, $B_0 - \Delta B$, where ΔB is a small drop in field resulting from the electronic shielding effect. Consequently, the spins will not resonate at a frequency of $\omega_0 = \gamma B_0$ but at $\omega_c = \gamma(B_0 - \Delta B)$. The more electrons there are around the nucleus of the atom, the greater the shielding effect will be. The small difference in frequency, $\omega_0 - \omega_c$, caused by the shielding is called the *chemical shift.*

The exact chemical shift observed is characteristic of the chemical group that the nucleus is in. For example, a ^{1}H nucleus in an O-H chemical group will have a different electron cloud to the ^{1}H nuclei in, say, a C-H$_3$ chemical group. It will therefore resonate at a slightly different frequency when placed in a strong magnetic field. For example, Fig. 1-3, *B* shows the basic ^{1}H NMR spectrum of ethanol. These effects are small; e.g., the chemical shift frequency difference between the ^{1}H nuclei of water molecules and lipid molecules in biologic tissues is only approximately 200 Hz when the sample is placed in a 1.5T magnet in which ^{1}H nuclei resonate at around 63 MHz (Fig. 1-3, *C*). Nevertheless, with strong (>8T) and homogeneous magnets, differences of less than 0.1 Hz (one part in a billion!) can be detected on some solutions. Herein lies the power of NMR spectroscopy: we may take an unknown sample, place it in a magnet, and measure its frequency spectrum. This spectrum will then tell us what chemical groups the sample is made of and how much of each is in the sample. Furthermore, more subtle magnetic interactions cause additional perturbations in the spectrum. These perturbations provide additional information that allow us to establish which chemical groups are next to each other and what the bond angles and lengths between the groups are. With this type of information, we may determine the chemical structure of the solution. This unique capability has made NMR spectroscopy a mainstay of modern chemistry. Although the work is difficult, very complicated molecules that generate spectra consisting of literally hundreds of peaks can now be examined, and the structure of many complex biomolecules has been determined by means of NMR spectroscopic techniques.

Further discussion of spectroscopy is outside the scope of this text, and the reader is referred to the literature.[1-6] Suffice to say that it is on this base of spectroscopy that imaging is built. In biologic tissues, by far the most abundant NMR nuclei are the ^{1}H nuclei contained in molecules of water (approximately 66% of the body weight) and lipids. A spectrum of most human tissues usually consists of two resonances, one from fat and one from water, as shown in Fig. 1-3, *C*. Other ^{1}H-containing molecules (e.g., creatine, choline) are present only in millimolar concentrations (water is about 60 molar in body tissues, over 1 million times more concentrated). Because of its relative abundance, water gives by far the largest NMR signal from the human body, in fact so much signal that there is enough, when properly encoded, to form the wonderful high spatial resolution images you see in this book. For the remainder of this chapter, I shall concentrate almost exclusively on MRI of water in the human body. The reader may be aware that it is possible to produce NMR images using other nuclei in the body, such as sodium and phosphate. However, because of the lower abundance of these nuclei in tissue, the spatial resolution in the result-

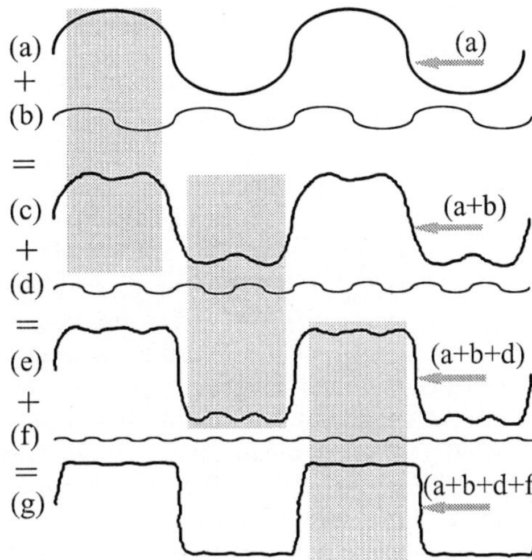

Fig. 1-4 This illustrates Fourier's theorem, which states that any periodic waveform, such as a square wave (g), can be generated from the sum of simple sinusoids of differing frequencies and amplitudes (a + b + d + f). Even "sharp"-looking waveforms can be made of a sum of "rounded"-looking waveforms.

ing images is relatively poor, and their clinical utility has not yet been established.

Fourier transform

Decoding complex time signals. Before we move on to NMR imaging, we require an understanding of one important mathematical tool. As described above, the NMR spectrum of a material can contain many frequency peaks. Consequently, the FID may be composed of several signals added together. The resultant FID is extremely complex, and it is not possible by simple visual inspection to say of what frequencies the FID is composed (or what the relative amplitudes of those signals are). We shall also see later that imaging is achieved by generating a large frequency range of signals that are added together to give a complex time signal. In both cases, some method of decoding these complex time signals into their component frequencies is required. This is achieved by the use of a mathematical relationship known as the *Fourier transform* (FT). The introduction of FT techniques revolutionized NMR spectroscopy in the early 1970s and is essential for modern NMR imaging. It is primarily for this work that Richard Ernst obtained the Nobel Prize in 1991.

Fourier's theorem. Fourier's theorem[15] states that *any periodic waveform can be produced by adding together the right combinations of simple sinusoidal waves.* For example, Fig. 1-4 illustrates how the addition of just four sinusoids of differing frequencies and amplitudes can approximate a square wave. Several sinusoids make a very good square wave. In a similar fashion, we can construct any waveform we like by adding together the right combinations of simple sine waves of appropriate frequencies and amplitudes. This is very convenient, since it is simple to build an electrical device that can produce a voltage that oscillates in a sine wave fashion with controlled and variable frequency. With several of these oscillators added together, we can synthesize any waveform we desire (e.g., a musical instrument referred to as a synthesizer does just this and can make many different waveforms of sounds by combining several different sinusoids). Mathematically, any periodic waveform, S(t), where (t) denotes this waveform to be a function of time, may be constructed by adding together n sinusoids, $a_n.\sin(n\pi f)$, where f is the frequency of that sine wave and a its amplitude:

$$S(t) = a_1.\sin(\pi f) + a_2.\sin(2\pi f) \qquad \textbf{(Eq.2)}$$
$$+ a_3.\sin(3\pi f) + a_4.\sin(4\pi f) + \cdots\cdots$$

We see then that the time wave may be related simply and mathematically to the sum of several waves of differing frequencies $(n\pi f)$ and amplitudes (a_n). This equation may be developed and manipulated under a set of well-defined rules,[15] leading to the FT. This transform takes a given time signal, e.g., the FID in NMR, and tells us what frequencies it is composed of. Further, now that we have a mathematical relation, we can use it both ways: not only can we construct any waveform from simple sine curves, but we may decompose any waveform into a set of its component sinusoids. The mathematical transform that works in this reverse sense is referred to as the *inverse Fourier transform (IFT)*.

We may use the FT to take our complicated NMR signal and decode it so that we know what frequencies it is composed of. For example, the FT of the square wave time signal in Fig. 1-4 would yield a frequency spectrum with four peaks in it. These four peaks correspond to the four frequencies of the four sinusoids that made up the square wave. The amplitudes of the four peaks represent the amplitudes of the four sine waves. Similarly, the IFT of the frequency spectrum would yield the square wave time signal again. Thus, we may use the FT to transform time into frequency, and vice versa. Since our square wave and our four-peak frequency spectrum are related through the FT (we may transform from one to the other), they are referred to as a *Fourier transform pair*. Note that these FT pairs are unique: only one particular time signal can produce a particular frequency spectrum, and vice versa.

Fourier transform pairs. Let us look at some typical examples of these FT pairs that are particularly useful in MRI. The transform pairs in the fol-

lowing example are illustrated in Fig. 1-5.

A sinusoid oscillating at a defined frequency will, upon Fourier transformation (FT), yield a frequency spectrum containing a single spike at that frequency (Fig. 1-5, *(a)*). This single spike is called a delta function. This spectrum tells us about the time signal: it says that the signal is made from one sine wave oscillating at a frequency f, and its height tells us how large that sine wave is, i.e., the signal intensity. In the reverse sense, the IFT of a delta function is a sine wave. The sine wave and a delta function thus constitute an FT pair. Fig. 1-5, *(b)* illustrates our square wave example, which produces a four-peak frequency spectrum. In Fig. 1-5, *(c)* the signal is complicated and hard to interpret. However, by looking at the spectrum obtained by FT, we can see that it is composed of several sinusoids of different frequencies and amplitudes. Later, we will see that it can be to our advantage to be able to "shape" the frequency profile of our spectrum. It turns out that a square-shaped frequency profile is produced by a sum of sinusoids that are sinc shaped (Fig. 1-5, *(d)*). Further, we may control the width of the square frequency profile by varying the duration of the sinc waveform. The shorter the time waveform, the wider is the frequency profile (Fig. 1-5, *(e)*), and vice versa (Fig. 1-5, *(f)*). This illustrates the inverse nature of the FT in that the wider the waveform in either the time or frequency domain, the narrower is the waveform in the other domain after the FT is performed. This inverse nature is apparent when we remember that for a given sine wave, $f = 1/t$ by definition (where t is the time for one full cycle of the sine wave).

The frequency spectrum of Fig. 1-5, *(g)* forms a half-circle in frequency space and was generated by FT of the very complicated time signal. This frequency spectrum would represent the projection of a circle (discussed later). A couple of these FT relationships are used in the following sections of this chapter.

Note that not all forms of MRI use Fourier techniques. However, the Fourier method makes it possible to be extremely efficient with regard to data collection, as we shall see later. Also, the FT is very amenable for implementation on a computer; in particular, there is a very fast algorithm, the fast Fourier transform (FFT), for calculating the Fourier transform extremely rapidly.[16]

Spin echo

Let us summarize briefly what has been said so far. In the most basic NMR experiments, an rf pulse is used to excite the spins in the sample. These excited spins precess in the magnetic field and induce an oscillating voltage, which can be detected in a receiver coil. The FT of this time signal or

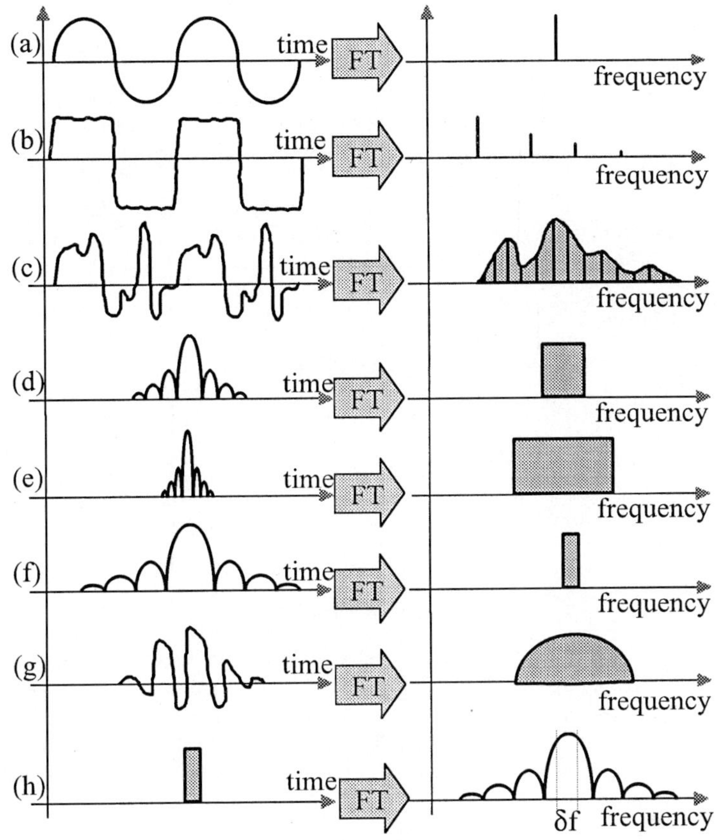

Fig. 1-5 Some Fourier transform pairs. The sinc pulse (d) that transforms into a square-shaped pulse is defined as sinc(x) = {sin(x)}/x.

FID produces the NMR spectrum. The spectrum tells us what frequencies the FID was composed of. If the sample is homogeneous and made principally of water, and is placed in a perfectly homogeneous magnetic field, all the ^{1}H nuclei will resonate at the same frequency, and the spectrum will be composed of one single peak corresponding to the resonant frequency of the water in that magnetic field. The signal will not last forever but will decay away under two distinct relaxation processes, T1 and T2, which are indicative of the environment of the nucleus.

However, the situation is not this ideal. A magnet is never perfectly homogeneous, and therefore the spins will never all resonate at exactly the same frequency: there will be a small distribution of frequencies corresponding to the degree of inhomogeneity in the magnet. For example, for ^{1}H nuclei in water in a 1.5T magnet, the resonant frequency is 63 MHz, and on a typical clinical magnet this will vary by a few tens of hertz across the bore of the magnet. It is very difficult to improve on this B_0 homogeneity of approximately 1 part in a million (1 ppm) and we have to live with it. Its effect, however, is to cause the FID to decay away

faster than T2 processes alone cause signal loss. This inhomogeneity decay mechanism is referred to as *T2** (T-two-star). Why does the signal decay away faster under T2* processes?

Magnet inhomogeneity and T2*. Spins tipped into the transverse plane will decay under T2 processes, as described above. We would represent this on the vector diagram (see Fig. 1-1) in the rotating reference frame as simply a shortening of the M_{xy} vector. As the vector shortens, less signal is induced in the receiver coil, and our signal thus decays away. So what happens when the magnetic field is inhomogeneous? As illustrated in Fig. 1-6, *(a)* and *(b)*, spins precessing slightly faster (S_{high}), which are in a slightly stronger part of the inhomogeneous magnetic field, move ahead of spins in a slightly-lower-strength magnetic field (S_{low}) (i.e., lower than B_0). We refer to the angle that the spin vector makes with the x-y axis as the *phase* of the spins. In the rotating frame of reference, we may then draw a vector diagram (Fig. 1-6) in which a positive phase is represented by the vector moving in the clockwise direction (away from spins resonating at B_0, which stay along the x axis). On the vector diagram the two groups of spins repre-

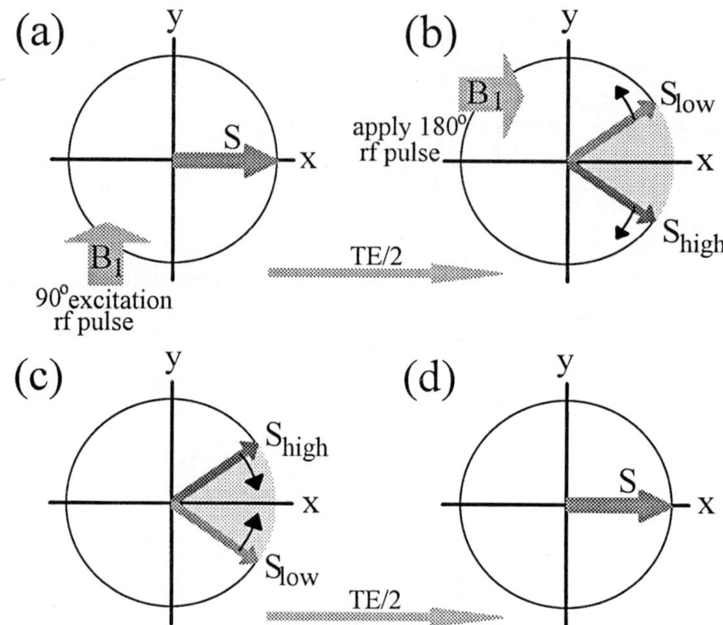

Fig. 1-6 (a), Transverse magnetization, S, which dephases under T2* decay **(b),** can be flipped around the x axis by the application of a 180-degree rf pulse. The clockwise dephasing spins are then moved behind the anticlockwise dephasing spins **(c),** and after an equal time (TE/2) the vectors will come together again **(d).** Note the small arrows indicating that the direction of dephasing stays the same for the spins in the rotating frame. This spin rephasing generates a spin echo.

sented by S_{high} and S_{low} *appear to move in opposite directions,* away from the x axis. In an inhomogeneous magnetic field, the spins thus "fan out" or *dephase* in the x-y plane, and when they are evenly distributed in the x-y plane there will be no net transverse magnetization (for each spin inducing a voltage, there is an opposite spin inducing the inverse voltage, which when coadded will cancel out). This T2* dephasing is added to the T2 dephasing that is already occurring, and thus makes the signal decay away even faster. So how can we measure T2 under these conditions, and how can we make the signal last longer so that we have more time to look at it?

Spin refocusing and spin echo. We may *refocus* or *rephase* the dephased spins by subsequent application of a 180-degree rf pulse (Fig. 1-7, A). The 180-degree inversion pulse is applied some time after the 90-degree pulse and serves to regenerate a signal called the *spin echo,* as illustrated. The 180-degree pulse applied in the direction of the x axis has the effect of flipping the spins around the x axis of the transverse plane so that the clockwise dephasing spins, S_{high}, which were originally ahead of the anticlockwise dephasing spins, S_{low}, are now behind the anticlockwise spins (see Fig. 1-6, C). In a time equal to that between the 90- and 180-degree pulses, the clockwise spins will catch up with the anticlockwise spins so that they are once again all pointing in the same direction (Fig. 1-6, D). On our vector diagram, we have flipped the vectors about the x axis, and they then continue to *move in the same direction* as before the 180-degree pulse was applied, so that they rephase along the x axis. We then say that they are *in phase.* Since all the spins now have the same orientation, there will be a net magnetization that will then decay away again as the fast spins once more move ahead of the slower spins. This rephased and dephased signal is called a spin echo and is in effect two FIDs placed back to back (Fig. 1-7, A). We may write this in a shorthand notation as a 90-180-echo pulse sequence. Further echoes may be generated by subsequent application of more 180-degree pulses; this would then be termed a *multiecho* sequence (90-180-echo$_1$–180-echo$_2$, and so forth). Two more things may be noted about these spin echoes.

TE, T2 measurement and T2 contrast. First, there is a period of time between the first 90-degree excitation pulse and the spin echo (the *time to echo,* or *TE*) that we may use to spatially encode the spins with gradient pulses, as we shall see later. Second, the spin echoes cannot be produced indefinitely, but decrease in amplitude as TE increases as a result of T2 decay. We may illustrate

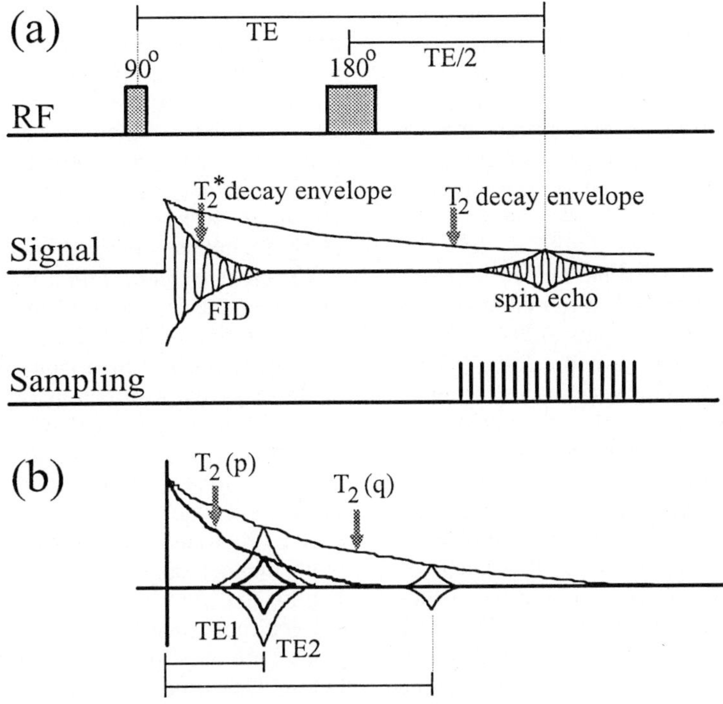

Fig. 1-7 (a), A basic 90-180-echo pulse sequence. Increasing TE increases the T2 weighting on the echo. **(b),** Samples with short T2s (T2(p)) have proportionally more T2 weighting than samples with longer T2s (T2(q)) as TE is increased (from TE1 to TE2).

this by drawing a T2 decay "envelope" (Fig. 1-7, *A*). The echo amplitude is thus a function of T2, and we say that the echo is *T2 weighted.* The longer we make TE, the more the T2 weighting is on the echo. By measuring the amplitude of several such echoes with differing TE values, we may trace out the T2 decay envelope and thus measure T2. These features are summarized in Fig. 1-7. Of particular significance to MRI is that we may use this T2 weighting to distinguish between samples with differing T2 values, even though they have the same number of nuclei (i.e., the same initial amplitude of signal in the FID). If two samples have different T2s, the amount of T2 weighting on the echo obtained from each sample using a spin echo sequence with the same TE will be different. The sample with the shorter T2 would give less signal than a sample with a longer T2 (Fig. 1-7, *B*). Herein lies one of the most significant powers of NMR. Two materials may have essentially the same concentration or number of nuclei in a given volume, i.e., the same *spin density,* but because of the interaction of the nuclei with their environment, they may have differing T2 values, allowing us to distinguish between them. In effect, the T2 value

is telling us what the environment of the nuclei is, i.e., what the structure of the material is. We shall use this later to generate what is called *T2 contrast* on our images.

There is one very important distinction between T2 and T2*. The magnet inhomogeneity dephasing, T2*, is reversible (so that we can produce echoes by using additional rf pulses), whereas the T2 decay is irreversible (we cannot get back the energy the spins have lost to each other). Thus, after the T2 decay has occurred, the sample must be reexcited to generate new signal that we can use.

TR and T1 contrast. In a spectroscopy or imaging experiment, there is usually not enough signal in one single echo acquisition and we must co-add or average several echoes. Further, multiple echo acquisitions are required for two-dimensional spatial encoding to make images, as we shall see later. After a 90-180-echo acquisition, there is T1 recovery of the spins along the B_0 axis. The time we wait between each acquisition is called the *time to repetition,* or *TR.* If we require all of the signal to recover along B_0 before we reexcite the system, we must wait several T1s for the spins to realign along B_0. However, we may speed up our acquisition by not waiting several T1s. However, in doing this we are sacrificing some signal, since only that fraction of the magnetization that has recovered along the B_0 axis will be excited by the next spin echo pulse sequence. Consequently, the TR can be used to vary the amount of signal we excite between 90-180-echo pulse sequences by making it less than several T1s. We thus say that we are controlling the *T1 weighting* of the echo. T1 is itself a characteristic of the nuclear environment and is different from T2. It may thus also be used to distinguish between materials. For example, two materials may have the same T2 but differing T1 values. Materials having differing T1 values will thus recover to different degrees in a T1-weighted sequence and may be distinguished.

TR and TE variation thus allows us to control the T1 and T2 weighting on the echo, respectively. As mentioned previously, we may use a multiecho sequence to measure T2. However, if we wish to measure only T2, the sequence should use a long TR so that there is no T1 weighting on the echoes. If there were T1 weighting, it would not be easy to distinguish how much of the echo weighting was due solely to T2. Similarly, if we wish to measure T1, it is desirable to measure signal changes caused purely by T1. However, if we use a spin echo (which we need to produce images, as we shall see later), there is always some signal loss due to T2 decay, since in a practical sequence TE is never zero (in an imaging sequence on a clinical instrument, the minimum TE is typically 5 to 10 msec). So how do we go about actually measuring T1 independently of T2 decay?

T1 measurement and inversion recovery. T1 measurement is achieved by first inverting the magnetization with a 180-degree rf pulse (Fig. 1-8, *A*). This will cause the magnetization to now point in the negative z direction, where it will recover under T1 processes to point in the positive z direction (Fig. 1-8, *B*). Note that there is no T2 decay since none of the magnetization is in the transverse (x-y) plane (remember that T2 decay occurs only in the transverse plane). However, since there is no magnetization in the transverse plane, there is no signal for us to observe. To observe the signal, we must then tip the spins into the transverse plane with an rf pulse and generate a spin echo as before. The time between the inversion pulse and the spin echo sequence is called the *time from in-*

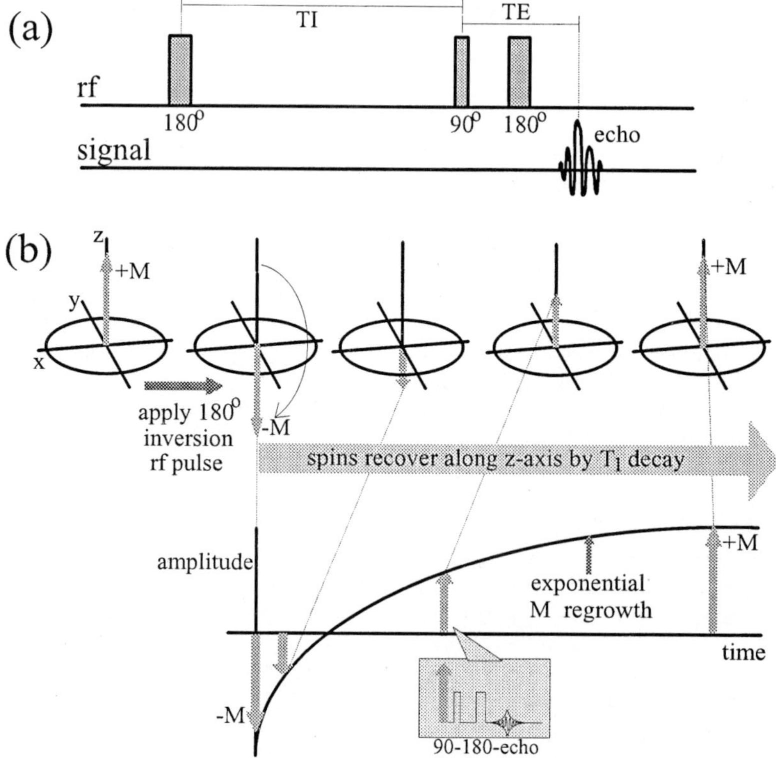

Fig. 1-8 (a), A basic inversion recovery pulse sequence and **(b)** its effect on the magnetization, M. The 180-degree pulse inverts M, which then decays under T1 relaxation and "grows back" along the z axis. By sampling M with a spin echo sequence after various inversion times, TI, we may map out the T1 relaxation curve.

version, or *TI*. If we wait for differing periods of time between the inversion pulse and the spin echo observation pulses, there will have occurred differing amounts of recovery of the magnetization along B_0. Consequently, the amplitude of the echo we observe will be modulated by the T1 relaxation. By collecting several echoes with differing TI values, we may map out the T1 recovery of the magnetization and thus measure T1.

NMR IMAGING

Having covered the basic physics of NMR, relaxation, and spin echoes, and after a brief introduction to the FT, we are now in a position to move on to the basics of MRI. An understanding of two tools is required: gradients and shaped rf pulses. We will then be in a position to understand how a basic imaging sequence works before moving on to more advanced imaging concepts and a discussion of the signal-to-noise ratio in the MRI experiment.

Gradients

Magnetic field gradients are applied to a sample in a homogeneous magnet field (B_0) using a set of gradient coils placed inside the magnet. A gradient coil consists of a set of current-carrying wires arranged so that they produce a small and linear magnetic field gradient. The gradient alters the main magnetic field so that, instead of being constant at B_0 across the magnet diameter, it now varies in a linear fashion from $B_0 + \Delta B$ to $B_0 - \Delta B$ (and is still B_0 in the center of the magnet) (Fig. 1-9, *B*). The full gradient coil set usually consists of three coils that produce linear gradients separately in the x, y, and z spatial directions so that all space may be encoded, as we shall see later. As a matter of convention, the z direction is defined as parallel to B_0, and this will be assumed for the rest of this chapter. Each gradient is connected to its own power supply so that the current passing through it (and hence the slope or strength of the gradient) may be controlled independently.

Frequency encoding in one spatial dimension

The effect of the gradient is illustrated in Fig. 1-9. Without application of a gradient, the spins will all precess at the same frequency in B_0 (Fig. 1-9, *A*). With the gradient applied (Fig. 1-9, *B*), the spins in different parts of the magnet along the gradient will be in slightly differing field strengths and will thus resonate at slightly different frequencies. Since we have arranged the gradient to be linear, the frequency at which the spins resonate will be directly proportional to their spatial position (Fig. 1-9, *C*). Consequently, by measuring the frequency at which the spins resonate, we can tell where they

are along the gradient. This is the central key to producing NMR images: by using the gradient, we may "encode" the FID, or more usually the echo, so that the signals it contains are dependent on the spatial position of the spins in the magnet.

The spatial encoding provided by the gradient is effected by simply turning on the gradient during the formation of the echo (Fig. 1-10). The echo is then said to be *frequency encoded*. In effect, we are using the gradient to "read" the echo, and thus we refer to this gradient as the *read gradient*. The FT of the signal obtained will thus produce a spectrum showing which frequencies are present in the signal (see Fig. 1-5, *[g]*). The height of the signal at each frequency corresponds to the number of nuclei contributing to the signal at each frequency. The echo we measure is digitized or sampled for use with a computer. If we sample the echo with 128 points, the FT will produce a spectrum consisting of 128 discrete frequencies. Since each frequency corresponds directly to a point in space, we may redraw the spectrum by "joining the dots" to produce a projection of the object that was placed in the gradient (Fig. 1-9, *[d]*). This one-dimensional projection of the object onto a spatial axis is analogous to the standard projection obtained in the x-ray CT experiment.

Note here that the effect of the gradient is very

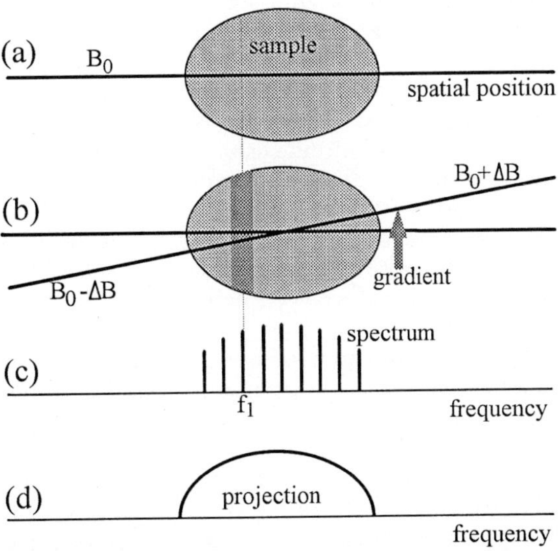

Fig. 1-9 (a), A homogeneous water sample placed in a static field B_0 will resonate at a single frequency. By applying a linear gradient **(b)** the resonance frequency will vary linearly along the sample **(c).** All the signal contributing to the frequency peak f_1 arises from that strip of material perpendicular to the gradient axis. By connecting the peaks of the frequency spectrum, a one-dimensional projection of the sample **(d)** is formed along the gradient axis.

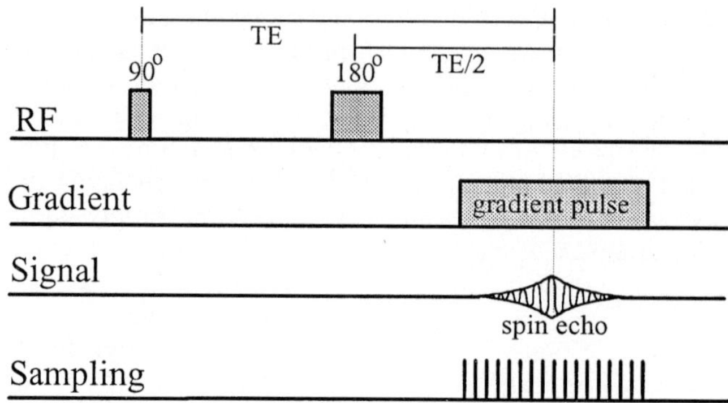

Fig. 1-10 Spatial encoding is achieved by sampling the spin echo during the application of a gradient pulse.

similar to that observed due to magnet inhomogeneity (above), i.e., it causes frequency differences. The difference, however, is that the magnet inhomogeneity is unwanted and essentially uncontrolled, while the gradient imposes a controlled and linear inhomogeneity that we require to encode space. Therefore, to be useful, our gradient must cause differences in frequency between adjacent sampling points in space that are larger than any frequency shift that may be due to magnet inhomogeneity. If the gradient does not impose a large enough frequency shift, a shift due to magnet inhomogeneity may be mistaken for a shift due to the gradient. In this case, our spatial encoding would be distorted, and the frequency shifts measured could not be assumed to be linearly proportional to the spatial dimension. This requirement that the gradient *dominate* the inhomogeneity frequency shifts defines a lower limit on the gradient strength that we need for imaging. Obviously, the larger the inhomogeneities in our magnet, the stronger gradients we need to produce undistorted images.

The region of space represented by each sample point in the frequency spectrum will be the *spatial resolution* of our projection. As we make the linear field gradient stronger, the signal will be spread out over a larger frequency range. Consequently, if we sample in the same way, the projection will be spread out over more sample points, and the spatial resolution is improved. However, if the signal is divided over more sample points, there must be less signal per point. Consequently, we cannot improve the spatial resolution indefinitely without running out of signal. The spatial resolution achievable will be limited by the amount of signal we can generate, which is in turn determined primarily by the number of spins in the sample, i.e., by the concentration of the water in the tissue in clinical ^{1}H imaging.

Encoding two spatial dimensions

A frequency projection as described above contains one-dimensional spatial information along one spatial axis defined by the read gradient. By combinations of x, y, and z gradients applied simultaneously, the projection may have any orientation in space as desired. (For example, two gradients of the same amplitude, say x and y, applied together will add vectorially to produce a resultant summed projection gradient at 45 degrees to both x and y axis.) Our next goal is to somehow use these one-dimensional projections to collect sufficient information for construction of a two-dimensional image. It is not possible to use an x and then a y gradient to encode the echo to form an x-y image, because our projection is a frequency encoding device that cannot tell which gradient has produced a frequency change. For example, if we measured a frequency shift of 10 Hz, we would not know whether that was in the x or y direction without additional information.

A similar problem is encountered when we give directions to each other. Suppose I want to tell you to move from where you are sitting now, at point P, to another point Q in the room you are sitting in (Fig. 1-11). If I asked you to move 5 m in a straight line from point P to Q, you would not know which direction to move in and could end up at any point on the circumference of a circle of radius 5 m centered on point P. To move you to a specific point on that circle, I must provide a second piece of information. One possibility is to use compass style coordinates: e.g., face east and turn 53 degrees north. The second piece of information provided in this case is an angle that will unambiguously move you to the right point in space, provided that point P is fixed in space. Such a coordinate system, which uses a length and an angle, is referred to as a polar coordinate system.

Alternatively, we may describe the position of

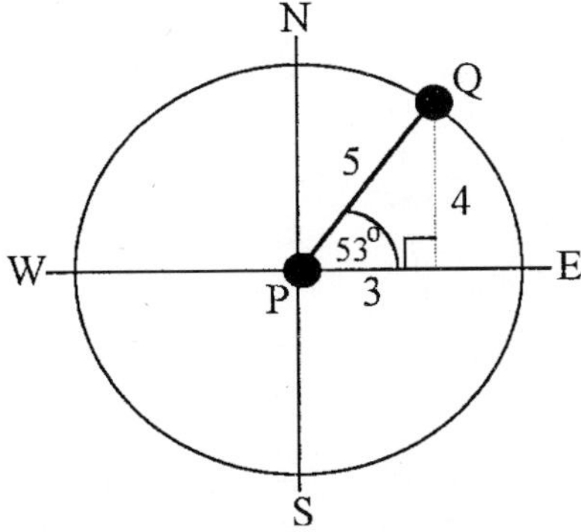

Fig. 1-11 To move from point P to Q requires two pieces of information: either the angle and length of the P-Q vector (polar coordinates) or the length of the projections of the P-Q vector onto the N-S and W-E axis (cartesian coordinates).

point Q relative to point P in two-dimensional space using two perpendicular spatial measurements. For example, I could tell you to move 3 m due east and then 4 m due north to get you from point P to point Q. This may be familiar as a vector notation, where each spatial length is associated with a direction. To achieve the direction encoding, we define a coordinate system with two perpendicular axes x and y, and make all movements relative to these axes. Mapping out space in a squarelike or maplike fashion like this is referred to as a cartesian coordinate system.

Going back to our imaging, we can also encode space in a polar or cartesian fashion. Our x gradient, used as a read gradient, can encode one spatial dimension in frequency. We cannot again use *solely* frequency to encode in the y direction, or the x and y measurements will be indistinct. Our example gives us two alternatives for our second measurement. First, we may incorporate an angular measurement; this forms the basis of *projection-reconstruction imaging*. Alternatively, the second spatial dimension can be encoded by using the y gradient to affect the phase of the signal. These *phase encoding* methods are used almost exclusively in modern clinical MRI.

Projection-reconstruction imaging

Using a polar coordinate system, images may be formed in a manner similar to that used to produce CT images. In CT a series of projections are collected at a variety of projection angles to the object. These projections are then used to reconstruct a two-dimensional image via a projection-reconstruction algorithm.[17] In MRI, our projection or read gradient is generated by a combination of two gradients of varied amplitudes, say x and y, so that the resultant read gradient produces projec-

tions at different angles in the x-y plane. An image may then be reconstructed from these projections using algorithms similar to those used in CT. Although projection-reconstruction methods were initially used for planar MRI (and in some special applications remain preferable), they were quickly superseded by phase encoding methods (described in the next section). Currently, nearly all commercial imaging machines use phase encoded imaging methods because of increased efficiency and flexibility in the imaging sequences.

Phase encoded MRI

An understanding of frequency encoded projections is usually easily grasped because of familiarity with analogous CT techniques. However, phase encoding is not usually familiar to the nonphysicist and is often the most poorly understood part of basic MRI physics. Jump ahead momentarily and look at Fig. 1-17, a three-dimensional phase encoding imaging sequence. Note that it is very similar to Fig. 1-10 with only the addition of phase encoding gradient pulses illustrated as boxes with ladder style rungs. These extra gradient pulses encode the other spatial dimensions, and we shall see how they do this.

In an effort to explain phase encoding, I will show how a frequency encoding gradient is actually a type of phase encoding gradient. Indeed, *all* gradients are phase encoding gradients, and it is the phase changes these gradients produce that we use to encode space. However, there are subtle differences in the way we can do the phase encoding that can have a profound effect on how the signal is manipulated and on the way that the manipulation is carried out; indeed, I shall show that frequency encoding is simply a particular way of phase encoding. First, let us go right back to basics and make sure we know what phase actually is.

What is phase?. As described above, most of us are familiar with the use of an angle to describe the locus of a vector that is fixed at one end to an origin, as in Fig. 1-12, *A*. This angle is called the *phase angle*. Given the length of the vector and the phase angle, we can draw in the vector. We are also familiar with sine waves (Fig. 1-12, *B*). We know that if the sine wave amplitude is zero at 0 degrees, the first half or hump of the sine wave spans 180 degrees, and so on. We also know that a cosine and sine wave are identical except that they are shifted by 90 degrees to one another; i.e., at t = 0, the sine wave is at 0 degrees and the cosine at 90 degrees (the top of the first hump). We call these degree measurements the *phase* of the wave, and refer to the difference in phase between two waves as the *phase shift* between the waves.

These two pictorial representations (Fig. 1-12)

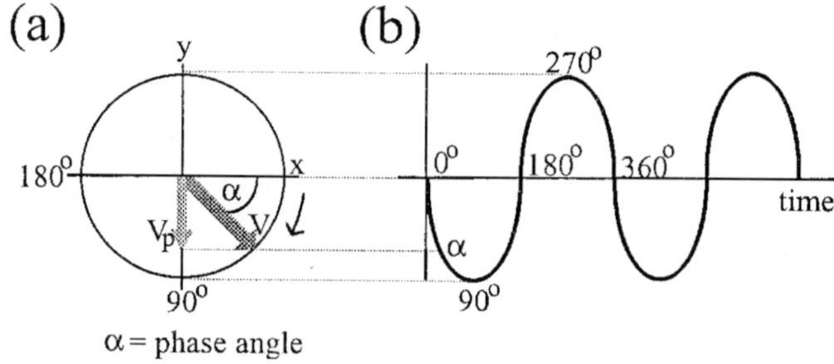

Fig. 1-12 A, The position of a vector, V, rotating around a fixed point can be described by the phase angle. **B,** Phase angles associated with a sine wave plotted as a function of time. The representations of phase angle in **A** and **B** are equivalent: the sine wave maps out the amplitude of the projection of V onto the y axis, i.e., V_p, as a function of time as V rotates.

of what we understand to be the phase are equivalent. We can see this if we consider the projection of the vector, V_p, on the vertical y axis in Figure 1-12, A. As the vector rotates, this projection will simply increase and decrease in length along the y axis. If we plot the length of this projected vector as a function of time, we can plot out the sine wave; e.g., the top of the first hump on the sine wave corresponds to the vector pointing up along the y axis of Fig. 1-12, A, and both correspond to 90 degrees. The sine wave is in effect the time dependence graph of the motion of the point of the vector.

Fig. 1-12 can now be used to show that phase and frequency are intimately related. If in Fig. 1-12, B the full 360 degrees of the sine wave were produced in 1 sec, the frequency of the sine wave (or cycles per sec) would be 1 Hz (this is in fact how hertz is defined). In that 1 sec, the phase of the sine wave changed by 360 degrees. If the frequency of the wave doubled to 2 Hz, a full 360-degree cycle would take 0.5 sec. In this case the rate of change of the phase has also doubled: the vector rotated by 360 degrees in half the time. Herein lies the connection between the frequency and the phase: *frequency is the rate of change of the phase*, i.e.:

$$\omega = 2\pi f = \Delta\alpha/\Delta t, \qquad \text{(Eq.3)}$$

where $\Delta\alpha$ is the phase change (in radians) that occurs in a time Δt.

Frequency and phase encoding are consequently very similar, and we shall see in the following section that frequency encoding gradients and phase encoding gradients encode space in the same way.

Gradient pulses and phase shifts. So far we have an understanding of what we have called frequency encoding gradients. However, this does not tell us what is going on while the gradient is applied, but what has happened *after* the gradient has

been applied and the signal processed. Our echo is a signal in time, so *when we talk about frequency, we have already done the FT of this time signal.* So what does a gradient actually do when we turn it on *during* an NMR signal? What happens in the time domain?

The effect of a gradient during the signal accumulation is illustrated in Fig. 1-13. Let us consider just one point in the sample. Initially the excited spins are precessing at a frequency defined by B_0 (Fig. 1-13, A). When the gradient is turned on, in this case positive so that the magnetic field the spins experience is now a little higher at ($B_0 + \Delta B$), the spins will precess a little faster, i.e., at a higher frequency (Fig. 1-13, B). Then at time T we turn the gradient off. The spins will then precess at the original frequency dictated by B_0. During the gradient, we are clear that the frequency increased. However, it is clear from Fig. 1-13 that we can look at this another way. The application of the gradient pulse caused a phase change in the signal. This is evident from the illustration, in that the signal that had no gradient applied (Fig. 1-13, A) had 0 phase at time T, but if the gradient pulse is applied, there is a phase change at time T of $+\alpha$ (see Fig. 1-12, B). If the gradient pulse was applied for twice as long, the spins would precess for twice as long at the higher frequency. Further, the phase change at time T would be twice as big, i.e. $+2\alpha$. (See Fig. 1-12, C.) Thus, we see that increasing the time that the gradient is on increases the phase shift we obtain.

We also note that the same phase shift of $+2\alpha$ obtained in Fig. 1-13, C can also be effected by doubling the amplitude of the gradient pulse (instead of doubling the time it was on) (Fig. 1-13, E). Doubling the amplitude of the gradient will double the frequency at which the spins precess, and thus twice the phase shift will be generated in the same time. We may thus increase the ampli-

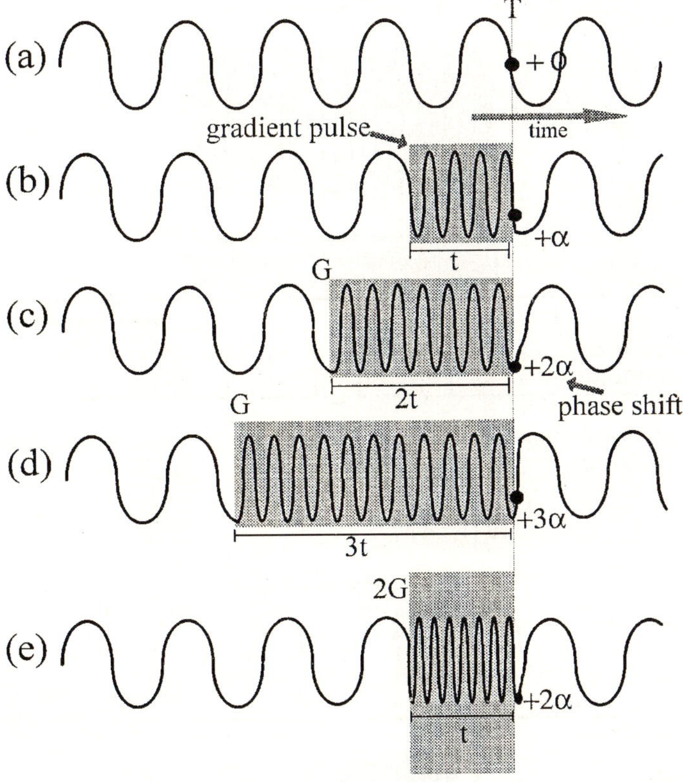

Fig. 1-13 The phase shifting effect of a gradient pulse. A gradient pulse of amplitude + G and duration t will increase the frequency of precessing spins **(b)**. When the gradient is turned off at time T, the spins will have acquired a phase shift, $+\alpha$, relative to that with no gradient applied **(a)**. Incrementing the gradient duration increments the phase shift **(c, d)**. The $+2\alpha$ phase shift in C can also be generated by doubling the gradient strength for the same time t **(e)**.

tude and/or the time the gradient pulse is applied to increase the phase shift.

Equivalence of frequency and phase encoding

Frequency encoding. Consider again the so-called frequency encoding gradient in Fig. 1-14. The echo signal is sampled during this read gradient, as illustrated. Instead of considering the entire pulse as changing the frequency, we may look at what has happened to the signal after each sample point, i.e., after each portion of the gradient. After the first sample point, there has been applied a small piece of gradient that will cause a small phase shift, $+\alpha$. After the second data point a $+2\alpha$ phase shift has been applied, then $+3\alpha$, and so on to collect N sample points. The read gradient is thus incrementing the phase shift of the signal. What we are measuring, therefore, is *the rate at which the gradient causes the phase to change,* which we now know is equivalent to frequency. However, by examining the phase shifts, we are considering something that changes as a function of time; i.e., we are thinking in the time domain

(and have not yet done the FT to the frequency domain).

Phase encoding. We could do this encoding in a different fashion. We could simply collect each sample point one at a time, as shown in Fig. 1-15. After collecting the first data point, we wait for T1 recovery (during TR) and repeat the experiment with the gradient on twice as long to collect the second data point. We then repeat again with three times the gradient to collect the third data point, and so on. Thus, in M separate experiments, we can collect M data points. We illustrate this in a shorthand notation, as shown at the bottom of Fig. 1-15.

Difference between phase and frequency encoding.

It is thus clear that both the frequency and phase encoding gradients are causing incremental phase shifts in the NMR signal. We name the two ways of affecting these phase shifts' frequency and phase encoding so that we may distinguish between them. In the frequency case, all the phase shifts we require are collected in a single echo. In

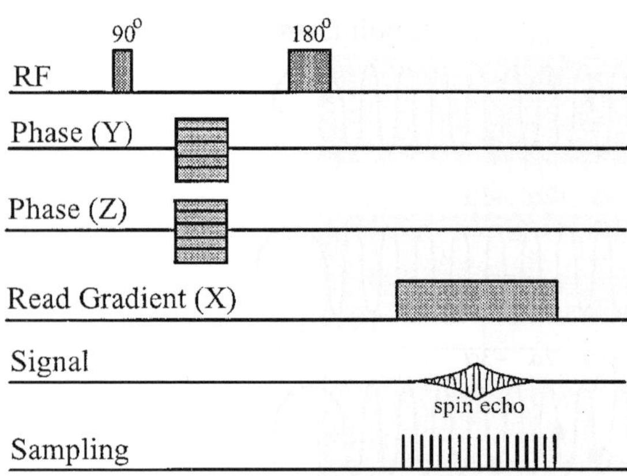

Fig. 1-17 A three-dimensional spin echo imaging pulse sequence using one read gradient and two phase encoding gradients.

phase changes. We do this by incrementing this third gradient as before, but for each increment of this third gradient, we increment the second phase encoding gradient over its full M increments. For each increment of the third gradient, the M increments measure the rate of change of the phase for the first phase encoding gradient. Then, each increment of the third gradient measures the rate of change of phase for the third spatial dimension independently. However, this is extremely time consuming, since for each sample point in the third dimension we must perform M experiments. An N × M × L three-dimensional matrix would thus require M × L experiments to collect, i.e., a minimum acquisition time of M × L × TR.

It is usually the case that multiple acquisitions are required to encode space. For example, we could encode three spatial dimensions by using three phase encoding gradients, which would then require a minimum acquisition time of N × L × M × TR, i.e., N times longer than when using a frequency encoding gradient for one of the dimensions. In a sense, then, the frequency encoding gradient is the "odd one out." Fortunately, the frequency gradient's "one shot" nature allows us to keep the total time required to collect an image N times shorter than it would have been were we restricted to purely phase encoding pulse sequences.

Because three-dimensional acquisitions are so time intensive they have found little clinical utility at the present time. Using a TR of 1 second, a typical 256 × 256 image matrix requires a 4-min acquisition time, while a 256 × 256 × 128 matrix would take 8 hours! For this reason, multislice methods are more often used (see later).

Phase encoding revisited. Now, let us look at phase encoding in a way that illustrates the differ-

ence between frequency and phase encoding in a more physical fashion. It may have become apparent that the difference between frequency and phase encoding is a matter of time, i.e., the time dimension or frame of reference in which we encode the data. Fig. 1-18 illustrates these reference frames. Consider our signal as a sine wave (ignoring decay processes) that we are going to sample with discrete sampling points. Fig. 1-18, *A* shows again the now familiar frequency encoding process: the wave is effectively stationary on the page, and our sample points are collected sequentially in time as we move from left to right across the page. We are moving the sample point with respect to the wave. In this way, N sample points can be collected in one echo.

Consider now Fig. 1-18, *B*. Suppose now we have only one sample point that is stationary (i.e., at the same point in time) across the page. This time, we may sample the wave by moving the wave across the page and across the sample point. Moving the wave across the sample point is achieved by using a gradient pulse to speed up (or slow down) the wave in increments before it reaches the sample point.

In effect, then, these two methods of measuring the rate of change of phase of the wave differ in the relative "motion" of the wave to the sample point; i.e., we may keep the wave fixed and sample along it, or keep the sample point fixed and move the wave over the sample point. Again, the advantage of having these two ways of encoding the data is that we may do both at the same time. If separate gradients are employed for each type of encoding, the encoding caused by each gradient is distinct.

Slice selection

We have so far described the use of frequency and phase encoding gradients for encoding spatial dimensions. In its present form, however, the two-dimensional imaging method would produce a two-dimensional image of the whole object, and there is no spatial discrimination in the third dimension. One way of imaging in that third dimension is to spatial encode it with a phase encoding gradient, but, as we have already seen, that can be very time consuming. Alternatively, we may arrange to excite only a thin slice or slab of material through the sample, and make a two-dimensional image of that slice. The technique used for this slice selection is described in the next section after a necessary introduction to selective rf pulses.

Shaped rf pulses. So far our discussions have all involved what are referred to as *"hard"* rf *pulses*. These pulses are relatively short (10 to 200 µsec) and will excite a large range of frequencies.

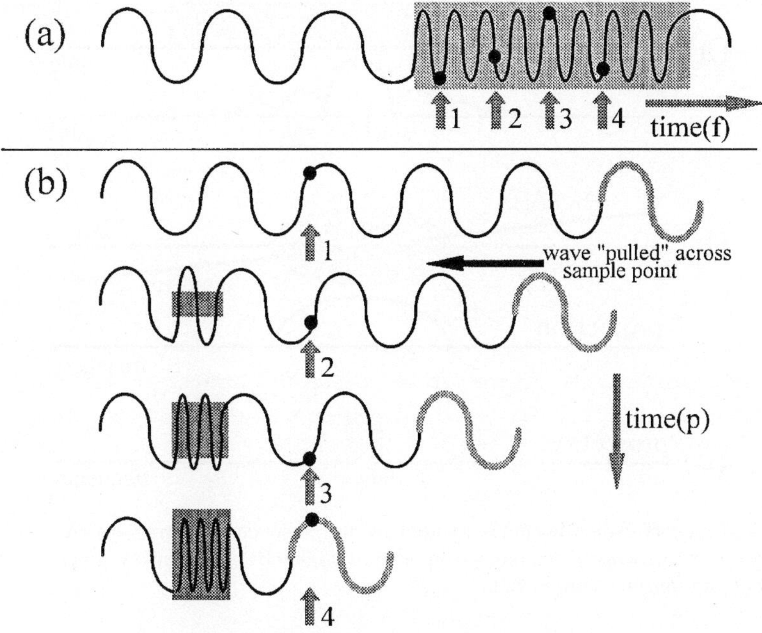

Fig. 1-18 A redrawing of Figure 1-16 illustrating the relative "motions" of the signal under frequency and phase encoding gradients. **A,** The wave is "stationary", and we move the sample point across the page, measuring phase increments in time across the page (time(f)). **B,** The sample point is stationary, and we move the wave over the sample point using a gradient pulse to "pull" it. The phase increments are then measured in time down the page (time(p)).

As seen above, a short square rf pulse excites a wide sinc-shaped region of frequency space many kilohertz wide (see Fig. 1-5, *H*). Since our sample is resonating over a relatively narrow range of frequency (at most a few hundreds of hertz), the excitation of the sample's frequency range is essentially homogeneous (i.e., over a small region at the central peak of the sinc frequency profile, which is then essentially flat, as marked in Fig. 1-5, *H* as δf).

Conversely, we have seen in Fig. 1-5, *F* that a sinc-shaped rf pulse produces a square-shaped frequency excitation profile. By controlling the time duration of the sinc rf pulse, we can control the width of the square frequency profile. The longer the sinc-shaped pulse in time, the narrower is the square frequency profile. In this way, we may use the FT relationship to tailor the rf excitation pulse so that only a desired range of frequencies of a defined shape are excited.

The amount of rf energy used to excite the sample is a function of the peak amplitude of the rf pulse and the length of time it is applied. This power is thus represented by the area of the rf pulse in our illustrations. If a certain area A of a square pulse is required to tip the spins by 90 degrees and the rf pulse is short, the amplitude of the rf pulse will be relatively large. Consequently, a large rf power supply capable of generating this peak amplitude is required. These pulses are thus called "hard." The shaped rf pulses, on the other hand, are relatively long (typically 2 to 4 msec). The peak amplitude of these pulses to maintain the same area A is thus proportionally smaller and relatively low. Hence, these pulses are referred to as *"soft" rf pulses.* We can use these soft pulses for exciting the NMR signal (instead of the hard 90-degree pulses) and simultaneously effect slice selection, as described in the next section.

Slice selective gradients. Consider what happens if we apply a soft rf pulse while a gradient, referred to as the *slice selection gradient,* is turned on. As seen above, the gradient will cause different parts of the sample in differing parts of the gradient to resonate at different frequencies. The shaped rf pulse will then excite only a small range of those frequencies. If we turn on the gradient so that the sample resonance is "spread out" over a few kilohertz frequency width, our rf pulse with a frequency width of only a few hundred hertz will excite only a small section of the sample, as shown in Fig. 1-19. Further, by changing the center frequency of our soft rf pulse (i.e., simply retuning the rf transmitter as you would a radio), we may

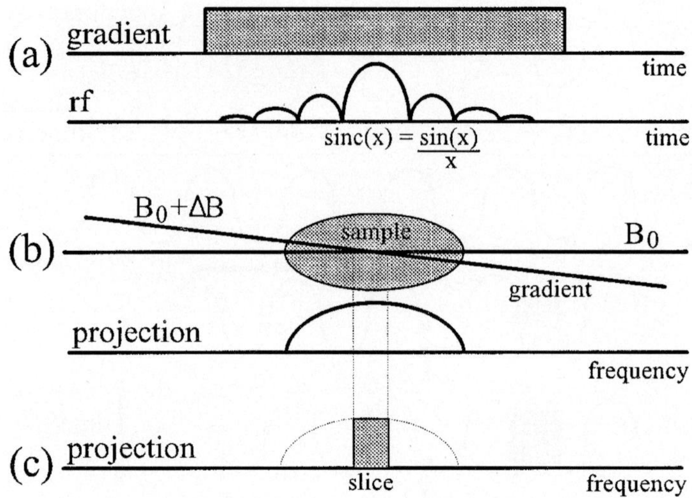

Fig. 1-19 A shaped rf excitation pulse applied in the presence of a gradient (**A**) excites only a narrow range of frequencies of the projection of the sample (**B**). This narrow frequency range constitutes a slice through the sample (**C**).

control exactly where along the gradient this slice is selected.

Using one of our three x, y, and z gradients, we now have a means of exciting only a thin slab of material within the sample. We may then use the remaining two gradients for frequency and phase encoding to produce a two-dimensional image of that slice.

Basic spin echo imaging sequence

We now have the necessary tools and components to produce a two-dimensional image of a slice through a sample. Fig. 1-20 shows a basic spin echo imaging sequence that will achieve this. Slice selection is achieved by a combination of soft rf pulses and the slice selection gradient. The two remaining gradients are used for frequency and phase encoding to produce the image. By suitable choice of which physical gradient (x, y, or z) is chosen for slice, frequency, and phase encoding, we may arrange that the imaged slice to be taken in any physical orientation. By using simultaneous combinations of the gradients, we may also arrange to image at oblique angles, greatly increasing the versatility of this imaging modality. Note that we choose to increment the amplitude of the phase encoding gradient (rather than its length) in order to increment its area. We do this so that we may keep TE constant during the image acquisition. Note also in Fig. 1-20 two gradient pulses (A and B) that are unfamiliar; for the sake of initial simplicity, these pulses were omitted. However, they are essential and must be included for the sequence to

work properly. The function of these two pulses is described below.

Slice rephasing gradient pulse. The slice selection portion of the pulse sequence consists of a gradient pulse in combination with a shaped rf pulse. The rf pulse excites the spins, and the gradient dephases the spins in order to excite only a narrow frequency range. However, the gradient is on during the excitation and will also affect even the spins we excite and dephase them. This dephasing of the signal we require will thus result in a signal loss if we simply turn off the gradient and observe. What we must do, therefore, is rephase the excited spins before observation. This is achieved by reversing the sign of the slice gradient, i.e., area A on Fig. 1-20. So how much rephasing do we need (i.e., how big should the slice rephase gradient area be)? We may naively imagine that at the beginning of the rf pulse there is no transverse magnetization and thus no dephasing. During the rf pulse the spins are tipped slowly into the xy plane, so that at its end all the spins are in the x-y plane at 90 degrees to the z axis and being maximally dephased by the gradient. Thus, halfway through the pulse the spins are only at 45 degrees to the z axis, and the gradient will have only half the dephasing effect on them. We can see, then, that on average the gradient will have only half the effect on the spins that it would have had had the spins been fully in the transverse plane during the whole gradient pulse. Consequently, the area of the gradient rephasing pulse needs to be set at one half that of the slice dephasing gradient pulse.

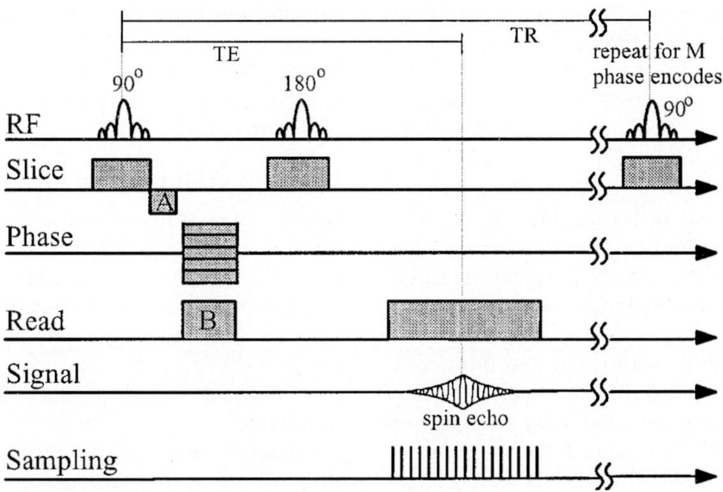

Fig. 1-20 A complete basic spin echo imaging sequence. An additional slice rephasing gradient pulse (A) and a read dephasing gradient pulse (B) are also required (see text).

Read dephasing gradient pulse. There is also an additional read gradient pulse applied in the interval between the 90- and 180-degree rf pulses (area B in Fig. 1-20). The effect of this pulse is to dephase the spins so that the echo is formed in the middle of the read gradient pulse. Why do we need to do this? As we have seen, a 90-180-pulse sequence produces a spin echo that we wish to encode with a gradient. If, however, we simply turn on a read gradient after the 180-degree pulse, it will affect the spins extremely rapidly (since the applied gradient is much stronger than the inhomogeneity gradients causing the T2* dephasing). We would thus see a gradient-generated FID produced immediately after we turned the gradient on. Ideally, we could simply sample this FID and transform it to make the image. There is, however, a very practical problem that prohibits the use of this FID: it turns out to be impossible to turn on a gradient instantly. Rather, they have an associated rise time (time to fully turn on) that on clinical scanners can be quite long (400 to 1000 μsec and limited by the gradient's inductance). The gradient is thus changing during the beginning of the FID and is not properly encoded. This would lead to image distortions after straightforward FT. For this reason, we pre-dephase the signal on one side of the 180-degree pulse with a read dephase pulse of area B. The effect of this dephase gradient is then canceled out (the spins rephased) on the other side of the 180-degree pulse by the first half of the read gradient (of equal area B). The second half of the read gradient (again of area B) then serves to again dephase the signal, resulting now in an echo that is formed in the middle of the read gra-

dient. The full echo is then properly sampled with the read gradient fully on, and the resultant image will be undistorted.

Multislice and multiecho imaging

Our basic imaging sequence will collect one image with a defined TR and TE in a minimum acquisition time of M × TR. However, we note here that there is often a lot of "unused" time in our sequence of events. Because T1 and T2 are often so different, we typically use TE values ranging from 15 to 150 msec and TR values ranging from 200 to 5000 msec, depending on the image contrast we require. A TE of 30 msec and a TR of 1 to 2 seconds is extremely commonplace. If the gradient and rf pulsing occurs in 30 msec and the TR is 2 seconds, 1.97 seconds is effectively unused. It turns out that we can use this time very efficiently. If we required several slices through the sample, we could acquire them as sequential and separate image acquisitions. However, we may more efficiently interleave these multiple slice acquisitions. Since each slice excitation does not affect the rest of the sample, we may, during TR, excite and examine other slices. Several slices may be excited and examined in the TR period, and the total image acquisition interleaved. The extra slices are obtained in the same time it took to acquire a single slice. We can do this provided that our slice selective pulses are good and there is no overlap of the slices, which would otherwise distort the images. To ensure this, a small gap is usually left between the slices. Each slice may then relax after excitation as it would have done in the single slice imaging case. The number of slices we can interleave in this fashion obviously depends on the relative TR and TE choices, but is often 10 to 30.

Similarly, we may increase our imaging efficiency through using this spare TR time to collect multiple echoes by following our initial 90-180-rf pulse excitation sequence by subsequent 180-degree pulses. In this way, two or more images may be collected with differing TE values, i.e., with different T2 weightings. The images will thus have different contrast, which may be required clinically to distinguish different pathologic conditions.

We may also combine multiecho and multislice sequencing in the TR period. The collection of two echoes (short TE, 30 msec, and long TE, 100 to 150 msec) from 4 to 20 slices form a common clinical imaging protocol. This allows us to be extremely efficient in our data collection procedure, and a very large amount of data may be collected in a reasonable time (60 to 100 images is not uncommon in a 1-hour imaging examination).

Controlling image contrast

Now that we have a basic spin echo imaging sequence, we may use it to obtain images of varying contrast, depending on the pathologies we are looking for. This is achieved by judicious choice of TE and TR. The effects of the various TE and TR weightings on the images are summarized in Table 1-1.

Throughout the rest of this book, you will see typical TR and TE values with the images that are used clinically to best highlight the particular features in those images that the clinician is interested in.

Inversion recovery imaging

Improved T1 contrast can be obtained in images using inversion recovery imaging pulse sequences, and may also be used to measure T1 itself. As described above, an inversion recovery sequence involves the insertion of an inversion pulse at a controlled time, TI, before a standard spin echo acquisition. Consequently, we do exactly the same to generate an inversion recovery image by simply placing an inversion pulse in front of the basic spin echo imaging pulse sequence. Although sometimes

offering improved T1 contrast in images, inversion recovery sequences are relatively long (since TI is added and TR is required to be long) and are often clinically avoided when T1-weighted images will suffice.

Gradient echo imaging

Instead of a spin echo, we may alternatively use what is called a *gradient echo* to generate an image. Fig. 1-21 shows a gradient echo pulse sequence, where it can be seen that the difference between that and a spin echo pulse sequence is that the 180-degree pulse has been replaced by a *gradient reversal,* which produces the echo. How does this work?

Gradient reversal spin rephasing. The first section of the read gradient serves to dephase the spins, as previously described, and potential signal rapidly dephases away under this gradient. To illustrate this, we again consider two groups of spins that are in a higher (S_{high}) and lower (S_{low}) magnetic field (relative to B_0) as determined by the linear gradient (see Fig. 1-6). To rephase the signal, we have seen that we may flip the spins with a 180-degree pulse so that S_{high} are moved behind S_{low} and catch up with them, so rephasing the signal. Alternatively, we may reverse the sign of the read gradient. The effect of this is illustrated in Fig. 1-22. Imagine that our S_{high} spins were precessing at a frequency 100 Hz larger (positive) than ω_0. They will thus dephase on the vector diagram in the positive phase direction (clockwise) (Fig. 1-22, *B*). (Remember that frequency is equivalent to rate of change of phase; thus, the vector corresponding to the higher frequency will have a bigger phase angle at a given time, i.e., the rate of change of the phase is larger.) If then the gradient is reversed, the spins will now precess at a frequency 100 Hz lower (negative) than ω_0; i.e., the vector will experience the same rate of change of phase relative to B_0 but in the negative phase direction (Fig. 1-22, *C*). Consequently, the direction of the vectors is reversed and they rephase in a similar manner as before (Fig. 1-22, *D*). Effectively then, in the rotating reference frame, we have *changed the direction* in which our spin vectors are dephasing, using the gradient reversal.

Table 1-1 Image classification according to TE and TR controlled T1 and T2 weighting

TE	TR	Weightings	Image classification
Short	Long	No T2, no T1	Spin density
Long	Long	Some T2, no T1	T2 weighted
Short	Short	No T2, some T1	T1 weighted
Long	Short	Some T2, some T1	Mixed T1/T2 weighting

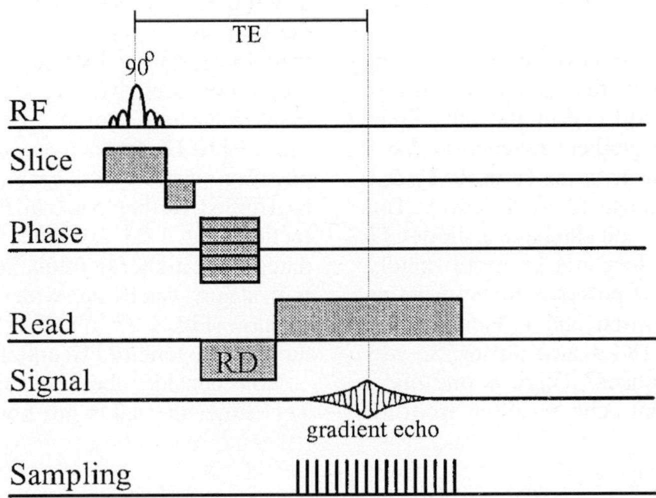

Fig. 1-21 A basic gradient echo imaging pulse sequence. *RD*, Read dephasing gradient.

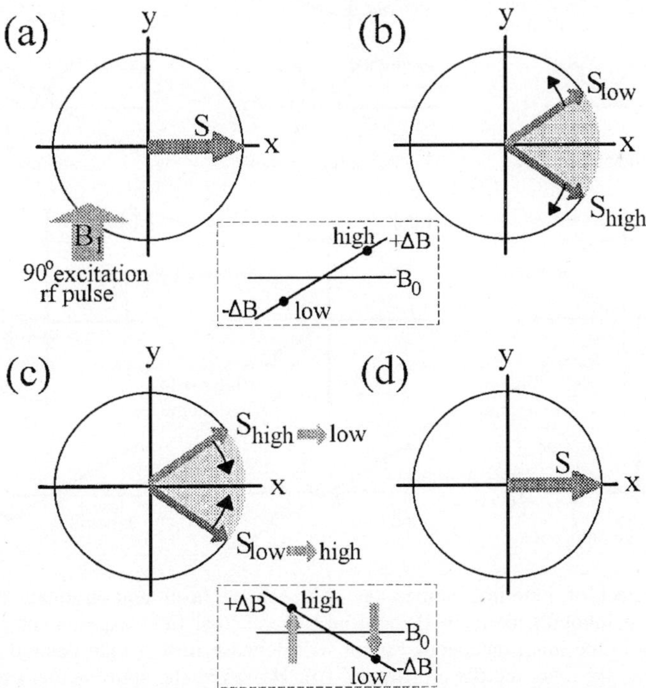

Fig. 1-22 Generation of a gradient echo. After the 90-degree excitation **(a),** spin vectors in the higher magnetic field dephase clockwise **(b).** When the gradient is reversed, as shown in the inset diagrams, spins in the higher field are now in the lower field and will dephase in the anticlockwise direction at the same rate (since the magnitude of the gradient offset relative to B_0 is the same). In effect then, the gradient reversal reverses the direction of the vectors **(c),** and the spins rephase **(d)** to constitute the gradient echo.

To reiterate this point, we see that in the rotating frame the effect of the spin echo is to flip the spin vectors, which then continue to move in the same direction. Alternatively, the gradient echo is formed by reversing the direction in which the vectors move.

Gradient versus spin echoes. The gradient and spin echoes appear to have the same end result, so when and why do we use one or the other? The major advantage of the gradient reversal is that it can be implemented much faster (1 to 400 μsec) than a 180-degree rf pulse (2 to 4 msec). This means that the gradient echo can have a shorter TE and can be used to collect images more rapidly. Second, the number of rf pulses is reduced, so reducing rf power deposition and reducing errors arising from imperfect 180-degree pulses. So why then do we use spin echoes? There is one major limitation to the gradient echo resulting from the

effects of magnet inhomogeneity. Let us suppose that we have a little inhomogeneity, resulting in the spins resonating $+10$ Hz faster than ω_0, and that we then apply the (positive) gradient causing, say, a $+100$ Hz frequency change from ω_0 for a particular point in space. Consider first the spin echo then formed by a 180-degree pulse. The spins in the inhomogeneity, $S_{high+inhomo}$, will dephase faster than they should, as shown in Fig. 1-23, *A* (i.e., $+110$ Hz faster than ω_0). However, after application of the 180-degree pulse, these spins will be flipped further back in the negative phase direction (Fig. 1-23, *B*). Since they continue to resonate a little higher in frequency, still $+110$ Hz, they will again catch up with the other spins and rephase (Fig. 1-23, *C*). The 10 Hz shift caused by the inhomogeneity effectively cancels out.

Now consider the effect of a gradient reversal. This time, the spins are not flipped; instead, the

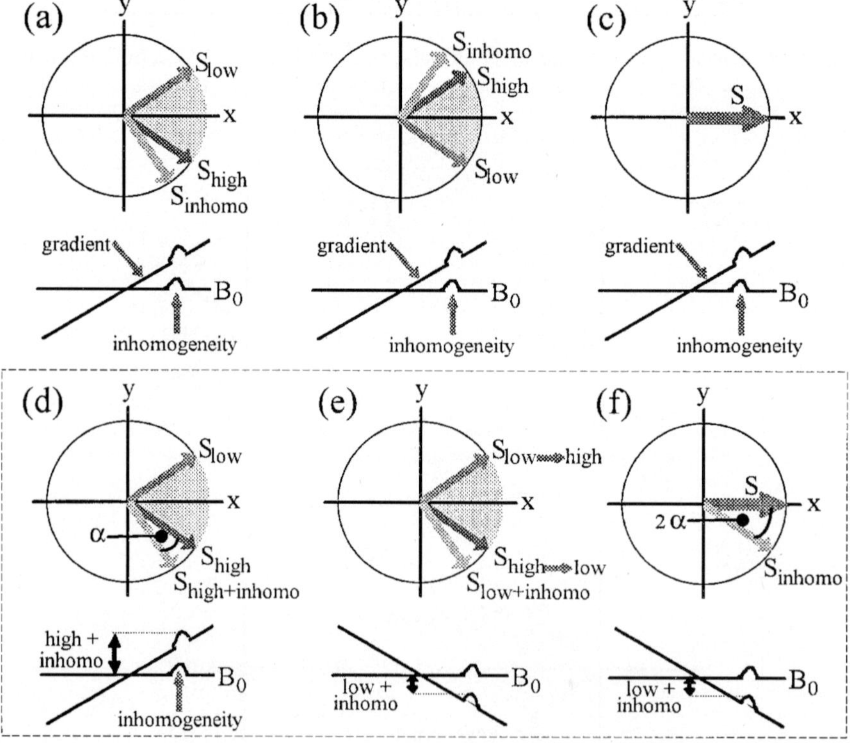

Fig. 1-23 The effect of inhomogeneities on spin echoes **(a-c)** and gradient echoes **(d-f)**. A positive "bump" or inhomogeneity in B_0 will add to the total field experienced by the spins (**A** and **D**), and spins in the inhomogeneous region will dephase further than desired (S_{inhomo}). After a 180-degree pulse, the spin vectors are flipped **(b)**. However, the spin vectors continue to move in the same direction and so rephase **(c)**, since the spins in the inhomogeneity rephase at the same rate as they dephased. However, after the gradient reversal **(e)**, the spins in the inhomogeneity will reverse direction (negative phase direction), but they will not rephase at the same rate because the inhomogeneity offset is still positive, i.e., high+inhomo $\neq$ low+inhomo. Consequently, they will not be in phase when the gradient echo is formed **(f)**, and any inhomogeneity dephasing, α, is doubled. In the text, high, low, and inhomo are exampled as $+100$, -100, and $+10$ Hz, respectively.

gradient changes from causing a $+100$ Hz frequency difference to causing a -100 Hz difference, i.e. the direction in which the vectors move is reversed as before (Fig. 1-23, *D* and *E*). However, the gradient inhomogeneity is still $+10$ Hz, so the spins in the inhomogeneity will resonate at $-100 + 10 = -90$ Hz. Consequently, during the rephasing part of the gradient echo, the spins in the inhomogeneity will have a different rate of change of phase when rephasing than when dephasing, and consequently will not come back together again after TE. In fact, if they dephase by effectively $+110$ Hz, then after rephasing by -90 Hz there will remain a $+20$ Hz discrepancy. Generally, an α inhomogeneity shift will result in a 2α total rephasing error for the gradient echo (Fig. 1-23, *F*). The gradient echo has thus doubled the frequency shift arising from the inhomogeneity. When the inhomogeneity frequency shift is larger than the frequency width of an image pixel, this leads to a misregistration of the signal in the image, and it is distorted.

The gradient strength must be strong enough to dominate the inhomogeneity frequency shifts so that the image is not blurred. This sets the lower limit on the gradient strength we require. The gradient strength itself is limited by physical parameters involving power requirements and the currents the gradients can carry without being destroyed. Consequently, we may not be able to dominate the larger inhomogeneities that may arise, in particular from susceptibility effects, as described below. In these cases, spin echo methods are preferable to gradient echo methods since they are less sensitive to B_0 inhomogeneities.

Magnet inhomogeneity and susceptibility. Magnetic field inhomogeneities are a limiting factor in NMR spectroscopy and imaging. Efforts are undertaken to make the magnets we use as homogeneous as possible. Clinically, however, an additional problem will always create magnetic field inhomogeneity, namely, *susceptibility* effects. Magnetic fields do not permeate all materials homogeneously. Different materials resist the penetration of the magnetic field to different degrees. The ease with which a magnetic field can pass through a material is characterized by its susceptibility. Consider, then, two materials placed in close contact that have differing susceptibilities. The magnetic field lines will be more concentrated (closer together) in one material than the field lines in the other material. Since magnetic field lines must be continuous, a small magnetic field gradient exists at the transition point between the two materials. This small gradient is effectively an inhomogeneity in the magnetic field, caused by the sample, which cannot be eliminated. The more interfaces there are, i.e., the more heterogeneous

the sample, the larger is the potential for susceptibility gradients. (Because of this, spectroscopists often arrange for their samples to be homogeneous.) Fortunately, most tissues in the human body have similar susceptibilities, and this effect is small. However, there is a particularly large susceptibility gradient at air-water interfaces, such as those existing in the lungs, stomach, trachea, and mouth. Images are distorted in these areas, and the effect is much greater on gradient echo images than on spin echo images. Very often, then, the magnet inhomogeneities we observe arise from the sample itself, and we do not gain by having more homogeneous magnets.

Clinical utility of gradient echoes. The dephasing due to B_0 inhomogeneities is the principal factor limiting the clinical utility of gradient echo imaging and can cause severe image distortion, particularly in regions where there are large susceptibility differences between tissues. Susceptibility effects also increase with B_0, and thus gradient echo imaging becomes increasingly difficult at high fields. Consequently, spin echo imaging remains the mainstay of modern clinical MRI, with gradient echoes being used for scout images (for fast set-up of the patient), for high speed imaging when clinically essential (in which case we must live with the image distortions), and of course for applications where we wish to highlight susceptibility variations.

Important pelvic imaging pulse sequences

There are literally hundreds of imaging techniques and pulse sequences that could now be discussed using our basic understanding. These include multiple techniques for performing high speed, microscopic, perfusion, diffusion, chemical shift, gated, solid, flow, and functional imaging, to name but a few. A discussion of all these methods is outside the scope of this chapter. However, within the context of this text on pelvic imaging, there are two important sequences that warrant some discussion, since they will be utilized in many of the studies described in the following chapters.

Water/fat chemical shift "artifact". As described so far, we have only considered NMR imaging using the NMR signal arising from the ^{1}H resonance from water in the human body. The NMR spectrum of water consists of a single resonance peak. However, there happen to be two major ^{1}H resonances observed from most body tissues: one arising from the water and one from the ^{1}H protons in lipids or mobile body fat (see Fig. 1-3, *C*). These two resonances are separated by a field-dependent frequency difference that at 1.5T is approximately 200 Hz.

This fat resonance has a twofold consequence:

(1) the generation of a chemical shift artifact on standard images and (2) provision of the opportunity of being able to produce separate images of the water and fat content in the body, as outlined below.

Chemical shift "artifact." I have described how the NMR image is a map of the frequency dependence of the NMR signal obtained when a magnetic field gradient is applied. Each pixel in the image thus has an associated frequency width, which is typically around 100 to 150 Hz. Since our fat resonance is shifted relative to the water resonance by 200 Hz, the image generated from the fat resonance will also be shifted by 200 Hz, i.e., by approximately 1 to 2 pixels. The fat image is thus displaced relative to the water image by a small amount and misregistered on the image. This effect is known as a chemical shift artifact and can be somewhat disruptive when one is interpreting images: the shifted fat image may sometimes overlie parts of the water image we wish to see. Sometimes it is not even clear if a small bright region in a particular image, for example, is water or fat, and thus in the right place or not. Care must be taken in these circumstances. Note here that the frequency difference between the fat and water resonances is directly proportional to the applied field, B_0, and thus this artifact is largest at high field strengths. Also, this effect is only significant in 2DFT imaging in the read gradient direction, i.e., we do not see a chemical shift artifact in the phase encoding direction.

Fat/water imaging. In many areas of the body, in particular the breasts and lower abdomen, there can be so much fat that it is difficult to distinguish the water signals. Generally, the water image is clinically far more informative than the fat image. Sometimes, however, it may be desirable to image just the fat. In this regard, several techniques are available for arranging to separate the fat and water images by exploiting either the frequency difference between the two resonances or the difference in their relaxation times.

Relaxation contrast. The T1 of fat is significantly shorter than that of water. Consequently, a heavily T1-weighted image (short TR) will weight the image toward fat content. Further, an inversion recovery sequence can be used with the inversion time chosen to null the fat signal in preference to the water signal. However, the lipids have a range of T1 relaxation times, thus reducing the effectiveness of this method.

Suppression/excitation. A suitably tailored rf pulse (one that excites a narrow frequency range) can be used to either excite or suppress only one of the resonances, since there is a frequency separation between them. Then, for example, we may arrange to form an image of either the fat or water content separately. Accurate control of the rf pulse is required, and thus good homogeneous rf coils are usually necessary. Also, good magnet homogeneity is required to ensure good separation of the fat/water resonances.

Segmented imaging sequences. As described so far, our basic imaging technique involves the collection of M suitably phase encoded echoes to construct an N × M image matrix. One phase encoded echo is collected after each excitation, i.e. after each TR. However, if we could collect more than one phase encoded echo within each TR, we would be able to collect all of our image data in fewer acquisitions and so decrease the total image acquisition time.

We may collect more than one phase encoded echo in each TR by using a multiecho sequence, as described above. There, we acquired several echoes within each TR, which consequently had differing T2 weightings. Alternatively, we may collect several echoes as before, but this time apply the appropriate phase encoding gradient pulse before each echo is collected. In this way we can typically collect two, four, eight, or 16 phase encoded echoes within each excitation (TR) and thus obtain our image two, four, eight, or 16 times faster, respectively. On clinical scanners the gradient performance usually limits us to obtaining eight or 16 echoes in each TR, since the echoes must be collected within roughly T2 (after which there is no signal left to encode). A common version of this form of imaging sequence is called fast spin echo (FSE) imaging. Although the images are collected faster, there is a penalty of reduced SNR (since less signal is collected), which is usually traded for a slight decrease in spatial resolution. Further, the image has a "composite" T2 weighting, since echoes are collected with different effective TEs. Nevertheless, such sequences have become very important for many applications where fast scans (a few seconds) are required to reduce motion artifacts and to perform time course studies, particularly in body imaging. FSE is also desirable rather than gradient echo fast scanning because of the reduced susceptibility artifacts, also extremely important for body imaging.

The idea of collecting more than one echo in each excitation was taken to its extreme early in the development of MRI. In the echo planar imaging (EPI) technique,[7] all the phase encoded echoes are collected in one excitation as quickly as in 30 to 40 msec. This is currently the fastest way of obtaining images and in particular has great potential application for real time imaging of the heart. However, very specialized hardware is required for this technique, in particular rapidly switching gradients. It is only recently that commercial imaging machines have had gradients of sufficient quality to allow an approach toward EPI. FSE is thus effectively a useful commercial compromise.

Hardware requirements

The detailed hardware design and construction considerations for MRI are beyond the scope of this chapter. Suffice it to say that the patient is placed in a large (usually 1-m bore) homogeneous magnet that is usually resistive (an electromagnet) or superconducting (a helium-cooled superconducting wire). The superconducting magnets have better homogeneity and can achieve higher field strengths for a given bore diameter but are more expensive. Incorporated just inside the central bore of the magnet are three orthogonal gradient coils interfaced to power supplies and gradient waveform control boards. A computer programs the imaging sequence into the waveform boards and initiates the image acquisition.

An rf coil is placed around the patient and interfaced to the rf transmitter/receiver electronics. A large power supply is required for the transmitter. The receiver digitizes the signal and passes it to a computer for processing, analysis, photography, and storage. For in-depth discussions of NMR hardware, the reader is referred to the literature.[7]

SIGNAL AND NOISE IN MRI

In the NMR experiment, there is a defined amount of signal available from the resonant nuclei within the sample, and it is our goal to utilize this signal most efficiently in order to generate the most useful clinical images. The following sections discuss those factors that control the signal and the noise in the NMR experiment. The hope is to impart to the reader a feeling for those parameters that influence the NMR image, how they interact, and how each may be manipulated in order to maximize image quality with respect to the particular information required of the image.

Signal-to-noise ratio

The signal in the NMR experiment is a small current induced in a receiver coil by an oscillating magnetic field generated by the excited resonant nuclei in the sample. This current is amplified, digitized, and processed to form the NMR image. In previous sections we saw that the amount of signal we can generate depends primarily on the number of resonant nuclei in the sample. The signal itself is coherent and linearly additive; i.e., if we add n units of signal, s, together we may expect the resultant signal to be n times larger:

$$(s + s + s + s \cdots)_n = ns \qquad \text{(Eq.4)}$$

Noise, on the other hand, is incoherent and is not linearly additive. It can be shown statistically that if n noise signals, N, are coadded, the resultant noise adds together as the square root of n:

$$(N + N + N + N \cdots)_n = N\sqrt{n}. \qquad \text{(Eq.5)}$$

The ratio of the signal to the noise is then the *signal-to-noise ratio (SNR)*, as previously mentioned. We thus see that if we have a signal with associated noise, we may coadd or average many such signals with noise together, whereupon the signal will increase in magnitude faster than the noise. This process is referred to as averaging and is a method of improving the SNR.

What is the noise? The noise arises primarily from two sources: the sample and the rf electronics. Random thermally generated motions of the electrons in the NMR electronics generate a random noise current that will add to the signal we wish to measure. This noise is minimized by careful electronic design and the use of low-noise-generating components, so that most of the noise arises from the intrinsic resistance of the NMR receiver coil. This may then be in principle eliminated by using supercooled rf coils so that their resistance is zero. Although supercooled coils can be difficult to construct, no noise would arise from the coil. However, there is a second noise source that is the sample itself.

Simplistically, we may imagine biologic tissues as large bags of water containing moving electrolytes or moving charges. When placed inside a large magnetic field, these moving charges will themselves generate random currents in the NMR receiver coil that add to the noise in the coil. We cannot eliminate this noise without removing the sample. Furthermore, this effect increases with the static magnetic field strength B_0. In practice, then, we design our hardware and minimize the noise arising from it until this noise is smaller than that arising from the sample. The dominant noise source is then the sample. Thus, in a practical MRI experiment, we have a fixed amount of signal available and a minimum to which we can reduce the noise, both of which are determined by the sample. It is then our goal to optimize our use of this signal.

Factors controlling signal-to-noise ratio

To a first approximation, the SNR in the MRI experiment is related to several physical and variable parameters[7]:

$$\text{SNR} \propto C \cdot (T2/T1)^{1/2} \cdot (1/r) \cdot f^{7/4} \cdot t^{1/2} \cdot (x,y,z) \qquad \text{(Eq.6)}$$

where C = an imaging efficiency factor, r = rf receiver coil radius, f = frequency, t = total acquisition time, and x,y,z = the spatial dimension of an image voxel.

The following sections briefly discuss each of the variables in equation 6 in terms of their impact on the MRI experiment and the ways in which we may optimize their contribution to the SNR.

Field strength. The signal available in the NMR experiment from a fixed number of resonant nuclei is proportional to $f^{7/4}$. Since the frequency increases linearly with B_0, the higher the magnetic field strength we use for the NMR experiment, the better the SNR we can achieve in a given time. For NMR spectroscopy this is certainly the case, and there has been a rapid drive toward the use of higher field strengths, and commercially available magnets currently reach field strengths of 14.2T with small-diameter magnets (5 cm). In a similar fashion, large-diameter magnets (100 cm) suitable for clinical use have evolved from the first low-field resistive type of 0.05 to 0.5T to the 2T superconducting whole body magnets of the present day. Although not yet clinically approved, 4T whole body magnets are presently being evaluated, and there exists the possibility of even higher-field whole body instruments.

However, each increment in the field strength of, say, 0.5T represents a considerable technical challenge that produces a relatively small increase in the SNR. Concurrent with the improved SNR achieved by increasing the field strength are several compromising factors.

Increased rf power requirements. The rf power required increases as the square of B_0. Presently, a commercial 1.5T whole body instrument uses 16-kW rf power supplies. A 12T whole body instrument would require up to 1-MW rf power supplies! The nature or occurrence of detrimental effects of relatively low rf power exposures currently remains unclear, and federal guidelines limit the rf power that can be used for clinical MRI. What is certain is that very large amounts of rf power are harmful and lead primarily to local heating in body tissues. Rf power requirements are consequently a real concern and may limit the ability to image at high field strengths.

Increased cost. The cost of development, construction, and maintenance of higher-field magnets increases rapidly with increasing field strength and is an obvious concern with regard to clinical efficacy. It is yet to be determined whether the improvement in image quality and utility is worth the increased cost, which ultimately will be paid by the patient.

Increased fringe field/siting problems. Higher-field magnets invariably become larger and heavier and have larger-ranging fringe fields, which may cause problems regarding attracting metal objects and affecting pacemakers, etc. Although various shielding strategies exist for reducing the fringe field of the magnets, these invariably lead to increased cost and may significantly increase the size and weight of the magnet.

Increased susceptibility effects. Magnetic susceptibility artifacts also increase with field strength and cause problems, especially in areas where there are air-liquid interfaces, e.g., lungs and abdomen. Generally, high-field imaging is beneficial for head and extremity imaging, and lower- or mid-field imaging is more suited for body imaging. We may find ultimately that radiology departments contain both low- and high-field machines, as a few presently do.

Rf coil design/construction/efficiency. As the field strength increases, so does the resonant frequency of the resonant nuclei in the sample; consequently, the rf transmitter and receiver coils must tune to this higher frequency. This requirement compromises the design of the rf coil and may somewhat reduce its efficiency, resulting in possible losses in the theoretically achievable SNR. It must be hoped that these problems are soluble and that these losses will be minimal.

Rf penetration. In 1978, it was predicted that MRI would not be feasible on a human body scale above a frequency of 10 MHz, because the rf energy would be absorbed by the sample and not penetrate all the way through the body tissue.[7] An image of the body would then be dark in the middle. These effects have proved extremely difficult to model and predict, primarily because of the complex heterogeneous nature of the body tissues, as borne out by the fact that we are presently imaging quite satisfactorily at 63 MHz. Although it is not yet clear at just what frequency this will ultimately be problematic, it may prove a major concern for high-field body imaging.

Biomagnetic effects. It is also extremely difficult to model and predict the effects of strong static magnetic fields on biologic tissues. Certainly, long-term exposure to very high magnetic fields can be harmful, but whether or not short-term exposure to medium field strengths has any detrimental effect is not clear. Federal guidelines exist to limit clinical use of high field strengths until appropriate studies have been performed. This may represent a major area for research should the trend toward the use of higher field magnets continue.

Gradient echo (fast) imaging. Gradient echo imaging techniques are more prone to susceptibility and B_0 inhomogeneity problems than spin echo imaging techniques, and consequently the workhorse of modern MRI is spin echo imaging. However, there is a necessity for gradient echo–based rapid imaging techniques for imaging, for example, the beating heart in real time and performing real time contrast wash-in/wash-out perfusion imaging experiments. Gradient echo methods become increasingly difficult to apply as the field strength increases and may ultimately be limited in their effectiveness to relatively low field strengths ($<2T$).

Considering the factors that may compromise high-field imaging, it is evident that a drive toward higher field magnets may not be warranted. Concerns regarding static field and rf exposure will be balanced by a patient risk-benefit ratio in a similar fashion to that presently used with regard to imaging with ionizing radiation. The effectiveness and utility of the several 4T whole body magnets presently under evaluation will determine the course of these events. It currently appears that higher fields (2 to 4T) may be most suitable for head and extremity imaging, while lower fields (0.1 to 1T) may be best for body imaging. Ultimately, relatively wealthy radiology departments may cater for both these regimens separately, whereas departments with smaller financial resources and/or smaller patient caseloads may compromise with one intermediate (1 to 2T) instrument.

Rf coil design and size

Coil size. The SNR varies inversely with the sensitive volume of the rf receiver coil. The noise in the NMR signal is not spatially localized and contributes to all voxels in the image, while the signal in each voxel arises from only that voxel and no other part of the sample. If we consider one voxel in an image, we may reduce the noise contribution to that voxel by reducing the size of the coil, i.e., reducing the size of the region from which the noise originates without changing the signal from the voxel. Reducing the size of the coil thus has the effect of reducing the noise in order to improve the SNR (contrary to frequent opinion, reducing the coil size does not increase the signal but reduces the noise). The size of the region the coil can interrogate will be referred to as its field of view (FOV).

Coil design. Given a particular coil size, the geometric design and construction of the coil can affect the SNR. There are many possible coil designs presently available, and the reader is referred to the literature. With careful coil design, signal losses can be minimized to a few percent. At higher fields where coil design becomes more difficult, this signal loss may be larger. However, these losses are not the most significant with regard to SNR, and with care may be minimized. By far the largest controlling factor with regard to SNR is the overall coil size.

This discussion is restricted to two general coil types: volume coils and surface coils. Volume coils encompass a complete section of the body, e.g., the head, the body, or a limb, and thus collect noise from that whole piece of tissue. Very often, however, we are interested only in some feature near the surface of the body, e.g., the eye, the heart, the spine, or a peripheral tumor. In these cases, a surface coil is optimal since it restricts the region from which noise is collected. A surface coil, in its most basic form, is simply a circular loop of wire of radius r.

Phased array coils. The improved SNR achieved through surface coils has inspired the development of a new range of NMR coils called *phased array* coils.[18] The idea is as follows: if a surface coil has improved SNR over a larger coil but a decreased FOV, we may regain the FOV by placing several surface coils in an array spanning the same FOV while maintaining the sensitivity of the smaller surface coils. In practice, this is limited by the fact that coplanar surface coils will normally interact with each other through inductive coupling and the image will be severely distorted. Further, each surface coil must have its own receiver and amplifier hardware to keep the signals from each coil distinct. These difficulties have recently been overcome by a careful coil arrangement and electronic design to eliminate interactions, resulting in phased array coils. As a result of this, we may choose to collect data from any or all of the surface coils in the phased array *simultaneously*. For example, if, instead of one 20-cm diameter surface coil, we used four 10-cm diameter coils arranged to cover approximately the same area as the 20-cm coil, we might expect to roughly improve the SNR by a factor of 2. One may then ask what the limit of such an approach may be: if we used 100 very small surface coils, each 2 cm in diameter, to again cover approximately the same FOV, could we expect a tenfold improvement in the SNR? In principle, yes. However, the trade-off here is that there is a decrease in the penetration depth of the coil array compared with the single coil. As shown in Fig. 1-24, we may expect a 20-cm diameter coil to produce a useful excitation to a depth of roughly one coil diameter (20 cm). The smaller coils, however, will be sensitive only to a depth of approximately 2 cm. Further, the array of 100 coils would require 100 separate receivers, which would be both cumbersome and expensive. Phased array coils thus appear most useful for examining regions close to the surface of the body where a relatively large FOV is required, in particular for examining the spine. They are now commercially available from General Electric, and we may expect arrays of up to eight coils giving SNR improvements of factors of 2 to 4.

Imaging sequence efficiency. The efficiency of

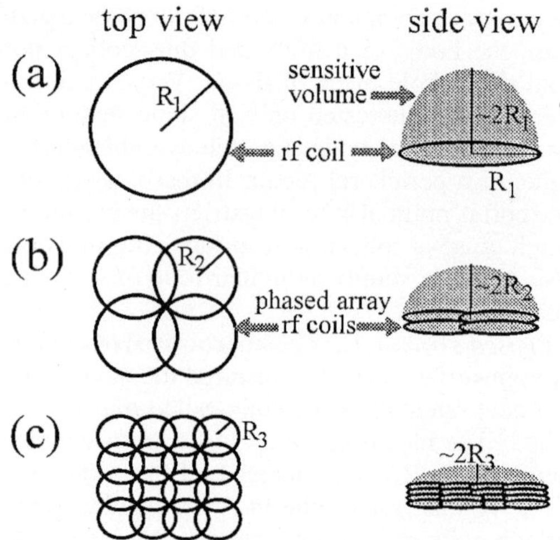

Fig. 1-24 A single surface coil excites a hemispherical volume of space (**A**). As the number of coils constituting a phased array covering approximately the same area as the single surface coils increases, the penetration depth (and hence hemispherical volume) decreases (**B** and **C**).

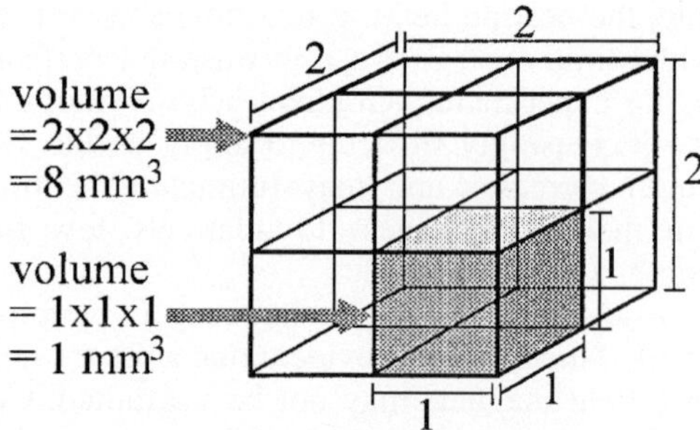

Fig. 1-25 A factor of 2 reduction in each spatial dimension of a cube results in an eightfold decrease in the volume of the cube.

the imaging sequence employed, C, will also dictate the available SNR we can achieve. However, these differences are relatively small (a few percent), and often our exact choice of imaging sequence is clinically determined by image contrast/information requirements. Other hardware or software factors may also lead to signal loss but may be minimized with careful pulse sequence design and hardware construction. These include imperfect rf pulses and gradient switching eddy current distortions, and can generally be kept down to a few percent.

Acquisition time. The SNR can be improved by averaging data accumulations. However, this quickly becomes very prohibitive with respect to the total imaging time, since the SNR improvement is proportional to the square of the acquisition time. For example, a doubling of the SNR requires an increase in the acquisition time of four, while a fivefold increase in the SNR requires a 25-fold increase in the acquisition time. Clinically, it is accepted practice to keep the total patient examination time to 1 to 2 hours, which often limits the number of averages we may use.

Relaxation times. The T1 and T2 relaxation times also affect the SNR we can achieve. Clinically, we cannot vary these parameters: obviously, they are fixed by the patient. However, given the T1 and T2 ranges in the body tissues, we must optimize the TE and TR of the imaging sequence with respect to the SNR. However, the constraint of

maximizing the SNR must be balanced against the image contrast we require and the total imaging time. Maximal SNR is obtained by using a very short TE (so that there is no T2 decay) and a long TR (so that the magnetization has returned under T1 relaxation to be aligned with the B_0 axis—this occurs after approximately 4 to 5 times T1). However, with a short TE there is no T2 contrast, and with a long TR there is no T1 contrast, both of which may be desirable in a clinical image to obtain good tissue discrimination. The object is therefore to use the minimal T2 and T1 weighting necessary to be clinically useful for tissue discrimination so that the SNR is reduced by the smallest amount possible.

Spatial resolution. The spatial resolution we require in the NMR image is the most expensive consideration with respect to the SNR. We must remember that the image is composed of an array of voxels that are three-dimensional entities. Clinically, we often speak of the image FOV (usually the same in the two dimensions of the image plane) and the slice width. Dividing the FOV by the number of sample points in each dimension gives us the lengths of two sides of each image voxel (x and y), with the slice thickness providing the third dimension (z). Suppose we have an image spatial resolution of 2 × 2 × 2 mm that we obtained in 1 minute, and we wish to simply "halve" this resolution while maintaining the SNR. At first thought the "halving" doesn't make this sound as if it would be very detrimental to the image quality. However, since the spatial resolution is three-dimensional, we would be required to halve the resolution in all three dimensions to 1 × 1 × 1 mm. As Fig. 1-25 illustrates, our voxel volume is now eight times smaller than it was originally and we have eight times less signal than before in each image voxel. If we used averaging to restore our SNR to that we had at the lower resolution, our imaging time would increase from 1 minute to 1 hour (since SNR is proportional to $\sqrt{t}$), and all we did was "halve" the resolution! In this example, we have assumed an isotropic spatial resolution, and so we may replace (x,y,z) in equation 6 with x^3. It is this cubic relationship that is the largest factor in equation 6. Improvements in spatial resolution are consequently very expensive with regard to the SNR.

In nearly all MRI studies the slice width is considerably larger (three to 10 times) than the in-plane spatial resolution. This practice is adopted to improve the SNR so that it produces reasonable-quality images and is often effective, leading to only a small and acceptable image blurring. This is helped by the fact that most tissues have considerable two-dimensional symmetry over regions of 1 to 5 mm.

Clinical decisions

So where does all this leave us, especially with regard to making clinical imaging decisions and maximizing the SNR? Which of the several factors described above have the most significant effect with regard to SNR, and which do we have reasonable control over?

1. The magnet will be of a fixed field strength and acquired primarily under financial constraints. This magnet will determine the maximum amount of signal that can be obtained from the sample. We then have to use this fixed amount of signal as efficiently as possible.
2. The T1 and T2 relaxation times are fixed by the sample in clinical imaging; we cannot alter the patient. Necessary T1 and T2 weighting may be desirable for good tissue discrimination and will degrade the SNR, depending on the contrast required to discriminate the tissues. These losses can usually be kept relatively low.
3. Similarly, losses due to imaging sequence efficiency will be determined by the type of sequence we need to produce the required contrast or image information. Again, these losses may be relatively small.
4. Although averaging may be used to increase the SNR, it quickly becomes very expensive with regard to total acquisition time because of the square root nature of the SNR improvement from coadding signals. Clinically, we are limited by considerations of patient tolerance. If patients are very ill, it is often difficult to keep them in the magnet for more than 1 hour while collecting useful data.
5. As a result of the cubic nature of the SNR dependence on the isotropic spatial resolu-

tion, this consideration is by far the most determining factor with regard to the SNR achievable in the images.
6. Reduction of the coil size is the most practical method available for improving the SNR in an image. For example, the reduction in size from a 60-cm diameter body imaging coil to a 6-cm diameter surface coil results in a 10-fold increase in the SNR. This improvement in the SNR may be traded for improved spatial resolution or decreased imaging time. The trade-off here is a reduced FOV as a result of the use of smaller receiver coil. This often restricts us to imaging some small portion of the patient, and most often to features relatively close to the surface of the body.

Clinically, then, we can make the following decisions:

1. The magnet (field strength), T1 and T2 relaxation times (the patient), and imaging sequence (clinical information) required are in most cases predetermined. Also, we prefer to minimize our total data acquisition time to under 1 hour.
2. We then choose the rf receiver coil size required to optimally encompass the clinical region of interest we wish to examine on the patient.
3. We choose the TE and TR desirable for suitable image contrast as dictated by the suspected clinical diagnosis, and select the spatial resolution desired.
4. These choices, in conjunction with the number of averages used, will result in an image with a particular SNR that may or may not be of useful quality. If not, we must then either increase the data acquisition time (often undesirable) or, most often, reduce the spatial resolution in the image. Since an isotropic spatial resolution increase has the largest (cubic) effect on the SNR, a relatively small decrease should usually be sufficient to correct the situation and produce useful images.

ACKNOWLEDGMENTS
The author gratefully acknowledges the patience of Dr. C. Hutchinson and Dr. P. Gibbs in laboring through this manuscript.

REFERENCES

1. Abragam A: *The principles of nuclear magnetism,* Oxford, 1961, Clarendon Press.
2. Ferrar TC, Becker ED: *Pulse and Fourier transform NMR,* New York, 1971, Academic Press.
3. Slichter CP: *Principles of magnetic resonance,* New York, 1978, Springer-Verlag.

4. Gadian DG: *Nuclear magnetic resonance and its applications to living systems,* Oxford, 1982, Oxford University Press.

5. Harris RK: *Nuclear resonance spectroscopy,* U.K., 1986, Longmans.

6. Ernst RR, Bodenhausen G, Wokaun A: *Principles of nuclear magnetic resonance in one and two dimensions,* Oxford, 1987, Clarendon Press.

7. Mansfield P, Morris PG: *NMR imaging in biomedicine.* Adv Mag Res, Suppl 2. New York, 1982, Academic Press.

8. Morris PG: *Nuclear magnetic resonance imaging in medicine and biology.* Oxford, 1986, Clarendon Press.

9. Foster MA, Hutchinson JMS: *Practical NMR imaging,* Oxford, 1987, IRL Press.

10. Stark DD, Bradley WG: *Magnetic resonance imaging,* ed 1, St. Louis, 1988, Mosby–Year Book.

11. Partain CL, Price RR, Patton JA, et al: *Magnetic resonance imaging,* Philadelphia, 1988, WB Saunders.

12. Wehrli FW, Shaw D, Kneeland JB: *Biomedical magnetic resonance imaging.* 1988, VCH Publishers.

13. Bleaney BI, Bleaney B: *Electricity and magnetism,* ed 3, Oxford, 1978, Oxford University Press.

14. Blackband SJ: *NMR imaging: an appraisal of the present and the future.* In Anderson JH, editor: *Innovations in diagnostic radiology,* Berlin, 1989, Springer-Verlag.

15. Bracewell RM: *The Fourier transform and its applications,* New York, 1965, McGraw-Hill.

16. Brigham EO: *The fast Fourier transform,* NJ, 1974, Prentice-Hall.

17. Herman GT: *Image reconstruction from projections: the fundamentals of computerised tomography. Computer science and applied mathematics,* 1980, Academic Press.

18. Roemer PB, Edelstein WA, Hayes CE, et al: *Magn Reson Med* 16:192, 1990.

2 Normal Magnetic Resonance Imaging Anatomy

Clare M.C. Tempany

Magnetic resonance imaging (MRI) provides the most detailed view of the female pelvic anatomy of any imaging modality currently available. Owing to the inherent tissue characterization properties and the multiplanar combination of T1- and T2-weighted MR images, the normal anatomy can be well delineated. This chapter reviews the normal MR appearance, on the major pulse sequences, of the following organs of the pelvis: (1) reproductive tract, (2) urinary tract, (3) gastrointestinal tract, and (4) musculoskeletal system, including the pelvic floor anatomy.

GENERAL STRUCTURE OF THE PELVIS

The pelvis is divided into two parts, the true and false pelvis, by the pelvic brim or iliopectineal line; the upper portion is the false pelvis. Thus, the true pelvis begins at the level of the sacral promontory, the iliopectineal lines on either side, and the crest of the pubic bones anteriorly. These lines form an angle of about 50 degrees with the horizontal. The pelvic cavity is bounded inferiorly by the pelvic outlet, which is made up of the pubic symphysis and arch and tip of the coccyx. Compared with the male pelvis, the female pelvis has lighter bones and less distinct muscle impressions, the cavity is larger, the sacral promontory is less prominent, the pubic arch is about 90 degrees (the male is about 60 to 70 degrees), and the inlet and outlet are larger and more oval in shape.

REPRODUCTIVE TRACT
Vagina

Structure. The vagina is a fibromuscular sheath that has a well-developed venous plexus in its walls. It has three layers: the mucosa, muscularis, and adventitia.[1] The walls are normally in apposition, and the inner lining is made up of folds of epithelium in ridges or rugae, which run in a circumferential manner from two longitudinal columns. This rugal formation, allows for significant distention, as seen in cases of hematometra.

The vagina is surrounded by several important structures: the urethra anteriorly, the rectum posteriorly, and the cervix superiorly. Histologically, it is lined by squamous epithelium that is continuous above over the vaginal portion of the cervix. The lymphatic drainage of the lower third is to the external iliac nodes, and of the upper two thirds to the internal iliac nodes.[2]

The upper third of the vagina is supported by the levator ani muscles, the middle third is attached to the lower portion of the cardinal ligaments, and the lower third is supported by the urogenital diaphragm and perineal body.

MR appearance. T2-weighted images allow for clear identification of the vagina itself and differentiation of its layers. The inner mucosal surfaces are usually apposed, and in between them there may be a thin layer of fluid or mucus. The vagina is best visualized in the axial plane, using T2-weighted images (Fig. 2-1). On T1-weighted images it appears, as on computed tomographic (CT) scans, often indistinguishable from the urethra, with similar signal intensity to skeletal muscle and no evidence of the different layers (Fig. 2-2). It is usually collapsed and sandwiched between the urethra and bladder anteriorly and rectum posteriorly (Fig. 2-2, *A*). These are all seen together as an H-shaped layer of high T2-weighted signal intensity (Figs. 2-1 and 2-3). The muscular wall of the vagina surrounds the inner H layer as a layer of low T2 signal intensity. The morphology of the flattened H shape allows differentiation from the adjacent urethra and rectum. The shape changes, however, becoming more ovoid and wider at the

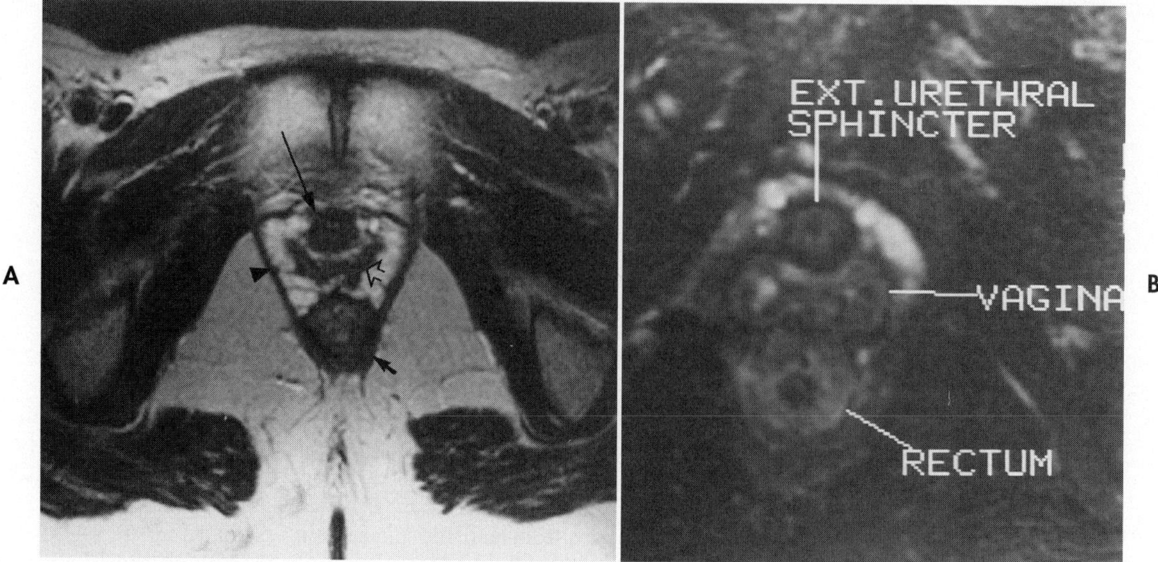

Fig. 2-1 Axial T2-weighted images of the lower pelvis, showing the vagina *(open black arrow)*, urethra *(long black arrow)*, perivaginal venous plexus *(black arrowhead)*, and rectum *(black arrow)*, both without **(A)** and with **(B)** fat suppression. Both images were obtained with the pelvic phased array coil.

level of the fornices. The presence of a tampon allows for easy distinction of the vaginal cavity (Fig. 2-4); this can also be useful in the sagittal plane, where the tissues of the lower pelvis come very close and are often indistinguishable (Fig. 2-5). As the axial plane images progress cephalad, the vaginal fornices become apparent as a widening of the H cavity. The outer wall of the fornices become less well defined, and they are surrounded by the high T2 signal vascular plexus. As the vaginal vault ends at the level of the fornices, the cervical stroma becomes evident in cross-section (Fig. 2-6). The external os of the cervix extends down into the vagina, which surrounds it with its lateral fornices (Figs. 2-7 and 2-8).

The perivaginal venous plexus lies beyond the vaginal cavity itself (see Figs. 2-1 and 2-3). This plexus is seen as a layer of high T2 signal intensity that forms a ring around the entire vagina, and extends anteriorly and posteriorly around the urethra and rectal orifices. It is of variable thickness, being under hormonal stimulation, and can reach thicknesses of up to 10 mm, especially in the secretory phase of menstruation, in patients on exogenous estrogen, and most especially during pregnancy, when it is thickest.

Cervix

Structure. The cervix is the lowest portion of the uterus that protrudes into the vagina surrounded by the vaginal fornices, which divide the cervix into the supravaginal and vaginal portions. The vaginal portion or exocervix is covered by squamous cell epithelium, and at its center is the external os. This is connected to the isthmus of the uterus at the internal os by the cervical canal. This canal measures 8 mm at its widest point and is lined by multiple mucosal folds called plicae palmatae.

The internal os is the beginning of the cervix; this is demarcated by a histologic change where the epithelium changes from glandular to columnar epithelium. The cervical stroma is a mixture of fibrous, muscular, and elastic tissue. The upper isthmus portion is 60% muscular, forming a sphincter; lower down, the stroma is predominantly fibrous.[3]

MR appearance. Morphologically the cervix appears as a discrete round mass. It has, in keeping with its tissue make-up, a very typical appearance on T2-weighted images (Fig. 2-8). As first described by Hricak et al, there are three layers of the cervix visible on T2-weighted images.[4] It appears as a very low signal intensity ring or "donut" with a central lumen of high signal intensity (Fig. 2-8), surrounded by an outer layer of intermediate signal intensity. The low signal intensity ring represents the dense fibrous stroma of the cervical canal, which is continuous with the junctional zone of the uterus. The high T2-weighted signal stripe represents the central endocervix containing glandular fluid, mucus, and the plicae palmatae.[5]

Text continued on p. 41.

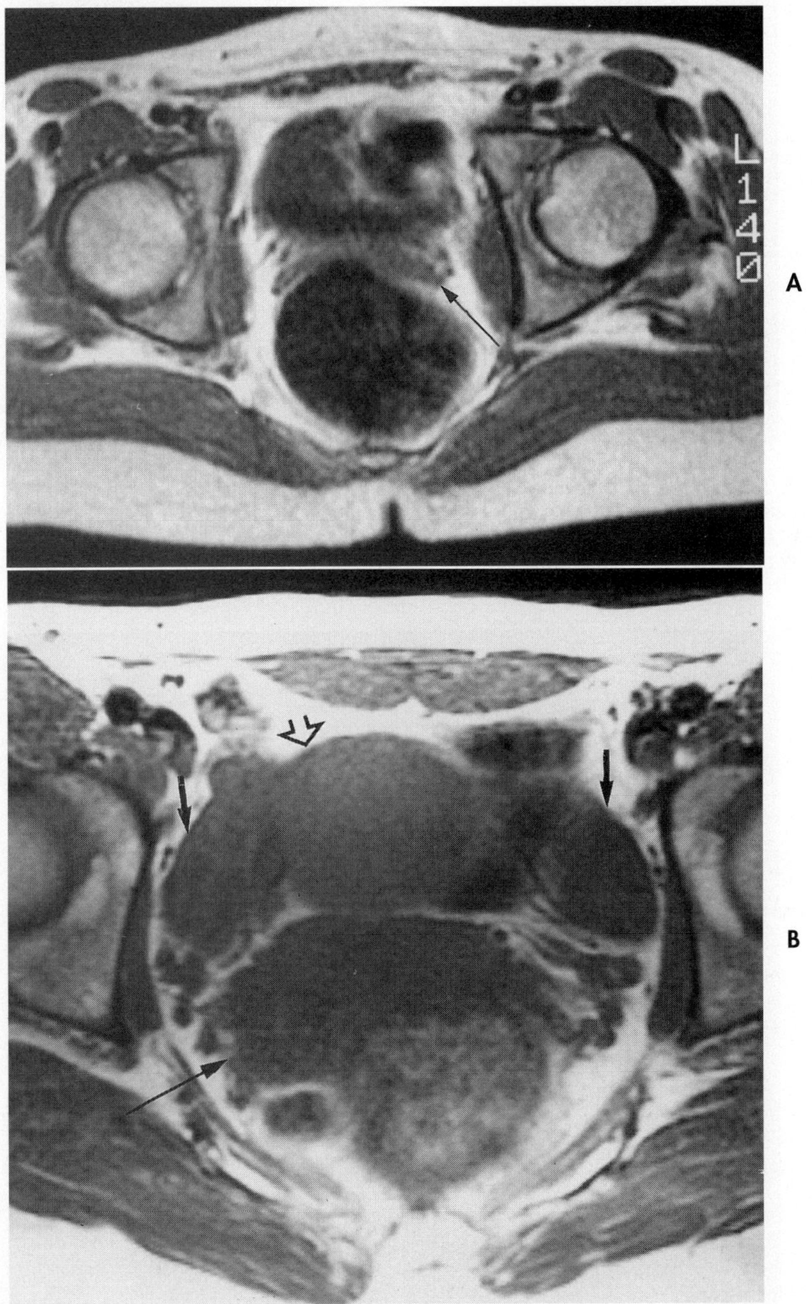

Fig. 2-2 Axial T1-weighted images of the upper vagina, only evident by its location and characteristic shape. **A,** An axial T1-weighted image, with the body coil of the vagina *(long black arrow)* between the bladder and the rectum. It is collapsed and sandwiched between the urethra, bladder, and rectum, forming a flat, ovoid-shaped structure. **B,** The signal intensity of the vaginal fornices *(long black arrow),* uterus *(open black arrow),* and ovaries *(short black arrows)* are all the same as skeletal muscle on this T1-weighted image with the phased array coil.

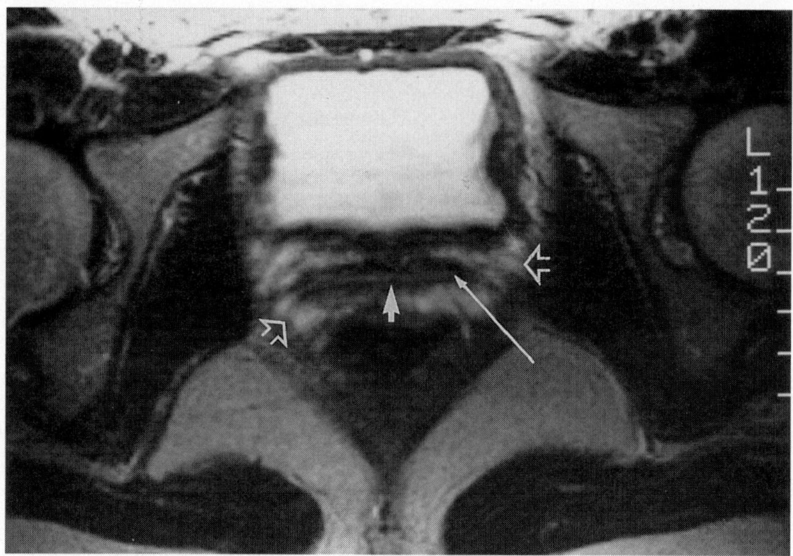

Fig. 2-3 Axial fast spin echo (FSE) T2-weighted image with the phased array coil, at the same level as the image in Fig. 2-2A, shows the typical signal of the vagina and its layers, the central mucosa *(long white arrow),* outer muscularis *(short white arrow),* and perivaginal venous plexus *(open white arrows).*

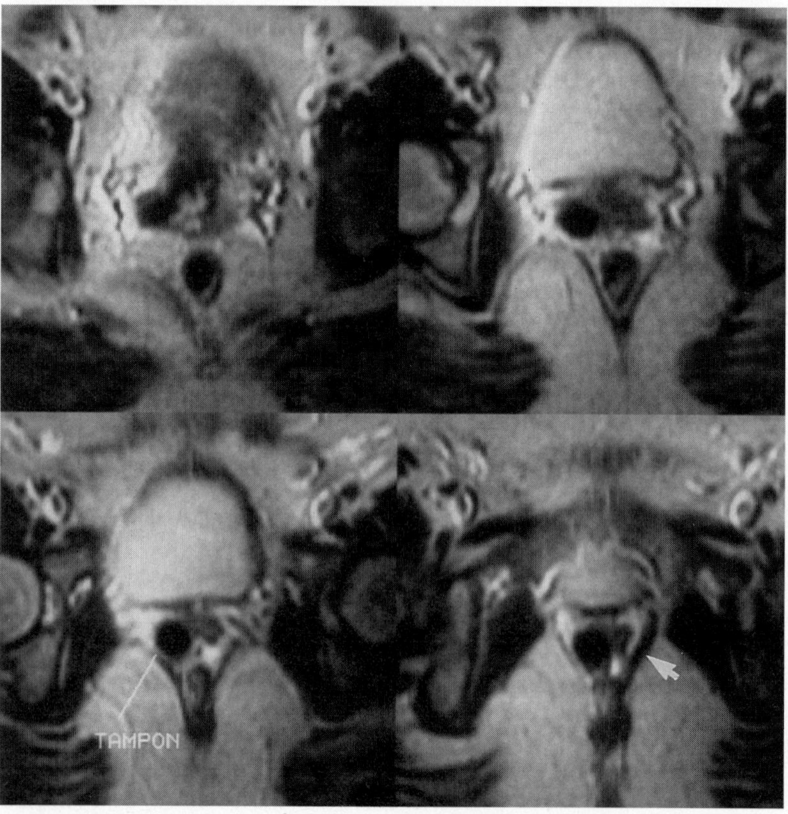

Fig. 2-4 Four axial CSE T2-weighted images (TR 2000, TE 80 msec) of the vagina with a tampon allow for easy identification of the cavity, especially at the different levels; the cavity can be followed inferiorly. Note the chemical shift artifact causing false thickening of the levator muscle on the left *(white arrow).*

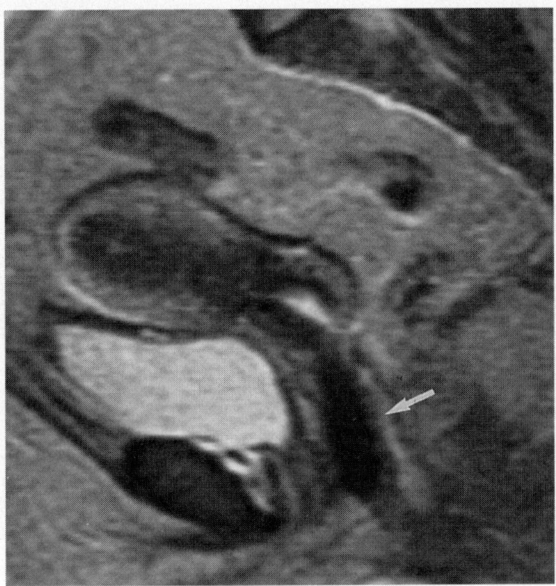

Fig. 2-5 Sagittal T2-weighted images (TR 2000, TE 80 msec). The tampon *(white arrow)* can also be useful in this plane where the tissues of the lower pelvis come very close and are often indistinguishable.

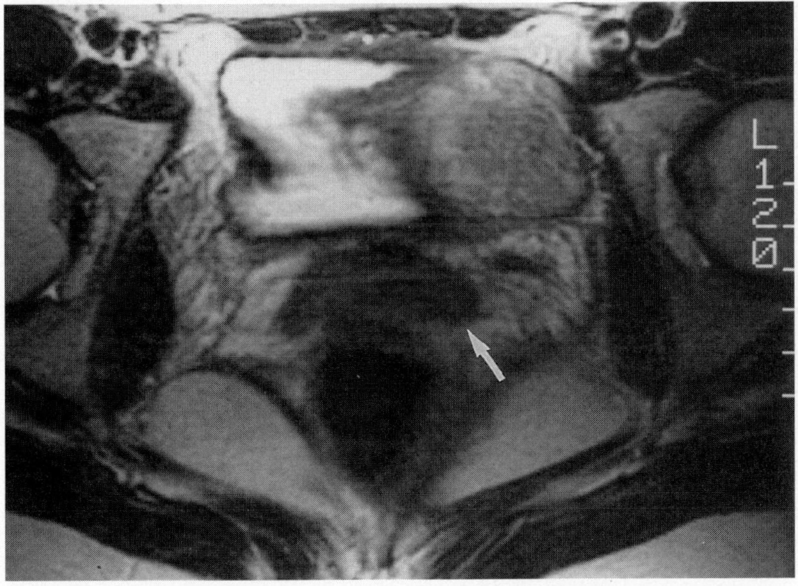

Fig. 2-6 Axial T2-weighted FSE images (TR 4000, TE effective 108 msec), with the phased array coil, show the uppermost portion of the vaginal vault at the level of the fornices *(white arrows).*

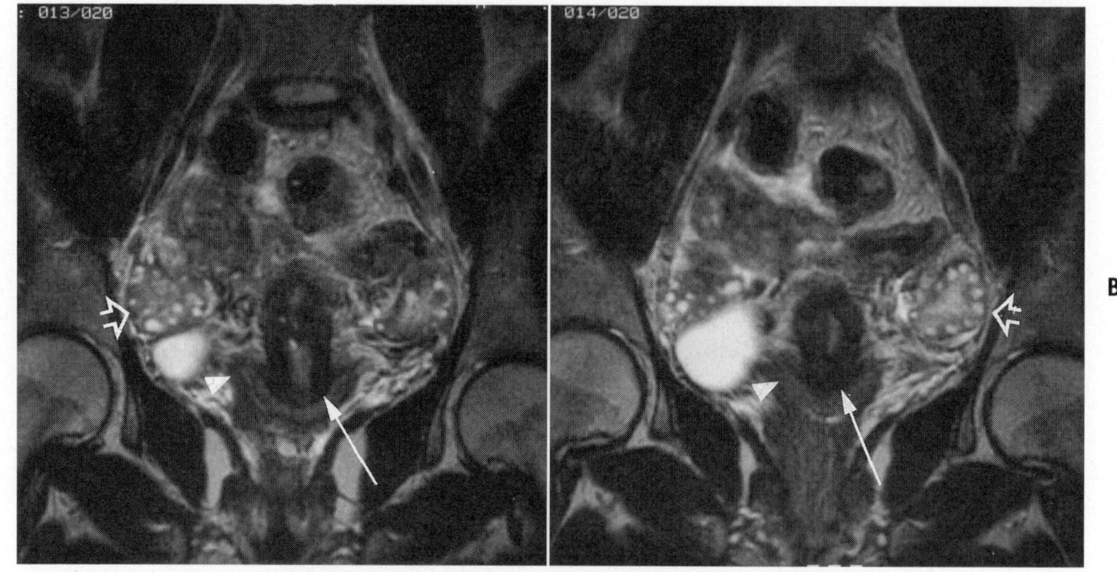

Fig. 2-7 Two coronal FSE T2-weighted images, with the phased array coil, 5 mm apart (TR 4000, TE effective 108). Both **A,** the more posterior, and **B** show the external os of the cervix *(long white arrow)* and the lateral fornices of the vagina *(white arrowhead);* the right and left ovaries are seen *(open white arrow)*. Note the normal appearance of the ovarian stroma with the surrounding follicles on the left.

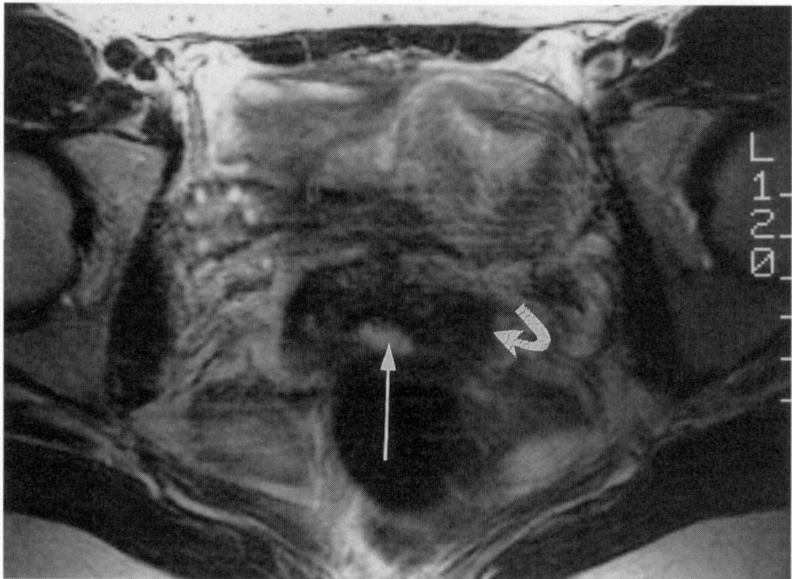

Fig. 2-8 Seen 1 cm higher than in Fig. 2-6, the external os of the cervix *(curved white arrow)* is visible on these T2-weighted images as a very low signal intensity ring or "donut" with a central lumen of high signal intensity *(long white arrow),* which represents the central endocervix containing fluid or mucus.

The fibromuscular stroma has two layers, an inner one that is the very low signal intensity layer, and the outer intermediate layer, which is now routinely seen on fast spin echo (FSE) images.[6] When detailed histologic correlation of the different layers was performed, it was found that the outer layer differs from the inner one only in that it has a lower percentage nuclear area (number of cells per unit volume); there was no difference in the composition of collagen, extracellular matrix, or basement membrane glycoproteins.[5]

The standard axial plane T2-weighted images normally depict the cervix clearly (Fig. 2-8). However, it may occasionally be necessary to obtain true cross-sectional images from the external to internal os. These may be obtained by an off-axis imaging plane, localized from a sagittal image. These will allow for a true cross-sectional assessment of the cervical stroma and canal with transaxial images through the cervical ring. The external os is defined as the lowermost portion of the endocervical canal, with the exocervix surrounded by the vaginal vault or fornices. The sagittal and coronal planes allow for visualization of the external os with the anterior and posterior lips of the cervix (Figs. 2-7 and 2-9). It can be clearly separated from the fornices of the vagina by its characteristic low signal. Nabothian cysts (benign simple cysts of the exocervix) are frequently seen; they are small (usually less than 2 cm) and best seen on T2-weighted images. Occasionally, even the plicae palmatae of the endocervical canal can be distinguished (Fig. 2-10).

The lymphatic drainage of the cervix is effected through four efferent channels (1) to the external iliac and obturator nodes, (2) to the hypogastric and common iliac nodes, (3) to the sacral nodes, and (4) to the nodes of the posterior wall of the bladder.

Ligaments of the cervix. The supravaginal cervix is suspended from the lateral pelvic side wall by the cardinal ligaments of Mackenrodt, which pass from the cervix out to the side wall and merge with the connective tissue surrounding the internal iliac vessels. The ureters pass through the middle of these ligaments. Interestingly, the ligaments may be pulled down in uterine prolapse, and lead to kinking and obstruction of the ureters.

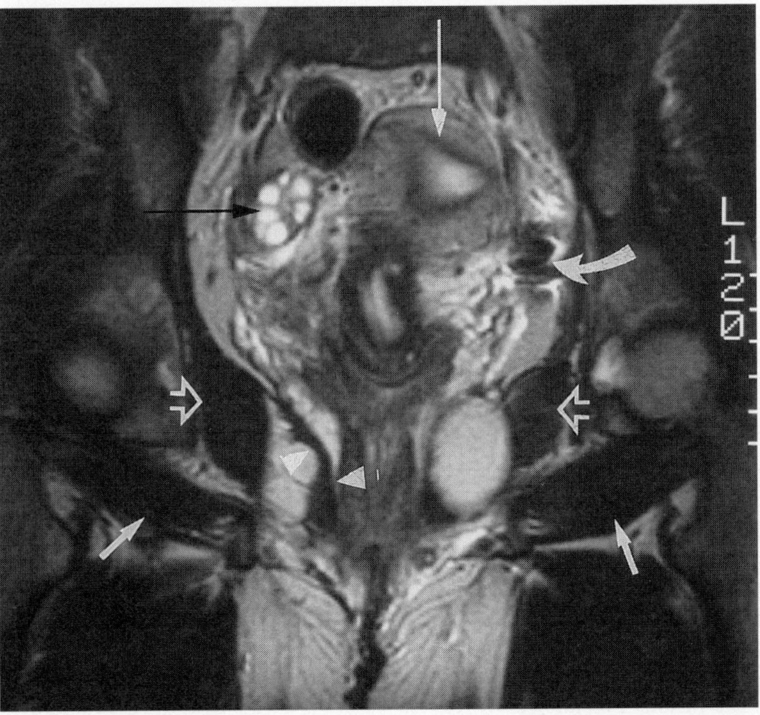

Fig. 2-9 FSE T2-weighted coronal image with the phased array coil, showing the external os with the fornices of the vagina surrounding the low signal cervix. The levator muscles supporting the lateral vaginal walls can be seen extending from the pelvic side wall *(white arrowheads)* and the muscles of the pelvic side walls, the obturator internus *(open white arrow)* and externus *(short white arrow)*. Note the uterus *(long white arrow)* and right ovary *(long black arrow)* superiorly. Of interest, there has been a left oophorectomy, and a surgical clip can be seen with the typical local field distortion and artifact *(curved white arrow)*.

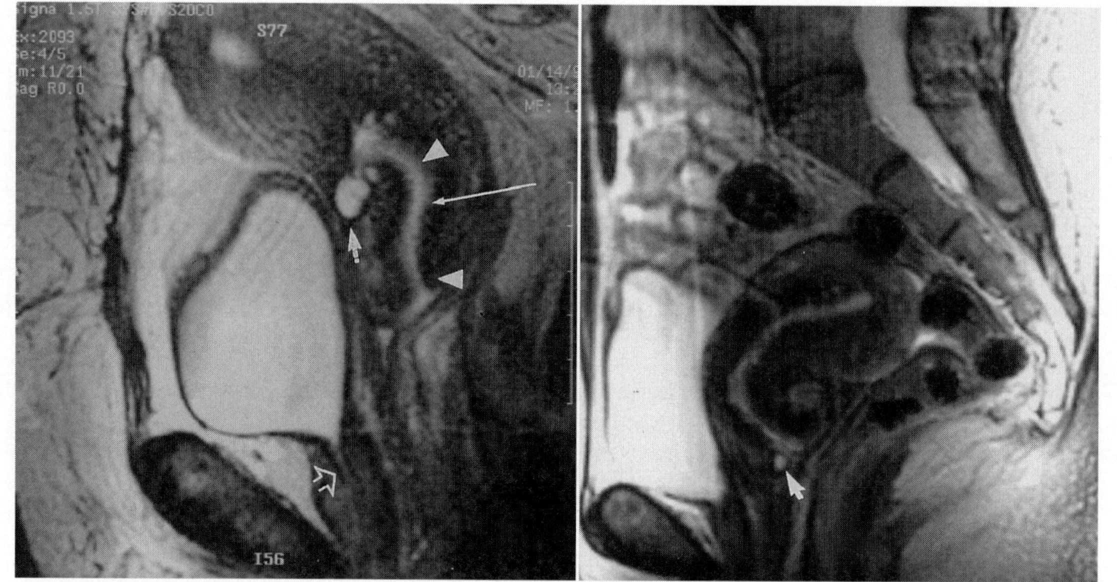

Fig. 2-10 A, Sagittal FSE T2-weighted image showing the full length of the cervical canal, from the internal to the external os *(white arrowheads).* A nabothian cyst is seen in the cervix *(short white arrow).* The plica palmatae can be seen in the endocervical canal *(long white arrow).* The bladder neck and external urethral sphincter can be seen with the urethra *(open white arrow)* in the normal closed or apposed condition. **B,** This sagittal T2-weighted image of a 48-year-old woman shows the cervical canal in this retroflexed uterus, with a small nabothian cyst at the external os *(white arrow).* Note that the zones of the uterus are not clearly defined in this perimenopausal woman.

Anteriorly, the supravaginal cervix is suspended from the posterior aspect of the pubic bone by the pubocervical ligament. This ligament also surrounds the internal urethral sphincter. Posteriorly, the cervix is connected to the sacrum (at sacral levels 2 to 4) by the uterosacral ligaments, one on either side of the rectum. These are a common site of tumor spread from the cervix. All these ligaments unite to form a continuous sheet of connective tissue across the pelvic floor.

Uterus

The uterus is a pear-shaped organ that averages about 7 to 9 cm in length. It varies in size, according to age, being largest during the reproductive years and smallest in childhood and after menopause. It is divided into the fundus, body, and cervix, the fallopian tubes enter the superolateral corners (cornua), and the fundus lies above this level. The body narrows down at the isthmus, which is a narrowed region between the body and the cervix. This area is the lower uterine segment of pregnancy and has less well developed muscle than the body, allowing for the enlargement and stretching during pregnancy. The vagina begins externally about halfway down the cervical canal. The internal os is the junction between the body and isthmus of the uterus. The mucosal surface of the isthmus is the same as the endometrium of the body of the uterus. The internal os opens into the cervical canal, which ends at the external os into the vagina.

Position. The normal uterus lies anterior to the cervix, forming an angle of 170 degrees at the internal os. This is the normal anteflexed uterus. Anteversion is when the cervix forms a 90-degree angle with the vagina; the uterus is then horizontal (Fig. 2-11). Retrodisplacement is either of two positions, retroflexion or retroversion. In retroversion the angle of the cervix is backward and upward (Fig. 2-12). In retroflexion the body of the uterus is backward compared with the cervix (Fig. 2-13).

Structure. The uterine fundus and body are covered by a layer of visceral peritoneum. Posteriorly the peritoneum reflects down deeply to the rectum, forming the rectouterine pouch (pouch of Douglas), which extends down to the level of the posterior fornix of the vagina; anteriorly, however, the vesicovaginal pouch is not so deep. The pouch of Douglas is a common place for dependent fluid or metastases to collect (Fig. 2-11). At the level of

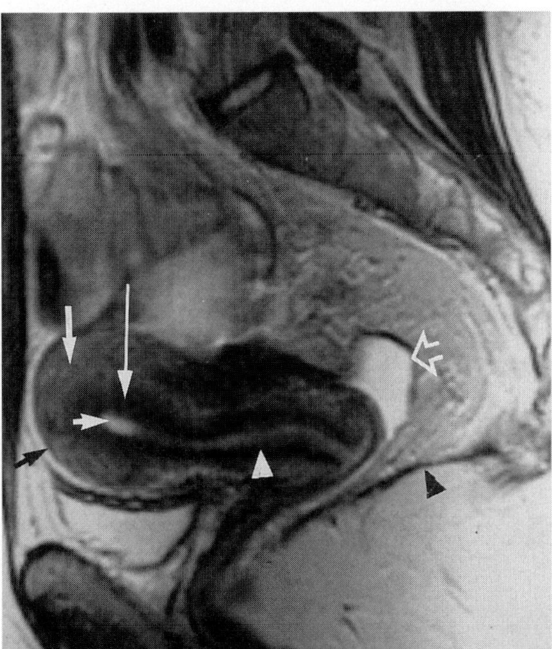

Fig. 2-11 Sagittal T2-weighted image with the phased array coil of the anteverted uterus, showing the normal T2 appearance of the uterine layers, the endometrium *(short white arrow)*, the junctional zone *(long white arrow)*, and the continuation of the junctional zone into the cervical canal. The myometrium *(white arrow)* and subserosal layer *(black arrow)* are also seen. A small collection of fluid *(open white arrow)* is seen in the pouch of Douglas. Note the plicae palmatae *(white arrowhead)* of the endocervical canal, and a portion of the pubococcygeal muscle extending from the tip of the coccyx *(black arrowhead)*.

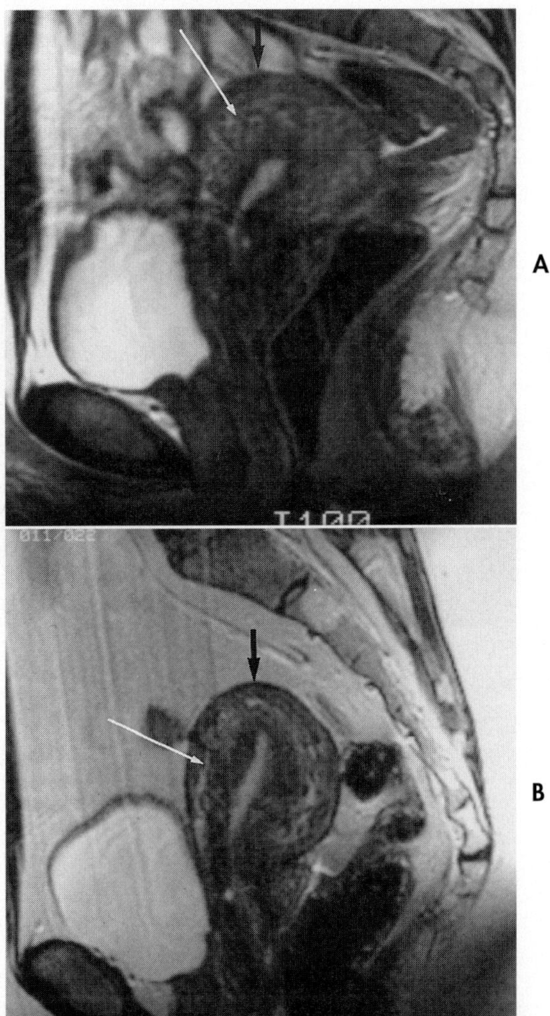

Fig. 2-12 A and **B,** Sagittal FSE T2-weighted images with the phased array coil, showing retroverted uterus, with all the uterine layers again evident. On these images the stratum vasculare *(long white arrow)* of the myometrium and subserosa *(black arrows)* can be identified. The anteroposterior relationships of the three organs (urethra, vagina, and rectum) can be seen to the level of the perineum.

the isthmus of the fallopian tubes is the insertion of the round ligament (Fig. 2-14) or muscle that passes down to the labia majora.

Histologically, there are four layers of the uterus: the endometrium, subendometrium, stratum vasculare, the subserosal layer.[7] The endometrium is a layer of variable thickness made up of endometrial glands called the stratum functionale and basale. These glands interdigitate with the myometrium. The two layers are often in apposition, with a thin layer of fluid, mucus, or blood between them. Beyond this is the subendometrial layer of smooth muscle. The next layer is the stratum vasculare, where the arcuate vessels run through the myometrium. The last layer is the subserosal muscle.

Deep to the peritoneal covering is the serosal layer, which covers the myometrium. There is a subserosal lamina layer made up of smooth muscle bundles.

MR appearance. The body and fundus of the uterus contain four distinct zonal layers that can be characterized clearly on T2-weighted images (see Figs. 2-10 to 2-14). The layers that are evident are, from the outside in, the serosal layer, myometrium, junctional zone, and endometrial cavity. The outermost or serosal surface is usually distinct from the myometrium. It may be seen on the higher-resolution, phased array T2-weighted images as a thin dark line (see Figs. 2-11 and 2-12).

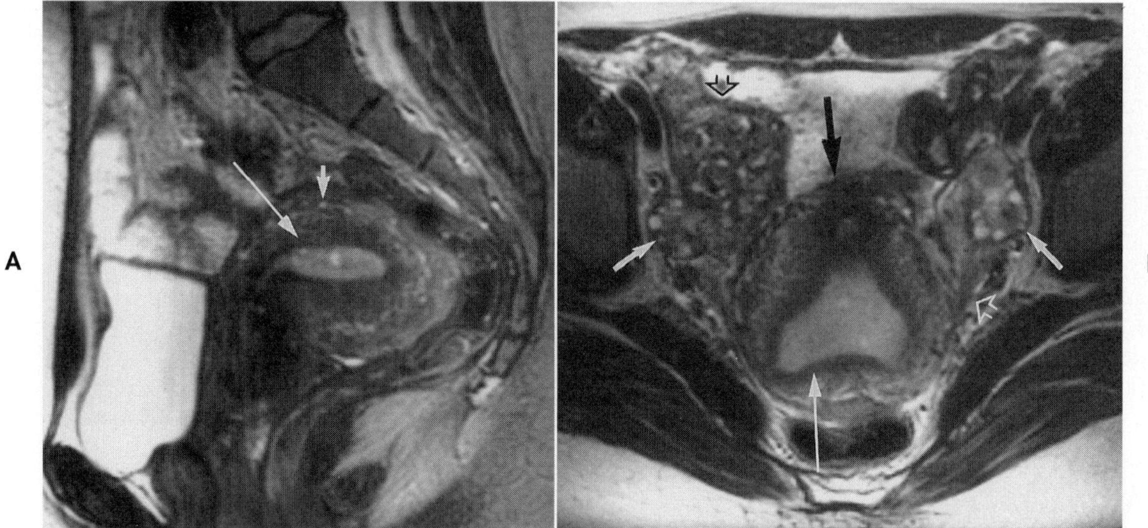

Fig. 2-13 Images of a 31-year-old woman, with the phased array coil, using FSE (TR 4000, TE effective 102 msec). **A,** Sagittal T2-weighted image shows a retroflexed uterus with normal zonal architecture, the junctional zone *(long white arrow)*, and the stratum vasculare *(short white arrow)*. **B,** Image of the same patient in the axial plane shows extreme retroflexion, allowing full visualization of the entire endometrial cavity surrounded by the junctional zone *(long white arrow)*, extending to the endocervical canal *(black arrow)* on one image. The ovarian ligament *(open white arrow)* can be seen on the left. The two ovaries *(short white arrows)* are seen anteriorly with several small follicles in each. The cecum *(open black arrow)* is also seen anterior to the right ovary.

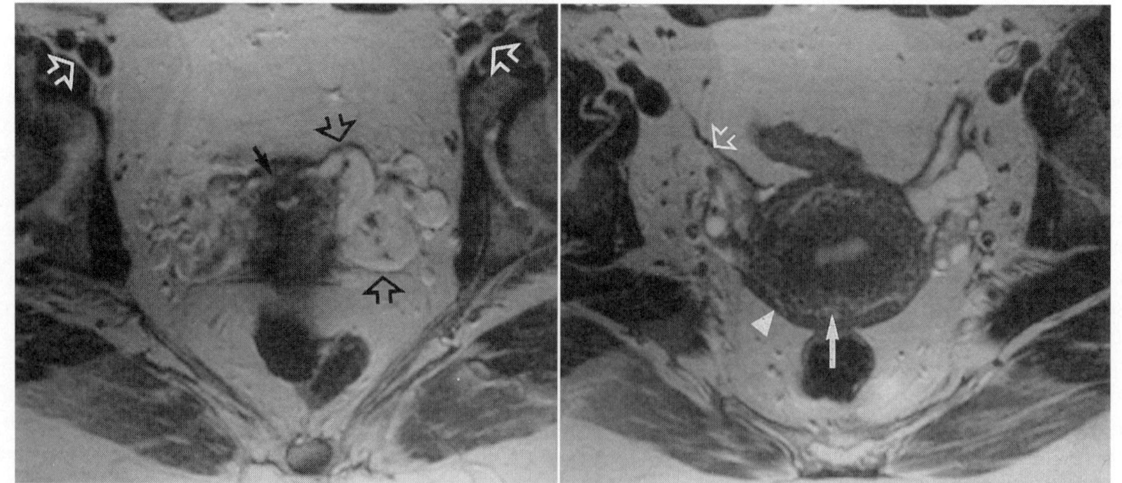

Fig. 2-14 Axial FSE T2-weighted images through the cervix and uterus with the phased array coil. **A** shows the cervix *(short black arrow)* and parametrial vessels *(open black arrows)*. The normal external iliac vessels *(open white arrows)* with central flow void are identified. **B** A more cephalad transaxial image shows the uterus in cross-section. The vascular layer with the arcuate vessels *(short white arrow)* and the subserosa *(white arrowhead)* are seen. The round ligament of the uterus is seen on the right *(open white arrow)*.

Both the myometrium and endometrial cavities are under hormonal stimulation and will therefore have varying MR appearances, depending on the phase of the menstrual cycle and the menstrual status (pre- or postmenopause) of the patient.

Myometrium. In premenopausal women in the follicular phase of the cycle, the myometrium has a relatively diffuse intermediate signal intensity on T2-weighted images (see Figs. 2-10 to 2-14). In the secretory phase of the cycle the myometrial signal increases diffusely with increasing fluid content and increased vascular flow. The higher signal may be inhomogeneous, and foci of higher signal may be seen corresponding to the increased tissue water and vascular perfusion. In postmenopausal women the myometrium no longer shows these cyclic changes and is usually diffusely low in signal on T2-weighted images. As the patient ages further, the uterus atrophies and decreases in overall size.

Interesting work has been done to correlate the MR signal of the myometrium and its histologic counterpart. Brown et al found that the myometrium has three layers, the inner third of which is the junctional zone.[8] The myometrium proper begins when the junctional zone ends at the level of the arcuate arteries, the stratum vasculare; the third layer is the subserosal layer (see Figs. 2-12 and 2-14).

The myometrial signal is normally intermediate to high signal on T2-weighted images but does change with the menstrual cycle. It increases in signal in the secretory phase, with changes in signal due to increased blood flow, increased water content, and congestion. The myometrial signal may even change during a single examination. It may show transient bulges and areas of lower signal. These have been described by Togashi et al and are thought to represent uterine contractions.[9] It is important to differentiate this normal finding from uterine leiomyomas or adenomyosis.

Junctional zone. The middle layer of the uterus, or junctional zone, represents the basal layer of the myometrium (see Figs. 2-11 to 2-14). It is composed of longitudinally oriented smooth muscle.[8] It is in fact two layers, the inner compact portion and the outer transitional portion that blends into the myometrium proper; the muscle is less compact in this area.[8] The junctional zone measures on average 5 mm, about half the thickness of the rest of the myometrium. It is a thin, low signal intensity line between the endometrium and myometrium on T2-weighted images. The low signal may be accounted for by the compact nature of the muscle bundles with little extracellular space. There is a difference in the nuclear area (number of cells per unit volume) in the junctional zone, which

is higher than the remaining myometrium.[10] The interface with the endometrium is sharp, but that with the myometrium is less well defined. The uterine arcuate arteries are at the level of this transition from junctional zone to stratum vasculare of the myometrium proper (see Fig. 2-14). The junctional zone is routinely visible and a continuous line in premenopausal women (see Figs. 2-10 to 2-14). It extends from the endocervical canal up around the body and fundus. This layer does not undergo hormonal stimulation and does not change during the menstrual cycle. It is, however, inconsistent, and if present may be incomplete in postmenopausal women. With the progressive atrophy and progressive drop in signal intensity of the myometrium, the junctional zone becomes less apparent (see Fig. 2-10).

Endometrium. The signal of the endometrial cavity is high on T2-weighted images, which show it best in the sagittal plane (see Figs. 2-10 to 2-13). At standard T2-weighted parameters, the signal contribution from blood, fluid, and the glandular layers themselves cannot be separated. This corresponds to the echogenic stripe seen on sonography and the low attenuation seen on CT.

The endometrium is usually thinnest just after menses, and progressively thickens toward ovulation and into the secretory phase. The cavity reaches its maximum thickness just before menses. In premenopausal women, it cycles, ranging in thickness from 3 to 5 mm. It is significantly wider in the secretory phase than in the follicular phase.[11] In women taking birth control pills, it no longer cycles and remains very thin (approximately 1 mm) throughout the "cycle." This measurement should be taken from T2-weighted images in the sagittal plane in the body of the uterus, taking in both layers, excluding the dark signal junctional zone. These correlates closely with ultrasonographic studies of the echogenic line of the endometrial cavity.[12] In postmenopausal women the endometrium atrophies, no longer undergoing monthly hormonal stimulation. The endometrial stripe becomes progressively thinner as the patient ages, with average thicknesses of 2 to 3 mm. Thus, in a postmenopausal woman who is not taking exogenous hormones, such as estrogen replacement, it should measure no more than 2 to 3 mm.

An exception at this age is the woman who is taking exogenous estrogen therapy. This therapy maintains the hormonal stimulation to the uterus, with consequential increased signal within the myometrium and increased thickening of the endometrial cavity. The postmenopausal woman on estrogen therapy may have an endometrial cavity measuring as much as 1 cm in thickness. Thus, it is important when imaging these patients to determine not only the menstrual status but also whether they are receiving exogenous estrogen therapy.

Serosal layer. This layer can now be routinely be seen on phased array MR images. It can be distorted by chemical shift artifacts, which can make one side appear thicker than the other.

The lymphatic drainage of the uterus is via three networks from the endometrium, myometrium, and superficial subperitoneal surface. The channels pass out in the broad ligament folds to the pelvic side wall and then into the iliac chain of nodes. Some of the drainage passes out with the round ligament down to the inguinal nodes; two of the lower channels drain into the parametrial nodes lateral to the ureter. A few channels drain posteriorly along the uterosacral ligament to the sacral nodes.[1]

Ovaries

The ovaries are normally located in the space formed just below the angle of the common iliac artery and vein bifurcation. They are typically against the pelvic side wall, anterior to the internal iliac vessels and ureter. This is the most common location for the ovaries in nulliparous women. In multiparous women the ovaries may be laterally placed or more superior or inferior in location. The ovaries are at the end of the fallopian tube's infundibulum, and are surrounded by the fimbriae and suspended from the uterus by the ovarian ligament (see Fig. 2-13, *B*).

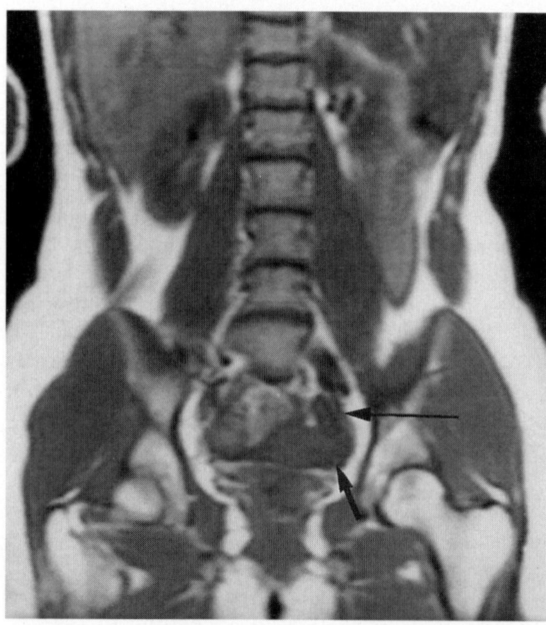

Fig. 2-15 Large field of view coronal T1-weighted image shows the uterus *(short black arrow)* and broad ligament. By following the ligament out laterally, the ovaries are identified *(long black arrow)*.

To locate the ovaries on MR, the coronal scan can be helpful (Fig. 2-15). The axial scans are the most reliable (Fig. 2-16). Using body coil technology at 0.35T, MR was found to identify up to 87% of the adenexa bilaterally in normal patients.[13] With phased array techniques at 1.5T, this figure is likely nowadays to be considerably higher. The coronal images can be very helpful by identifying the uterus and the broad ligaments that lead out to the ovaries (Fig. 2-17). The sagittal T2-weighted images are also useful for identifying the ovaries, as the angle inferior to the iliac bifurcation can usually be clearly seen in one plane (Fig. 2-18). The sagittal plane images should always cover the center of the pelvis from side wall to side wall, as the ovaries can lie almost anywhere in the pelvis, especially in patients who have undergone hysterectomy (Fig. 2-19).

The normal ovary, best identified on T2-weighted images, has a very typical appearance, with an "almond" shape and with multiple small, high signal intensity follicles identified around the central stroma (see Fig. 2-16). In normal cases, the outer boundary or capsule of the ovary can be clearly defined surrounding the discrete, well-defined follicles (see Fig. 2-16). The ovaries involute and atrophy in postmenopausal women and, as the patient ages, become more difficult to identify on a routine basis. While the increased resolution offered currently from the phased array coil in MRI should help reduce this problem, it is relatively common not to identify the ovaries in elderly women. However, it is nearly always possible to identify the ovaries in all premenopausal women.

URINARY TRACT

The urinary tract consisting of the urethra, bladder, and distal ureters, is routinely well delineated on MR images. The distal urethra has a very typical appearance on T2-weighted images.[14] The muscular layers of the external urethral sphincter can be seen. At the level of the perineum and just below the bladder base, the urethra is a round or funnel-shaped structure that consists of layers of longitudinal and circular muscle (see Fig. 2-1). In continent females the central lumen of the urethra is apposed or closed and may be seen only as a very small focus of high signal intensity on T2-weighted images. The high signal intensity represents fluid within the apposed layers of the urethra. In women with incontinent sphincters the lumen is wide and the funnel shape of the unapposed lumen is seen on T2-weighted images. The bladder is clearly identified on T1- and T2-weighted images, with the typical signal intensity of fluid identified (Fig. 2-20). The boundaries and outer layer of the bladder are best identified on T1-

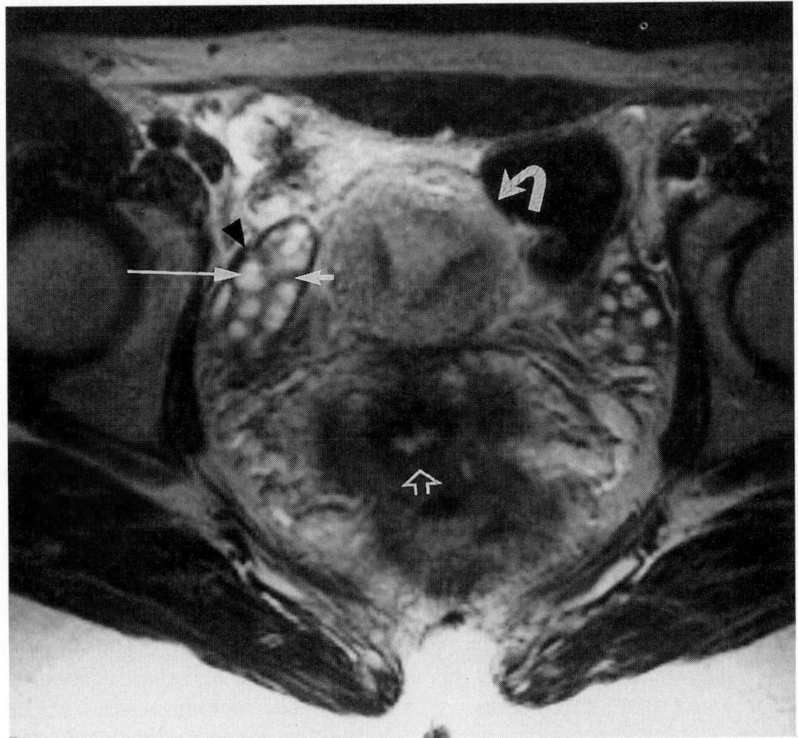

Fig. 2-16 Axial FSE T2-weighted image of the normal ovaries. The image of the right ovary shows several normal follicles *(long white arrow)*, the ovarian stroma *(short white arrow)*, and the capsule of the ovary *(black arrowhead)*. An anteflexed uterine body *(curved white arrow)* and the cervix *(open white arrow)* posteriorly are also identified.

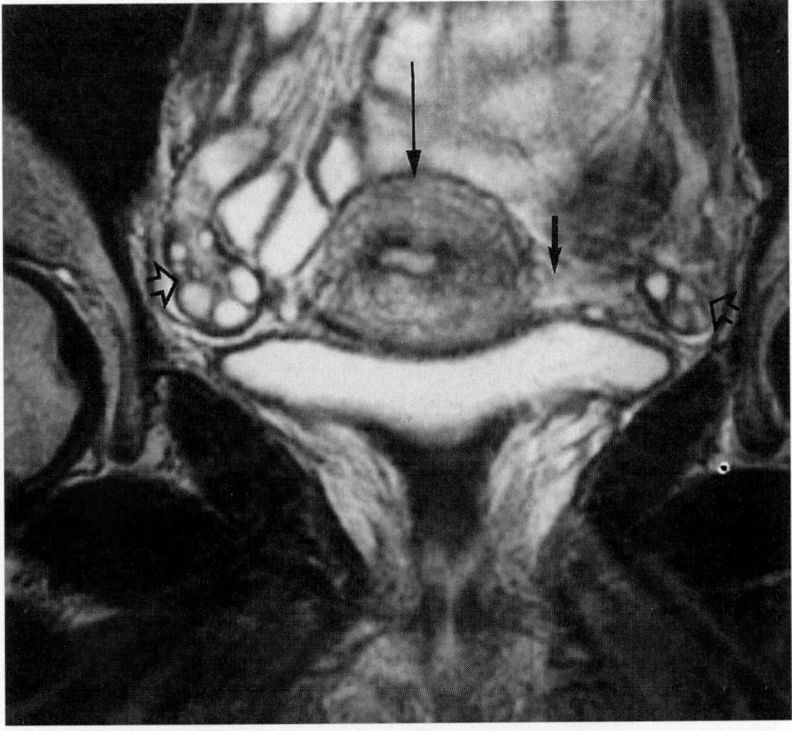

Fig. 2-17 Coronal FSE T2-weighted image of the normal ovaries, showing the two ovaries *(open black arrows)* on either side of the uterus *(long black arrow)* and part of the broad ligament *(short black arrow)* on the left.

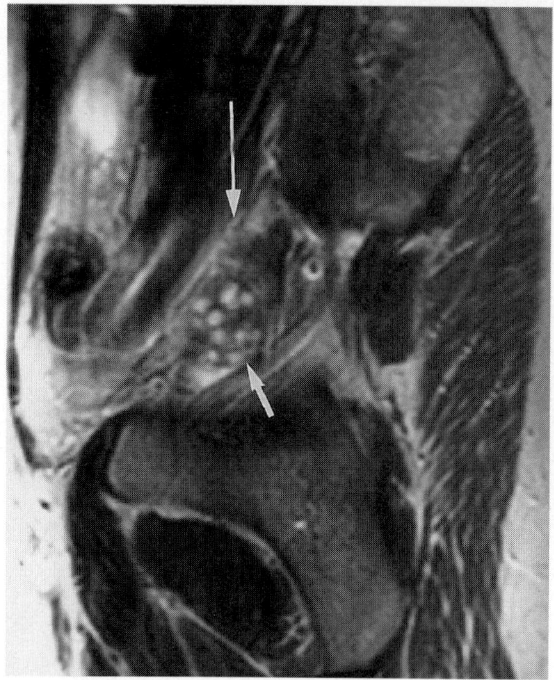

Fig. 2-18 Sagittal T2-weighted FSE image (TR 4000 msec, TE effective 102 msec) of a 30-year-old woman, with the phased array coil showing the left ovary *(short white arrow)* in the angle inferior to the bifurcation of the iliac vessels *(long white arrow).*

weighted images using the perivesicle fat for contrast (see Fig. 2-2).

The urethral orifices can be seen indirectly by identifying a jet phenomenon or turbulence within the urine in the bladder (Fig. 2-20). The ureters can be identified in the pelvis as small, high signal intensity tubular structures on either side of the pelvis on T2-weighted images. In the axial plane the ureters can be followed through the retroperitoneum to the renal hilus.

The external urethral sphincter can be shown on the coronal and sagittal images, demonstrating the length and width of the entire muscle layers (see Figs. 2-10 and 2-20). The coronal plane shows the relative length that lies above and below the urogenital diaphragm. As in the vagina, there is a venous plexus surrounding the sphincter.

GASTROINTESTINAL TRACT

The rectum, sigmoid, and descending colon with loops of small bowel are routinely visualized in the pelvis. The rectum, at the level of the vagina and urethra, is clearly seen surrounded by the muscles of the levator sling (see Figs. 2-1, 2-3, 2-4, 2-9, 2-11, 2-23, and 2-24). These muscles are bounded by the fat of the ischiorectal fossa. The rectosigmoid junction can routinely be identified at the point where the cross-sectional lumen of the rec-

Fig. 2-19 Four sagittal T2-weighted images (TR 2500 msec, TE 100 msec) with the body coil, after injection of gadolinium, show a normal left ovary *(white arrows)* just above the vaginal cuff in this 38-year-old patient who has had a hysterectomy. Note the low signal of the concentrated gadolinium in the bladder anteriorly.

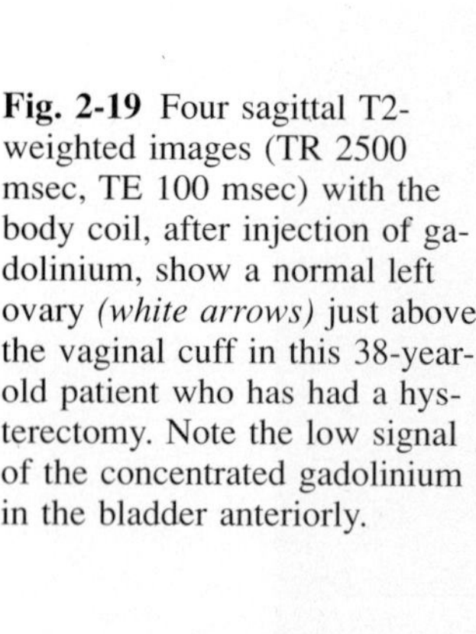

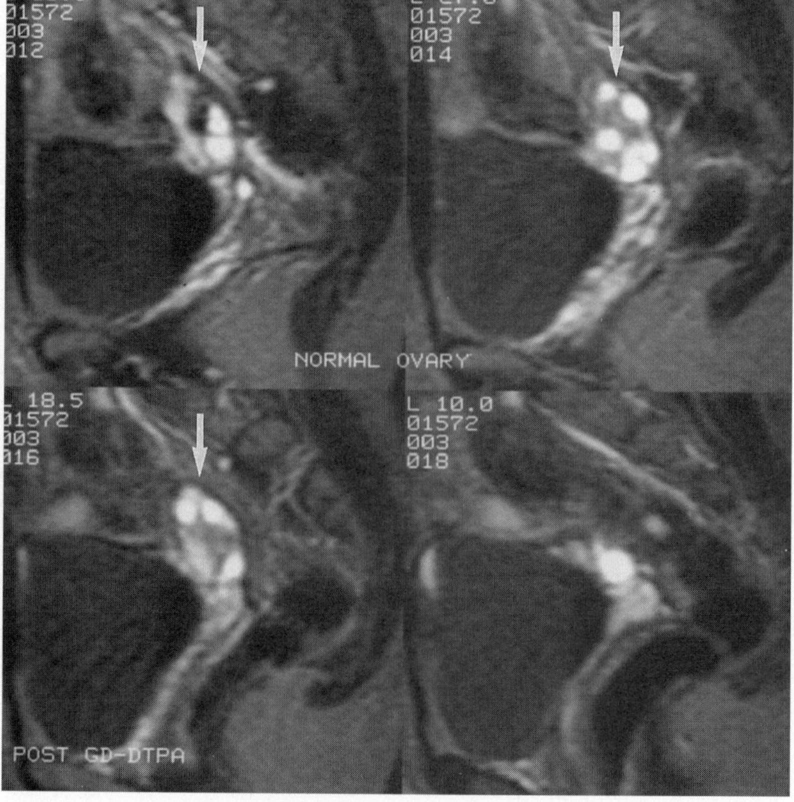

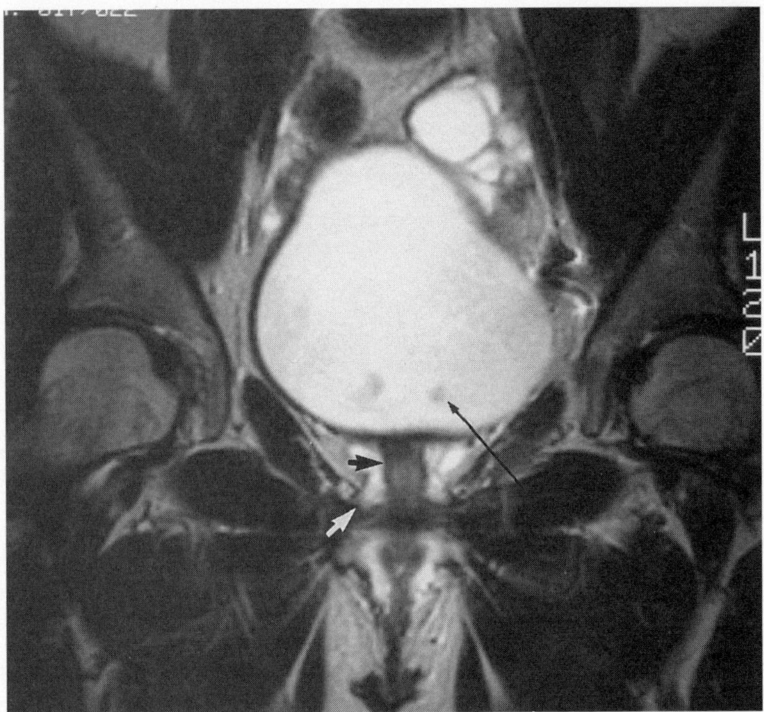

Fig. 2-20 Coronal T2-weighted image with the phased array coil, showing the typical appearance of a full bladder. Note the foci of low signal *(long black arrow)* in the bladder, which is likely due to the jet phenomenon or turbulence from the ureteral orifices. The external urethral sphincter *(short black arrow)* is seen, along with the length and width of the entire muscle layers with the relative length above and below the urogenital diaphragm. Note that, as in the vagina, there is a venous plexus *(white arrow)* surrounding the sphincter.

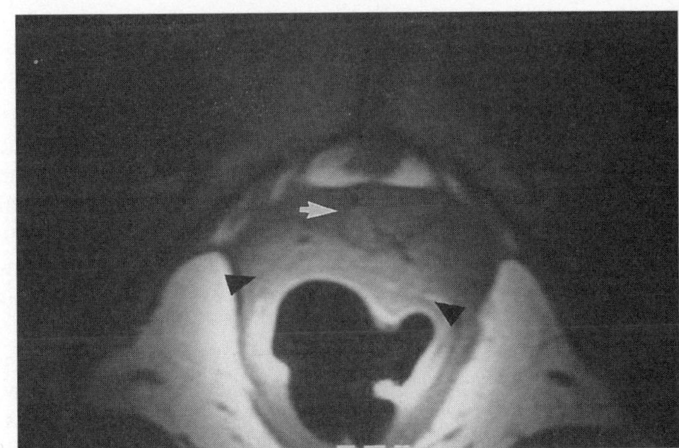

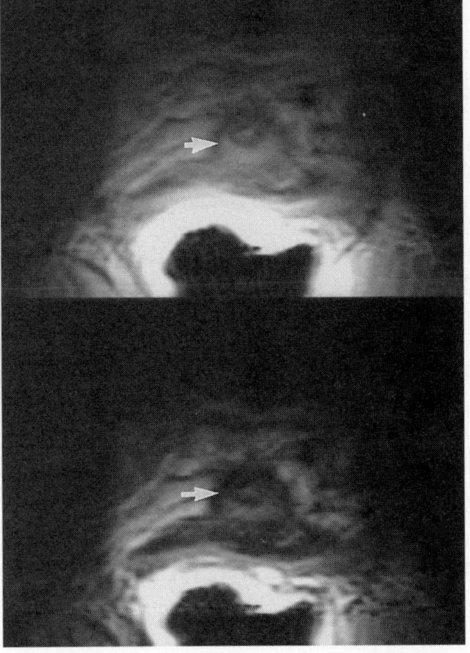

Fig. 2-21 A, Axial T1-weighted image (TR 600, TE 20) of a 33-year-old woman with an endorectal coil shows a normal urethra *(white arrow)* anterior to the vagina *(black arrowheads).* **B,** Axial proton density (TR 3000, TE 20 msec) and **C,** T2-weighted (TR 3000, TE 20 msec) images of the patient in Figure 2-20, showing the urethral sphincter.

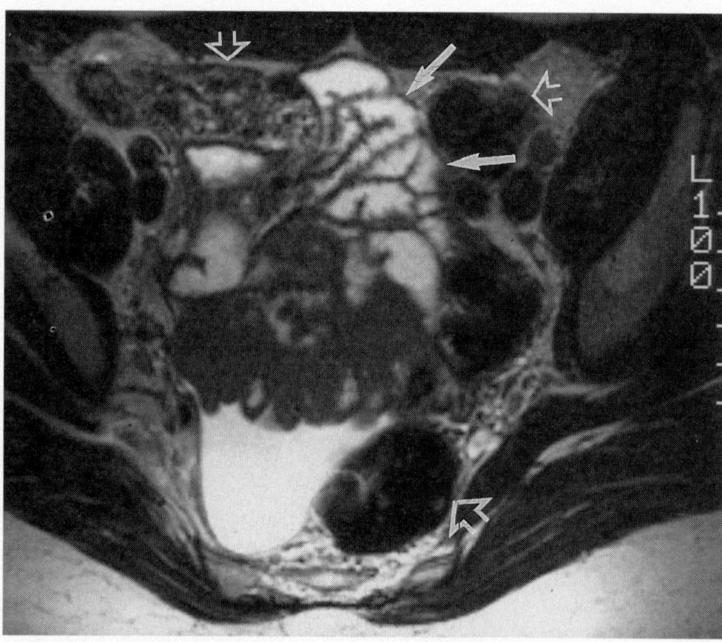

Fig. 2-22 Axial T2-weighted FSE image with the phased array coil shows clear visualization of fluid-filled small bowel loops *(white arrows)* in the pelvis. The large bowel loops filled with air and stool *(open white arrows)* have a more heterogeneous appearance.

tum changes its orientation, progressing anteriorly into the sigmoid (Fig. 2-22). The sagittal plane images show the relationship of the rectosigmoid to the uterus and the pouch of Douglas (see Fig. 2-11). The lower rectal and anal regions can also be distinguished from the other pelvic structures on these images. The MRI appearance of bowel loops is variable, depending on their content. The low signal intensity air (on T1- and T2-weighted images) is often helpful for identifying the internal lumen and determining whether the structure is in fact a bowel loop. Fecal matter has a heterogeneous appearance on T2-weighted images (Fig. 2-22) and, particularly on gradient echo images, can demonstrate a strong T2* appearance with "blooming" artifact from the air-stool interfaces. The loops of small bowel may be fluid or fat filled and thus have the corresponding signal intensities on T1- and T2-weighted sequences (Fig. 2-22). The use of glucagon intramuscularly prior to imaging helps considerably to reduce bowel peristalsis and thus improve bowel wall and lumen definition. Oral contrast agents help visualize the bowel lumen considerably (see the chapter on MR techniques, Chapter 3).

MUSCULOSKELETAL TRACT

As in all musculoskeletal imaging, MRI offers a unique opportunity to visualize the bone marrow,

cortex, and joints. When imaging the pelvis, it is routinely possible to examine the sacroiliac and hip joints with clear depiction of the pelvic floor, side wall, and gluteal muscles. The coronal T1- and T2-weighted images show the sacroiliac joints better than in the axial plane, which can be limited because of the oblique orientation. The coronal T1- and T2-weighted images show the normal low signal intensity line of the joint and cortical surfaces of the sacroiliac bones (Figs. 2-23 and 2-24). As the sacroiliac joint is an oblique joint, an oblique coronal plane may be useful to angle through the joint itself in a true coronal position. The coronal and axial T1- and T2-weighted images also show the hip joints clearly and should always be examined for evidence of pathology, such as avascular necrosis.

The inherent tissue contrast of MRI provides a unique opportunity to examine the bone marrow. This can be seen with ease on T1-weighted images, which, because of the high signal intensity of fat, show the marrow fat clearly. The marrow of the pelvis ages, like other sites in the axial skeleton with progressive replacement by fat marrow, as the patient ages. Younger women (20 to 40 years of age) may have a heterogeneous appearance of the marrow on T1-weighted images, with islands of fat and hematopoietic red marrow interspersed. The normal aging process and normal aging patterns on

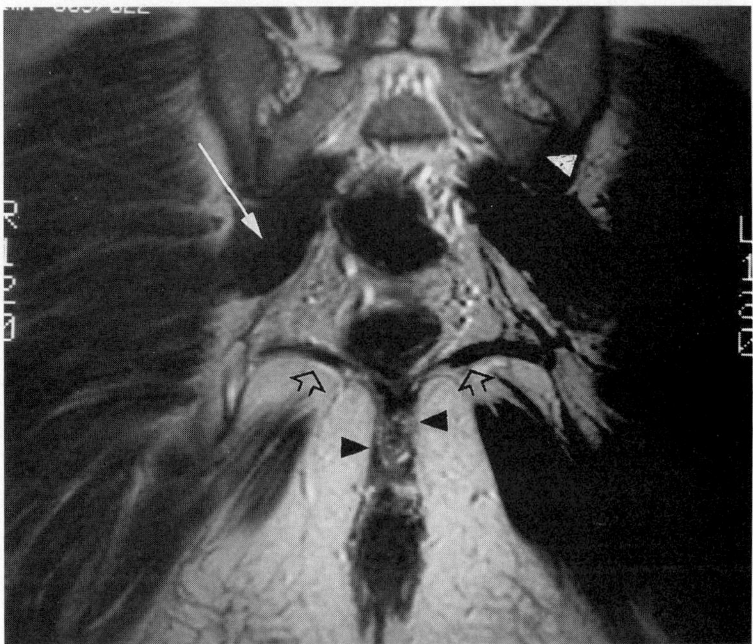

Fig. 2-23 Coronal T2-weighted FSE image of a normal 26-year-old woman with the phased array coil, showing the anatomy of the posterior pelvis. The piriform muscles *(long white arrow)* are seen bilaterally; the puborectalis *(open black arrows)* portion of the levator ani sling surrounding the lower rectum is shown with the anal canal *(black arrowheads)* below it. The left sacroiliac joint *(white arrowhead)* is also identified.

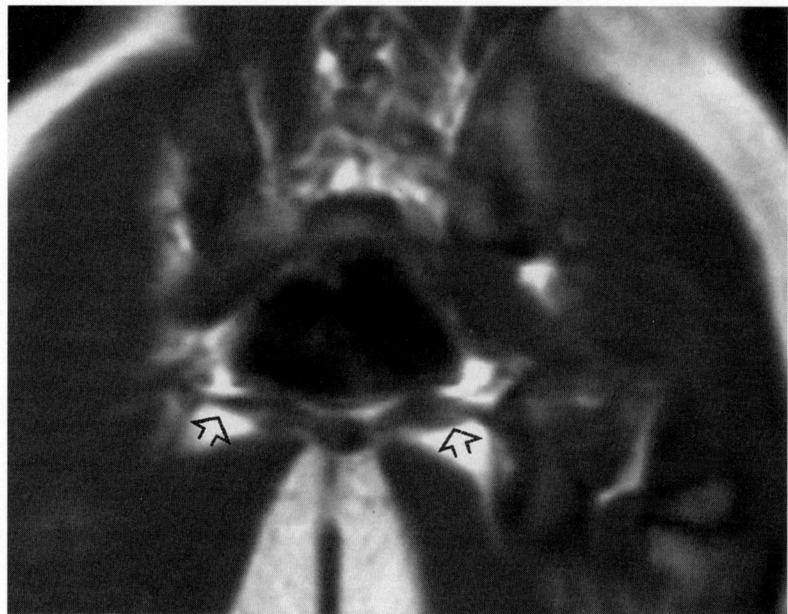

Fig. 2-24 Coronal T1-weighted image of a 2-year-old girl shows similar posterior pelvic anatomy. The levator muscle is seen bilaterally with a paucity of fat, typical of the pediatric patient.

T1-weighted MRI have been described, with progressive fat replacement commencing typically at sites of maximal weight bearing, e.g., the superior acetabular surface.[15] The marrow of the femur and intertrochanteric regions can also be assessed, and the normal trabecular markings clearly seen (see Fig. 2-17). These are best visualized on T1-weighted images, with abnormal pathology best

demonstrated and characterized on a combination of T1- and T2-weighted images. Fat-suppressed images may be very helpful in this area, particularly in assessing the bone marrow.

The neural foramina of the sacrum are clearly visualized in coronal and oblique coronal images. It is often possible to visualize the nerve roots as they exit the sacral foramen to form the sacral and femoral nerves. For specific visualization of these nerve roots, the oblique coronal plane is recommended. The T2-weighted pulse sequence with fat suppression is best to demonstrate the nerve roots, as they have a high signal intensity on T2 corresponding to the arachnoid sleeve containing cerebrospinal fluid as the nerve roots exit the foramen. The sciatic nerve and its course can be followed over the piriform muscle posteriorly and through the sacrosciatic notch into the posterior aspect of the thigh. The axial plane T1- and T2-weighted images are best for this definition, and side-to-side comparison of the size of the neurovascular bundles is useful. The superior gluteal artery and vein pass through the sacrosciatic notch along with the sciatic nerve. The nerve on a T1-weighted image appears as an isointense structure, with the signal void of the vessel often seen in association with it.

The piriform muscles are seen posteriorly as triangular muscular structures with typical signal intensities associated. On T1-weighted images, they are isointense to the remaining soft tissues within the pelvis. On T2-weighted images, they have a diffuse low signal intensity associated with the muscle bundles (see Fig. 2-23). The individual muscles of the pelvis can be clearly identified in varying planes, again with typical muscle signal intensities noted (see Fig. 2-23).

PELVIC FLOOR ANATOMY

The muscles and ligaments of the pelvic floor form a supportive sling that suspend the pelvic organs from the anterior urethra to the posterior rectum (see Figs. 2-1, 2-3, 2-4, 2-9, 2-11, 2-23, and 2-24). These muscles and ligaments are very important for maintaining the integrity of the pelvis and continence of the bladder and rectum. These muscles lie superior to the urogenital diaphragm, which consists of a fascial layer extending across the perineum.

The levator muscle sling consists of an extensive network of multiple muscle components that surround each of the major midline organs. The pubovaginal muscle surrounds the lateral walls of the vagina and the urethra, securing them to the posterior aspect of the pubic bone. The puborectal muscle (puborectal sling) extends from the back of the pubic bone around the lateral walls of the rectum, surrounding the external sphincter (see Fig. 2-23). This muscle has a wide origin off the superior pubic rami bilaterally. The pubococcygeal muscle is the longest component of the pelvic floor muscles and a major supporting structure (see Fig. 2-11). The levator ani muscles are best visualized in the coronal or sagittal planes; they can be distinguished in these planes from the normal mus-

cular walls of the pelvic organs. The function of these muscles can be seen on the dynamic gradient echo images as the patient is imaged in different stages of pelvic floor straining.[16] A line extending from the most inferior aspect of the symphysis pubis to the distal tip of the coccyx, the pubococcygeal line, is used for reference in cases of evaluation of pelvic floor descent. This is found on the sagittal images, and the relationship of the bladder floor, external os, and inferior rectum to the line can be determined. This assessment is particularly useful prior to surgical intervention. Axial T2-weighted images may show asymmetry in size of the levator muscles, which is most often artifactual. This is due to the chemical shift artifact, in the frequency encoding direction (see Fig. 2-4).

Imaging of the major organ systems within the pelvis can be performed simply and easily by a combination of T1- and T2-weighted images. The genital tract can be clearly visualized with T2-weighted images, which are essential for the characterization of organs, allowing clear differentiation among each of them.

REFERENCES

1. Sedlis A, Robboy SJ: *Disease of the vagina.* In Kurman R, editor: *Blaustein's pathology of the female genital tract,* ed 3, New York, Springer-Verlag, pp 98-101.
2. LLewelyn-Jones D: *Anatomy of the female genital tract.* In *Fundamentals of obstetrics and gynecology,* vol II, London, Farber & Farber, pp 24-36.
3. Ferenczy A, Winkler B: *Anatomy and histology of the cervix.* In Kurman R, editor: *Blaustein's pathology of the female genital tract,* ed 3, New York, Springer-Verlag, pp 141-145.
4. Hricak H, Alpers C, Crooks LE, Sheldon PE: Magnetic resonance of the female pelvis: initial experience, *AJR* 141:1119-1128, 1983.
5. Scoutt LM, McCauley TR, Flynn SD, et al: Zonal anatomy of the cervix: correlation of MR imaging and histological examination of hysterectomy specimens, *Radiology* 186: 159-162, 1993.
6. Smith RC, Reinhold CR, McCauley TR, et al: Multicoil high resolution fast spin-echo MR imaging of the female pelvis, *Radiology* 184:671-676, 1992.
7. Schwalm H, Dubrauszky V: The structure of the musculature of the human uterus: muscles and connective tissue, *Am J Obstet Gynecol* 94:391-404, 1966.
8. Brown HK, Stoll BS, Nicosia SV, et al: Uterine junctional zone: correlation between histological findings and MR imaging, *Radiology* 179:409-413, 1991.
9. Togashi K, Kawakami S, Kimura I, et al: Uterine contractions: possible diagnostic pitfall at MR imaging, *J Magn Reson Imaging* 3:889-893, 1993.
10. Scoutt LM, Flynn SD, Luthringer DJ, et al: Junctional zone of the uterus: correlation of MR imaging and histological examination of hysterectomy specimens, *Radiology* 179: 403-407, 1991.
11. McCarthy S, Taubert C, Gore J: Female pelvic anatomy: MR assessment of variations during the menstrual cycle and with use of oral contraceptives, *Radiology* 160:111-123, 1986.

12. Fleischer AC, Kalemeris GC, Machin JE, et al: Sonographic depiction of normal and abnormal endometrium with histopathological correlation, *J Ultrasound Med* 5: 445-452, 1986.

13. Dooms GC, Hricak H, Tscholakoff D: Adenexal structures: MR imaging, *Radiology* 158:639-646, 1986.

14. Hricak H, Secaf E, Buckley DW, et al: Female urethra: MR imaging, *Radiology* 178(2):527-535, 1991.

15. Ricci C, Cova M, Kang YS, et al: *Radiology* 177:83-88, 1990.

16. Yang A, Mostwin JL, Rosenshein NB, et al: Pelvic floor descent in women: dynamic evaluation with fast MR imaging and cinematic display, *Radiology* 179:25-33, 1991.

3 MRI Techniques and Protocols

Clare M.C. Tempany

This chapter reviews the different ways to image the pelvis using MR, covering the types of MR coils, and pulse sequences, and the use of contrast agents. The choice of which sequence and coils to use depends on the clinical question to be answered, an important step in protocol planning. Such decisions are based on which combination of possibilities are indicated. Is the study a high spatial resolution, small field of view (FOV) study? If so, it requires dedicated surface coil work. Alternatively, for a large FOV, medium spatial resolution examination, the body coil is excellent. It is desirable to keep examination times as short as possible. Thus, it is important to have a clear imaging protocol planned before the examination begins. This chapter reviews the currently available clinical sequences, outlines their uses, and suggests specific protocols based on common clinical questions. Appendices 3-1 to 3-3 provide detailed protocol parameters.

PATIENT PREPARATION

Before imaging, it is useful to obtain several important clinical details from the patient or her referring doctor. The appearance of the pelvic organs varies according to the patient's menstrual status and hormonal medications, so a detailed review of

the gynecologic history is helpful.[1] The clinical history and purpose of the imaging study are standard prerequisites. For MR examinations of the female pelvis, these details should be recorded prior to imaging (see box below). It is useful to know whether the patient has any devices or foreign bodies in the pelvis, such as an intrauterine device (IUD) (Fig. 3-1). The data can be obtained by a standardized questionnaire or in an interview by the radiologist or technologist. These questions should be asked along with the routine pre-MRI screening questions, such as whether the patient has a pacemaker, brain aneurysm clips, or inner ear implants.

It is not necessary for the patient to undergo any form of bowel preparation before the examination. It is helpful if she empties her bladder beforehand. This will help her tolerate the procedure longer; a full bladder is not usually necessary for imaging. If it is necessary to see the bladder wall, it will usually be at least partially filled by the end of the examination, so the bladder sequences can be done then, or the patient can start with a partially filled bladder. Occasionally, it may be helpful to have the patient insert a tampon in the vagina if imaging of

---

USEFUL CLINICAL DATA TO OBTAIN BEFORE IMAGING THE PELVIS

1. What is the patient's menstrual status: pre- or postmenopausal? What was the date of the last menstrual period? Could the patient be pregnant?
2. Is the patient taking any form of exogenous hormone therapy, such as estrogen or birth control pills?
3. Has there been any prior pelvic surgery, including a dilatation and curettage? Or radiation therapy? If so, when?
4. Does the patient have any foreign objects in the pelvis, such as a tampon, intrauterine device (IUD), or cervical ring pessary?
5. Is the patient diabetic? Does she have a pheochromocytoma or any contraindication to glucagon?

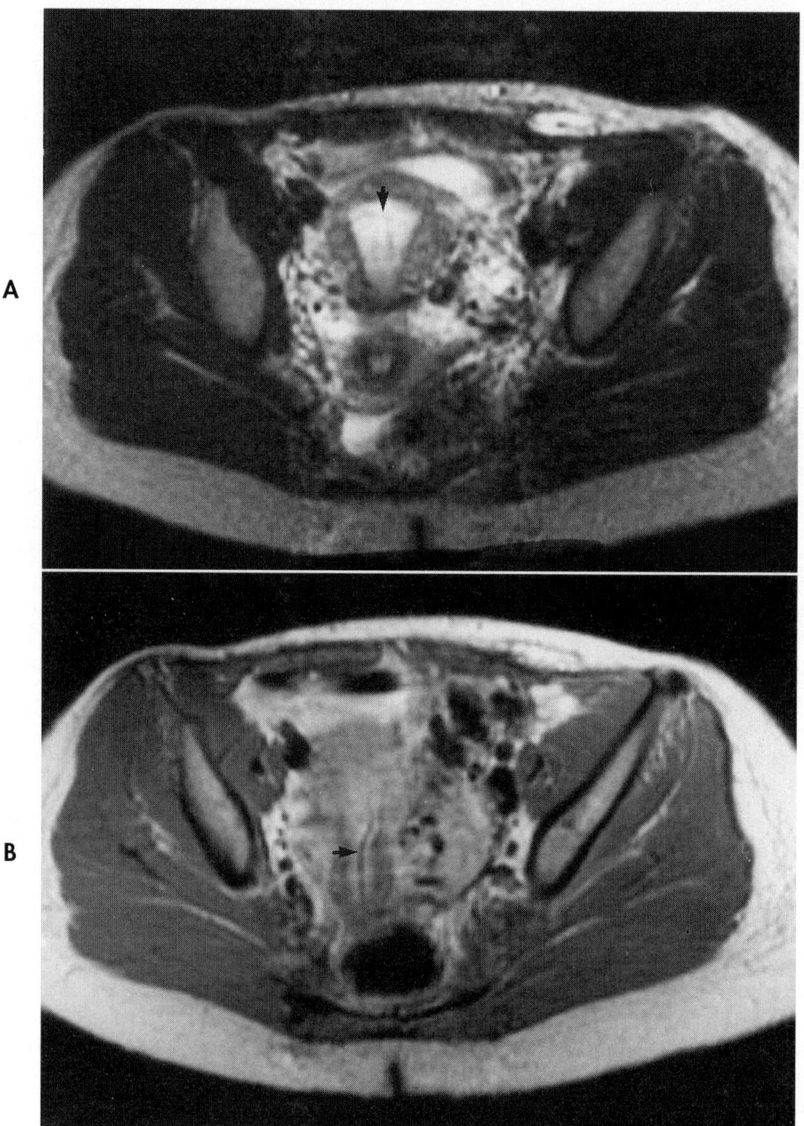

Fig. 3-1 Axial T2-weighted image showing the appearance of an intrauterine device (IUD) in (**A**) the uterine cavity *(black arrow)* and (**B**) the endocervical canal *(black arrow)*.

the vaginal walls is required (Fig. 3-2). This is not routinely done but can be useful as a means of separating the anterior and posterior walls clearly. The tampon will not cause a significant artifact and will appear as an area of signal void, due to air, on all pulse sequences. However, it may cause an artifact on the fast gradient echo sequences, and so is not recommended routinely.

CONTRAST AGENTS
Intravenous contrast media

Intravenous (IV) gadolinium contrast media can be helpful in many situations of pelvic imaging (Fig. 3-3). Gadopentetate dimeglumine or gadolinium diethylenetriaminepentaacetic acid (Gd-DTPA) was the first of these agents to be approved for use in MRI; consequently, most of the work in the literature has been performed with this medium. The role of contrast-enhanced images in the pelvis varies according to the pathology or suspected lesion under examination. In general, Gd-DTPA is a safe, nontoxic contrast medium that is well tolerated, even by patients with renal insufficiency. It is often used when iodinated contrast for computed tomography (CT) is contraindicated. Specific indications are discussed in more detail in the organ-specific chapters. These should be carefully reviewed, as it has been shown that in many

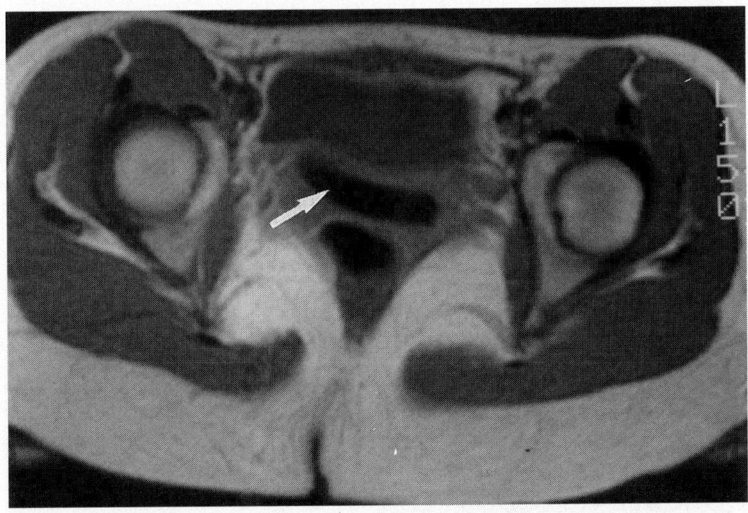

Fig. 3-2 Axial T1-weighted image showing the appearance of a vaginal tampon *(white arrow)*, which can be used to depict the vaginal cavity.

instances the T2-weighted images are adequate and the post-contrast T1-weighted images may not provide significantly more information.[2]

Administration methods. When IV contrast is to be given, the method of administration should be planned: whether the agent is to be given as a bolus, with scans obtained dynamically, or simply as a routine injection with postcontrast T1 spin echo images obtained. The preferred method is to give the contrast in a bolus fashion. The maximum recommended dose of Gd-DTPA for pelvic imaging is 0.1 mmol/kg.[2-4]

If the patient is to receive the contrast in a bolus fashion, it is useful to have an IV line sited connected to a 100-ml bag of normal saline before the examination starts. The gadolinium can then be easily administered with the patient in the scanner, and the dynamic images can be obtained immediately after the injection has been given. Currently, the IV injection is usually given by hand, but power injector pumps are becoming available and will allow for standardized rates of injection.

When a contrast medium is to be given in a bolus, it is followed by rapidly acquired gradient echo images such as a fast multiplanar spoiled gradient recalled (FMSPGR) echo sequence or a FLASH sequence. These images are obtained in a very short time, currently about 10 to 20 seconds, using the gradient echo techniques. Even faster images in milliseconds can be obtained with the echo planar units. Alternatively, after gradual hand injection, a repeat T1-weighted sequence is obtained, either with or without fat suppression. The advantage of fat suppression is to allow for clear visualization of the areas of tissue enhancement. Without suppressing the fat, an area of gadolinium en-

hancement may reach the same high signal as fat on the T1-weighted sequence; thus, the fat will be indistinguishable from the enhancement. Similar T1-weighted image parameters should be used before and after the injection, to allow for true detection of enhancement. A very short TE is recommended to allow for maximum contrast enhancement. The pre- and post-contrast images should all be filmed with the same window and width levels. It may occasionally be necessary to measure the signal intensity changes, as one measures Hounsfield number changes on CT. However, this is not usually required, as the dynamic images will generally clearly display the enhancement pattern, if present.

Gastrointestinal contrast agents

Several bowel contrast agents are currently under investigation, including air, water, barium, and MR-specific agents such as perflurocarbons. Bowel contrast agents can be divided into positive and negative ones, depending on the signal in the bowel lumen, which will be either increased (positive) or decreased (negative) on T1- and/or T2-weighted sequences. The negative agents may prove the better of the two, as they allow for differentiation between the bowel lumen and adjacent lesions or tumors, which often have high signal intensity on T2-weighted images.

The first agent approved by the Food and Drug Administration (FDA) is perfluorooctybromide or Imagent (Perflubron), which provides a negative contrast in the bowel lumen on all pulse sequences. In the phase III clinical trials, this agent was tested in 127 patients and found to be highly effective in darkening the bowel signal.[5] Another phase III trial

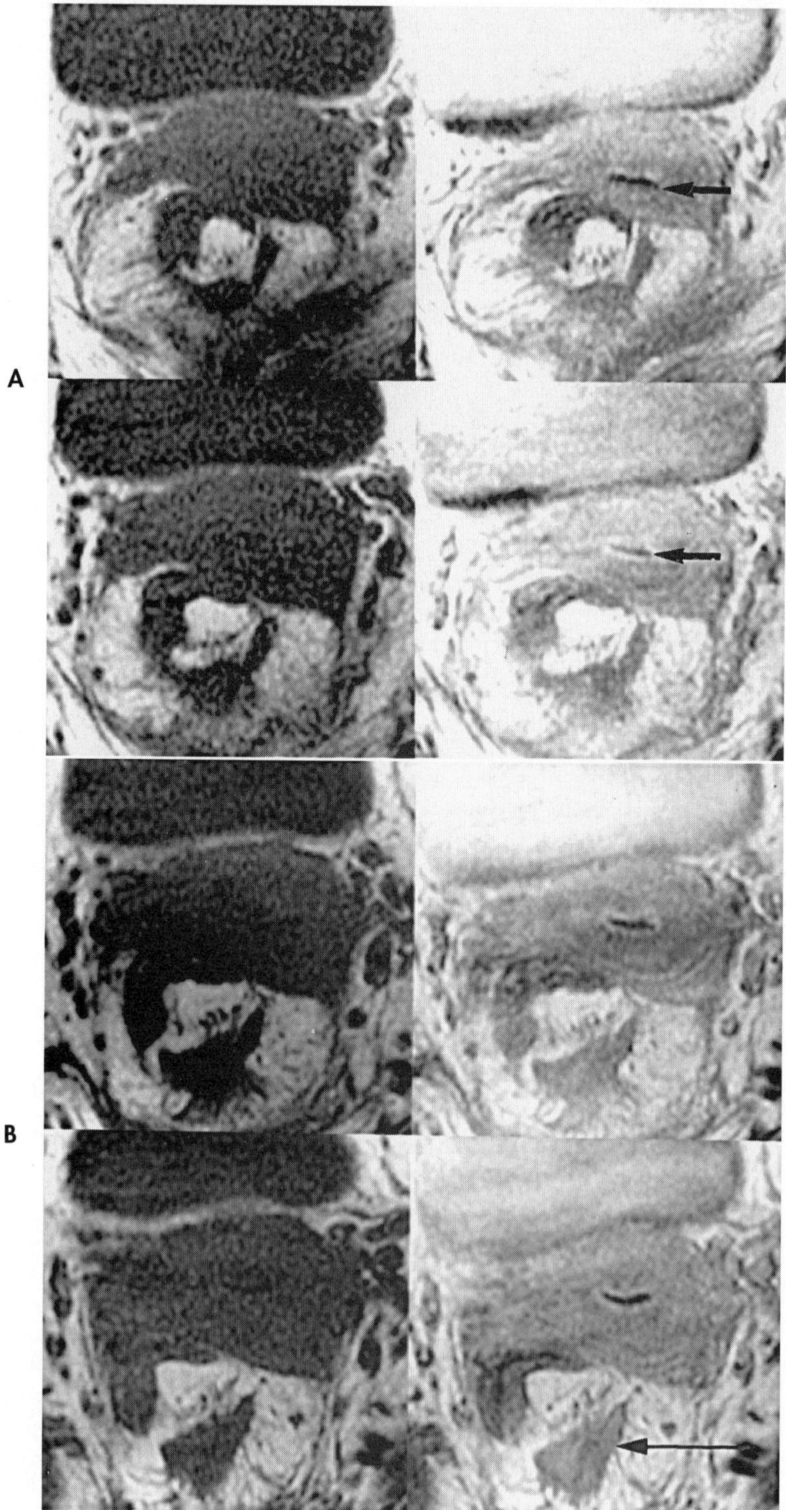

Fig. 3-3 A series of axial T1-weighted images before *(left)* and after *(right)* injection of 10 ml of Gd-DTPA. These show the normal enhancing pattern of the vagina **(A)**, cervical stroma **(B)**, and myometrium **(C).** Note the enhancement in the fluid collection posteriorly in this postoperative patient.

demonstrated the advantage of glucagon when used with this agent; significantly less phase encoding artifact was seen with glucagon than without it.[6] There are several potential advantages to using a bowel contrast agent for pelvic imaging. For example, in the evaluation of women with endometriosis, implants may occur along the bowel walls and cause adhesions; thus, visualization of the bowel lumen and walls may be very helpful. Similarly, they are useful when one is looking for peritoneal implants from carcinomatosis, such as ovarian cancer metastases. The clinical applications of oral contrast in the pelvis remain to be demonstrated fully.

Other groups have used oral and rectal barium to provide a negative MR contrast agent, especially useful on T1-weighted images. Barium has the advantage of being freely available in all radiology departments, and is well proven to be safe and acceptable to patients.[7] It has the added advantage that MRI can be performed after the patient has had an upper gastrointestinal examination or barium enema. In some cases, it may be important to visualize the rectal wall and lumen; this can be done by insufflating air into the rectum via a rubber catheter. This is best done with the patient in the left lateral position on the scanner table and then imaging the patient prone, so that the air will stay in the rectum.

RECEIVER COIL CHOICES

The selection of coil type is based on two important parameters: (1) the size of the area to be imaged and (2) the degree of spatial resolution required to answer the clinical questions. For wide coverage and average resolution, the body coil is most frequently used; at the opposite extreme, small volume and high resolution, the endoluminal or 3- or 5-inch diameter surface coils may be utilized.

The most commonly used coil is the standard *transmit/receive body coil.* There are many advantages and few disadvantages to the use of this coil. It can accommodate most patients without difficulty. The average scanner table allows for body weights of up to 136 kilograms and the bore of the 1.5T units is 50 cm in diameter. The major advantage of this coil over the other localized coils is its wide range of coverage (see Figs. 3-1 and 3-2). Not only does it allow for excellent imaging of the pelvis, but if necessary it is possible to scan the entire abdomen with the same spatial resolution. This may be the case when, for example, the study consists of assessment of a malignancy requiring full abdominopelvic staging. Another example is in the evaluation of ovarian vein thrombosis when it is necessary to scan up to the renal hilus.

The body coil is a transmit/receive coil and thus

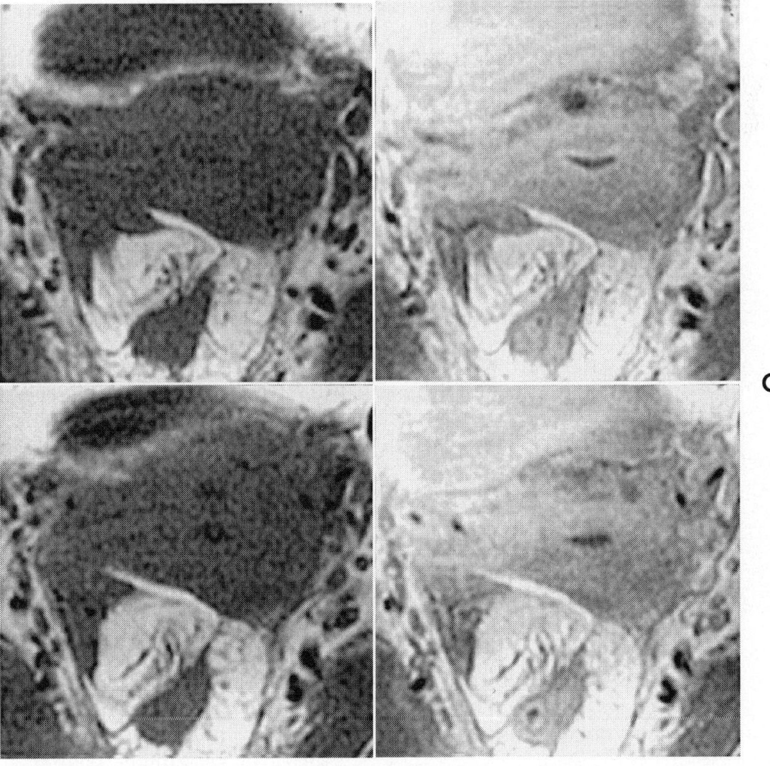

Fig. 3-3, cont'd For legend see opposite page.

provides a homogeneous magnetic field with good signal-to-noise ratios. It is, however, limited in its spatial resolution. The smallest FOV recommended is 25 cm (one half the diameter of the coil). It is not recommended to use slice thicknesses of less than 5 mm or matrices greater than 256. The body coil is useful, as it does not require sophisticated operator input for set-up and prescription of a standard protocol.

Surface coil imaging is much more operator dependent, because it always requires greater supervision and monitoring to ensure that the appropriate area is scanned and the highest spatial resolution obtained.

The second most popular coil used for pelvic imaging is the relatively new *pelvic phased array coil,* a coil arrangement first described by Roemer et al.[8] This consists of four coils, two anterior and two posterior, each with separate receiver channels, digitizers, and memory, arranged in an array to allow for simultaneous signal acquisition and spatial encoding from all four coils, resulting in one high resolution image. These surface coils are small in diameter (5 inches) and allow for higher signal-to-noise ratios.[9] They are arranged in an external frame, which is placed around the pelvis like

to a diaper (Fig. 3-4). The anterior coils lie on the patient's lower anterior pelvic wall. The anterior and posterior coils must be aligned according to the external markers: i.e., the center of the anterior coil must match that of the posterior coil. The external Velcro wraps are then applied to ensure that the coils remain in position.

There are several physical constraints in using these coils. The patient cannot be too large: in obese or pregnant patients, it will not be possible to receive signal from the center of the pelvis. In these cases, the increased signal-to-noise advantage of the coil will be lost, owing to a drop in signal at the center of the imaging volume. Also, if the patient has a protuberant lower abdomen or pelvis, it will not be possible to balance the coils on the anterior pelvic wall. Likewise, the suspected lesion should not be too large, as the area of coverage is limited to approximately 20 cm from the center of the coils. Depending on the body habitus of the patient, these coils may be used for different applications. For example, in a thin patient they may be used to image the upper abdomen, e.g., kidneys, the adrenals, and the pancreas. A significant disadvantage is the increased phase encoding artifact due to the anterior coils that are lying on the patient's pelvis and therefore move with the patient as she breathes (Fig. 3-5). The image reconstruction time can be longer than with the body coil alone, as the demand on the memory and computer hardware is greater.

The phased array coils can, by way of an external adapter, be used in combination with an en-

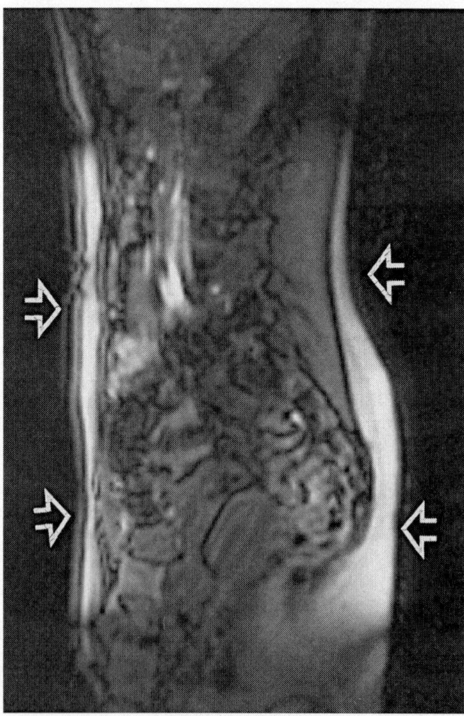

Fig. 3-4 Sagittal fast gradient echo localizer scan shows the high signal adjacent to the surface of all four coils *(open white arrows)* in the phased array arrangement. This scan allows for the demonstration of the coil's position and resultant field of view (FOV).

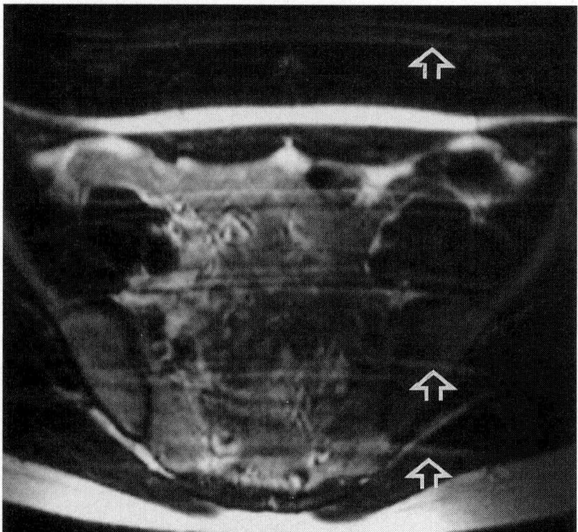

Fig. 3-5 Axial fast spin echo (FSE) T2-weighted image with the phased array coil, showing the phase encoding ghost artifacts *(open white arrows)* that arise from the fat and are misregistered in the image, which was obtained without saturation pulses.

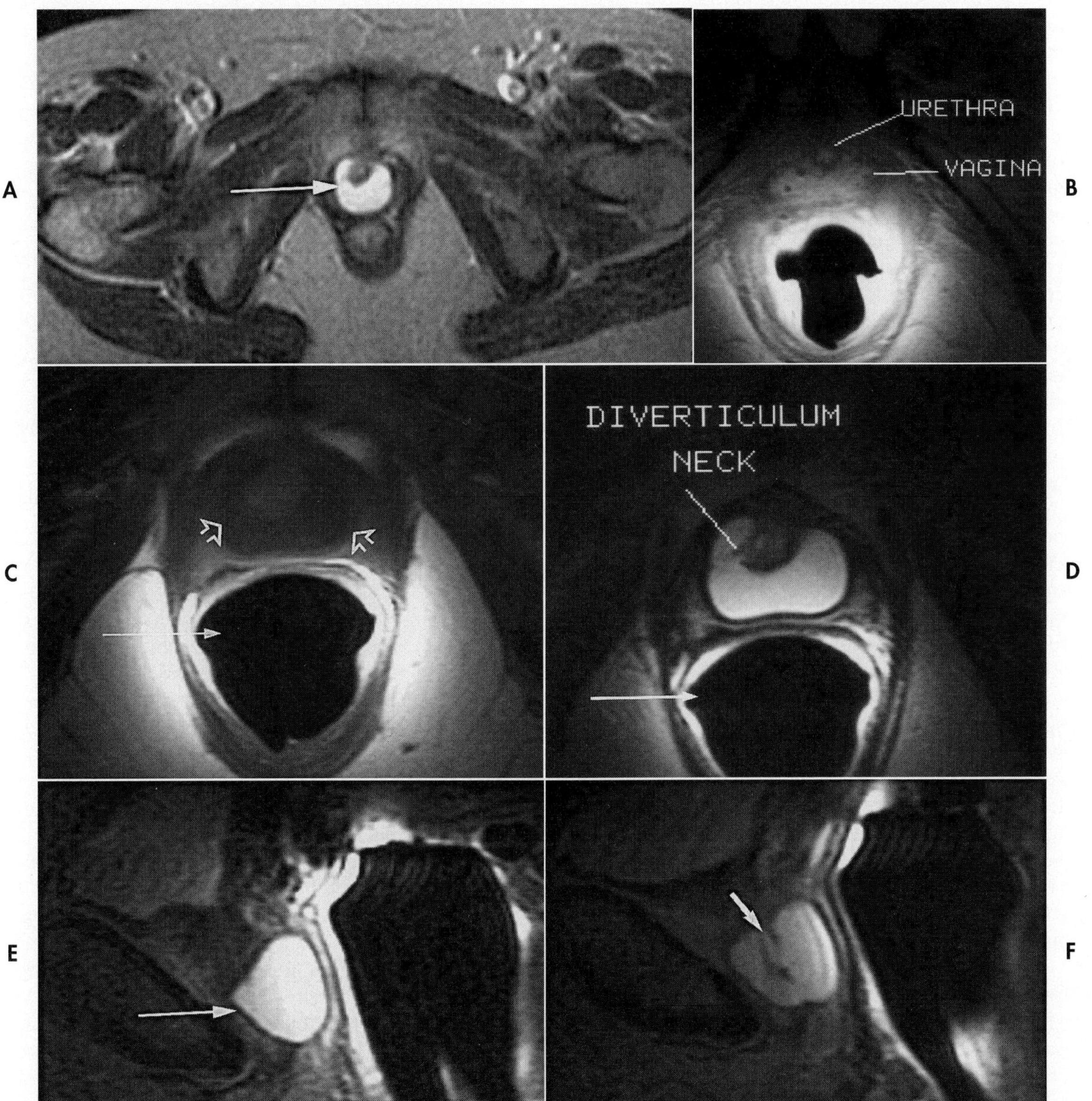

Fig. 3-6 Multiple images of a patient with a urethral diverticulum, showing the improved resolution obtained with the endorectal coil. **A,** Axial T2-weighted image of the lower pelvis obtained with the body coil shows a cystic abnormality *(long white arrow)* in the region of the urethra. **B,** Axial proton density image at the level of the perineum shows the urethra and vagina. **C,** Axial T1-weighted image more cephalad shows a low signal mass surrounding the posterior aspect of the urethra *(open white arrows);* the coil filled with air is in the rectum *(long white arrow).* **D,** Axial T2-weighted image now shows the cystic fluid-filled diverticulum, with its neck originating off the right lateral aspect of the urethra. **E** and **F,** Sagittal images with the coil in the rectum show the relationship of the diverticulum *(long white arrow)* to the bladder and its origin *(short white arrow).*

doluminal coil, such as the recently FDA-approved *cervical* or *rectal coils*. This will allow for five coils to work together, to provide the advantage of local high resolution and the wider field of imaging with the phased array coverage. The signal acquisition will be much more uniform with the five coils than with a single endoluminal coil.

The endoluminal coils alone allow for high resolution imaging of the adjacent areas, including the urethra (Fig. 3-6). Both are placed in the rectum and are designed slightly differently to view the cervix or rectal wall. Intravaginal coils have also been found to provide good-quality images of the cervix, vaginal wall, and parametrium.[10] They operate by the same design and principle as the endorectal coil used for prostate imaging. All of these coils are "receive" only coils with small FOVs. They all have a rapid drop-off of signal away from the center of the coil. The cervical coil is placed in the rectum, and a latex balloon is inflated to ensure close apposition of the coil to the anterior rectal wall, as close to the cervix as possible. There is an external steering device that can be used to direct the coil to the cervix. The optimal positioning of the coil close to the cervix can be difficult, as the cervix is mobile and not always in the same position in every patient. A local rectal coil can provide very high resolution images of the urethra, which can show the sphincter and external urethra (Fig. 3-6). This can be advantageous when imaging urethral pathology, such as urethral diverticula. The advantage lies not so much in the diagnostic yield, which is high, but in the guide provided to surgical intervention. As in Fig. 3-6, the high resolution surface coil images allow for the neck of the diverticulum to be seen and surgery performed to unroof the diverticulum and close its neck.

The other coils used to image the pelvis are the 3- or 5-inch coils used either singly or paired in a Helmholtz arrangement. These do not have the same signal-to-noise advantages of the phased array, but they are more readily available and considerably cheaper. They are best used for small lesions and local evaluation.

MOTION SUPPRESSION AND ARTIFACT REDUCTION TECHNIQUES
General techniques for all coil types

The most common artifacts on pelvic MR images are the phase encoding or ghost artifacts (see Figs. 3-5 and 3-7). These are so called because they appear most often in the direction of the phase encoding gradient. As the phase encoding steps take longer than the frequency encoding steps, they are more susceptible to interference from interval motion. The main sources of motion in the pelvis

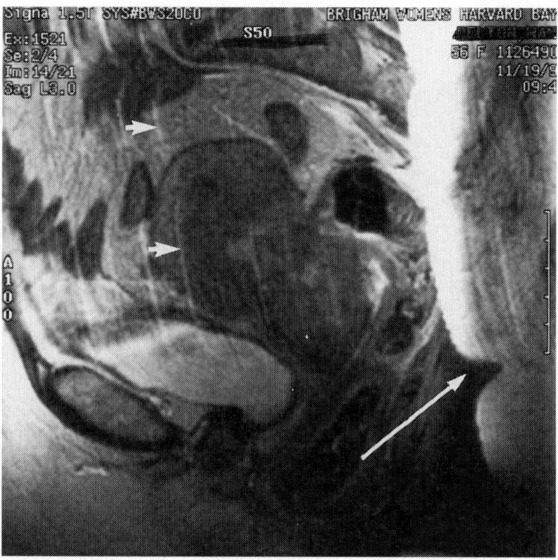

Fig. 3-7 Sagittal T2-weighted FSE image showing a wrap-around artifact *(long white arrow)* resulting from too small a FOV. There are also multiple phase encoding artifacts *(short white arrows)*.

come from bowel peristalsis, vascular pulsations, respiration, and motion from the bladder, anterior abdominal wall and the patient herself.

There are several ways to reduce these ghost artifacts that can be used in all body imaging sequences. Glucagon, a gastrointestinal hypotonic agent, is recommended for all pelvic imaging whenever possible to reduce bowel motion (Fig. 3-8). The image blurring from bowel peristalsis can be a significant problem in the pelvis, especially when there are a large number of small bowel loops lying deep in the pelvis. The most common route of administration is intramuscular with a dose of 1 mg; this allows the effect of the glucagon to last about 20 to 30 minutes.

To reduce the motion from the patient's anterior abdominal wall and respiration, it is useful to have a compression band placed around her; this will splint the abdominal wall. Alternatively, the patient can lie prone on the table if this is comfortable. Respiratory compensation (Exorcist) is a useful technique to reduce respiratory motion. It uses a separate external belt or "bellows" placed around the patient's abdomen, and the phase encoding steps are acquired in a ordered fashion to reduce the interference from the patient's breathing.

The patient should be asked to empty her bladder before the examination, because a full bladder causes not only discomfort but also increased artifact, both from its motion and from chemical shift on the T2-weighted images.

The use of spatial presaturation pulses on T1-

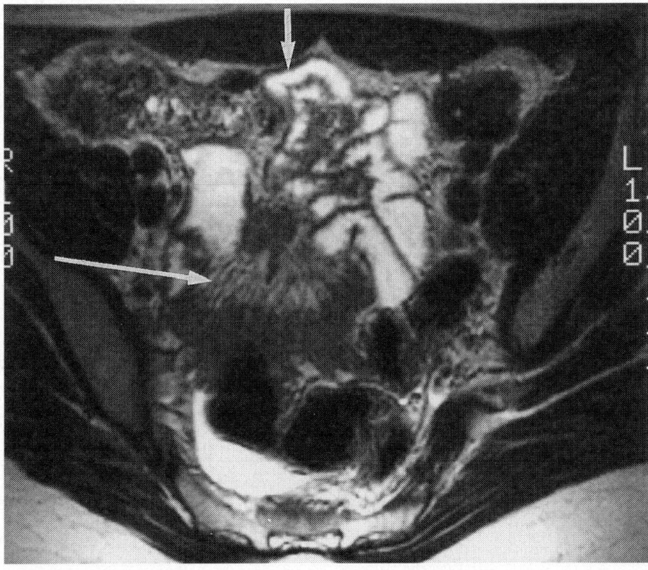

Fig. 3-8 Axial FSE T2-weighted image with the phased array coil shows the advantage of glucagon. The small bowel can be seen clearly *(short white arrow),* as can the mesentery *(long white arrow).* There are no artifacts from peristalsis, which has been completely suppressed.

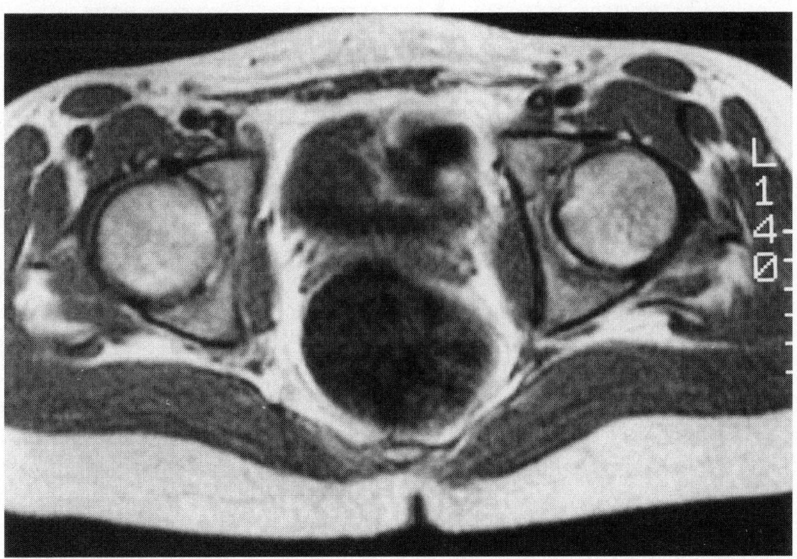

Fig. 3-9 Axial T1-weighted image of the lower pelvis (TR 600, TE 20 msec). This was obtained with superior and inferior saturation pulses to allow for good flow void in the normal iliac vessels. It also shows the sharp contrast between the bladder, rectum, and vagina and the very high signal fat. This contrast allows for clear delineation of the organ borders. The normal fat in the marrow space is also seen clearly on this sequence.

weighted images, will help reduce the flow-related artifacts from the arteries and veins as they flow through the pelvis (Fig. 3-9). These are additional radiofrequency (rf) pulses placed outside the imaging volume in any of the six planes (e.g., anterior and posterior), usually superior and inferior, to saturate the spins moving into the imaging volume.

Specific coil improvement techniques

Phased array coils. There are several very useful tips to help improve image quality when using these coils; most of these come from the work of McCarthy et al.[11,12] The first most useful tip is to reduce the signal from the anterior and posterior fat. This is necessary because, owing to the signal profile of the locally placed coils, the anterior and posterior fat will be high signal, both on T1-weighted images and, more importantly, on T2-weighted fast spin echo (FSE) sequences. This high signal can cause considerable artifact in the phase encoding direction (see Figs. 3-5 and 3-7). A solution to this problem is to carefully place anterior and posterior saturation pulses (Fig. 3-10). To do this, it is necessary to have a quick "localizer" sequence in the sagittal plane. The anterior and posterior boundaries can then be defined and the locations for the pulses determined. It is also useful to swap the phase and frequency encoding gradient directions, placing the phase encoding gradient from right to left in the axial plane.

A single coil failure can occur and will be apparent on the initial large FOV sagittal image as an area of signal loss (Fig. 3-11). If this is not appreciated and imaging is continued, the resultant images will show the dramatic signal loss. All may not be lost, however, as the remaining three coils can compensate to a degree, and reasonable signal may be present.

Endoluminal coils. With endoluminal coils, the correct positioning of the coil is critical. The coil position can be determined from a fast scan localizer after placement. The coil should also be inflated with an adequate amount of air to ensure correct "seating" adjacent to the organ of interest. Intramuscular glucagon is very helpful to reduce the phase encoding artifact at the coil surface. The images need to be filmed carefully. The window and width levels should be altered for each image and adjusted for the coil's profile. It can occasionally be helpful to use an "intensity correction" technique, which will average out the signal differences across the range in each image. This can be done either during or after image processing.

Pulse sequences

When imaging the pelvis, many of the standard pulse sequences are used, these include T1- and T2-weighted sequences. The T1-weighted images are usually acquired via conventional spin echo

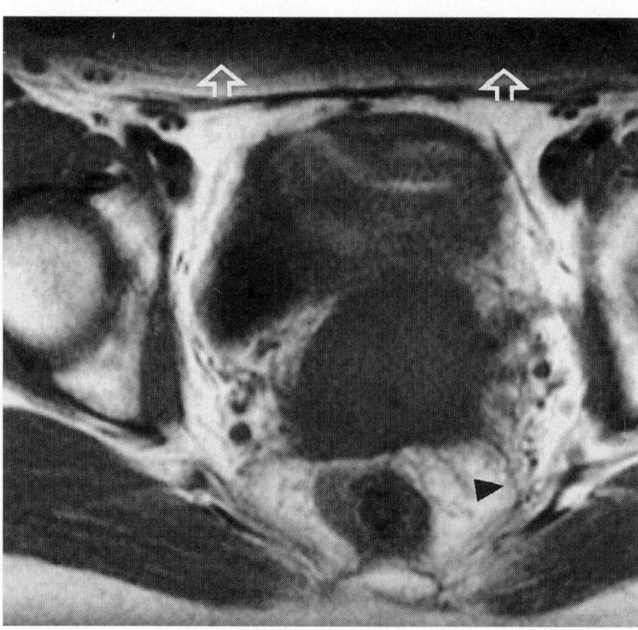

Fig. 3-10 Axial T1-weighted image of a patient with cervical carcinoma shows the cervical enlargement and infiltration and thickening of the uterosacral ligament on the left *(black arrowhead).* Note the saturation pulse anteriorly *(open white arrows),* which reduces the signal of the fat.

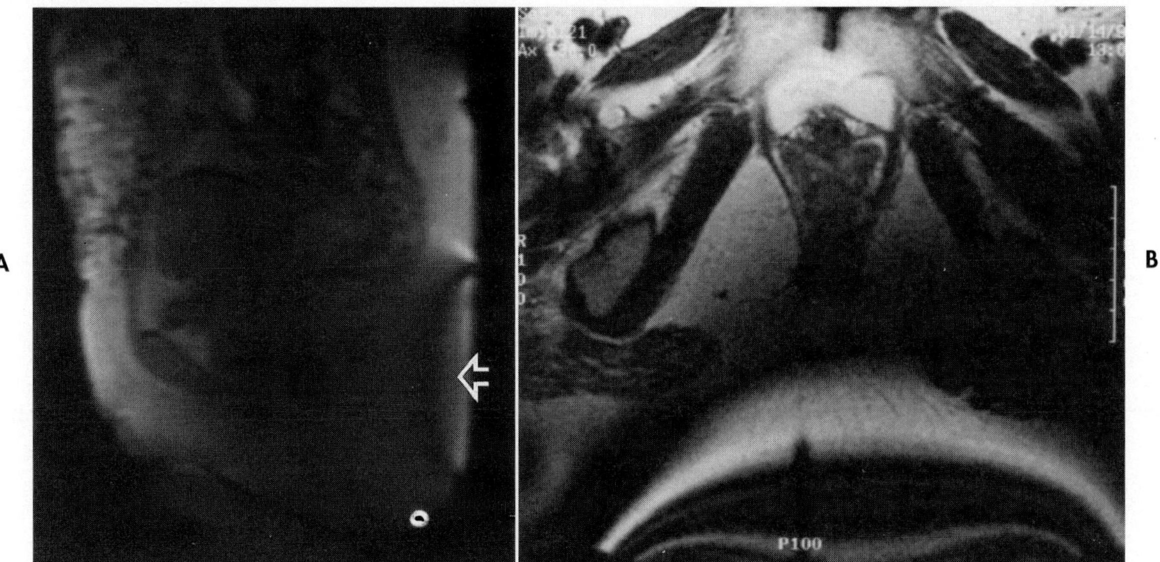

Fig. 3-11 Phased array coil failure. **A,** Sagittal fast gradient echo localizer scan shows the high signal adjacent to the surface of three of the coils in the phased array arrangement. This scan shows the loss of signal adjacent to the posterior inferior coil *(open white arrow),* which is due to coil failure. **B,** Axial FSE T2-weighted image shows the artifact arising from the failed coil, with no signal posteriorly.

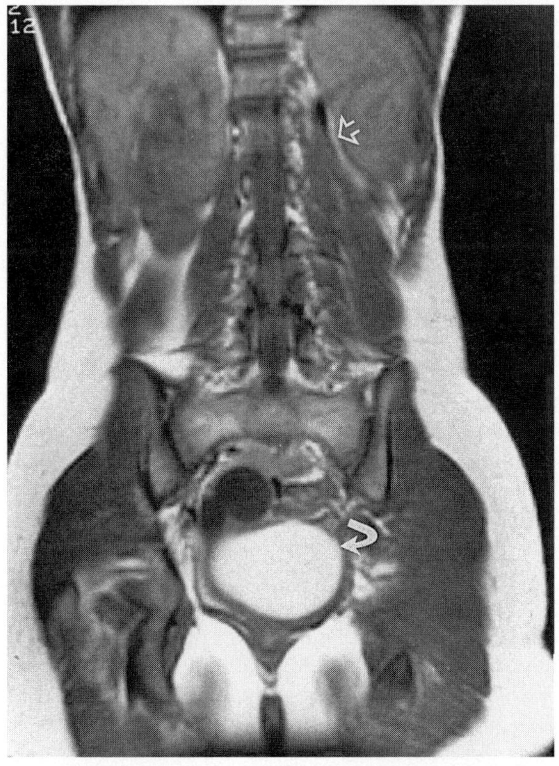

Fig. 3-12 Coronal T1-weighted image used for localization purposes and anatomic survey, including the upper abdomen. This shows agenesis of the left kidney *(open white arrow)* in this patient with hematometra *(curved white arrow).*

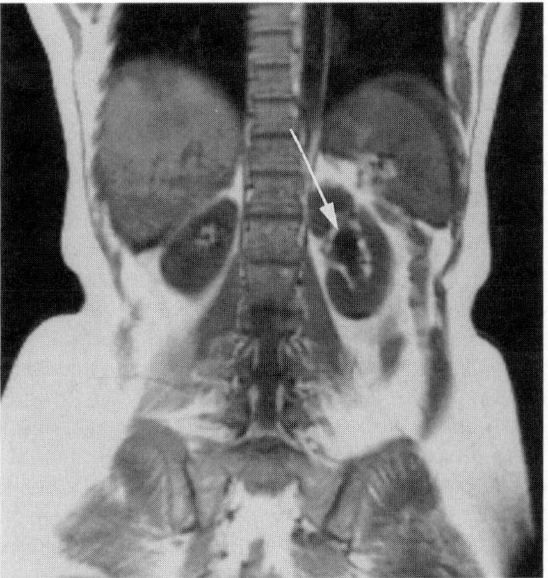

Fig. 3-13 Coronal T1-weighted image showing mild hydronephrosis of the kidney, seen on the left side *(long white arrow).*

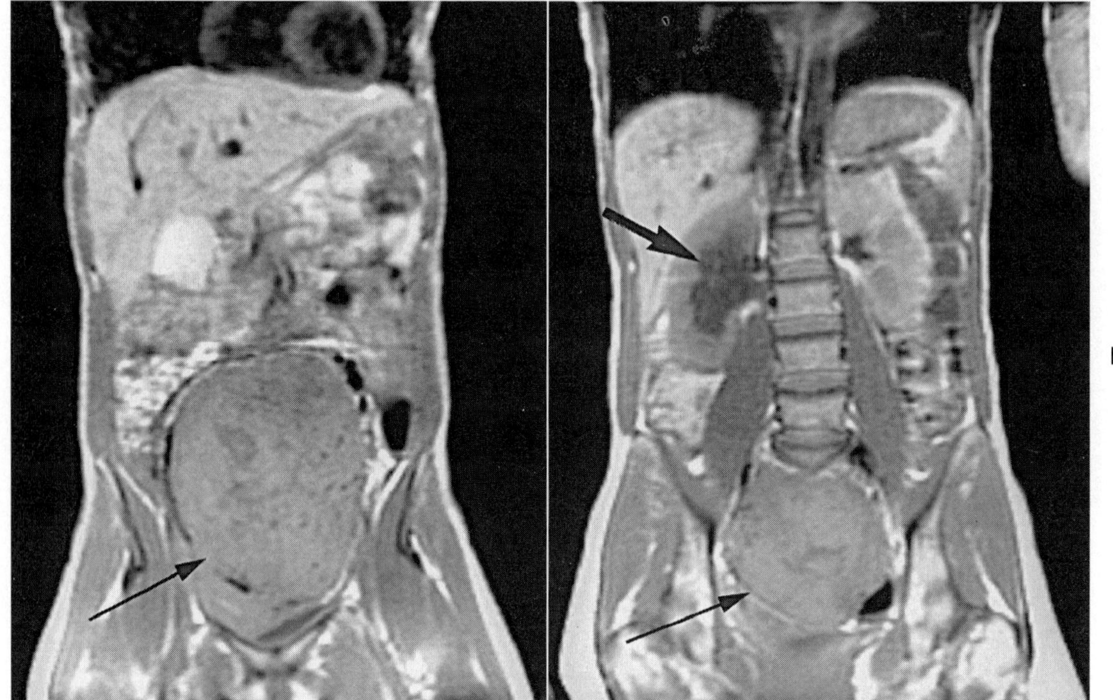

Fig. 3-14 A, Coronal T1-weighted images used for localization purposes and anatomic survey, including the upper abdomen. In this case, there is a very large mass arising in the pelvis *(long black arrow).* **B,** There is resultant hydronephrosis of the kidney on the right side *(large black arrow).*

(CSE) and, now more commonly, the FSE technique. Occasionally, a fat-suppressed sequence can be helpful, as is one of the flow-sensitive sequences such as an angiographic or gradient echo sequence.

Spin echo pulse sequences. These sequences consist of a single 90-degree pulse followed by one or more 180-degree refocusing pulses. They are used to obtain either T1- or T2-weighted images. The T1-weighted spin echo sequence is very much a standard sequence obtained in pelvic imaging. A coronal plane T1-weighted sequence is a good first sequence, which when obtained with a large FOV of 40 to 48 cm will display the pelvic and abdominal landmarks clearly (Figs. 3-12 and 3-13). One important reason to obtain this at a large FOV is to visualize the kidneys. It is important to document the presence or absence of congenital anomalies (see Fig. 3-12). Also, in patients with malignancies, the ureter may often be involved, with resultant hydronephrosis (Fig. 3-14).

After the coronal T1-weighted spin echo sequence, a similar sequence in the axial plane is useful. The high T1 signal of the fat in the pelvis provides strong contrast to the outline of the pelvic organs. It is a very useful sequence for assessing

the degree of invasion of the pelvic fat and parametria by local tumors (Fig. 3-10). When this is obtained with spatial presaturation pulses placed superiorly and inferiorly, the pelvic vessels will exhibit a normal flow void thus allowing for clear differentiation of vessels from lymph nodes (Figs. 3-15 and 3-16).

T1-weighted images are also very useful for assessment of bone marrow and skeletal abnormalities, and for defining the morphology of any abnormality. They are also very good for examination of the bone marrow for metastases or other pathologies. The coronal and axial planes allow for detailed examination of the sacroiliac and hip joints, important sites of pelvic pain. As we need to reduce exam times, this coronal T1-weighted sequence can be replaced by a gradient echo sequence such as spoiled gradient echo sequence (FSPGR), which can be obtained in about 50 seconds and provides almost equivalent information (Fig. 3-17).

T2 spin echo and fast spin echo. These T2-weighted sequences are essential for evaluating the female genital organs. At 1.5T a long TR (2000 msec and greater) will allow for clear visualization of the normal zonal anatomy of the uterus and cer-

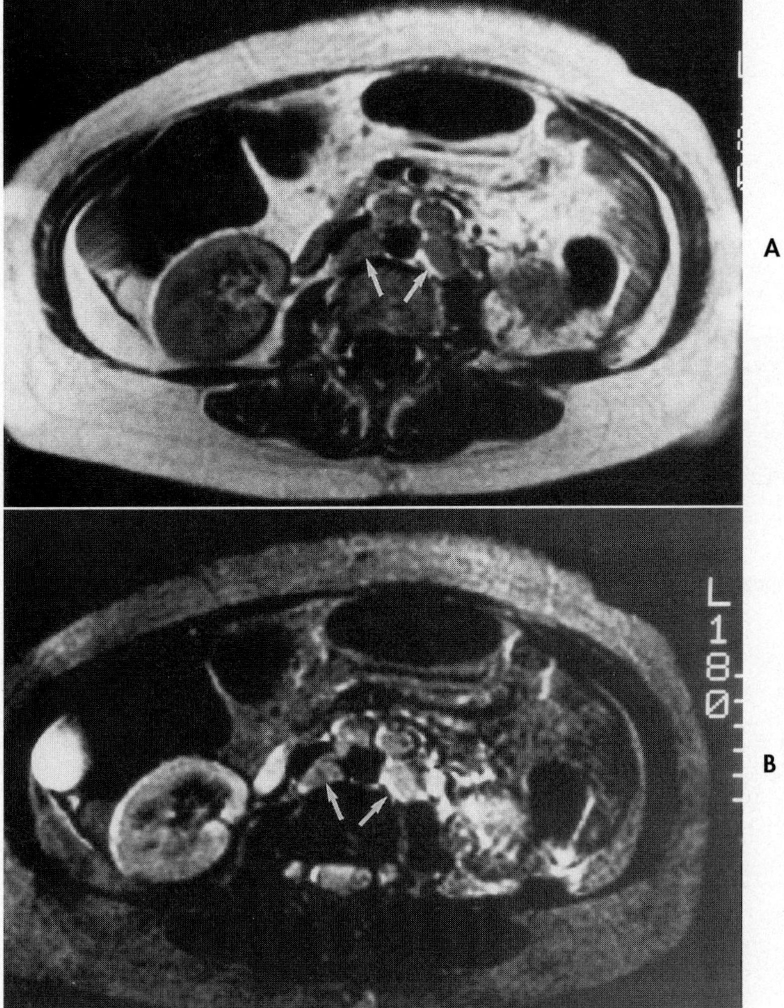

Fig. 3-15 Axial images in a patient with metastatic lymph nodes. **A,** Axial T1-weighted image with spatial presaturation shows the nodes *(white arrows)* beside the aorta and inferior vena cava. **B,** T2-weighted image shows the increased signal within these metastatic nodes, typical of active disease states. This high signal increases the conspicuity of these nodes.

vix and visualization of the ovaries. T2-weighted images are the cornerstone of pelvic imaging; often they alone are diagnostic. They should be obtained in conjunction with T1-weighted images, as these are needed for true tissue characterization.

FSE is a mixture of spin echo and echo planar techniques. The FSE sequences use multiple 180-degree refocusing pulses (like spin echo sequences) during the T2 decay, to acquire multiple phase encode signals, one per 180 pulse (as in echo planar sequences). This approach was first described by Hennig and colleagues, who developed the RARE (rapid acquisition with relaxation en-

hancement) technique.[13] If there are 16 refocusing pulses, the scan acquisition time will be reduced by a factor of 16. This allows for the matrix and number of signal averages to be increased, thus improving the signal to noise and resolution. The T2 contrast can be manipulated and a single or double echo sequence obtained. Most often, a single echo sequence will be sufficient for pelvic imaging, as there is no need for a proton density image.

One of the major advantages to using FSE sequences in the pelvis is that several different imaging planes can be obtained. For uterine imaging the sagittal plane is the best to show the zonal

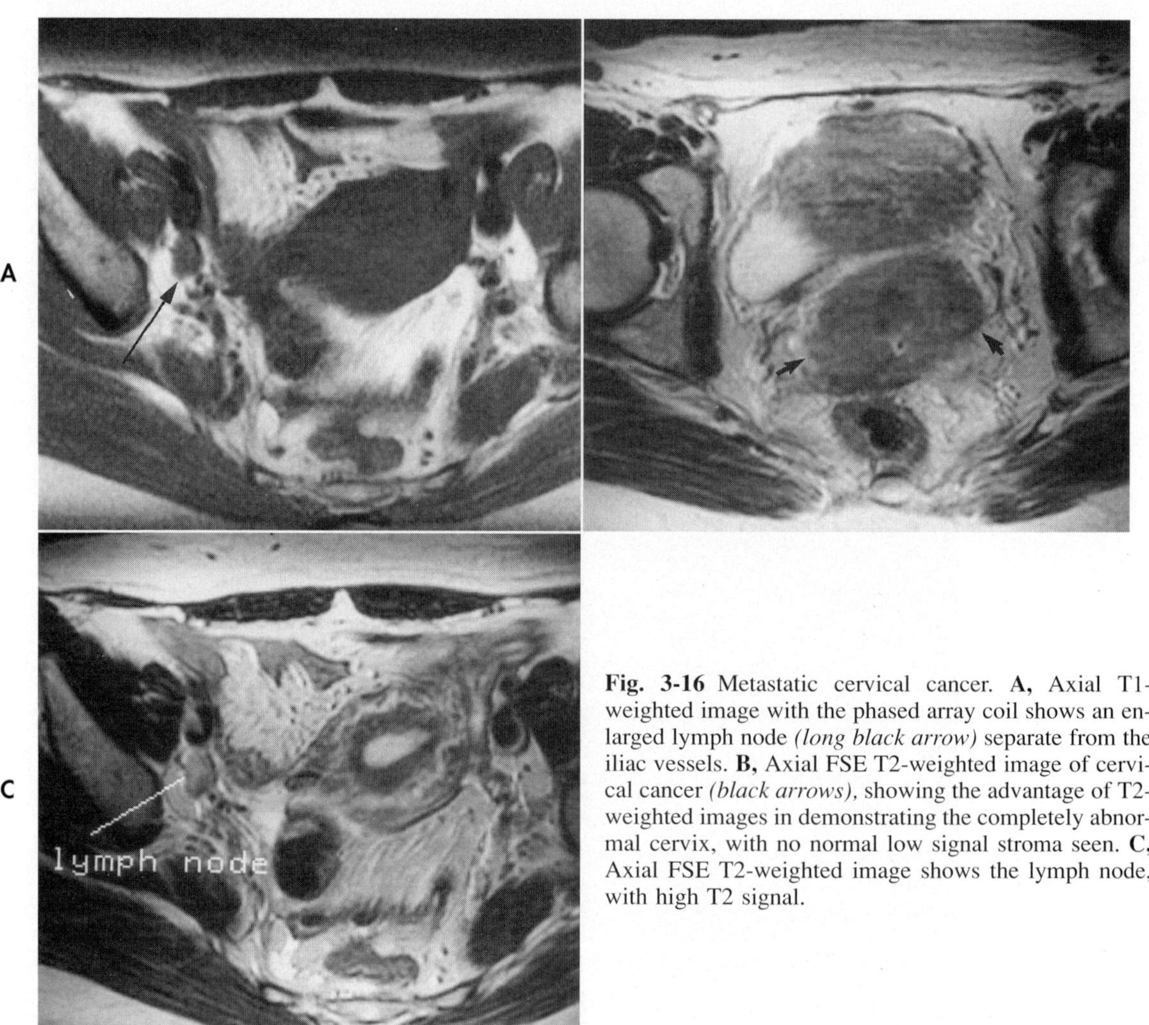

Fig. 3-16 Metastatic cervical cancer. **A,** Axial T1-weighted image with the phased array coil shows an enlarged lymph node *(long black arrow)* separate from the iliac vessels. **B,** Axial FSE T2-weighted image of cervical cancer *(black arrows),* showing the advantage of T2-weighted images in demonstrating the completely abnormal cervix, with no normal low signal stroma seen. **C,** Axial FSE T2-weighted image shows the lymph node, with high T2 signal.

anatomy, and this is often complemented by an axial or coronal plane. To visualize the cervix the standard axial plane is often adequate, but a true axial image of the cervix can be obtained using an off-axial plane. This plane is best found from the sagittal image, with the plane perpendicular to the long axis of the uterus or cervix (Figs. 3-18 and 3-19).[14]

Fat suppression sequences. There are several varieties of fat suppression techniques. Inversion recovery, chemical shift imaging, opposed phase imaging, and Dixon techniques are some of these. Each has advantages and disadvantages, discussion of which is beyond the scope of this chapter. One important feature to be aware of is that, as in the pelvis, we are using these techniques to differentiate fat from blood. It is important to use a sequence that will suppress the signal only from fat and not from blood. This can happen with some

of the inversion recovery sequences, such as the *short tau inversion recovery (STIR)* sequence (Fig. 3-20). In the case illustrated, the pattern of the suppressed tissue helps differentiate the typical central fat from the peripheral blood of the hemorrhagic cyst. The *chemical shift technique* uses a frequency-selective presaturation pulse to suppress signal from either fat or water. This is probably one of the easiest ones to use on the GE units (Fig. 3-21), as it is simply selected from the menu of imaging options. Inversion recovery sequences are spin echo techniques with a 180-degree pulse preceding the 90-degree excitation pulse. Other techniques require more sophisticated manipulation of the sequences.

Vascular sequences. MR angiographic methods may be used in the pelvis to visualize the deep tortuous pelvic vessels, which can be difficult to image using other techniques. The two- and three-

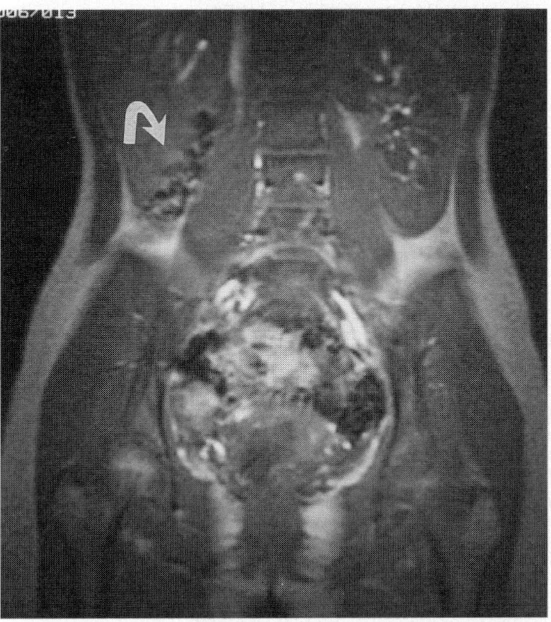

Fig. 3-17 A fast gradient echo technique for localization can be obtained in less than 30 seconds. This image, which shows the agenesis of the kidney on the right, was obtained with the pelvic phased array coil, demonstrating that adequate signal of the upper abdomen can be obtained.

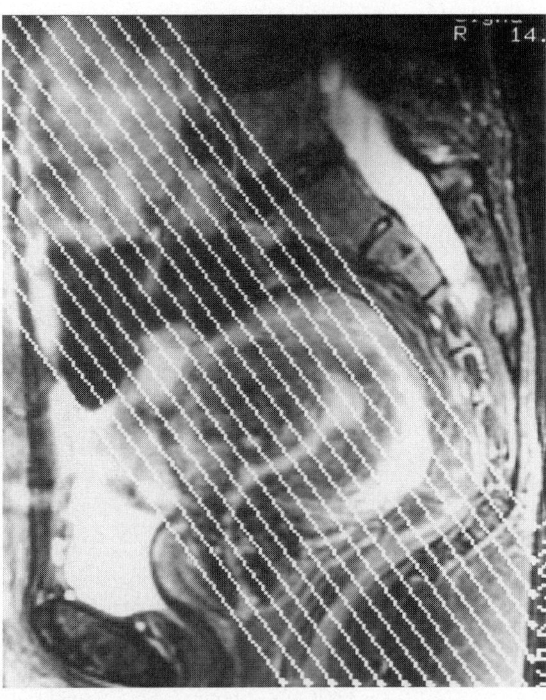

Fig. 3-18 Sagittal image showing the oblique coronal plane used to image the uterine cavity transaxially. These images allow for the entire junctional zone to be examined all through the body of the uterus.

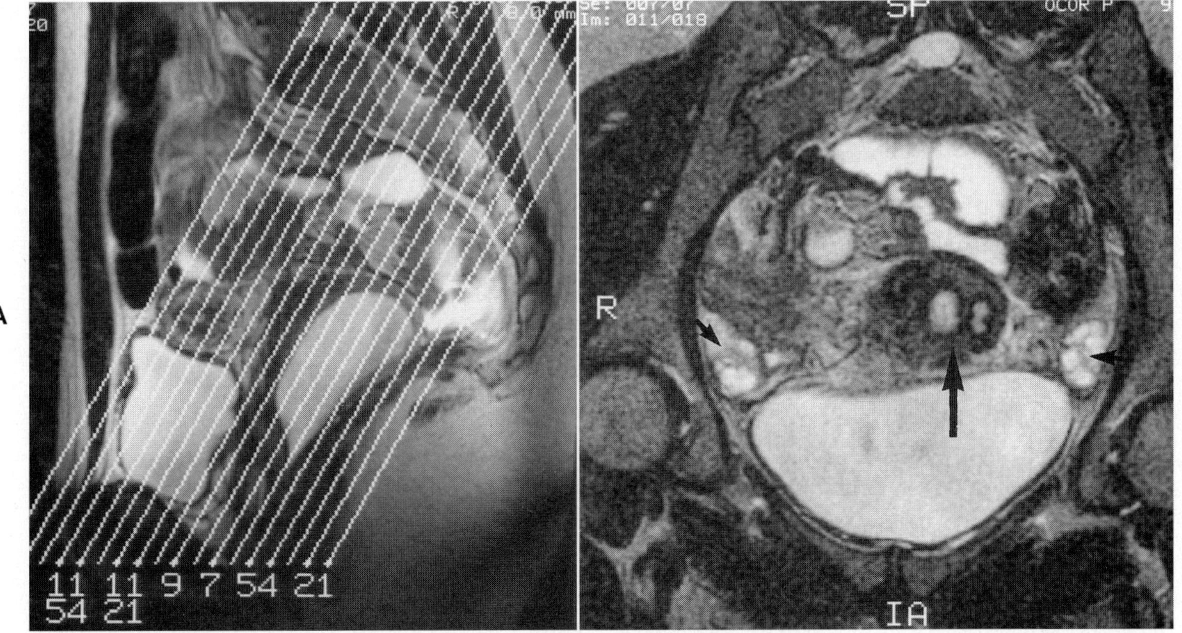

Fig. 3-19 A, A sagittal FSE T2-weighted image with the phased array coil is used to find the correct transaxial plane for the cervical canal. **B,** The resultant oblique coronal FSE image showing a true cross-section of the cervix *(black arrow),* in this case revealing two cervices in this patient with uterine didelphysis. The two ovaries are also seen in this image *(short black arrows).*

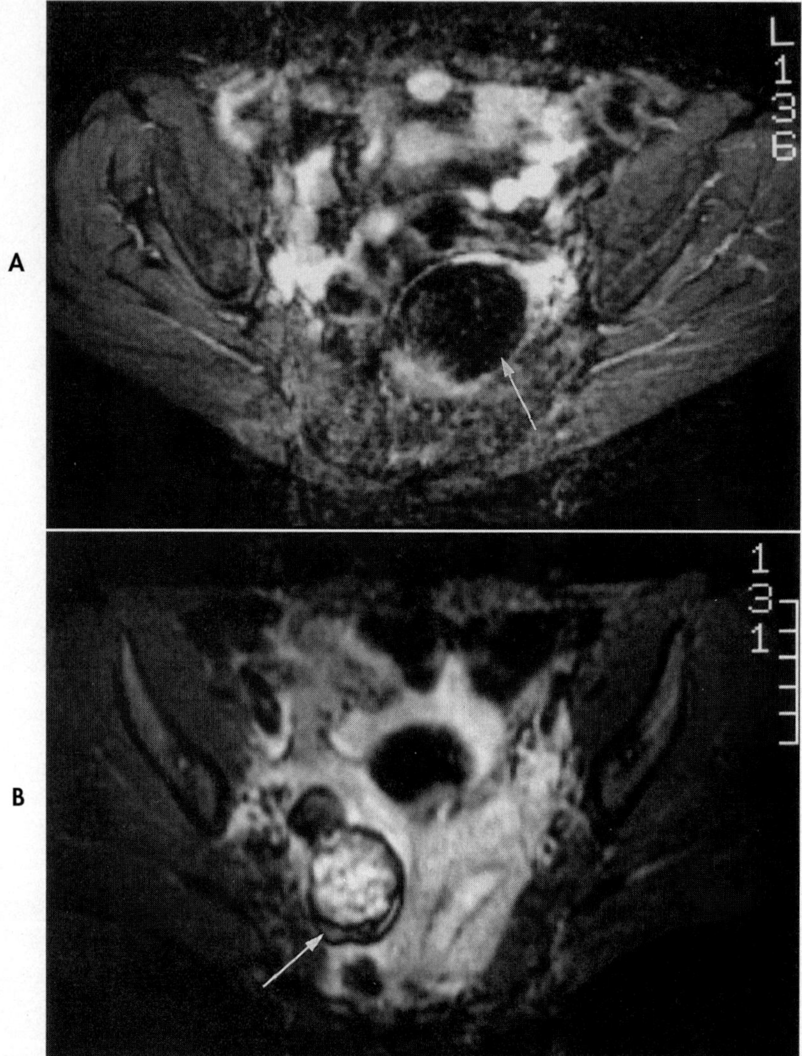

Fig. 3-20 A, Axial short tau inversion recovery (STIR) image of a patient with a left-sided teratoma *(long white arrow)*. The entire lesion suppresses, owing to the high fat content. **B,** The same sequence (STIR) causes suppression of the outer rim of this hemorrhagic cyst, which does not contain fat. The T1 of the hemorrhagic wall is similar to that of the fat in this case and therefore suppresses also.

dimensional time of flight (TOF) and phase contrast (PC) techniques are both useful. Both of these are better when obtained with the phased array coils, compared with the body coil, because of the increased signal. MRA or MRV images are very useful in the pelvis, as invasive methods are difficult and vascular anatomy is useful for surgical planning. The flow can be assessed using gradient echo techniques such as GRASS (gradient recalled acquisition in the steady state) images, which are

fast and easy to obtain and may be done with breath holding, as a single slice, or in a group without breath holding (Fig. 3-22).

Current MR techniques for imaging the pelvis are very powerful and adaptable. They require attention to detail and careful suppression of artifacts. Several approaches have been outlined in this chapter. The reader is advised to review the radiology literature regularly to keep up to date with this ever-improving imaging technology.

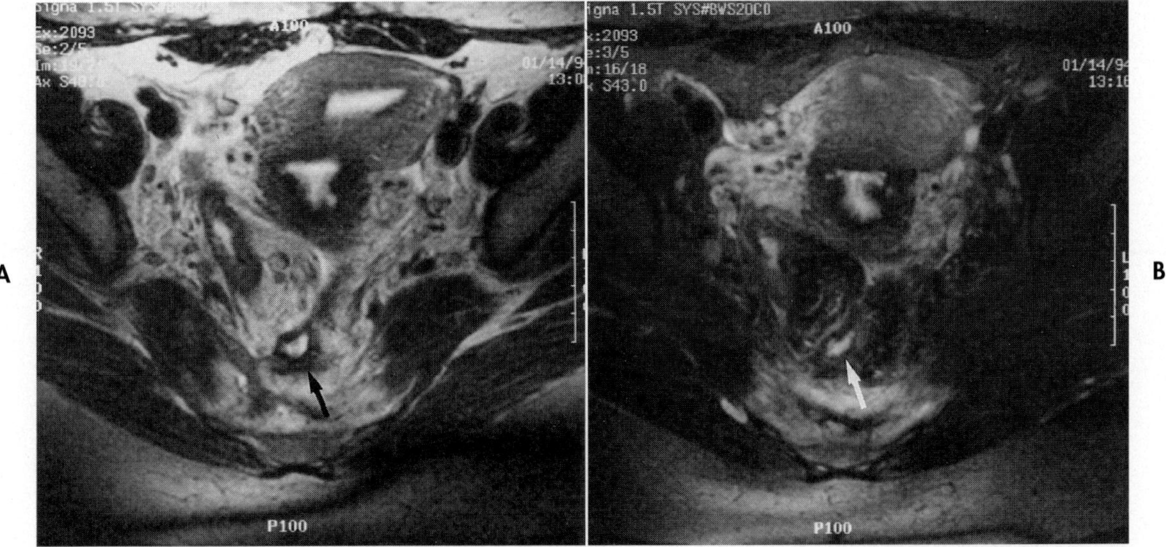

Fig. 3-21 Axial FSE images of the pelvis, without fat suppression **(A)** and with fat suppression **(B)**, illustrate the different appearances of the two. This patient, who had had a total colectomy and ileoanal pull-through, had a small fluid collection posteriorly *(black and white arrows)*.

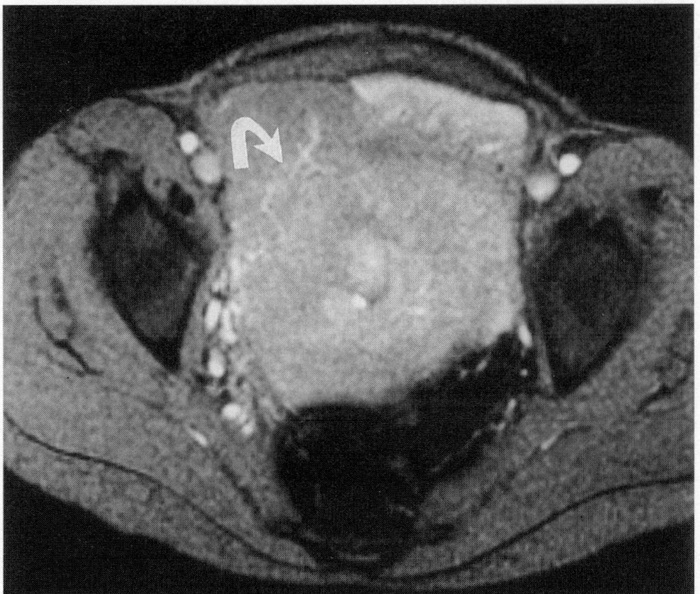

Fig. 3-22 Single-slice, breath-hold, axial gradient echo image (TR 33 msec, TE 13 msec, flip angle 30), showing neovascularization in an ovarian neoplasm *(curved white arrow)*. The iliac vessels are patent.

Protocols for the Pelvic Phased Array Coils

	1	2	3	4	5
Coil	Pelvic PA	PA	PA†	PA	PA†
Plane	Sagittal	Axial	Axial	Sagittal/coronal	Axial
Pulse sequence	Fast SPGR	FSE SAT (S/I, and A/P*)	T1 SAT (S/I and A/P*)	FSE SAT (S/I and A/P*)	ME SAT (S/I and A/P*)
No. of echoes	1	1	1	1	1
Echo TL		16		8-16	
TE1/TE2	Min TE	104-126	Min	104-126	Min TE
TR	400	4500-4000	600	4500-4000	600
FOV (cm)	40-48	16-20	16-20	16-20	16-20
Slice thickness (mm)	5	4	4	4	10
Gap (mm)	1.5	1-2	1-2	1-2	2
Matrix	128	256/512	256/192	256/192	256/192
NEX (averges)	1	4	4	4	2
Frequency encoding dir.	S/1	A/P	A/P	R/L	R/L
Gd-DTPA	No	No	No	No	No
No. of slices	9	14	12		12
Time (min)	2-3	5	3.5	3.5	5
Center frequency	Mid	Water	Water	Water	Mid

One mg of glucagon prior to scanning with these coils is recommended.
*SAT pulses should be S/I and A/P. Localize off the sagittal SPGR sequence 1.
†T1-weighted images through the pelvis before and after administration of Gd-DTPA.

PA = phased Array, TE = echo time, TL = train length, TR = time to relaxation, S/I = superior/interior, Mid = midpoint, A/P = anterior/posterior, SAT = saturation, R/L = right/left.

MRI Protocols: Pelvis
Parameters for Use with the Body Coil

	1	2	3	4	5
		Pelvis	Pelvis	Pelvis	Pelvis
Plane	Coronal	Axial	Axial	Sagittal	Axial
Pulse sequence	ME	ME*	FSE+/− IR	FSE+/− IR	ME*
PSD	RCSAT	RCSAT	RC	RC	RCSAT
No. of echoes	1	1	1	1	1
Echo train			8	8	
TE1/TE2	Min TE	Min TE	102	102	Min TE
TR	600	600	4000	4000	600
FOV (cm)	48	To fit	To fit	To fit	Same as #2
Slice thickness (mm)	5	5-10	10	5	5
Gap (mm)	1.5	2	2	1	1
Matrix	256	256	192	192	192
NEX (averages)	2	2	2-4	4	2
Frequency encoding direction	S/I	R/L	R/L	R/L	S/I
Gd-DTPA	No	No	No	No	Yes
No. of slices	12	12	20	Cover area of interest	12
Approx. time (min)	5	5	3.12-6.24	3.5	5
Center frequency	Mid	Mid	Water	Water	Mid

*T1-weighted images through the pelvis before and after Gd-DTPA.
RCSAT = respiratory compensation, IR = inversion recovery.

MRI Protocols According to Clinical Diagnosis

I. **Mass lesion evaluation:** preferably, use phased array coils if available
1. Sagittal FSPGR or T2 CSE/FSE
2. Axial T2 CSE/FSE
3. Sagittal T2 CSE/FSE ± fat suppression
4. Axial GRASS
5. Axial T1 (fat suppression may be helpful)
6. Axial T1 with Gd-DTPA (fat suppression may be helpful) *Upper abdomen with body coil* (may be needed if there is a suspicion of malignancy with metastases)
7. Axial T1 with FAT SAT

II. **Uterine body abnormality,** e.g., fibroids, adenomyosis, endometrial cancer: use phased array coil
1. Sagittal FSPGR (localizer) or FSE
2. Sagittal T2 CSE/FSE
3. Oblique T2 CSE/FSE (perpendicular to uterine cavity)
4. Axial T1
5. Axial T1 with Gd-DTPA (for endometrial cancer)

III. **Congenital anomaly:** use phased array coil
1. Coronal T1 (large FOV)
2. Sagittal T2 CSE/FSE
3. Oblique T2 CSE/FSE (depends on orientation of uterus/vagina); may need more than one oblique
4. Axial T1

REFERENCES

1. Demas BE, Hricak H, Jaffe RB: Uterine MR imaging: effects of hormonal stimulation, *Radiology* 159:123-126, 1986.
2. Hricak H, Finck S, Honda G, Goranson H: MR imaging in the evaluation of benign uterine masses: value of gadopenetate dimeglumine–enhanced T1-weighted images, *AJR* 158:1043-1050, 1992.
3. Hirano Y, Kubo K, Hirai Y, et al: Preliminary experience with gadolinium-enhanced dynamic MR imaging for uterine neoplasms, *RadioGraphics* 12:243-256, 1992.
4. Yamashita Y, Takahashi M, Sawada T, et al: Carcinoma of the cervix: dynamic MR imaging, *Radiology* 82:643-648, 1992.
5. Mattrey RF, Trambert MA, Brown JJ, et al: Oral contrast agents of magnetic resonance imaging, result of phase III trials with Imagent (R) GI as an oral magnetic resonance contrast agent, *Invest Radiol* 26:S65-S66, 1991.
6. Brown JJ, Duncan JR, Heiken JP, et al: Pefl" uroctylbromide as a gastrointestinal contrast agent for MR Imaging: use with and without glucagon, *Radiology* 181:455-460, 1991.
7. Ros PR, Steinman RM, Torres GM, et al: The value of barium as a gastrointestinal contrast agent in MR imaging: a comparison study in normal volunteers *AJR* 157:761-767, 1991.
8. Roemer PB, Edelstein WA, Hayes CE, et al: The NMR phased array, *Magn Reson Med* 16:192-225, 1990.
9. Axel L: Surface coil magnetic resonance imaging, *J Comput Assist Tomogr* 8:381-384, 1984.
10. Baudouin CJ, Soutter WP, Gilderdale DJ, Coutts GA: Magnetic resonance imaging of the uterine cervix using an intravaginal coil, *Magn Reson Med* 24:196-203, 1992.
11. Smith RC, Reinhold C, McCauley TR, et al: Multicoil high-resolution fast spin echo MR imaging of the female pelvis, *Radiology* 184:671-675, 1992.
12. Mc Cauley TR, McCarthy S, Lange R: Pelvic phased array coil: Image quality assessment for spin-echo MR imaging, *Magn Reson Imaging* 10:513-522, 1992.
13. Hennig J, Nauteth A, Friedburg H: RARE imaging; a fast method for clinical MR, *Magn Reson Med* 3:823-833, 1986.
14. Baumgartner BR, Bernardino ME: MR imaging of the cervix: off-axial scan to improve visualization of zonal anatomy, *AJR* 153:1001-1002, 1989.

4 Congenital and Pediatric Disorders of the Müllerian and Genitourinary Systems

Part I: Anomalies of the müllerian system

Julia Fielding

Part II: Congenital and pediatric genitourinary disorders

Ronald A. Morton, Jr. *and* ***Clare M.C. Tempany***

This chapter reviews congenital anomalies of the pelvis. The first section discusses the female müllerian system with a full review of the embryology and imaging features of each of the forms of anomaly. The müllerian anomalies can be complex and difficult to evaluate, often requiring a multimodality approach. As we will illustrate, we feel that magnetic resonance imaging (MRI) provides a very complete evaluation of the entire müllerian system and should be the first-line imaging study in all young women with suspected müllerian anomalies.

The anomalies of the genitourinary system are less common but often as complex, again having multisystem manifestations. The second section of this chapter reviews the clinical and surgical perspective to these anomalies. MRI has been used in these patients particularly for surgical planning. The soft tissue detail and multiplanar capabilities highlight the unique role of MRI in this patient population.

Part I: Anomalies of the Müllerian System

Müllerian duct anomalies are rare in the general population, occurring with a frequency of 1 in 200 to 1 in 600.[1-5] In the population evaluated for in-

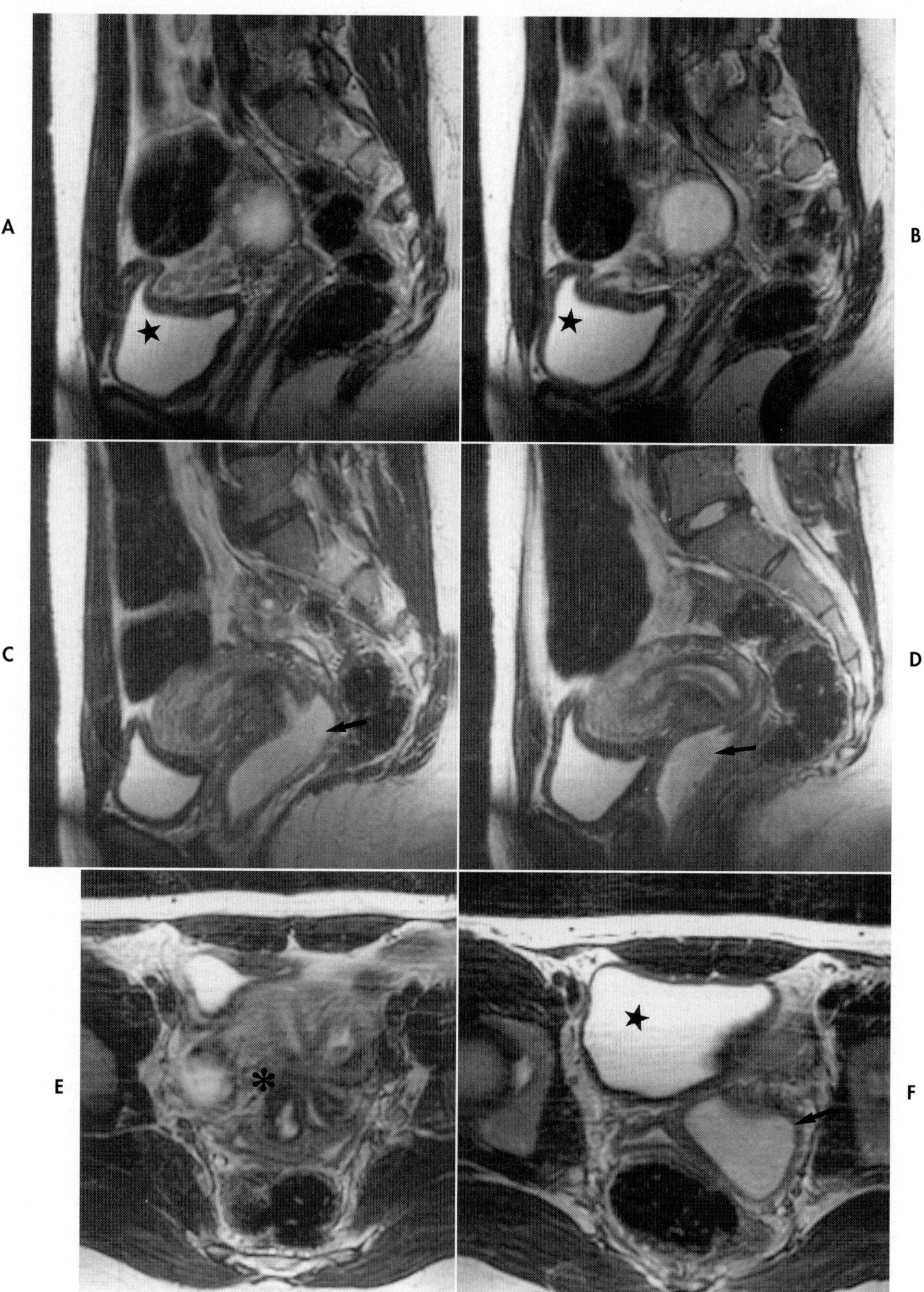

Fig. 4-1 Uterus didelphys, class III. Sagittal, consecutive **(A-D)** and axial **(E and F)** fast spin echo (FSE) T2-weighted (TR 4000, TE 102, ET 8) MR images obtained using the pelvic phased array coil demonstrate two cervices *(asterisk)* and obstruction of the left vagina *(arrow)*. The bladder is marked by a star.

fertility or repeated spontaneous abortions, the prevalence is much higher, occurring in 9% to 25%.[5-8] Imaging, including hysterosalpingography (HSG), endovaginal ultrasonography (EVS), and MRI, has in many cases either replaced or helped guide diagnostic laparoscopy in classifying the type of anomaly present. MRI is currently the imaging modality of choice because of its high accuracy and ability to evaluate the entire genitourinary tract.

EMBRYOLOGY AND PATHOGENESIS

The fallopian tubes, uterine cavity, cervix, and upper four fifths of the vagina arise from fusion of the paired müllerian ducts. The two ducts are hollow tubular structures that unite and fuse in the midline. After fusion, there is resorption of the midline septum, leaving a single uterine cavity. The distal portions of the ducts persist as the two fallopian tubes. The developmental process begins during the tenth to seventeenth weeks of gestation and extends until term.[9] Abnormalities may occur at any time during this period and are the result of failure of development, fusion, or recanalization.

Lack of fusion leads to the formation of duplicate structures. In the most extreme case, uterine didelphys (a double uterus) is formed (Fig. 4-1). The two uterine cavities and cervices are often accompanied by a vaginal septum. The septum may occlude one uterine cavity in up to 75% of cases, resulting in hematometrocolpos.[10] Near-complete fusion may result in only a small indentation along the superior surface of the uterine cavity. This is the arcuate uterus. The most common duplication anomaly is a bicornuate uterus, in which a myometrial or mixed myometrial and fibrous septum may completely or partially separate the uterine cavities (Fig. 4-2).

Failure of development of one müllerian duct results in a unicornuate uterus (Fig. 4-3). A rudimentary horn is often present, which may contain an endometrial lining. When no connection exists between the rudimentary horn and the main uterine cavity, obstruction, endometriosis, and even rupture can result.

When fusion occurs but there is failure of resorption at the midline, a septated uterus results (Fig. 4-4). With the exception of the diethylstilbestrol (DES)–related abnormalities, this is the most common müllerian anomaly. The septation may be partial, separating only the uterine cavities, or complete, extending into the cervix and sometimes the vagina. Both fenestrated and solid septa have been reported.

Complete failure of development of both müllerian ducts results in agenesis of the upper four fifths of the genital tract (Fig. 4-5).

The most common müllerian anomalies are currently those resulting from in utero exposure to DES. This synthetic estrogen was administered to more than 2 million women between 1948 and 1971, in most cases to prevent spontaneous abortion. Its use was discontinued when an increased incidence of vaginal clear cell adenocarcinoma was identified in daughters of women exposed to DES. Large national cohort studies have since been used to follow these women. In a review by Kaufman et al, it was reported that 69% of these patients had abnormal upper genital tracts.[11] Vaginal adenosis and cervical structural abnormalities were the most common anomalies; uterine and cervical hypoplasia were also seen to occur with increased frequency. HSG revealed an abnormal shape to the uterus in 61.5% of referred patients. In most cases, this was the so-called "T-shape" uterus or uterine constrictions. Irregular margins of the endometrial cavity were seen in 52%; these have been shown to be due to focal thickening of the myometrium.

Müllerian anomalies are accompanied by abnormalities in other organ systems in a high percentage of cases. In their study of 47 women with duplication of the uterus and cervix, Gilsanz and Cleveland found 31 patients with major genitourinary malformations.[12] These included cloacal abnormalities in 16 patients, exstrophic deformities in four, and renal malformations on the same side as an obstructed müllerian duct in 11 patients. The renal anomalies included nine cases of renal agenesis and two of ectopic insertion of the ureter. Renal anomalies, including agenesis, crossed fused renal ectopia, pelvic kidney, and duplication of the collecting system, have been reported by Buttram and Gibbons and others to occur in association with all classes of müllerian anomalies (Fig. 4-6).[6,13] Skeletal defects of the upper and lower extremities have been reported to occur in 10%, especially in the presence of vaginal agenesis.[14] There is a 6% incidence of associated cardiac, ophthalmologic, and otologic abnormalities.[15] Harger et al reported an increased level of antinuclear antibodies (ANA) in 11% of women with müllerian anomalies, compared with 2% of the normal population.[7] The significance of this finding is not yet apparent, but there is an an association of elevated ANA levels with collagen vascular diseases. Mayer-Rokitansky-Küster-Hauser (MRKH) syndrome consists of congenital absence of the uterus, cervix, and vagina (Fig. 4-7). This syndrome was recently subdivided into types A and B by Strubbe et al on the basis of a review of the radiologic and laparoscopic findings in 91 cases.[16] Both types of the syndrome are thought to be due to the presence of excess müllerian inhibiting factor. Laparoscopy reveals symmetric muscular bud and fal-

Text continued on p. 83.

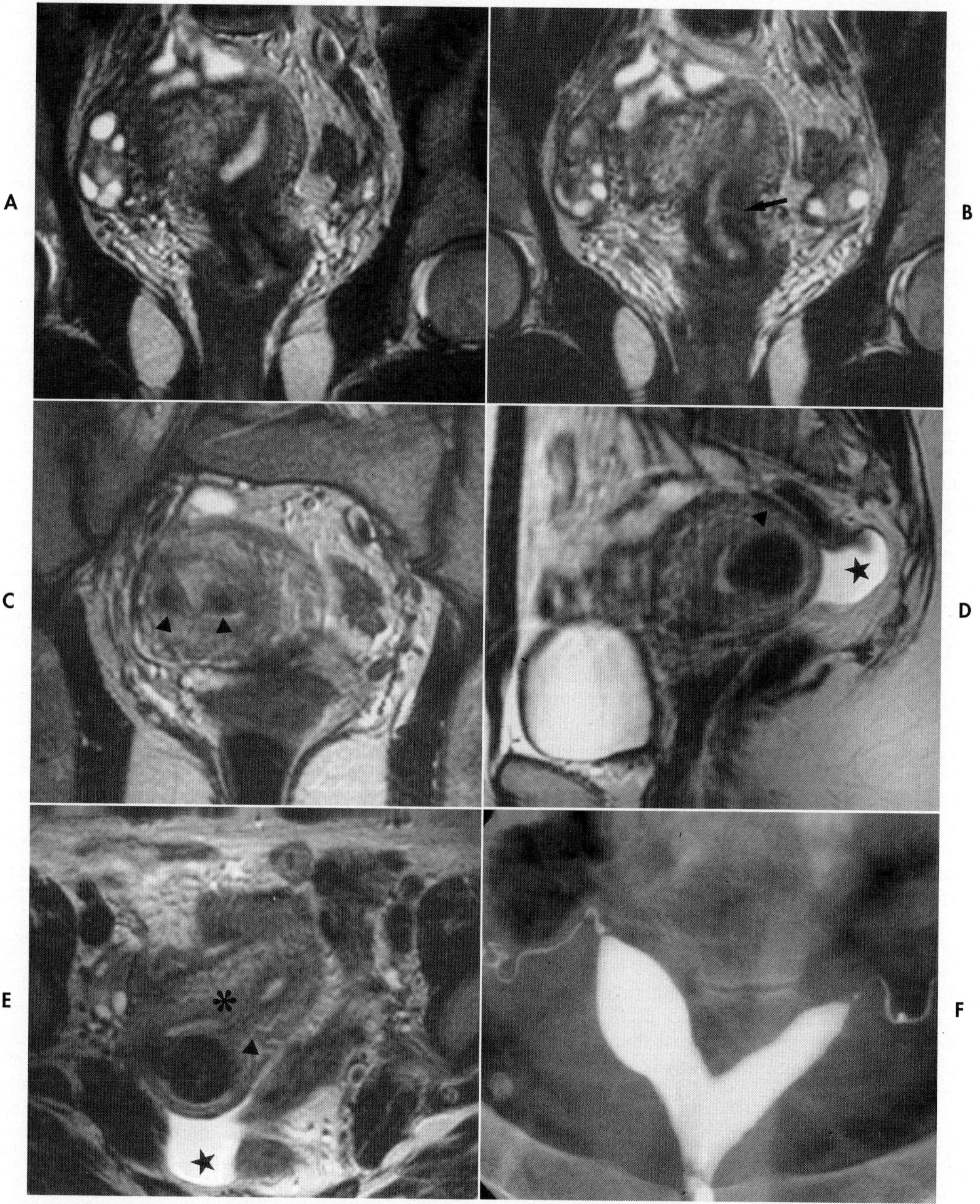

Fig. 4-2 Bicornuate uterus, class IV. Coronal **(A-C)**, sagittal **(D)**, and axial **(E)** FSE T2-weighted (TR 4000, TE 108, ET 8) MR images obtained using the pelvic phased array coil show a single cervix *(arrow)*, myometrial septum *(asterisk)*, and low-signal fibroids impressing upon the right endometrial cavity *(arrowheads)*. Free fluid is present in the cul-de-sac. The correlative hysterosalpinogram (HSG) **(F)** demonstrates uterine horns with an angle of divergence of 80 degrees, indeterminate for a bicornuate uterus.

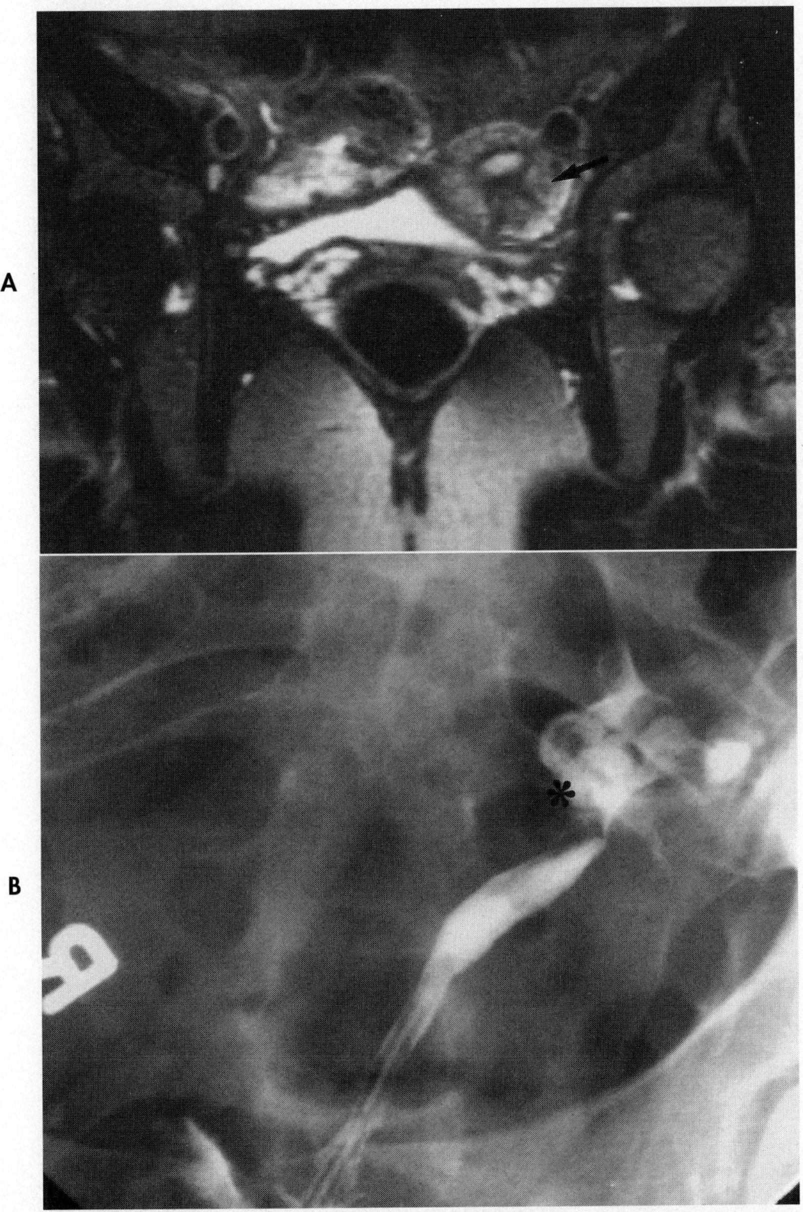

Fig. 4-3 Unicornuate uterus, class III. **A,** Coronal FSE T2-weighted (TR 4000, TE 102, ET 8) MR image with fat suppression demonstrates a solitary left uterine horn *(arrow)*. **B,** HSG of the same patient shows hydrosalpinx *(asterisk)*.

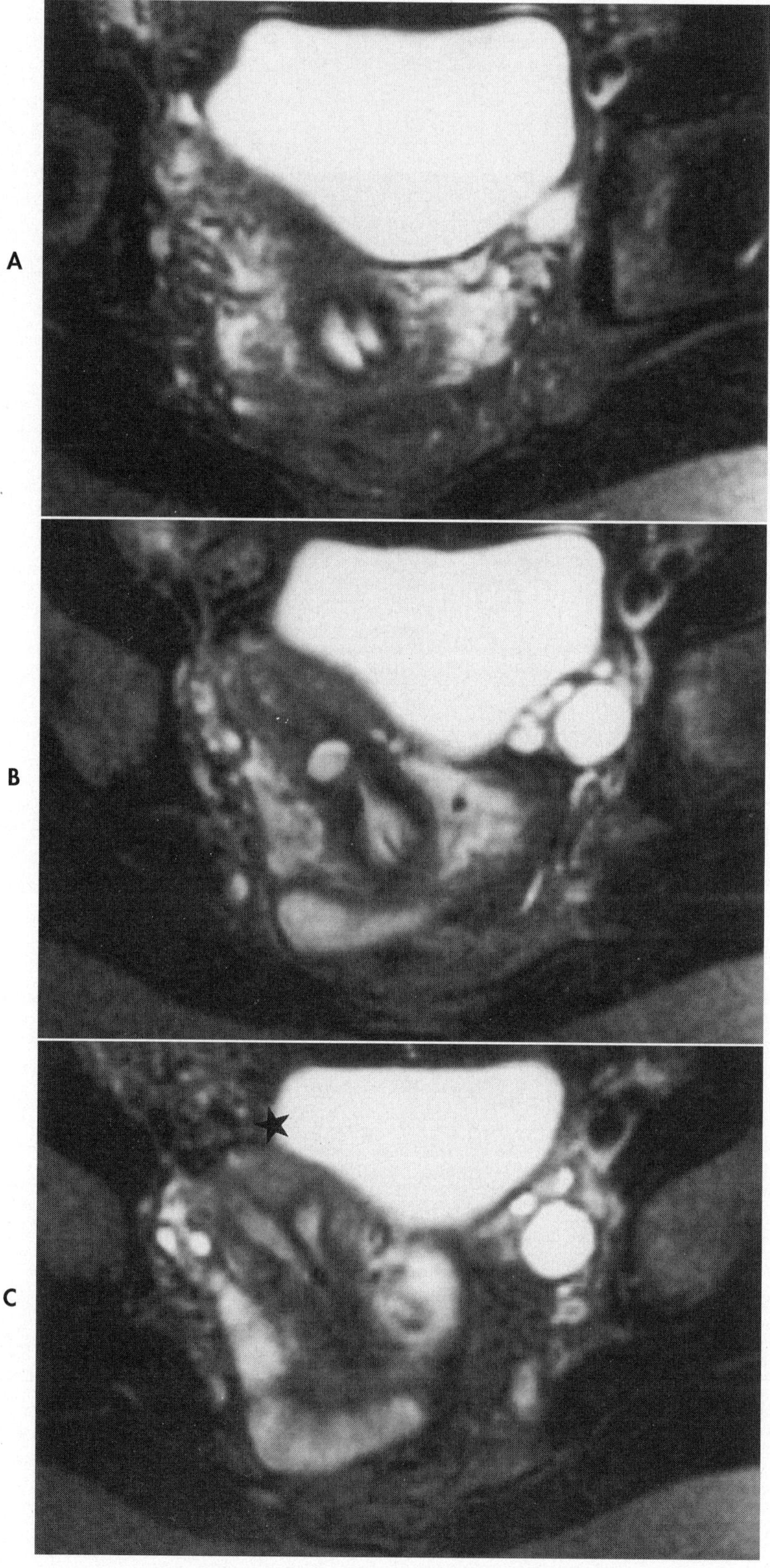

Fig. 4-4 For legend see opposite page.

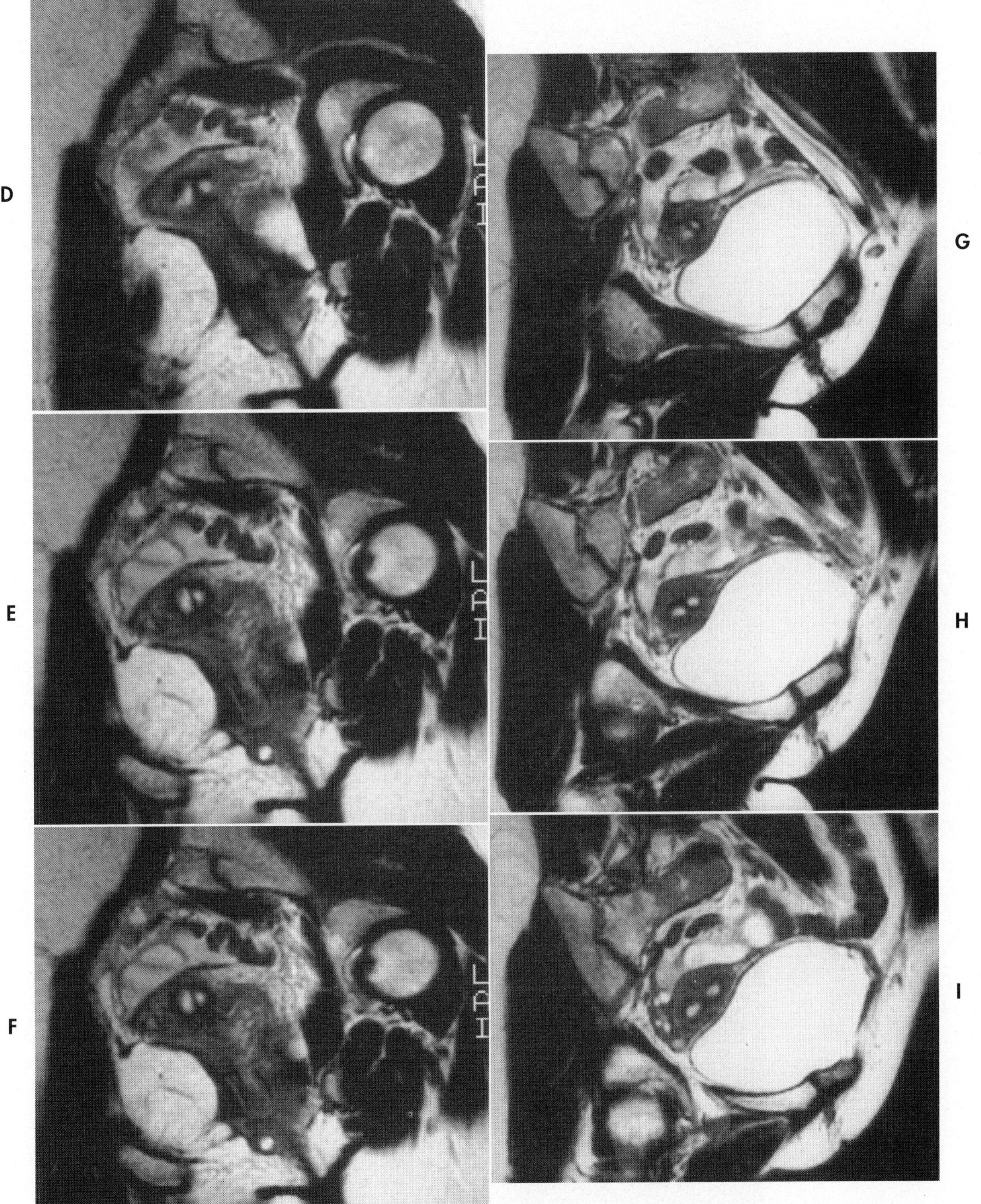

Fig. 4-4 Septated uterus, class V. Fat-suppressed axial **(A-C)** and consecutive, oblique coronal **(D-I)** FSE T2-weighted (TR 4000, TE 102, ET 8) MR images show normal external contour and size of the uterus *(star)* with a thin, low T2 signal septum separating two endometrial cavities. The inferior portion of the septum is fenestrated *(arrow)*.

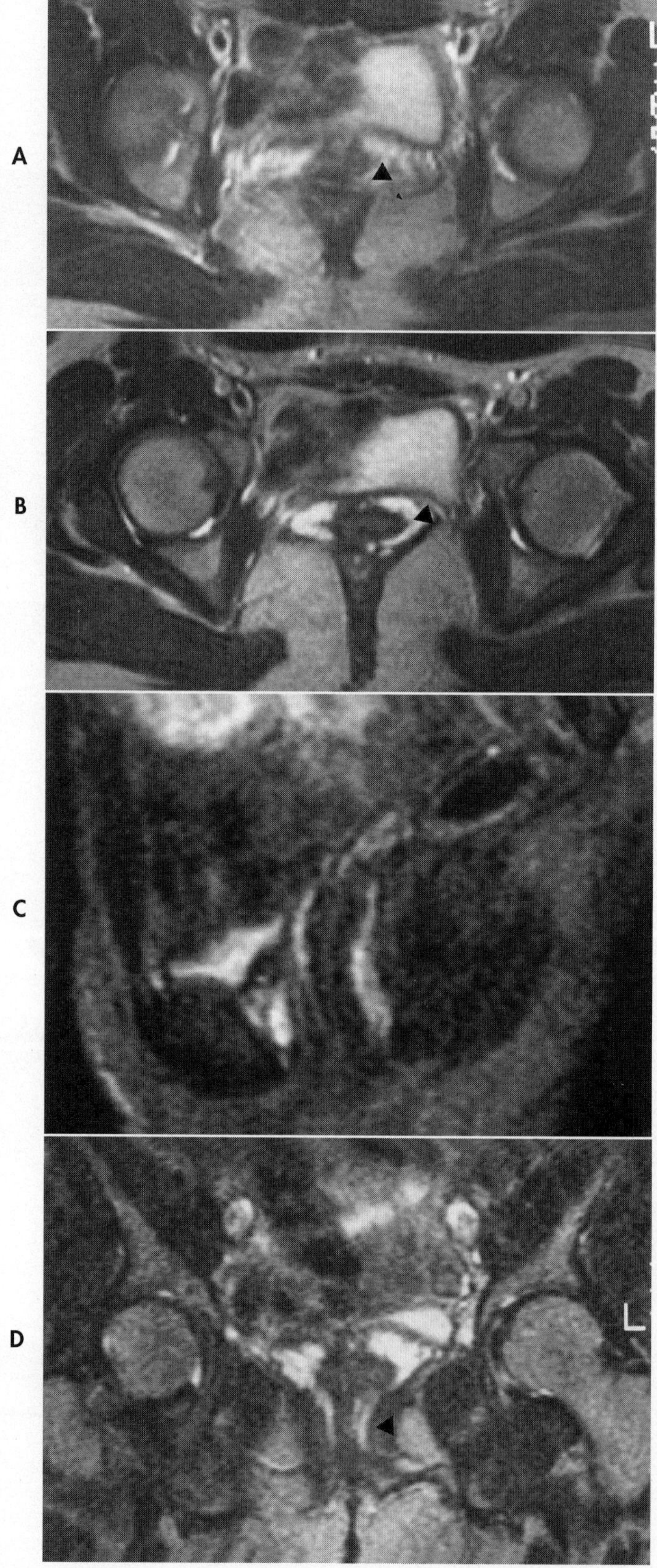

Fig. 4-5 Agenesis of the upper four fifths of the genital tract, class I. Axial (**A** and **B**), sagittal (**C**), and coronal (**D**) T2-weighted (TR 2700, TE 80) MR images show absence of the uterus, cervix, and upper two thirds of the vagina. The distal third of the vagina is formed by tissue derived from the urogenital sinus and is of normal appearance *(arrowhead)*.

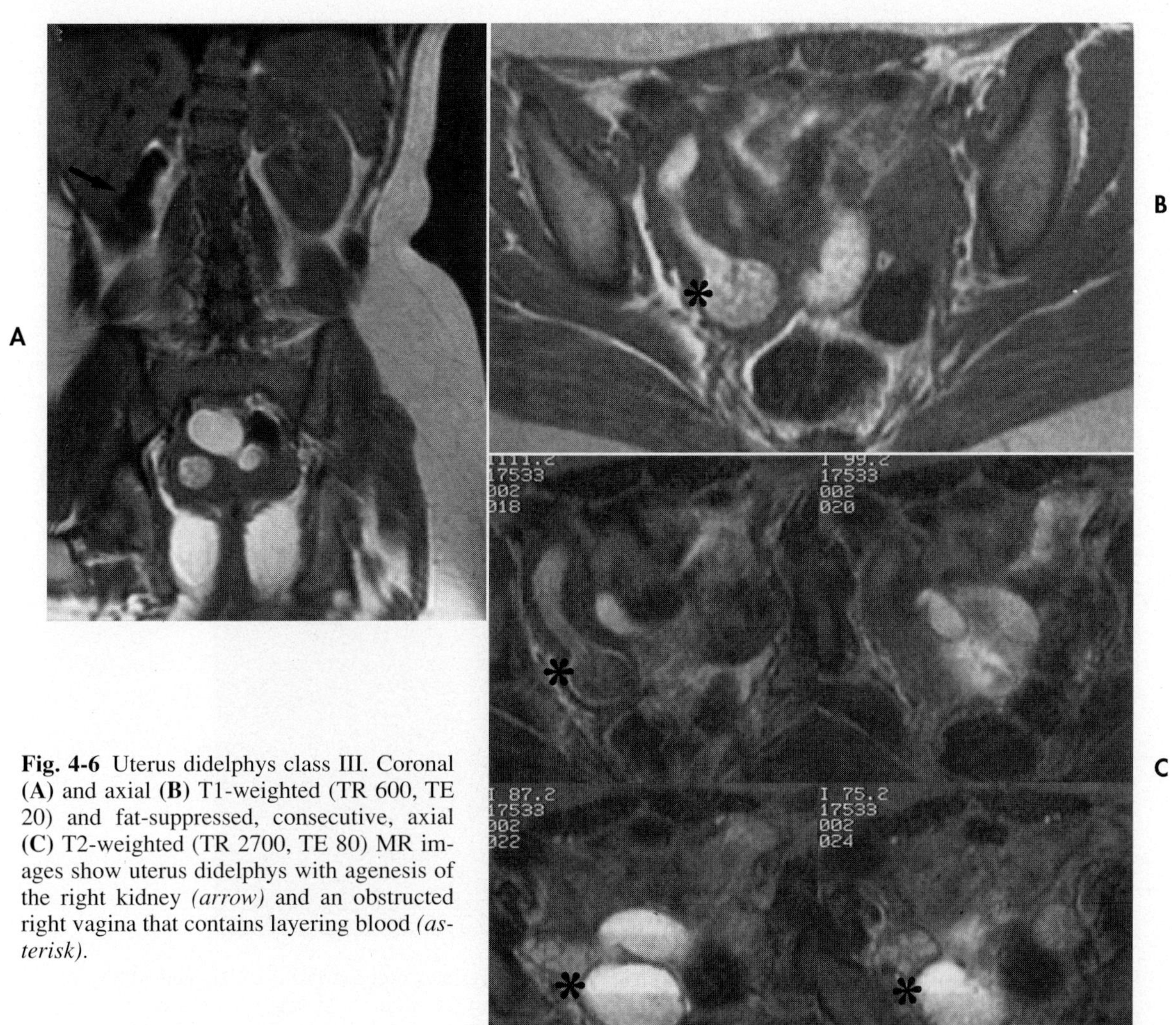

Fig. 4-6 Uterus didelphys class III. Coronal **(A)** and axial **(B)** T1-weighted (TR 600, TE 20) and fat-suppressed, consecutive, axial **(C)** T2-weighted (TR 2700, TE 80) MR images show uterus didelphys with agenesis of the right kidney *(arrow)* and an obstructed right vagina that contains layering blood *(asterisk)*.

lopian tube development in type A. In type B, there is asymmetric muscular bud or abnormal fallopian tube development. Only patients with type B have additional abnormalities of the kidneys and ovaries. There have been no reports of anomalies in organ systems other than the genital tract in women exposed to DES.

CLASSIFICATION OF MÜLLERIAN ANOMALIES

During 1988, in an attempt to standardize the reporting and treatment of müllerian anomalies, the American Fertility Society adopted a classification system developed by Buttram and Gibbons.[10,13] The patient's significant medical history is recorded, including fertility history, pregnancy outcomes, previous surgery, and genitourinary tract

infections. The radiologic study results, clinical findings, type of müllerian duct anomaly present, and estimated prognosis for future pregnancies are recorded (Fig. 4-8). Müllerian anomalies are divided into seven classes, based on degree of failure of normal development. The anomalies are separated into groups that have similar clinical presentations, treatments, and expected outcomes (see box on p. 84).

SYMPTOMATOLOGY

Women with müllerian duct anomalies may present with a wide range of symptoms extending from puberty through child-bearing years and into menopause.

Severe vaginal or pelvic pain, which may be cyclic, constant, or intermittent in nature, is a com-

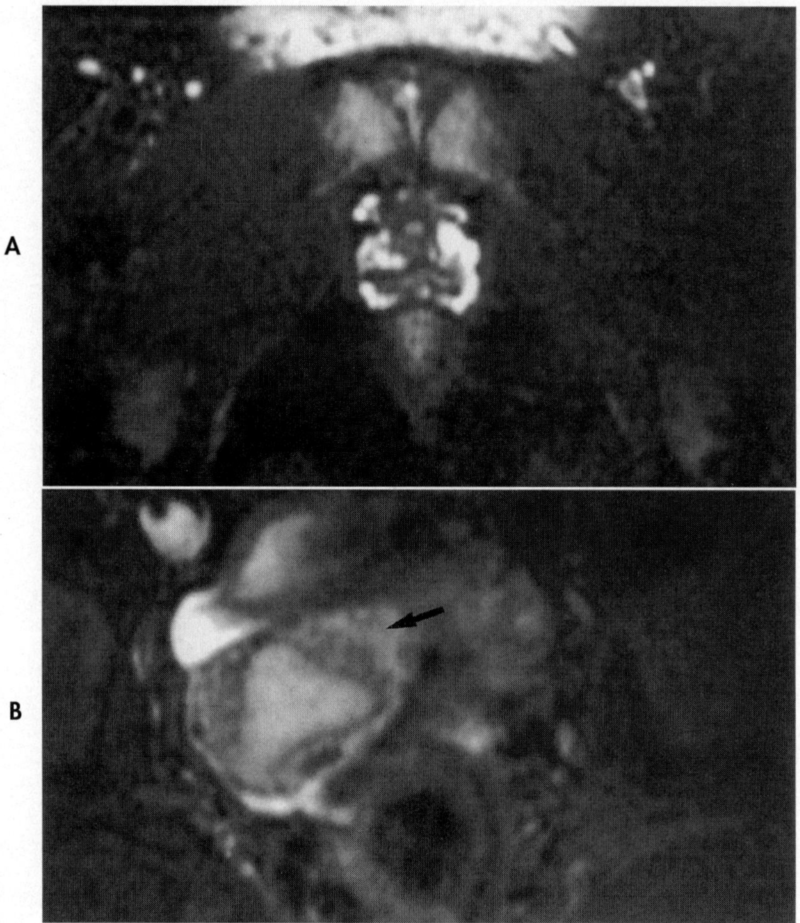

Fig. 4-7 Mayer-Rokitansky-Küster-Hauser variant. Axial **(A)** and coronal **(B)** T2-weighted (TR 2500, TE 80) fat-suppressed MR images demonstrate a normal vagina and small uterine cavity *(arrow)*. At surgery, only one fallopian tube was found.

CLASSIFICATION OF MÜLLERIAN DUCT ANOMALIES

Class I: Segmental müllerian agenesis or hypoplasia
   A. Vaginal
   B. Cervical
   C. Fundal
   D. Tubal
   E. Combined
Class II: Unicornuate uterus
   A1. Rudimentary horn contains endometrium and
       may (A1a) or may not (A1b) communicate with
       main uterine cavity
   A2. Rudimentary horn without endometrium
   B. No rudimentary horn

Class III: Uterus didelphys
Class IV: Bicornuate uterus
   A. Complete division to internal os
   B. Partial division
Class V: Septate
   A. Complete; two distinct cervices may be present
   B. Partial
Class VI: Arcuate
Class VII:
   Drug (diethylstilbestrol [DES]) related; includes
       T-shaped uterus, constricting bands, widening of
       lower two thirds of uterus, and other abnormalities

THE AMERICAN FERTILITY SOCIETY CLASSIFICATION OF MULLERIAN ANOMALIES

Patient's Name ____ Date __________ Chart # __________

Age _______ G _______ P _______ Sp Ab _______ VTP _______ Ectopic _______ Infertile Yes _______ No _______

Other Significant History (i.e. surgery, infection, etc.) ____

____

HSG __________ Sonography __________ Photography __________ Laparoscopy __________ Laparotomy __________

EXAMPLES

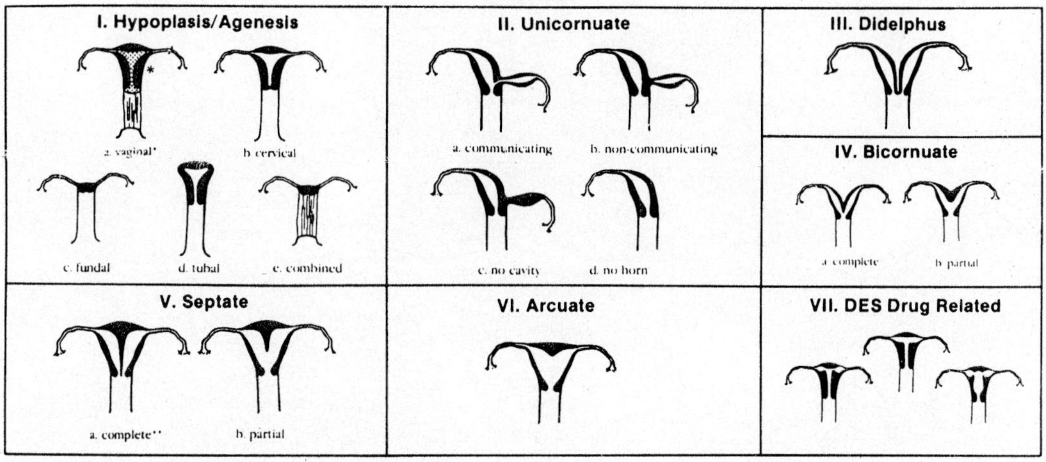

* Uterus may be normal or take a variety of abnormal forms.
** May have two distinct cervices

Type of Anomaly

Class I	__________	Class V	__________
Class II	__________	Class VI	__________
Class III	__________	Class VII	__________
Class IV	__________		

Treatment (Surgical Procedures): __________

____

____

Prognosis for Conception & Subsequent Viable Infant*

__________ Excellent (> 75%)

__________ Good (50-75%)

__________ Fair (25%-50%)

__________ Poor (< 25%)

*Based upon physician's judgment.

Recommended Followup Treatment: __________

____

____

Additional Findings: __________

____

____

Vagina: ____________________________________

Cervix: ____________________________________

Tubes: Right __________ Left __________

Kidneys: Right __________ Left __________

DRAWING

L   R

Property of
The American Fertility Society

For additional supply write to:
The American Fertility Society
2140 11th Avenue, South
Suite 200
Birmingham, Alabama 35205

Fig. 4-8 The American Fertility Society Classification of Müllerian Anomalies. (From the American Society of Fertility and Sterility; with permission.)

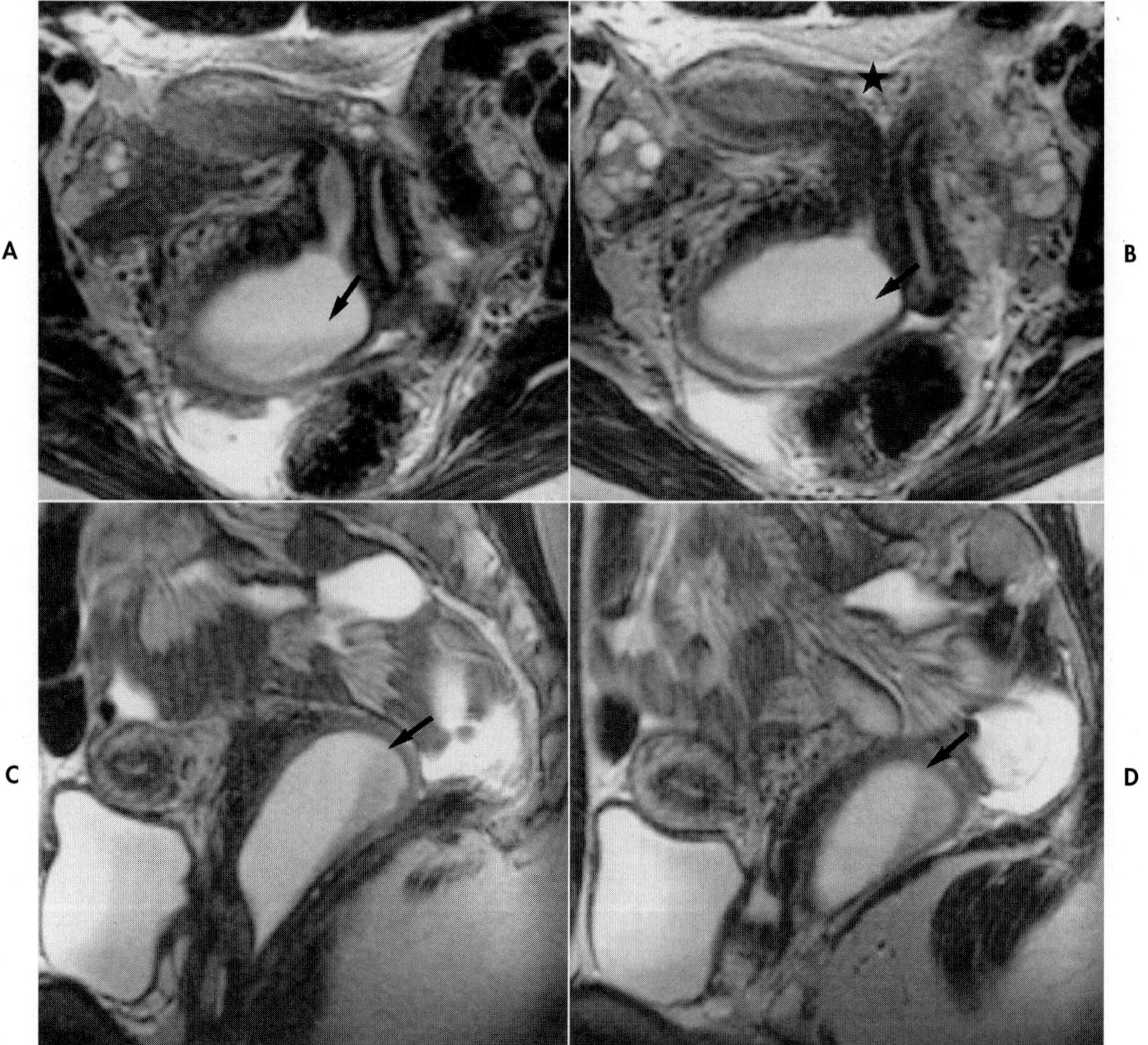

Fig. 4-9 Uterus didelphys class III. Axial (**A** and **B**) and sagittal (**C** and **D**) FSE T2-weighted (TR 4000, TE 102, ET 8) MR images reveal two uterine cavities *(star)* and a right vagina that is obstructed by a transverse septum and contains layering blood *(arrow)*. There is free fluid in the cul-de-sac.

mon complaint and is often the result of an obstructed müllerian duct system. In the case of a vaginal septum, blood accumulates proximally, causing the obstructed cavity to balloon and impress upon the adjacent nonobstructed system, often resulting in pain with intercourse (Fig. 4-9). A rudimentary uterine horn that is lined with endometrium and has no connection with the patent cavity can cause endometriosis.

Primary amenorrhea may be the result of imperforate hymen or uterine agenesis. The hymen arises from the müllerian tubercle at the level of the urogenital sinus. When the hymen is complete, hema-

tometrocolpos and pain often result (Fig. 4-10). This diagnosis can usually be excluded by physical examination. Most women with uterine agenesis have a normal female genotype and external genitalia. They are infertile. Hypomenorrhea can be due to the presence of a unicornuate uterus or a rudimentary horn as part of a bicornuate uterus.

Women with müllerian duct anomalies have an increased incidence of obstetric problems (25%) compared with the 10% rate in the normal population. The problems occur not in conception but in maintaining and delivering a pregnancy. There is an increased risk of spontaneous abortion, ab-

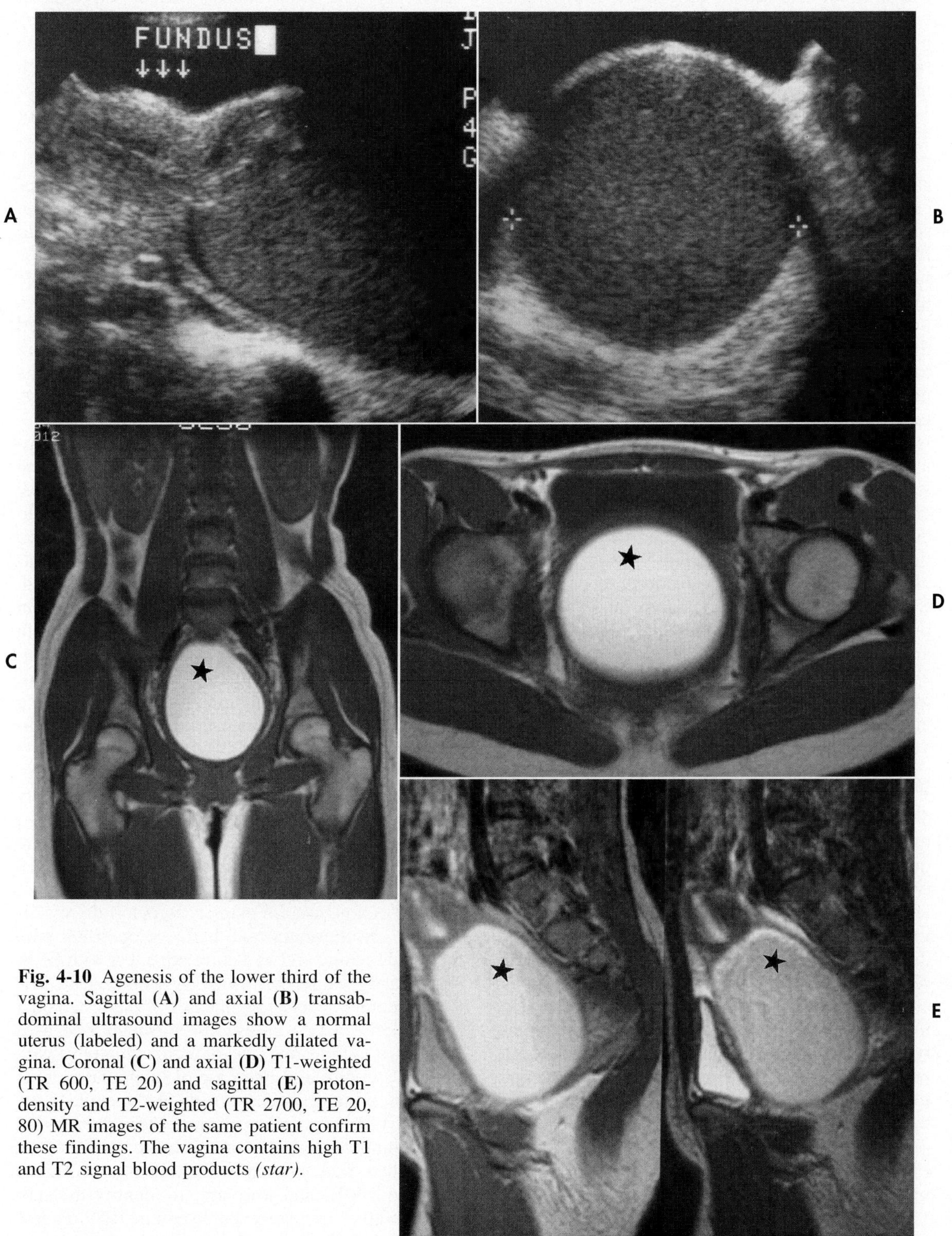

Fig. 4-10 Agenesis of the lower third of the vagina. Sagittal (**A**) and axial (**B**) transabdominal ultrasound images show a normal uterus (labeled) and a markedly dilated vagina. Coronal (**C**) and axial (**D**) T1-weighted (TR 600, TE 20) and sagittal (**E**) proton-density and T2-weighted (TR 2700, TE 20, 80) MR images of the same patient confirm these findings. The vagina contains high T1 and T2 signal blood products *(star)*.

normal fetal presentation, premature labor, dystocia, stillbirth, and ectopic pregnancy, which varies with the type of uterine anomaly. Buttram and Gibbons, in their review of müllerian duct anomalies, further subdivide pregnancy risks.[13] Patients with unicornuate uterus have a spontaneous abortion rate of 48% and a premature delivery rate of 17%. There is also an increased risk of intrauterine growth retardation. Uterus didelphys, probably because each cavity resembles a unicornuate uterus, causes the same complications and at nearly the same rates. Patients with bicornuate uteri suffer from a spontaneous abortion rate of 35% and a premature delivery rate of 23%. Septated uteri carry the highest rate of spontaneous abortion (67%) and premature delivery (33%). The high rate of abortion is thought to be due to the lack of vascularity in the fibrous septum; thus, a normal vascular supply to the developing pregnancy cannot be maintained. The more complete the septum, the higher is the rate of abortion. All müllerian anomalies are associated with higher rates of abnormal fetal presentations, especially breech, and dystocia. Golan et al also reported an increased risk of cervical incompetence resulting in second-trimester abortions.[17] Anomalies secondary to DES exposure are also associated with complications of pregnancy. Kaufman et al reported increased rates of ectopic pregnancies and preterm deliveries in patients with abnormally shaped uterine cavities.[11] No specific abnormality was identified as more likely to result in an adverse outcome. There is also thought to be an increased rate of infertility, although this has not yet been statistically proved.

IMAGING

The imaging procedure chosen for evaluation of müllerian duct anomalies should fulfill several requirements. It must be accurate in determining the type of anomaly present. This is especially important in the case of septate versus bicornuate uterus, in which prognosis and choice of therapy are very different. It should be able to assess accurately the remainder of the genitourinary tract for additional abnormalities. As there is a strong association of müllerian duct anomalies with renal anomalies, both kidneys should be visualized. A search should be made for other processes that may contribute to infertility, including endometriosis, occlusion of the fallopian tubes, and pelvic adhesions. The chosen procedure must be acceptable to the patient. Finally, it should provide the most useful package of information for the lowest reasonable cost.

For many years, HSG was used to identify and classify müllerian duct anomalies.[18] The advantages of the technique are its low cost and the ability to determine tubal patency and, in some cases,

identify peritubal adhesions that may contribute to infertility. The disadvantages include exposure to ionizing radiation and contrast agents, patient discomfort, and limitation of the examination to the inner surface of the genital tract. Assuming both cavities are opacified, HSG can differentiate septate from bicornuate uteri only when the angle of divergence between the uterine cavities is less than 75 degrees, which indicates a septated uterus. In addition, the kidneys cannot be evaluated. The accuracy of HSG in accurately classifying müllerian duct anomalies is reported to range from 50% to 92%.[19,20]

Ultrasonography has the ability to evaluate the uterus and ovaries from many planes. The external contour of the uterus can be assessed. In skilled hands, tubal patency can be evaluated by instilling saline into the uterus and directly visualizing its passage through the fallopian tubes. The kidneys can be easily and fully evaluated. Before the development of the endovaginal probe, transabdominal scanning was performed, often in association with HSG, to evaluate müllerian duct anomalies. In many cases, septate and bicornuate uteri could not be differentiated and the accuracy of the examination was compromised (Fig. 4-11). In a retrospective study of 68 patients by Malini et al, transabdominal ultrasonography was diagnostic in 28%, confirmatory of a known abnormality in 60%, and incorrect in 12%.[21] In a study of 63 patients performed by Reuter et al, the addition of transabdominal ultrasonography performed during the luteal phase of the menstrual cycle to HSG improved accuracy from 55% to 90%, with persistent difficulty in separating bicornuate from septate uteri.[19] The endovaginal probe has markedly improved visualization of female genital anatomy. In the study of Pellerito et al, EVS was accurate in classifying müllerian duct anomalies in 11 of 12 patients.[22]

MRI is now used in many centers to fully evaluate the genitourinary tract before proceeding with surgical therapy and as a correlative test with EVS. In an early study performed by Mintz et al, MR was accurate in six of eight cases of müllerian duct anomaly.[23] In two cases, MR misdiagnosed as a bicornuate uterus one case of uterus didelphys with vaginal septum and one case of bicornuate uterus without septum. These errors likely could have been avoided had slice thickness less than 8 mm and oblique imaging planes been used. Fedele et al studied five women with known unicornuate uteri with MRI and were able to identify the subclass in all.[24] In a study published in 1989, Fedele et al studied 18 women with müllerian duct anomalies diagnosed by hysterosalpingography with MRI.[25] To maximize accuracy, they employed ob-

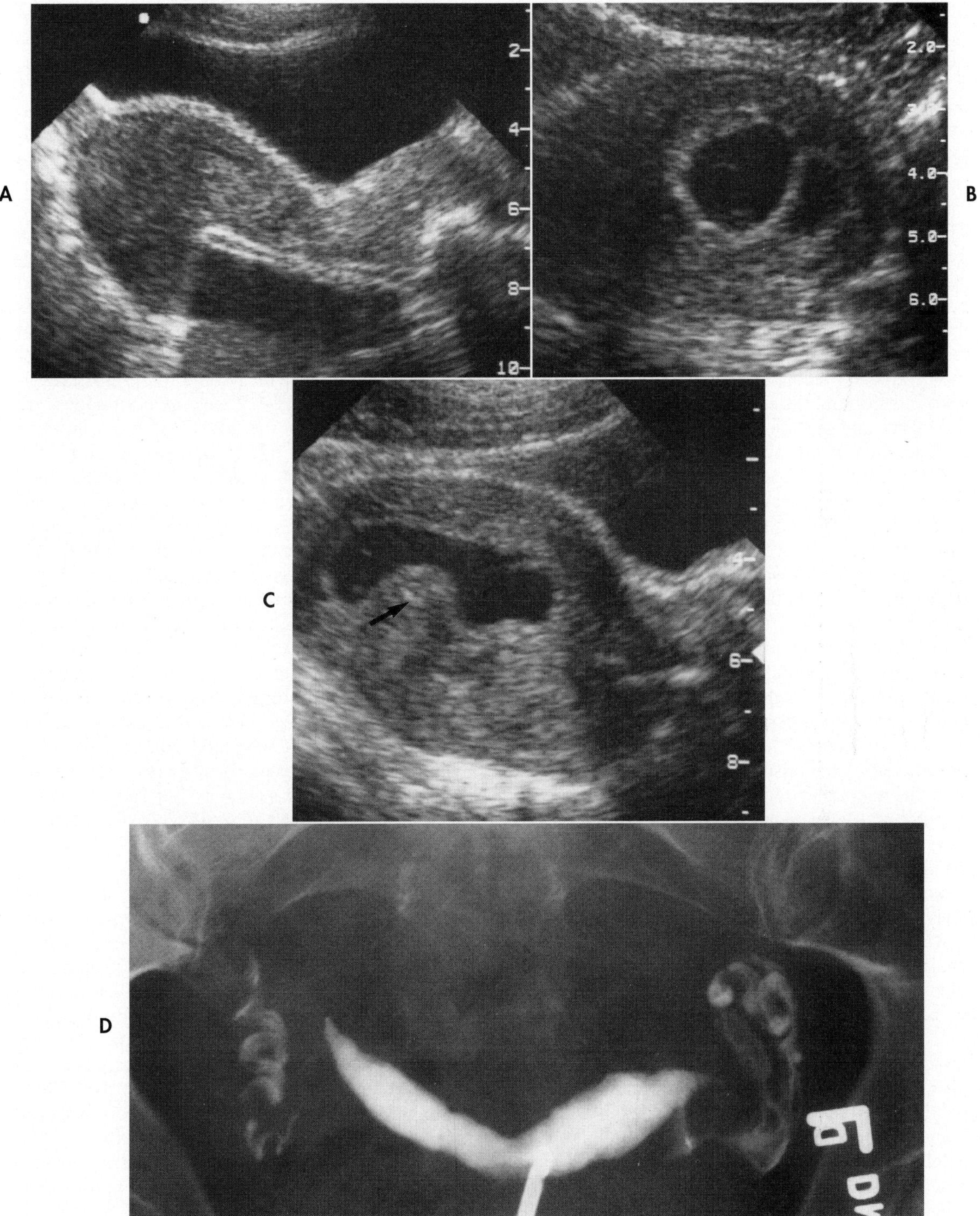

Fig. 4-11 Bicornuate uterus class IV. Sagittal (**A** and **C**) and transverse (**B**) transabdominal ultrasound images show two uterine cavities separated by a septum that contains myometrial tissue at its superior aspect *(arrow)*. Correlative HSG (**D**) demonstrates an angle of divergence of uterine horns of 110 degrees, which suggests a bicornuate rather than a septate uterus.

lique images paralleling the long axis of the uterine fundus, and imaged during the luteal phase of the menstrual cycle when the contour of the endometrial cavity should be most easily evaluated. MR was 100% accurate in classifying the type of uterine anomaly. In three cases, cervical prolongation of the septal spur was not identified. The authors reported that the configuration of the uterus in these three patients made identification of an optimal imaging plane for cervical anatomy difficult. They emphasized the necessity of evaluating the outer contour of the uterine cavity in accurately diagnosing septated uteri, as they found the tissue composition and signal of the septum to be variable. Carrington et al studied 29 patients with müllerian duct anomalies using MRI.[26] In their study, the parameters recorded were external fundal contour, intercornual distance, signal characteristics of the uterus and septum when present, and the ratio of endometrial to myometrial width. MR was 100% accurate in determining the type of müllerian duct anomaly present. Carrington et al identified three patients with bicornuate uteri in which a mixed fibrous and myometrial septum was present. Other gynecologic disease was identified in 10 patients. In the only study prospectively comparing EVS with MRI and cited above, Pellerito et al found MR 100% accurate in classification of 26 müllerian duct anomalies.[22] They reported a muscular component in the majority of uterine septi and recommended careful evaluation of the external uterine contour in classifying the anomaly present. MRI has also been successfully used to evaluate anomalies secondary to DES exposure. In a study of five patients, van Gils et al compared the results of MRI with those of HSG and found good correlation.[27] They demonstrated that the internal cavity irregularities were secondary to focal thickenings of myometrial tissue.

The cost of each medical test must be balanced against the usefulness of the information it provides. Costs vary regionally, by institution and with the expertise of the physician performing and interpreting the test. In the Northeastern United States, HSG costs $440.00, pelvic or endovaginal ultrasound $360.00, and MR examination of the pelvis $1050.00. The cost of a diagnostic laparoscopy is approximately $2000.00. The initial use of MRI may save the patient money and avoid laparoscopy, the combined cost of HSG, EVS, and laparoscopy being approximately $2800.00.

MRI TECHNIQUE

Examination of women with a suspected congenital anomaly is best performed using the highest resolution technique available. In the GE Signa system, this is the pelvic phased array (PPA) coil, which allows for high resolution images without significant loss in signal to noise. Careful attention to patient positioning is essential. The small fields of view (FOVs), 14 to 20 cm, allowed with the PPA coil leave little room for error. Glucagon (1 mg intramuscularly) is useful, as in other abdominal and pelvic studies, to diminish bowel peristalsis. External banding should also be performed to diminish respiratory motion. A complete examination usually requires 45 to 60 minutes.

The routine approach we use is to obtain a large FOV coronal T1-weighted image initially to visualize the kidneys. A second T1- or T2-weighted image is then obtained in the sagittal plane. From this set of images, locations are chosen for placement of saturation bands over the anterior and posterior abdominal wall fat, which serve to diminish respiratory artifact. Several T2-weighted images are then obtained. Since the advent of fast spin echo (FSE), we routinely use this pulse sequence with 192 phase encodes, 4- to 5-mm slice thickness and 2 to 4 signal averages to obtain images in the sagittal and axial planes. These are crucial images, since they enable evaluation of the external contour and zonal anatomy of the uterus, and visualize the ovaries. From the sagittal images, a third plane is chosen, either parallel to the long axis of the uterus or perpendicular to the uterine cavity, and a third T2-weighted sequence is performed (see Fig. 4-4). Fat saturation sequences can be useful in highlighting the endometrial cavity. We often obtain axial T1-weighted images to assess ovarian cysts or fibroids for the presence of hemorrhage. Gadolinium-DTPA is not routinely used but may be employed to assess possible adnexal masses.

MRI APPEARANCE

Agenesis of any part of the genitourinary tract, with the exception of the fallopian tubes, is easily evaluated by MRI.[28,29] Absence of the uterus is best seen on sagittal images, while absence of the cervix and/or proximal vagina is often more obvious on axial images. Hypoplasia of the uterus is often accompanied by thinning and decreased signal of the endometrium. In evaluating the unicornuate uterus, it is essential that the precise subtype of this class of anomalies be identified. Most women with communicating rudimentary horns require no treatment. The removal of a noncommunicating cavitary rudimentary horn or a noncavitary horn is often of benefit. On MRI the uterus is lateroflexed and banana-shaped. The presence of high T2 signal within the rudimentary horn indicates endometrial tissue. The uterus didelphys is recognized on MRI by the presence of two normal-sized uterine cavities and cervices with a longitudinal upper vaginal septum (Fig. 4-12). A transverse vaginal septum may obstruct one cavity, resulting in hematometrocolpos and hematosalpinx (Fig. 4-13). The features of a bicornuate uterus are increased intercornual distance, greater than 4 cm, with fundal concavity greater than 1 cm and a longitudinal septum (Fig. 4-14). The septum is usually formed of myometrial tissue that is of intermediate T1 and high T2 signal intensity. The inferior portion of the septum may be formed of fibrous tissue that of low T1 and T2 signal. The arcuate uterus has a normal convex or flat fundal contour and minimal indentation of the endometrial canal. There is no true septum. The septated uterus is of normal size and may have a flat, convex, or mildly concave outer contour, less than 1 cm. There should be one all-encompassing layer of myometrium and one junctional zone. The longitudinal septum may be complete, partial, or fenestrated. In most cases, it is formed of low T1 and T2 signal fibrous tissue, but the superior portion may be formed of myometrial tissue. Evaluation of the septum can best be carried out using a plane perpendicular to the short axis of the uterus.

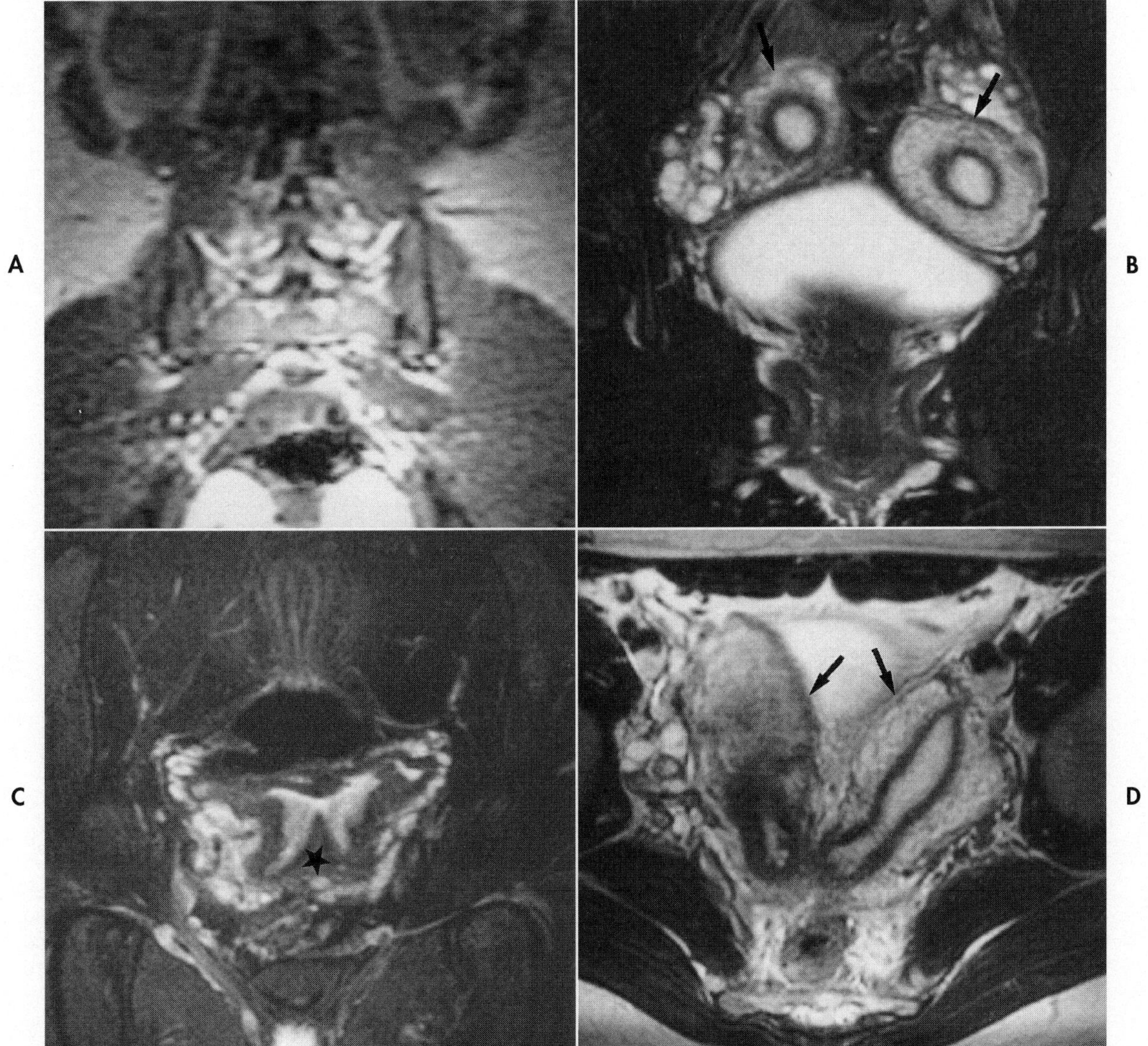

Fig. 4-12 Uterus didelphys, class III. Coronal (**A**) fast-spoiled gradient echo (TR 18, TE 5, FA 60 degrees) and fat-suppressed coronal (**B** and **C**) and axial (**D**) FSE T2-weighted (TR 4000, TE 102, ET 8) MR images were obtained using the pelvic phased array coil. The large field of view (FOV) coronal image (**A**) shows two kidneys. The high resolution T2-weighted images obtained with a 20-cm FOV clearly show two separate, complete uteri *(arrows)*, with a partially resected vaginal septum *(star)*.

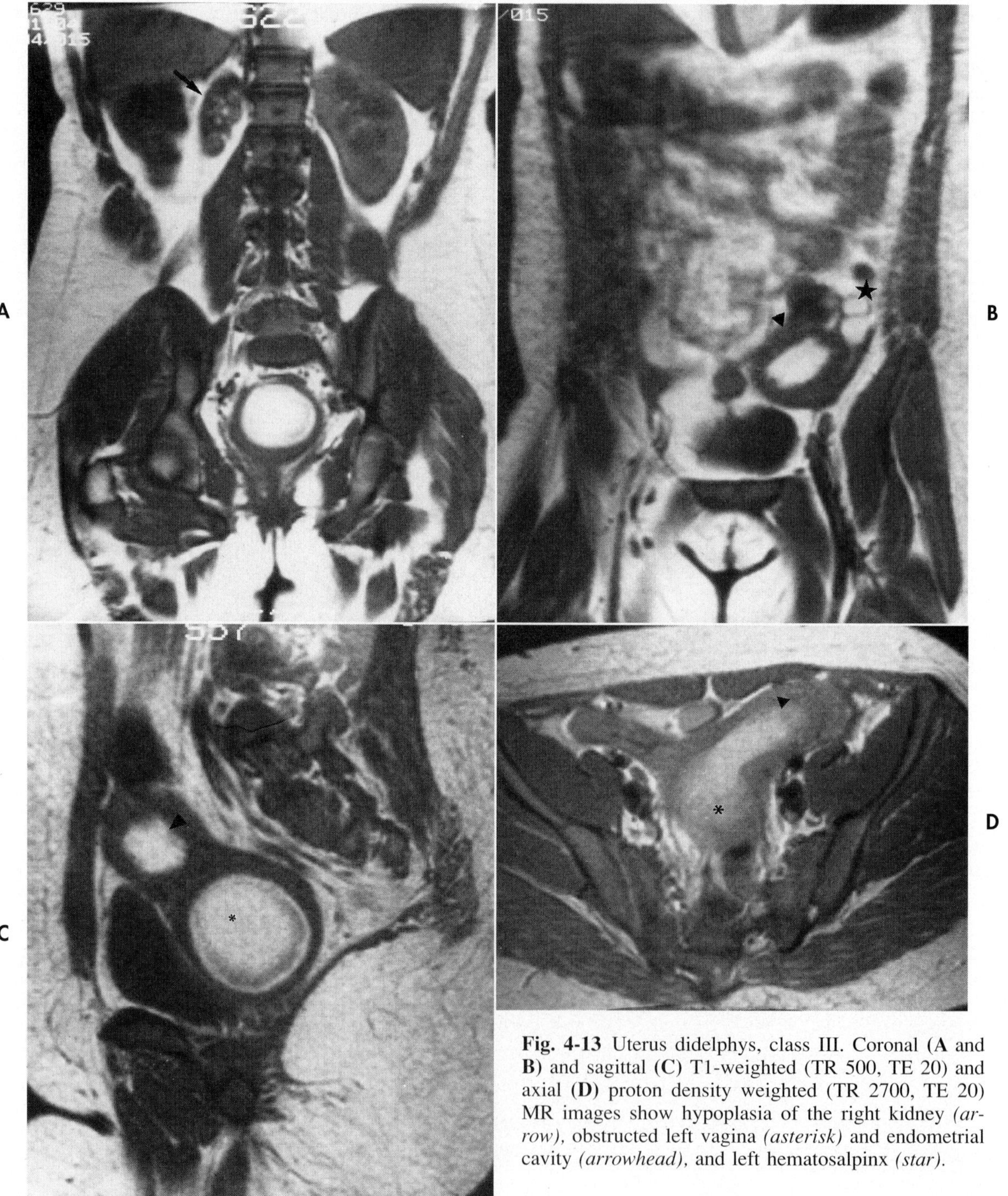

Fig. 4-13 Uterus didelphys, class III. Coronal (**A** and **B**) and sagittal (**C**) T1-weighted (TR 500, TE 20) and axial (**D**) proton density weighted (TR 2700, TE 20) MR images show hypoplasia of the right kidney *(arrow)*, obstructed left vagina *(asterisk)* and endometrial cavity *(arrowhead)*, and left hematosalpinx *(star)*.

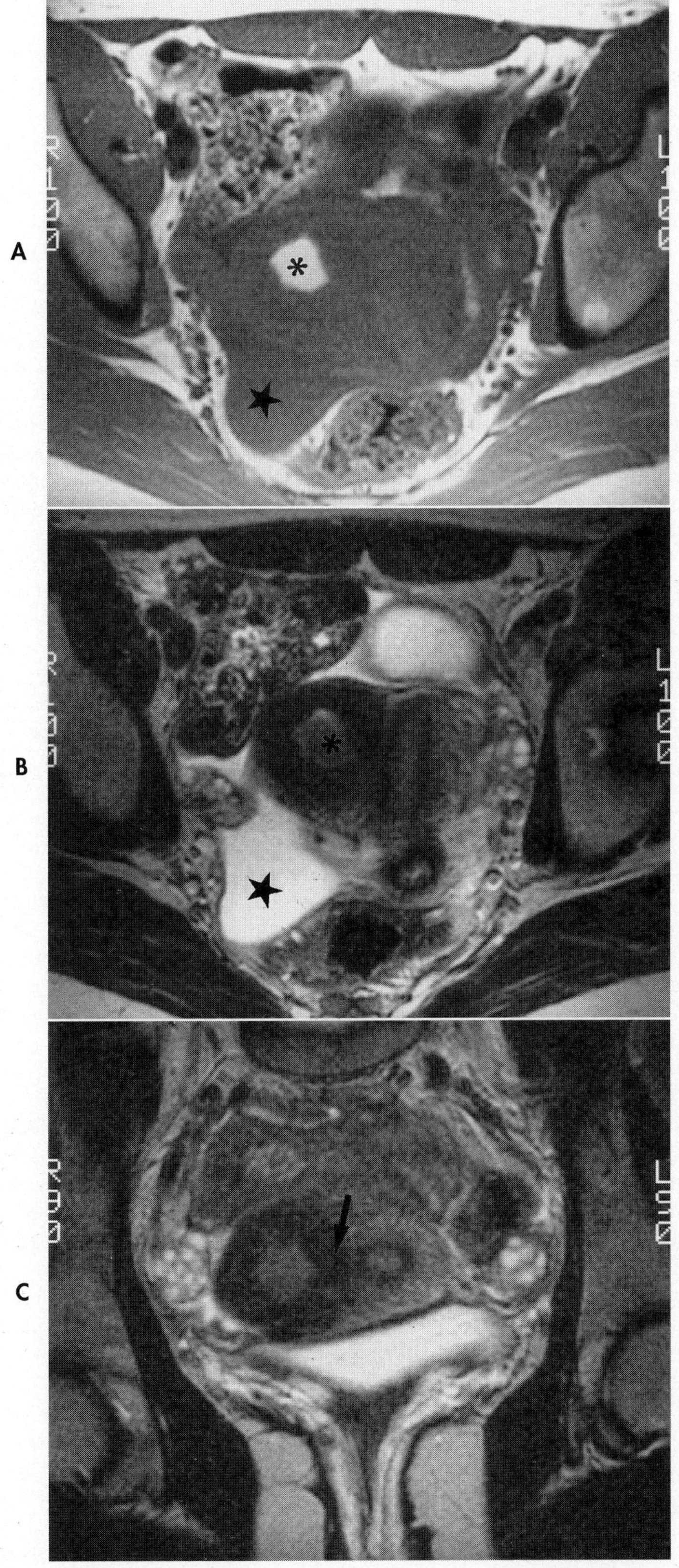

Fig. 4-14 Bicornuate uterus, class IV. Axial **(A)** T1-weighted (TR 600, TE 11) and axial **(B)** and coronal **(C)** FSE T2-weighted (TR 4000, TE 102, ET 8) MR images were obtained using the pelvic phased array coil. There is free fluid in the cul-de-sac *(star)* and a bicornuate uterus with myometrial septum *(arrow)* and obstructed right horn *(asterisk)*.

Abnormalities identified on MRI in women exposed in utero to DES include uterine and cervical hypoplasia, T-shaped uterus, constrictions of the uterine cavity, and hydrosalpinges. These are best identified on images that parallel the long axis of the uterus. Irregular margins of the endometrial cavity and diverticula of the fallopian tubes are beyond the resolution of MRI.

TREATMENT

Vaginal agenesis, class I-A, is often treated with a McIndoe procedure, in which a neovagina is created. Up to 50% of these patients will have an associated uterine anomaly or cervical agenesis that will require further surgical management. There is little effective treatment for the remainder of the class I anomalies. The unicornuate uterus, class II, is not treated. The associated rudimentary horns may be removed when obstruction or endometriosis occurs. The class III anomaly, uterus didelphys, is generally not repaired, with the exception of removal of an associated transverse vaginal septum. Thus, through correctly defining and diagnosing this anomaly by MRI, no abdominal or pelvic incisions will be necessary, as the septum can be removed transvaginally. A bicornuate uterus, class IV, is generally treated with a Strassman metroplasty. This is a transabdominal procedure that requires 2 to 3 hours of operating time, several days of recuperation in the hospital, and several weeks of rest at home. Conception must be delayed 6 months. The class V anomaly, septated uterus, is often treated with hysteroscopic metroplasty. This procedure requires less than 1 hour of operating time, and the patient returns home the same day. Patients are allowed to conceive 2 months after the procedure. The arcuate uterus, class VI, generally requires no treatment. There is currently no effective treatment for DES related, class VII, anomalies, although cerclage is often used to decrease the high rate of second-trimester abortion.

Thus, it can be seen that careful and accurate definition of the anomaly is essential. This can reduce the rate of abdominopelvic surgeries and lead to more accurate treatment protocols. The skill of the radiologist in the judicious use of the imaging modalities at his or her disposal can greatly influence patient outcome.

PART II: Congenital and Pediatric Genitourinary Disorders

MRI of the female pelvis in the pediatric age group is becoming a very useful modality. It is less dependent than ultrasonography on bowel and bladder status, and avoids the ionizing radiation and intravenous contrast of computed tomography (CT). The pediatric population presents a different set of diagnostic challenges from those of adults. This is because the lesions most frequently encountered are congenital, and the neoplasms that do occur are of a different origin from those seen in adults. Congenital anomalies of the pelvis can have devastating consequences for the female genitourinary tract. These are commonly manifested as problems with either continence, upper urinary tract function, or appearance or function of the genitalia. Classic bladder exstrophy and cloacal exstrophy are congenital anomalies that can greatly affect the genitourinary system and also the gastrointestinal tract. Fortunately, these and most other variants of the exstrophy-epispadias complex are rare. Although this group of disorders represents an orderly spectrum from mild epispadias to full cloacal exstrophy, classic bladder exstrophy is seen most commonly. This section discusses the embryology, anatomic defects, and radiologic evaluation of the exstrophy-epispadias complex, as well as other female pelvic anomalies, and the use of MRI in the evaluation and management of these patients.

PEDIATRIC IMAGING TECHNIQUES

MRI in young children frequently requires sedation. Thus, it is imperative that, depending on the presenting clinical situation, imaging planes and pulse sequences be selected before the start of the examination. These studies should also be performed as rapidly as possible. In general, pelvic studies are performed to assess abnormal anatomy, evaluate solitary structures that may or may not be in the midline, or evaluate paired structures. In most cases an ultrasound study will have been performed prior to MRI. In patients in whom simple cysts and/or simple fluid collections have been diagnosed by ultrasonography, MRI adds little to clinical management.[30] However, in cases of solid masses or variations in anatomy, MRI provides superior information to both ultrasonography and CT.[30,31] For midline structures the sagittal plane is most useful (Fig. 4-15). The rectus abdominis, pubic symphysis, bladder, vagina, cervix, uterus, rectum, and sacrum are all well visualized in the midline and parasagittal views.[32,33] The ovaries, musculoskeletal structures, and pelvic lymph node system with bilateral symmetry are best imaged in the axial plane. Coronal images are useful for defining the pelvic muscles and comparing their symmetry (Fig. 4-16). Also, in cases of neoplasia, the coronal plane is useful, where the superoinferior extent of the lesion can be identified, as well as the upper urinary tracts and lymph nodes.[32,33] A combination of T1- and T2-weighted sequences is usually needed. However, for structural variations,

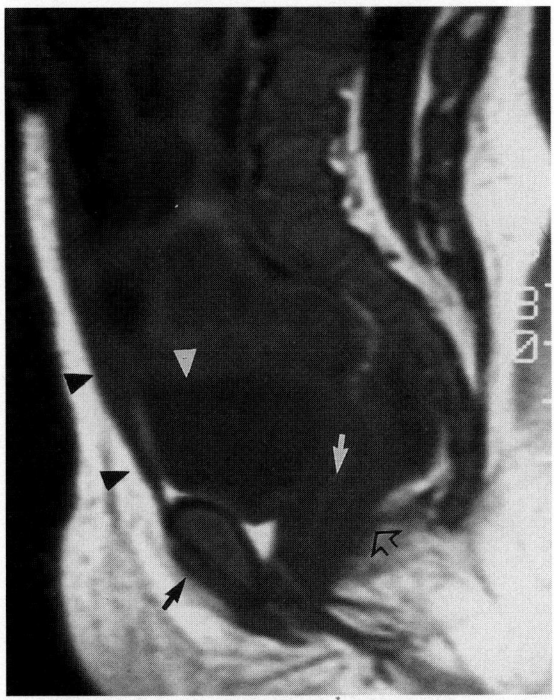

Fig. 4-15 T1-weighted image of a 1-year-old girl showing the normal pelvic anatomy in the sagittal plane: the pubic bone *(black arrow)*, anterior abdominal wall muscles *(black arrowheads)*, bladder *(white arrowhead)*, vagina *(white arrow)*, and rectum *(open black arrow)*. Also, the normal sacrum and coccyx can be seen posteriorly.

Fig. 4-16 A, Normal pelvis in a 2-year-old girl. The coronal plane T1-weighted image shows normal hip joints with the ossification centers *(white arrows)* well located within the hip joint. Also seen is the normal appearance of the full bladder *(white arrowheads)*. **B,** Posterior coronal T1-weighted image of the same patient shows the sacroiliac joint *(white arrow)* and one of the right sacral nerve roots *(long white arrow)*. The normal posterior pelvic floor muscles are seen, the pyriform *(open white arrow)* and levator ani sling *(small black arrows)* on either side. Note also the normal anorectal junction *(open black arrow)*.

multiplanar T1-weighted images alone may suffice because of their superior anatomic resolution. Lesions having a high blood and/or proteinaceous fluid content such as hemangiomas, lymphangiomas, and abscess collections which characteristically have high signal intensity on T2-weighted images. T2 images are also useful for identification of the ovaries.

SPECIFIC CLINICAL SITUATIONS

In patients presenting with ambiguous genitalia, it is imperative to make an accurate and prompt diagnosis. The genitogram is the study of choice for initial evaluation. However, in cases in which one or both gonads are nonpalpable, MRI can be helpful. Under these circumstances, two pieces of information, easily obtainable with MRI, are necessary for appropriate treatment: (1) the presence or absence of internal gonads, and (2) the presence or absence of a uterus.

For cystic lesions of the ovaries or pelvis, ultrasonography should be the initial study of choice. On MRI, simple cysts appear as thin-walled, low signal intensity lesions on T1 with high signal intensity on T2. Complex cysts, particularly those with proteinacous or blood content, can be characterized with a combination of T1 and T2-weighted images. For small cysts of the ovaries and small masses MRI, with the new phased array coils, has greater spatial resolution and allows for more detailed tissue characterization.[34]

Pelvic tumors are not very common in this patient population (see box on p. 96). MRI gives more detailed information than ultrasonography and can image lesions independent of the bladder.

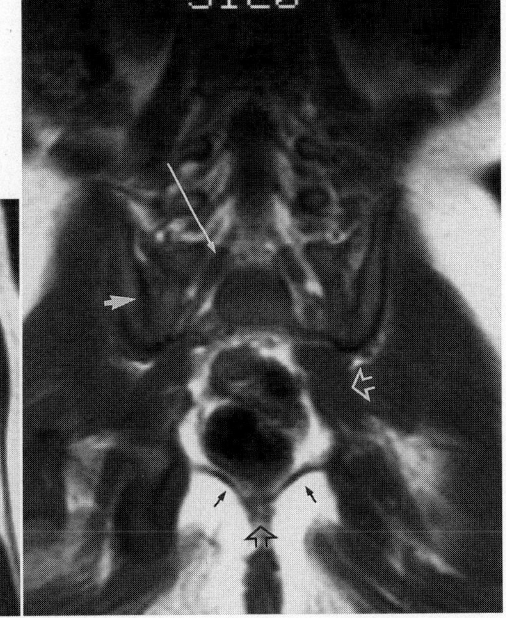

TUMORS FOUND IN THE PEDIATRIC FEMALE PELVIS

Neuroblastoma
Rhabdomyosarcoma
Chordoma
Neurofibromatosis
Lymphoma and leukemia
Xanthoma
Sacrococcygeal teratoma
Cystadenoma
Dermoid cyst
Gonadoblastoma
Transitional cell carcinoma of bladder
Leiomyosarcoma
Lymphohemangioma
Clear cell adenocarcinoma
Squamous cell carcinoma of uterus

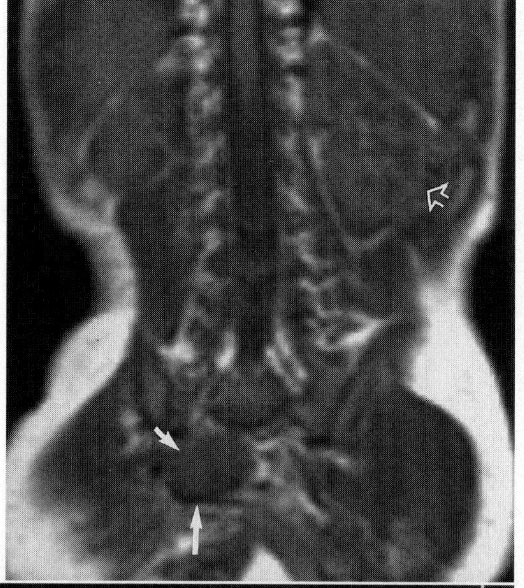

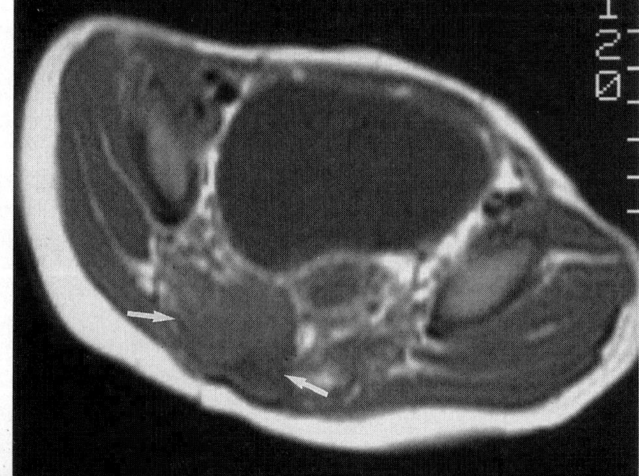

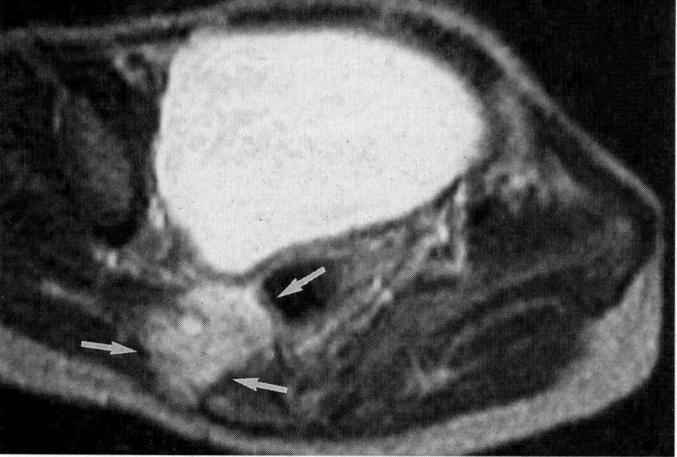

Fig. 4-17 A 2-year-old girl with a sacrococcygeal teratoma. **A,** coronal T1-weighted image shows the right posterior pelvic mass within the right pyriform muscle *(white arrows)*. Note the normal-appearing left kidney *(open white arrow)*. **B,** Axial T1-weighted and **(C)** T2-weighted images of the same patient show the right-sided tumor *(white arrows)* with the typical high signal on T2-weighted images and the invasive nature of the mass into the adjacent muscles.

These can be characterized as cystic, solid, or mixed with either modality. MRI demonstrates some ability to differentiate tissue type in these tumors. T1-weighted images provide anatomic details, and T2 images can be used to characterize the tissue to some degree and define borders between tumors and adjoining structures (Fig. 4-17). Several features have been used to suggest malignancy, such as heterogeneity of signal (especially on T2-weighted images), ill definition of tumor borders, and frank invasion into the adjacent structures.[35]

EXSTROPHY-EPISPADIAS COMPLEX
Embryology

The etiology of the exstrophy-epispadias complex is not fully understood. The cloacal membrane is a bilaminar layer at the caudal end of the germinal disc. Mesenchymal ingrowth between the layers of the cloacal membrane is responsible for the formation of the lower abdominal wall structures, anterior wall of the bladder, and genital tubercle. In 1964 Muecke, working on a chick embryo model, theorized that persistence of an abnormally large cloacal membrane prevents mesenchymal ingrowth, which in turn prevents normal midline apposition of lower abdominal structures.[36] Subsequent normal rupture of the cloacal membrane results in the exstrophy-epispadias complex.[36] The severity of the defect is dependent on the amount of abnormal cloacal membrane and the timing of cloacal membrane rupture. Smaller amounts of abnormal membrane result in lesser abnormalities (see box below), and early membrane rupture (prior to ingrowth of the urorectal septum) results in cloacal rather than bladder exstrophy, or epispadias.[37]

Thomalla et al produced exstrophy in chick embryos via early cloacal membrane ablation with a CO_2 laser.[38] This is evidence that early damage to the cell layer responsible for forming the cloacal membrane can result in cloacal exstrophy. Other theories have been presented to explain the exstrophy-epispadias complex, but since the above-mentioned models best fit the findings of

---

EXSTROPHY-EPISPADIAS COMPLEX VARIANTS

Pseudoexstrophy
Superior vesical fissure
Epispadias without exstrophy
Duplicate exstrophy
Covered exstrophy
Classic bladder exstrophy
Cloacal exstrophy

---

the full spectrum of disorders, they receive the most attention.

CLASSIC BLADDER EXSTROPHY

Exstrophy is one of the most serious anomalies of the genitourinary system in children with multisystem manifestations.[39] Because of this multisystem involvement, MR is a very useful imaging tool for full evaluation of patients with suspected exstrophy.

Musculoskeletal system

All exstrophy patients have a characteristic widening of the symphysis pubis (Figs. 4-18 and 4-19). In a review of congenital widening of the pubic symphysis, 91% of 89 patients also suffered from the exstrophy-epispadias complex.[40] Conditions other than exstrophy that may be associated with pubic diastasis include urethral duplication, diphallus, anorectal anomalies, and congenital hydro- and hematocolpos. Widening of the symphysis is the direct result of two pelvic anomalies that always accompany exstrophy. The innominate bones are rotated outward, in relation to the sagittal plane, along the sacroiliac joints. Second, there is outward rotation of the pubic rami at their junction with the ilium and ischium. In the most severe cases a third pelvic anomaly can occur, lateral displacement of the inferior aspects of the innominate bones, with the sacroiliac joints acting as the fulcrum.[41] Despite these obvious pelvic disturbances, exstrophy patients usually have a normal gait. Initially they may have a wide, waddling gait, but this corrects itself in early childhood. This suggests that from a musculoskeletal standpoint, there is little to be gained from pubic reapproximation during exstrophy closure.

In addition to these structural problems, there are a number of common musculofascial defects. There is diastasis of the inferior portion of the rectus, and a low-set umbilicus with an always present umbilical hernia. These umbilical hernias are usually of no functional significance, but if large they should be repaired at the time of exstrophy closure. In 11% of female patients with classic bladder exstrophy, there are inguinal hernias.[42] This has been attributed to lack of obliquity of the inguinal canal and poor development of the lower abdominal musculature. Bilateral inguinal exploration at the time of initial bladder closure has been advocated for these patients. Because of poor lower abdominal musculature, simple excision of the hernial sac is to be avoided. In addition to herniotomy, careful reconstruction of the floor of the inguinal canal is necessary to decrease the risk of recurrence. Another defect encountered, more commonly with cloacal exstrophy, is an omphalo-

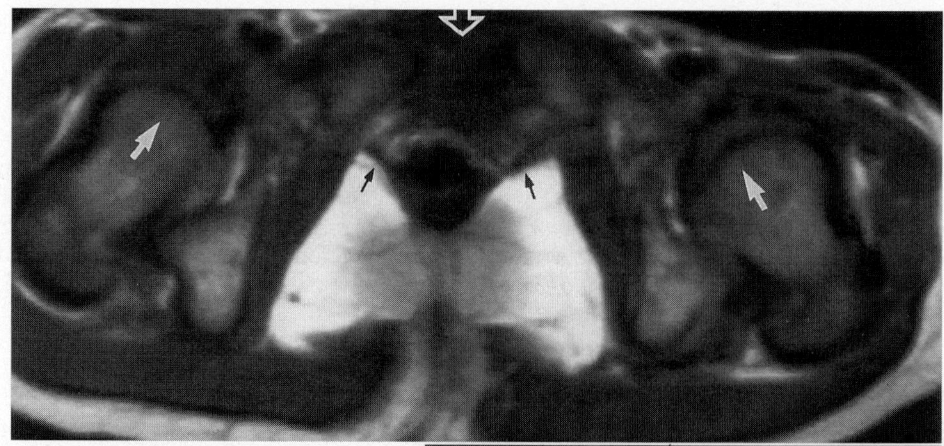

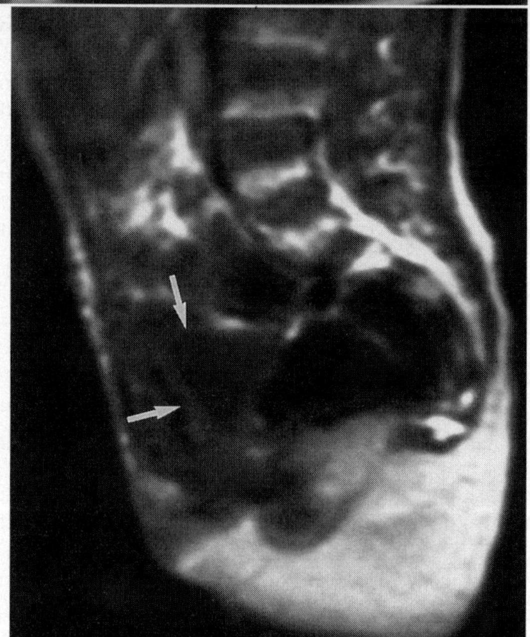

Fig. 4-18 Preoperative images of a 5-year-old girl with bladder exstrophy. **A,** Axial T1-weighted image shows the pubic diastasis *(open white arrow)* and abnormal alignment of the hip joints *(white arrows)*. Note also the typical anterior displacement of all the pelvic soft tissue structures and the thin levator ani slings bilaterally *(small black arrows)*. **B,** Sagittal T1-weighted image shows a small, thick-walled bladder *(white arrows)*.

cele; this can usually be handled at the time of initial closure.

Urinary tract

The upper urinary system is usually normal in these patients.[43] Abnormalities in form and number of the renal units have been reported but at no greater incidence than in the general population. The peritoneal pouch of Douglas is usually enlarged, forcing the ureters laterally and inferiorly. Because of this, the distal ureter approaches the ureteral orifice from an inferolateral position, resulting in little obliquity to the intramural ureteral tunnel. This is manifested as vesicoureteral reflux in essentially 100% of patients after bladder closure. The most distal segment of the ureter is almost always dilated; this has been attributed to edema, infection, and fibrosis of this segment. The

bladder is of small capacity, which may limit one's ability to perform a successful closure. The bladder mucosa may appear grossly normal to severely ulcerated. Even when the bladder mucosa appearance is grossly normal, microscopic abnormalities, including squamous metaplasia, cystitis cystica, cystitis glandularis, and acute and chronic inflammation, are common.[43]

Genital system

The urethra and vagina are short, the vagina is often stenotic, the clitoris is bifid, and the labia and mons are divergent. The uterus, ovaries, and fallopian tubes are normal.

A common problem encountered in adolescents after exstrophy closure is uterine prolapse. This can contribute significantly to the development of urinary incontinence. For this reason, iliac osteoto-

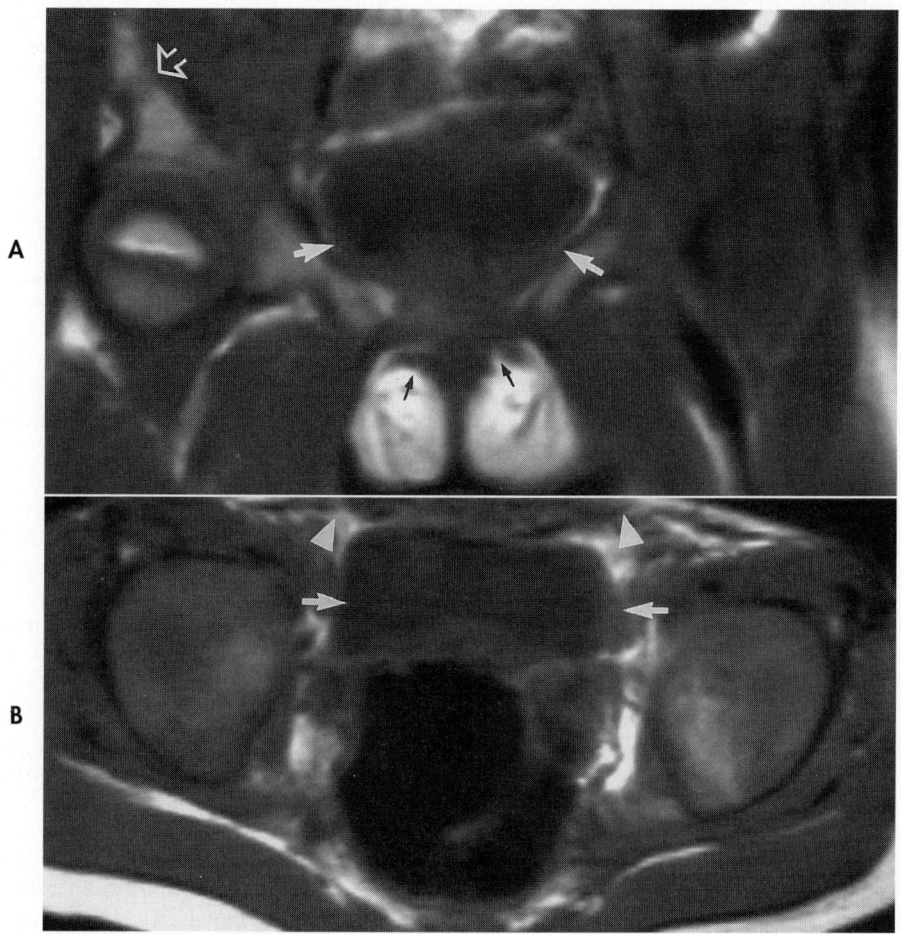

Fig. 4-19 Postoperative images of the same 5-year-old girl as in Fig. 4-18. **A,** Coronal T1-weighted image shows the now normal capacity bladder after repair *(white arrows)*. The levator sling muscles *(small black arrows)* at the base of the bladder can be seen particularly well in view of the pubic diastasis. The patient has had bilateral osteotomies *(open white arrow)*. **B,** Axial T1-weighted images show the postoperative findings of good bladder capacity *(white arrows)* and reasonable reapproximation of the anterior abdominal musculoskeletal structures *(white arrowheads)*.

mies have been advocated in all patients who undergo exstrophy closure in the first 48 to 72 hours of life.[41,43] The performance of osteotomies allows for placement of the urethra within the pelvic ring. This reduces the ureterovesical angle and facilitates urethral suspension and bladder neck plasty at a later date.

CLOACAL EXSTROPHY
Visceral anomalies

In cloacal exstrophy the presumed cloacal membrane insult leading to these defects occurs prior to division of the cloaca by the urorectal septum. This results in a constellation of characteristic visceral abnormalities. There is exstrophy of the bladder, which is bivalved by an exstrophied hindgut or cecum. The exstrophied bowel segment presents three or four orifices. The proximal orifice is the terminal ileum, of which there is often prolapse. The distal orifice is a blind-ending tailgut or distal colon. There are one or two flanking orifices that represent appendiceal orifices.[44]

Urinary tract

Upper urinary tract anomalies are the most common anomalies associated with cloacal exstrophy and were found in 66% of a series of 29 patients.[45] The anomalies included, in order of occurrence, pelvic kidney, unilateral renal agenesis, multicystic kidney, ureteral duplication, crossed fused renal ectopia, and distal ureteral atresia with hydroureteronephrosis.

Gastrointestinal tract

In the above-mentioned series, 46% of patients had gastrointestinal tract anomalies in addition to those inherent in the condition. Omphalocele, bowel malrotation, shortening, and duplication were the most common findings. Other anomalies included duodenal atresia and Meckel's diverticulum.[45] The anus lies abnormally far anteriorly, and its sphincter is often lax, permitting prolapse. This is due to the malposition of the anus with relation to the levator sling (see Fig. 4-18, *A*).

Other anomalies

Other systems that can be affected include the vertebral system (48%), lower extremities (26%), and central nervous system (CNS) (29%). The CNS lesions include myelomeningocele, meningocele, and lipomeningocele.

RADIOLOGIC EVALUATION

Preoperatively the upper urinary tracts of each patient are evaluated for hydronephrosis and anatomic defects. This is adequately done with ultrasonography. In the follow-up period, post–exstrophy closure MRI can be of particular use. In the female exstrophy patient, failure is most commonly due to urinary incontinence. The causes of incontinence can be poor outlet resistance, a small neurogenic bladder, or both.[46] MRI can be used to evaluate functional urethral length. Should this prove to be inadequate, a bladder neck plasty can be performed to improve continence. If this is not technically feasible, a continent urinary diversion is a viable alternative. On occasion, urethral length will be adequate, but support from the pelvic musculature may be inadequate. This is commonly associated with uterine prolapse. The occurrence of this situation can be decreased if iliac osteotomies are performed at the time of initial closure. On T1-weighted images the degree of muscular support in the midline can be evaluated as well as an intrapelvic position of the urethra (see Fig. 4-18, *A*).[47] If this is thought to be inadequate, a sling or some other procedure to provide urethral support can be performed, with correction of uterine prolapse at the same time. It has been noted that this procedure is technically easier in patients who were closed with osteotomies (J. Gearheart, personal communication). T1-weighted images in the sagittal plane provide an excellent evaluation of bladder size. The 5-year-old girl shown in Figs. 4-18 and 4-19 had severe urinary incontinence after undergoing bladder closure within the first 4 days of life. She was initially evaluated with ultrasonography and MRI, which demonstrated a small-capacity, thick-walled bladder (Fig. 4-18).

The closure was taken down and redone with osteotomies (Fig. 4-19). She is now 2 years post repeat exstrophy and has a 6- to 8-hour dry interval.

Anorectal anomalies

There are several types of anorectal anomalies, which can be seen alone or in combination with other multisystem anomalies. The four main types are ectopic anus, imperforate anus, rectal atresia, and anorectal stenosis.[48] The imperforate anus is characterized by a blind-ending pouch of distal colon with no fistula. (Fig. 4-20). MRI can be used to define the anomaly and the presence of any possible fistula, and to fully assess the musculoskeletal structures.

Postoperative evaluation

The patient with complex congenital anomalies often needs to undergo many surgical procedures on the many different organ systems involved. As the patient grows older, postoperative complications, such as the incontinence described in the young girl with bladder exstrophy, may develop. Other cases may be seen when patients develop masses or obstructions in the genitourinary or gastrointestinal systems. MRI offers a comprehensive imaging study that can assess all the organ systems and evaluate the postoperative anatomy much better than any other imaging study (Fig. 4-21). CT can define the bowel and urinary tract anatomy well, if these are both opacified clearly with both oral and intravenous contrast agents. Ultrasonography can evaluate the reproductive tract by combining the transabdominal and transvaginal approaches to assess any pelvic mass. However, only MRI offers the opportunity to evaluate all systems.

SUMMARY

MRI in female children has distinct advantages over ultrasonography and CT. It avoids the ionizing radiation of CT and provides more detailed anatomic information than ultrasonography without dependence on a full bladder for imaging. Ultrasonography is less expensive and more readily available in most places, and should remain the initial study of choice. However, in patients in whom further imaging is deemed necessary, MRI as opposed to CT should be given strong consideration. An exciting use of MRI is in follow-up of patients after bladder exstrophy closure. Incontinence is often the main problem, and MRI provides very useful information pertaining to the anatomic mechanisms of incontinence. Further studies to completely define the role of MRI in the evaluation of this condition are ongoing.

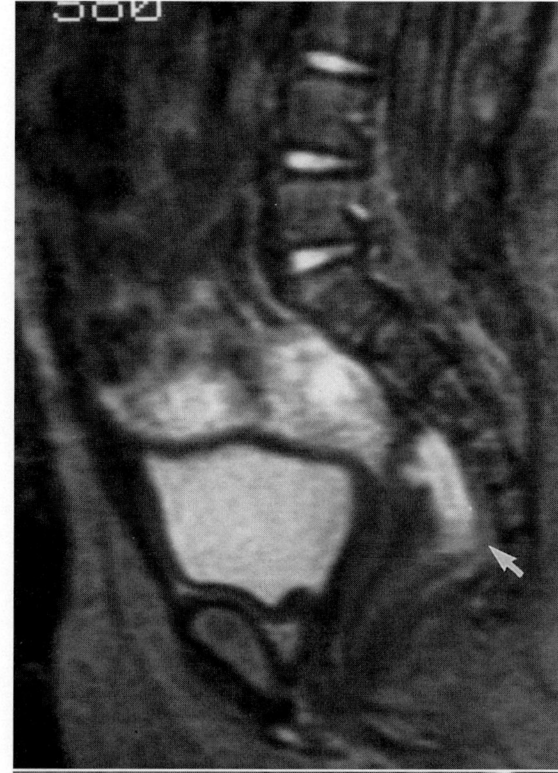

Fig. 4-20 **A,** A 1-year-old girl with imperforate anus. The T2-weighted sagittal image shows the blind-ending rectum *(white arrow)* and an otherwise normal-appearing pelvis with normal sacrococcygeal spine. **B** and **C,** A 6-month-old baby with a long anal stenosis. The sagittal T1-weighted image **(B)** shows the anal canal to be narrowed *(arrows)* for approximately 3 cm. The T2-weighted image **(C)** shows the same finding *(arrows)* but not as clearly.

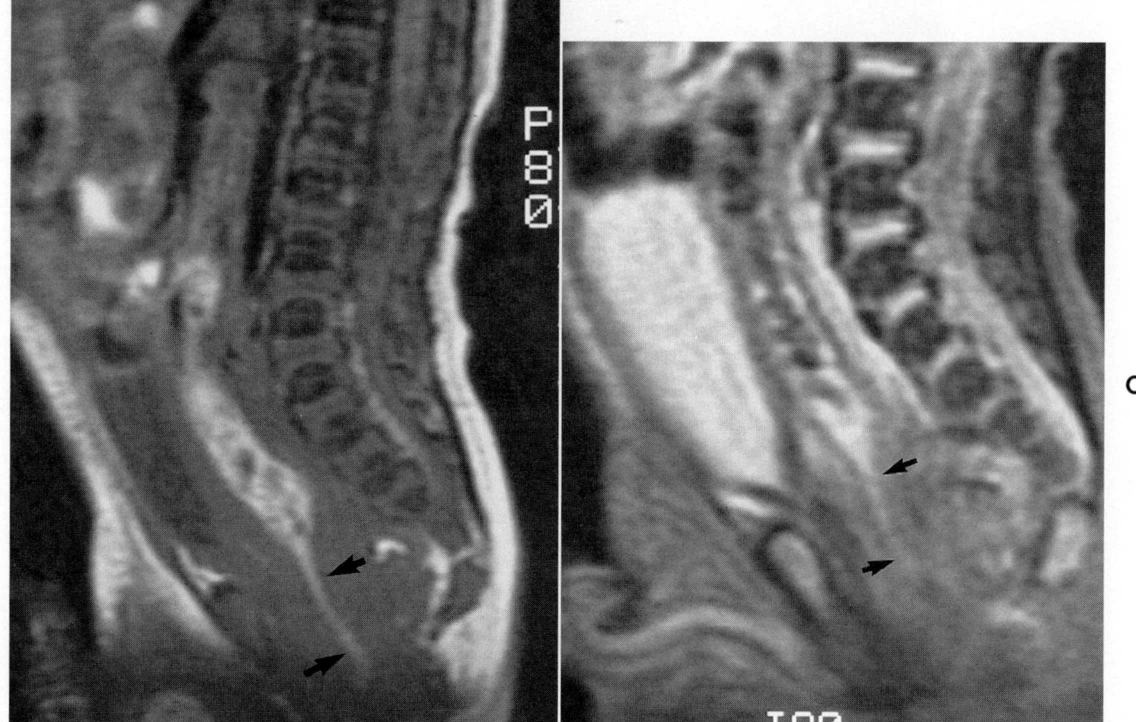

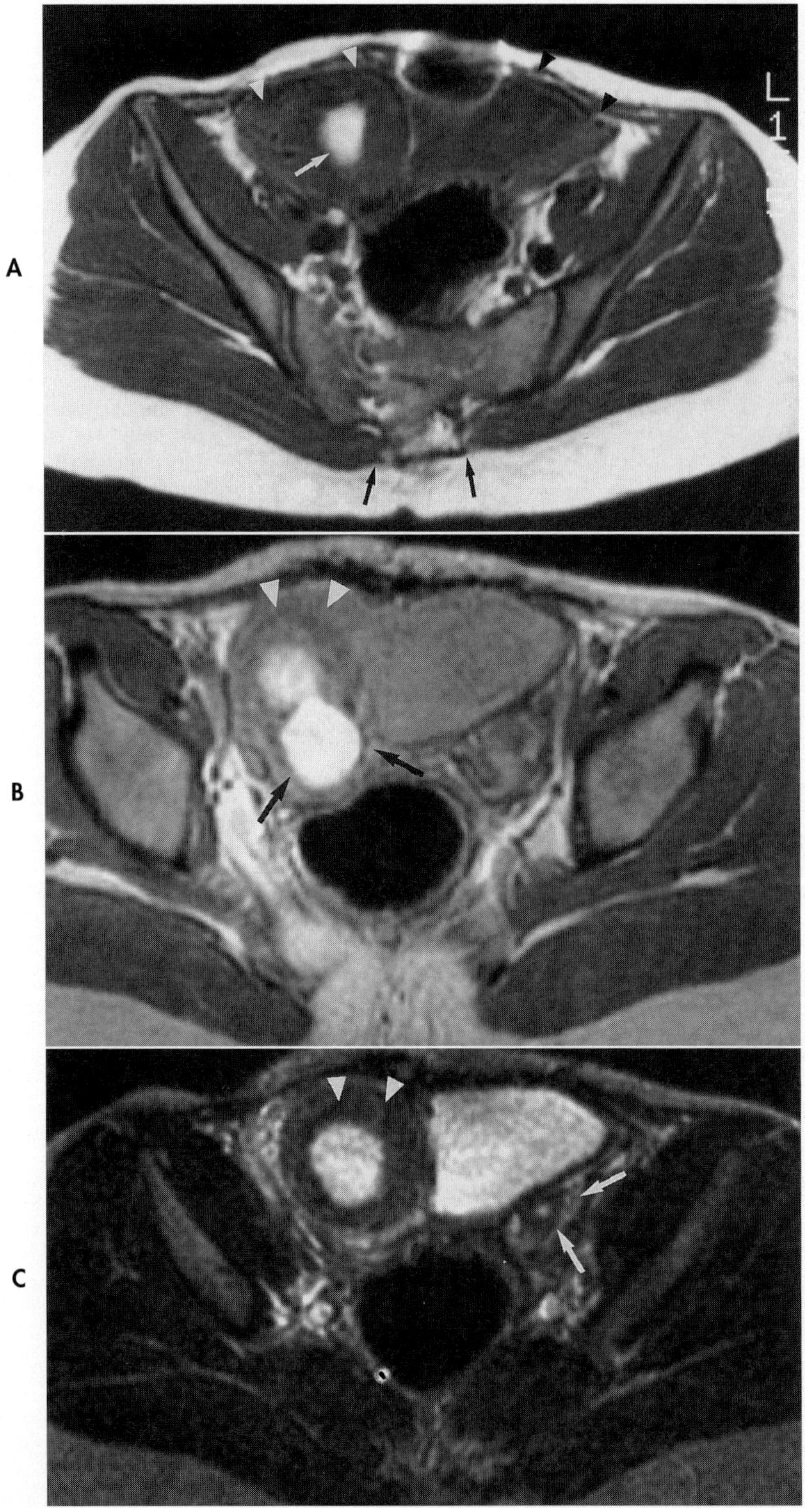

Fig. 4-21 For legend see opposite page.

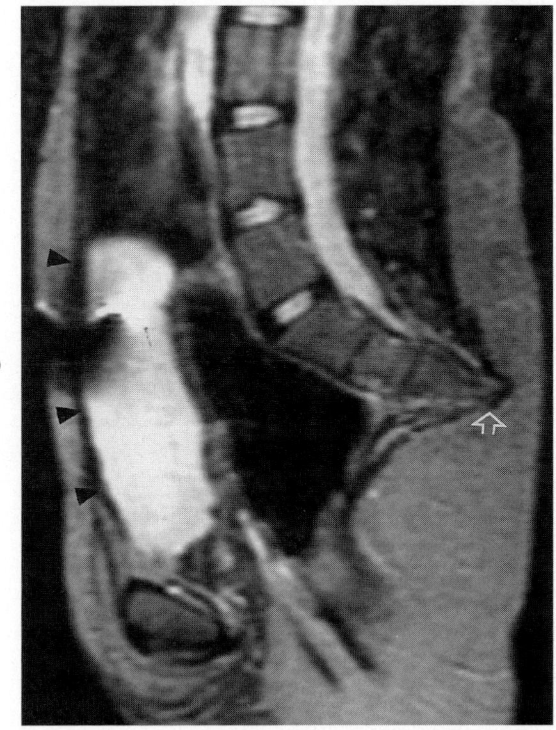

Fig. 4-21 A 19-year-old woman with a history of a complex anomaly, with previous urinary diversion and uterine didelphys, who presented with a pelvic mass. **A,** Axial T1-weighted image shows a right-sided uterine horn *(white arrowheads)* filled with high signal intensity blood *(white arrow)*. The bladder pouch is seen just to the left of midline beneath the surgical clip *(black arrowheads)*. Notice the sacral deformity posteriorly *(black arrows)*. **B,** Axial proton density and **(C)** T2-weighted images show the uterine horn on the right with typical zonal signal intensity *(white arrowheads)*. There is also a second collection of blood seen on the proton density image *(black arrows)*, posterior to the uterine body, representing an obstructed, blood-filled vagina. The rudimentary left uterine horn can now be identified, owing to its typical signal intensity on the T2-weighted image, just lateral to the bladder pouch *(white arrows)*. **D,** Midline sagittal T2-weighted image of the same patient shows the large-capacity urinary pouch *(black arrowheads)* anteriorly and the sacral agenesis posteriorly *(open white arrow)*.

REFERENCES

1. Rock JA, Schlaff WD: The obstetric consequences of uterovaginal anomalies, *Fertil Steril* 43:681-692, 1985.
2. Heinomen PK, Sarrikoski S, Pystynen P: Reproductive performance of women with uterine anomalies, *Acta Obstet Gynecol Scand* 61:157-162, 1982.
3. Gray SE, Roberta DK, Franklin RR: Fertility after metroplasty of the septate uterus, *J Reprod Med* 29:185-188, 1984.
4. Sorensen, SS: Estimated prevalence of müllerian anomalies, *Acta Obstet Gynecol Scand* 67:441-445, 1988.
5. Doyle MB: Magnetic resonance imaging in müllerian fusion defects, *J Reprod Med* 37:33-38, 1992.
6. Ansbacher R: Uterine anomalies and future pregnancies, *Clin Perinatol* 10:295-304, 1983.
7. Harger JH, Archer DF, Marchese SG, et al: Etiology of recurrent pregnancy losses and outcome of subsequent pregnancies, *Obstet Gynecol* 62:574-581, 1983.
8. Abramovici H, Faktor JH, Pascal B: Congenital uterine malformations as indication for cervical suture (cerclage) in habitual abortion and premature delivery, *Int J Fertil* 28:161-164, 1983.
9. Winfield AC, Wentz AC: *Congenital anomalies of the uterus and fallopian tubes.* In Winfield AC, Wentz AC, editors: *Diagnostic imaging in infertility,* ed 2, Baltimore, 1992, Williams & Wilkins, pp 57-74.
10. Buttram VC: Müllerian anomalies and their management, *Fertil Steril* 40:159-163, 1983.
11. Kaufman RH, Noller K, Adam E, et al: Upper genital tract abnormalities and pregnancy outcome in diethylstilbestrol-exposed progeny, *Am J Obstet Gynecol* 148:973-984, 1984.
12. Gilsanz V, Cleveland RH: Duplication of the müllerian ducts and genitourinary malformations. Part 1: The value of excretory urography, *Radiology* 144:793-796, 1982.
13. Buttram VC, Gibbons WE: Müllerian anomalies: a proposed classification (an analysis of 144 cases), *Fertil Steril* 32:40-46, 1979.
14. Seigler AM: Hysterosalpingography, *Fertil Steril* 40:139-158, 1983.
15. Pinsonneault O, Goldstein DP: Obstructing malformations of the uterus and vagina, *Fertil Steril* 44:241-247, 1985.
16. Strubbe EH, Willemsen WN, Lemmens JA et al: Mayer-Rokitansky-Küster-Hauser syndrome: distinction between two forms based on excretory urographic, sonographic, and laparoscopic findings, *AJR* 160:331-334, 1993.
17. Golan A, Wexler S, Segev E, et al: Cervical cerclage—its role in the pregnant anomalous uterus, *Int J Fertil* 35:164-170, 1990.
18. Zanetti E, Ferrari LR, Rossi G: Classification and radiographic features of uterine malformations: hysterosalpingographic study, *Br J Radiol* 51:161-170, 1978.
19. Reuter KL, Daly DC, Cohen SM: Septate versus bicornuate uteri: error in imaging diagnosis, *Radiology* 172:749-752, 1989.
20. Randolph JR, Ying YK, Maier DB, et al: Comparison of real-time ultrasonography, hysterosalpingography, and laparoscopy/hysteroscopy in the evaluation of uterine abnormalities and tubal patency, *Fertil Steril* 46:828-832, 1986.
21. Malini S, Valdes C, Malinak R: Sonographic diagnosis and classification of anomalies of the female genital tract, *J Ultrasound Med* 3:397-404, 1984.
22. Pellerito JS, McCarthy SM, Doule MB, et al: Diagnosis of uterine anomalies: relative accuracy of MR imaging, endovaginal sonography, and hysterosalpingography, *Radiology* 183:795-800, 1992.
23. Mintz MC, Thickman DI, Glussman DG, Kressel HY: MR evaluation of uterine anomalies, *AJR* 148:287-290, 1987.
24. Fedele L, Dorta M, Brioschi D, et al: Magnetic resonance imaging of unicornuate uterus, *Acta Obstet Gynecol Scand* 69:511-513, 1990.
25. Fedele L, Dorta M, Brioschi D, et al: Magnetic resonance evaluation of double uteri, *Obstet Gynecol* 74:844-847, 1989.
26. Carrington BM, Hricak H, Nuruddin RN, et al: Müllerian duct anomalies: MR imaging evaluation, *Radiology* 176:715-720, 1990.
27. Van Gils APG, Tham RTOTA, Falke THM, Peter AAW: Abnormalities of the uterus and cervix after diethylstilbestrol exposure: correlation of findings on MR and hysterosalpingography, *AJR* 153:1235-1238, 1989.

28. Woodward PJ, Wagner BJ, Farley TE: MR imaging in the evaluation of female infertility, *RadioGraphics* 13:293-310, 1993.

29. Olson MC, Posniak HV, Tempany CM, Dudiak CM: MR imaging of the female pelvic region, *RadioGraphics* 12:445-465, 1992.

30. Dietrich RB, Kangarloo H: Pelvic abnormalities in children: assessment with MR imaging, *Radiology* 163:367, 1987.

31. Dietrich RB, Kangarloo H: *Pediatric body imaging.* In Stark DD, Bradley WG Jr, editors: *Magnetic resonance imaging,* St. Louis, 1988, Mosby-Year Book, p 1436.

32. Fisher MR, Hricak H, Crooks LE: Urinary bladder MR imaging, *Radiology* 157:467-70, 1985.

33. Fisher MR, Hricak H, Tanagho EA: Urinary bladder MR imaging. Part 2: Neoplasm, *Radiology* 157:471-7, 1985.

34. Hricak H: MRI of the female pelvis: a review, *AJR* 146:1115-22, 1986.

35. Berquist TH, Ehman RL, King BF, et al: Value of MR imaging in differentiating benign from malignant soft-tissue masses: study of 95 lesions, *AJR* 155:1251-1255, 1990.

36. Muecke EC.: The role of the cloacal membrane in exstrophy: the first successful experimental study, *J Urol* 92:659, 1964.

37. Manzoni GA, Ransley PG, Hurwitz RS: Cloacal exstrophy and cloacal exstrophy variants: a proposed system of classification, *J Urol* 138:1065-8, 1987.

38. Thomalla JV Rudolph RA, Rink RC, Mitchell ME: Induction of cloacal exstrophy in the chick embryo using the CO_2 laser, *J Urol* 134:991-5, 1985.

39. White P, Lebowitz RL: Exstrophy of the bladder, *Radiol Clin North Am* 15:93-107, 1977.

40. Muecke EC, Currarino G: Symphysis: associated Clinical disorders and Roentgen anatomy of affected bony pelves. *AJR* 103:179-85, 1968.

41. Gokcora IH, Yazar T: Bilateral transverse iliac osteotomy in the correction of neonatal bladder exstrophy, *Int Surg* 74:123-5, 1989.

42. Gearheart JP, Jeffs RD: State of the art reconstructive surgery for bladder exstrophy at the Johns Hopkins Hospital, *Am J Dis Child* 143:1475-8, 1989.

43. Gearheart JP, Jeffs RD: *Exstrophy of the bladder, epispadias, and other bladder anomalies.* In Walsh PC, Retik AB, Stamey TA, Vaughan ED, editors: *Campbell's textbook of urology,* ed 6, Philadelphia, 1992, WB Saunders, p 1772.

44. Diamond DA, Jeffs RD: Cloacal exstrophy: a 22-year experience, *J Urol* 133:779-82, 1985.

45. Hurwitz RS, Manzoni GA, Ransley PG, Stephens FD: Cloacal exstrophy: a report of 34 cases, *J Urol* 138:1060-4, 1987.

46. Mitchell ME, Brito CG, Rink RC: Cloacal exstrophy reconstruction for urinary continence, *J Urol* 144:554-8, 1990.

47. Hricak H, Williams RD: Magnetic resonance imaging and its application in urology, *Urology* 23:442-54, 1984.

48. *Radiology of the newborn and young infant,* ed 2, Baltimore, 1980, Williams & Wilkins.

5 Vaginography

Richard A. Cooper

Techniques
Illustrations: cases 1-13
Discussion

Vaginography was described in the radiololgic literature in the early 1960s[1-3] and again in 1982.[4] Experience with vaginography has shown it to be an invaluable tool for assessing vaginal fistulas, far superior to a barium enema or small bowel study.

TECHNIQUES

If indicated, a scout film of the pelvis is obtained to check for residual contrast material from a previous examination. The patient lies supine on the fluoroscopic table, and a large Foley balloon catheter or barium enema catheter with balloon tip is placed in the vagina. The key to a successful vaginogram lies in stopping the contrast material from escaping via the introitus. To accomplish this, once the balloon is inflated, gentle traction is applied to the catheter so that the intravaginal balloon is snug against the vaginal orifice. The patient is then placed in a slight Trendelenburg position. Also, it may be helpful to wrap a towel around the catheter and push the towel firmly against the introitus. All of these techniques may be necessary to prevent leak of contrast material.

Water-soluble material should be used in case there is leakage into the peritoneal cavity or venous system. Although I have never seen venous intravasation during vaginography, there are cases in which the uterus has filled, and my experience with hysterosalpingography shows that venous opacification may then be the next step. Also, a thin, water-soluble solution is more likely to traverse a narrow fistulous track than is the more viscous barium. A case has been reported[5] in which a sigmoidovaginal fistula was seen on an enema study obtained with water-soluble contrast material but not on a barium enema examination.

The contrast material is introduced slowly into the vagina under fluoroscopic control. The vagina and any fistula will be visualized and appropriate spot radiographs obtained. It may be necessary to place the patient in oblique or lateral positions to see the track.

The procedure is painless and well received by the informed patient.

ILLUSTRATIONS

At Loyola University Medical Center, Maywood, Illinois, forty-seven vaginograms have been performed in patients suspected of passing feces, flatus, or urine via the vagina. Of these examinations, there were 22 true positive, 21 true negative, 0 false-positive, and four false-negative results, yielding a sensitivity of 85% and a specificity of 100%.

Figure 5-1 shows a normal vaginogram.

Case 1 is a 61-year-old patient who 18 months previously underwent a diverting colostomy because of diverticulitis. She also had a hysterectomy at that time. Several weeks after closure of the colostomy, the patient complained of passing feces per vagina. She was operated on to close the fistula and create another diverting colostomy. At this operation the fistula could not be located. The patient then underwent a negative upper gastrointestinal and small bowel examination, which was ordered because the clinicians now suspected a vaginal–small bowel fistula. A vaginogram (Fig. 5-2) shows a single 1 × 1 cm fistula from the posterior vaginal cuff to the rectum. The patient underwent repeat surgery, and the fistula was located and closed. The surgeons commented that without vaginographic guidance, the fistula was not initially found.

Case 2 is a 45-year-old patient who complained of feculent vaginal discharge 1 week after a hysterectomy was performed because of fibroids. A vaginogram (Fig. 5-3) shows a very small fistulous track from the vaginal dome to the anterior sigmoid colon.

Case 3 is a 68-year-old woman complaining of passing stool per vagina for 2 weeks. The vaginogram (Fig. 5-4) shows a huge cavity connecting the left vaginal fornix to the sigmoid colon. The cause of this fistula is unknown, but it is most likely secondary to diverticulitis.

Case 4 is a 54-year-old patient who complained of a foul-smelling vaginal discharge that consisted

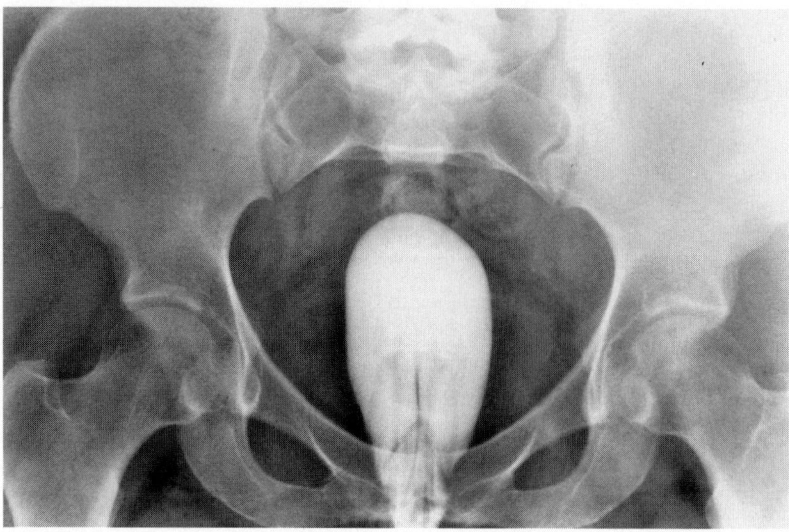

Fig. 5-1 This normal vaginogram shows contrast material confined to the distended vaginal vault.

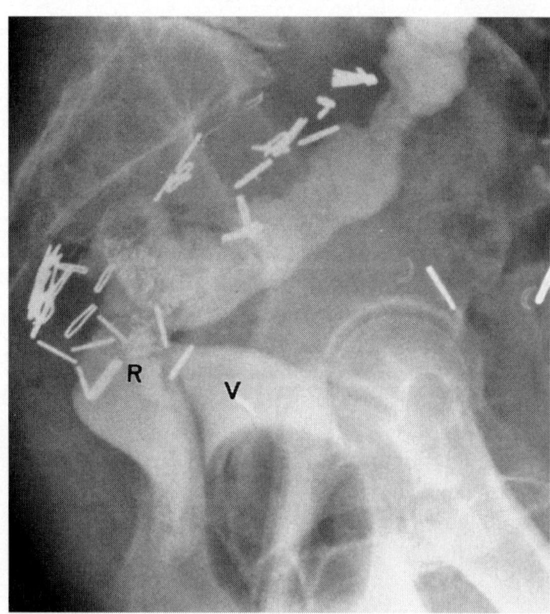

Fig. 5-2 Lateral film shows communication between the vagina *(V)* and the rectum *(R)*.

of both brownish liquid and gas. This began 3 weeks after abdominal hysterectomy and bilateral salpingo-oophorectomy was performed for ovarian carcinoma. The patient was also found to have ingested seeds in the vagina. A proctoscopy did not reveal a vaginal fistula. A barium enema examination was interpreted as normal, although, in retrospect, slight staining of the vaginal mucosa was probably present. Vaginography (Fig. 5-5) revealed copious flow of contrast material from the left side

of the vaginal cuff into the rectosigmoid colon. A second fistula was seen from the center of the vaginal cuff to the sigmoid colon. These findings were confirmed at surgery, and a two-stage repair was made.

Case 5 is a 76-year-old patient with a 3-year history of anterior resection and radiation therapy for rectosigmoid carcinoma. The carcinoma was attached to the vagina at the initial surgery. The patient was shown to have abdominal carcinomatosis 9 months previously. The patient now presented with a 13-day history of passing liquid stool per vagina. The clinicians ordered a vaginogram to locate a sigmoidovaginal fistula. However, an unexpected ileovaginal fistula was found (Fig. 5-6).

Case 6 is a 73-year-old patient with transitional cell carcinoma of the bladder who underwent surgery and radiation therapy. She was subsequently operated on for a small bowel obstruction secondary to adhesions. She then underwent abdominoperineal resection because of a malignant rectal polyp. At this surgery, many adhesions were found and several small bowel perforations occurred, resulting in resection of 14 cm of small intestine. Three days after surgery a feculent vaginal discharge began. Vaginography (Fig. 5-7) demonstrated a 1-mm wide fistulous track from the left fornix to the ileum. This track was probed at vaginal exploration. Over the next 3 months the patient underwent vaginography twice more to follow closure of the track. Interestingly, of two small bowel studies performed during this period, only one demonstrated the fistula.

Case 7 is a 37-year-old patient with a 3-week

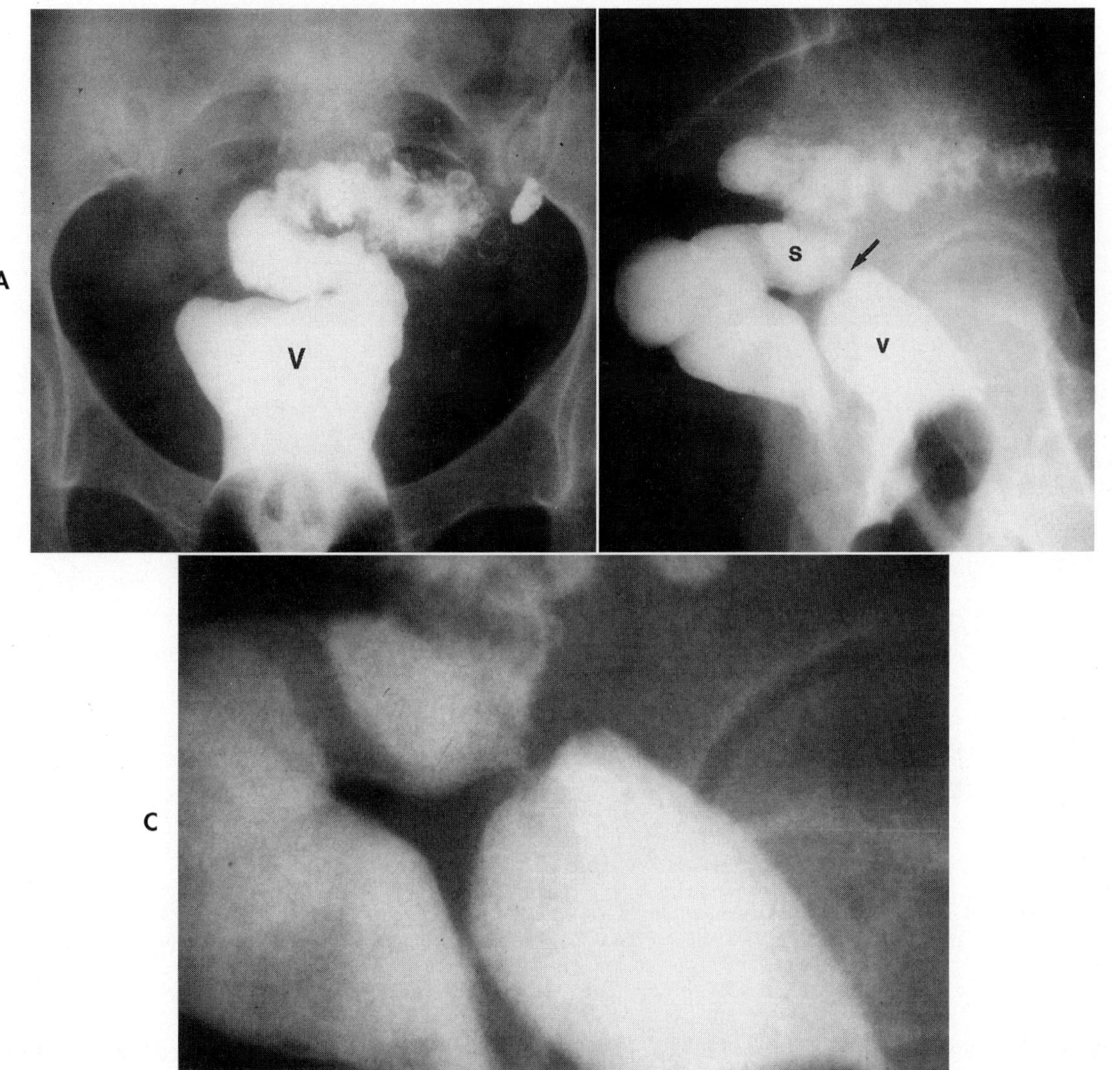

Fig. 5-3 A, Vaginogram, anteroposterior view, shows filling of the vagina *(V)* as well as the sigmoid. However, the track itself is not seen. **B,** The lateral view is necessary to delineate a single fistulous track *(arrow)* between the vagina *(V)* and the anterior sigmoid *(S)* that measures 5 mm in length and 2 mm in width. **C,** Close-up of the lateral view.

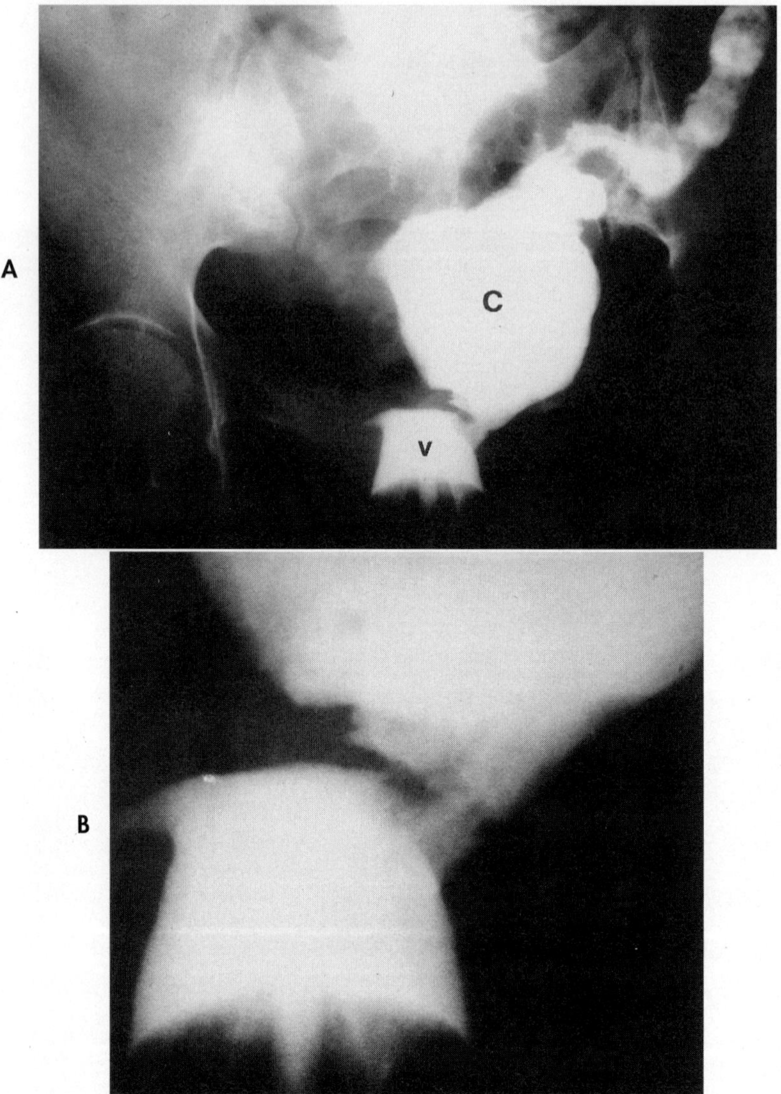

Fig. 5-4 A, There is a 9-cm diameter cavity *(C)* connecting the sigmoid colon to the left fornix of the vagina *(V).* **B,** Close-up view shows the connection to the vaginal fornix to be narrow.

history of passing urine per vagina. This began 4 weeks after a vaginal hysterectomy performed because of uterine fibroids. Intravenous pyelography (IVP) was ordered to demonstrate a vesicovaginal fistula, but the results were normal. A vaginogram (Fig. 5-8) shows filling of the bladder through a 1-mm wide fistula from the anterior, somewhat superior vagina.

Case 8 is a 51-year-old woman 6 months after total abdominal hysterectomy and bilateral salpingo-oophorectomy for cervical cancer. She had finished radiation therapy 1 month previously. She presented with a foul-smelling vaginal discharge of 1 week's duration. A vaginogram (Fig. 5-9) shows

a vesicovaginal fistula, as evidenced by spill from the dome of the vagina into an irregular pelvic cavity that communicates with the posterior bladder. Surgery confirmed the findings, and biopsies of the pelvis showed both radiation changes and metastatic cervical carcinoma.

Case 9 is a 37-year-old patient who underwent radiation therapy for cervical carcinoma. She complained of passing feces per vagina. The vaginogram (Fig. 5-10) shows both the anticipated rectovaginal fistula and an unsuspected vesicovaginal fistula.

Case 10 is a 73-year-old patient 1 month after coronary artery bypass grafting and 1 week after a

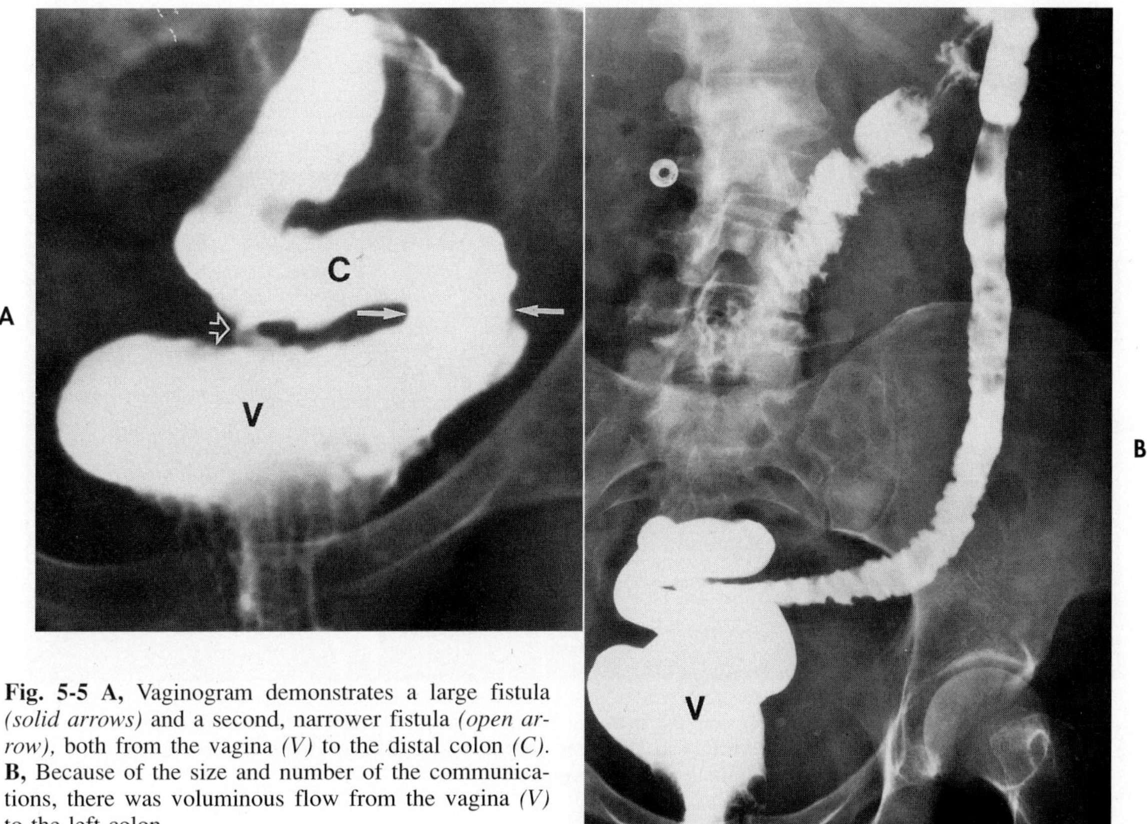

Fig. 5-5 A, Vaginogram demonstrates a large fistula *(solid arrows)* and a second, narrower fistula *(open arrow),* both from the vagina *(V)* to the distal colon *(C).* **B,** Because of the size and number of the communications, there was voluminous flow from the vagina *(V)* to the left colon.

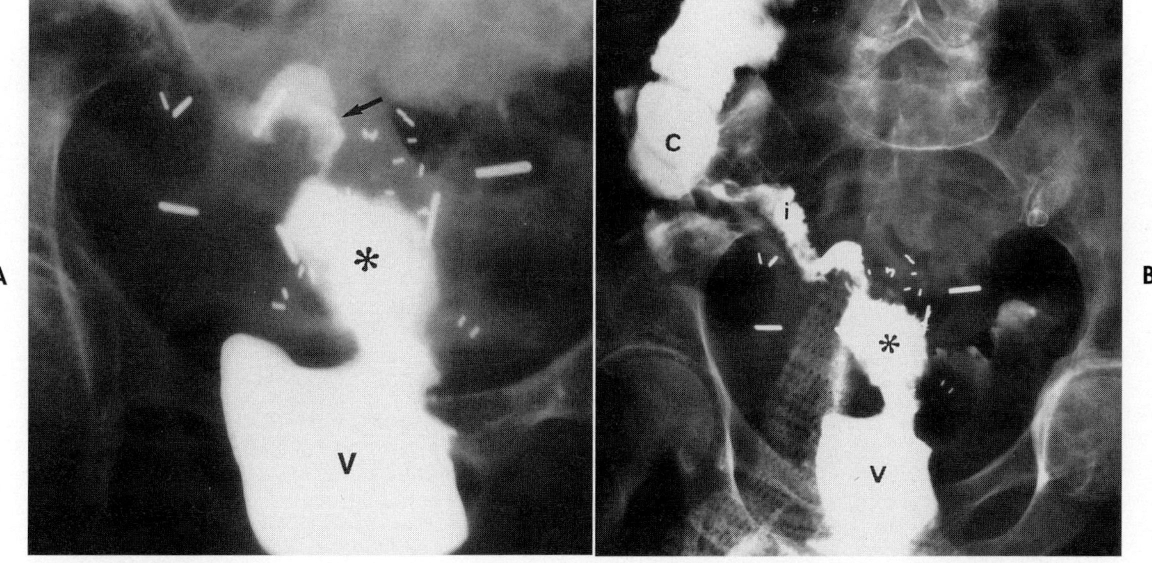

Fig. 5-6 A, Vaginogram shows an irregular cavity (*) communicating with the dome of the vaginal vault *(V).* The linear collection of barium *(arrow)* was initially thought to be an irregular extension of the cavity, but persistent fluoroscopy revealed it to be the terminal ileum. **B,** Examination shows contrast material spilling from the dome of the vagina *(V)* into an irregular 2 × 3 cm cavity (*) that communicates with the terminal ileum *(i).* The cecum *(C)* is now filled.

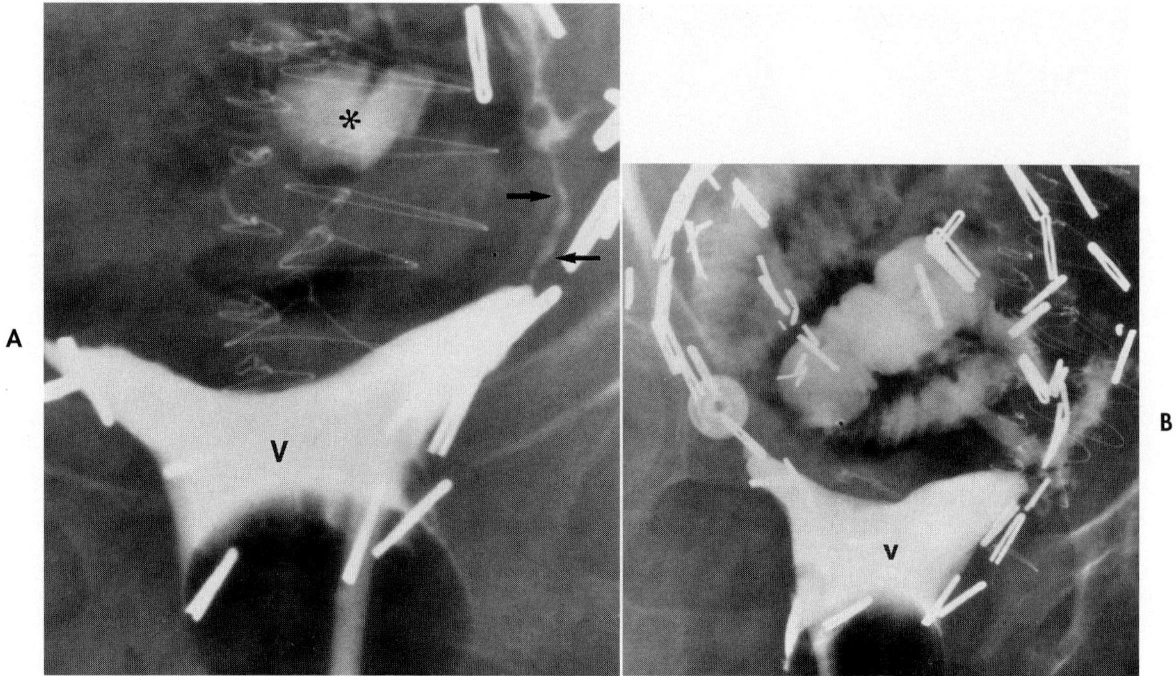

Fig. 5-7 A, Vaginogram shows contrast material filling a fistulous track *(arrows)* from the left fornix of the vagina *(V)* and resulting in slight staining of the small bowel (*). **B,** Several small bowel loops are now visualized along with the vagina *(V)*.

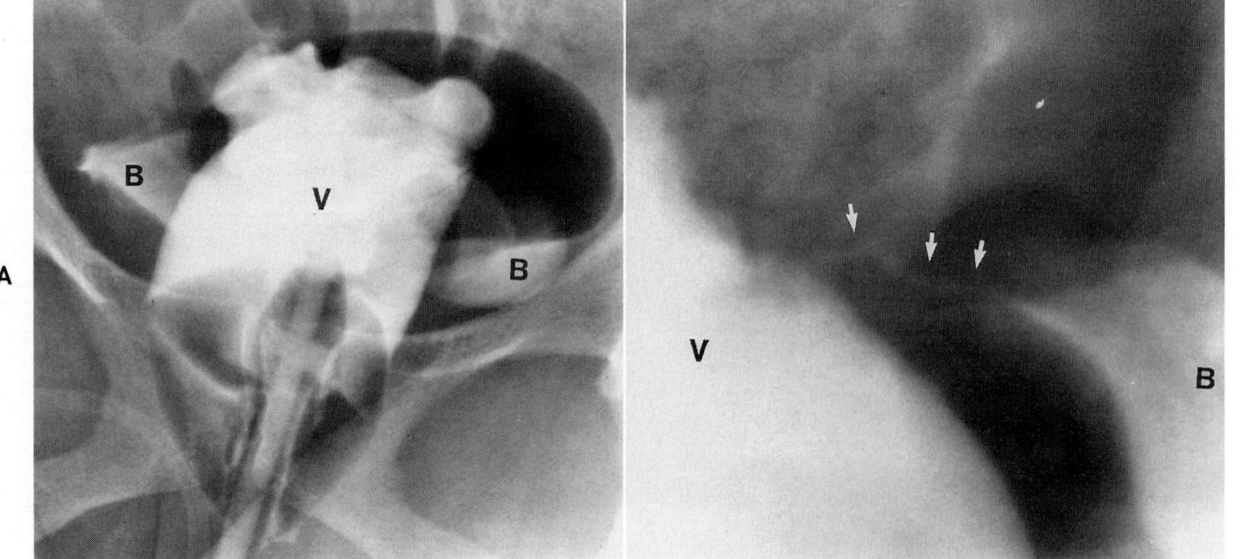

Fig. 5-8 A, Vaginogram, anteroposterior view, shows contrast material filling the bladder *(B)* from the vagina *(V)*. **B,** Coned-down oblique view shows the 1-mm wide × 2-cm long fistulous track *(arrows)*.

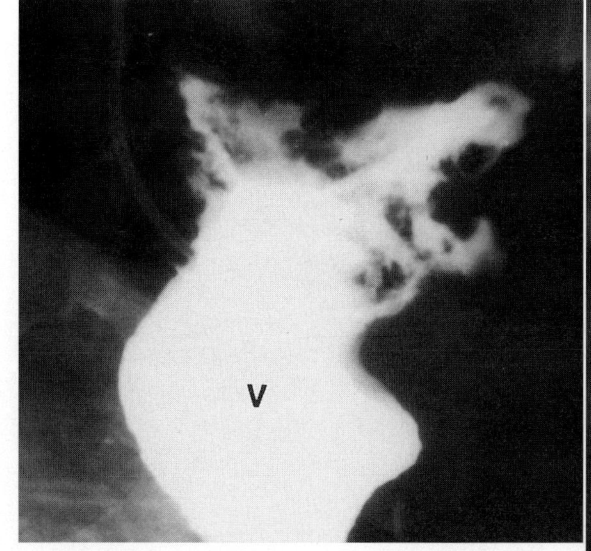

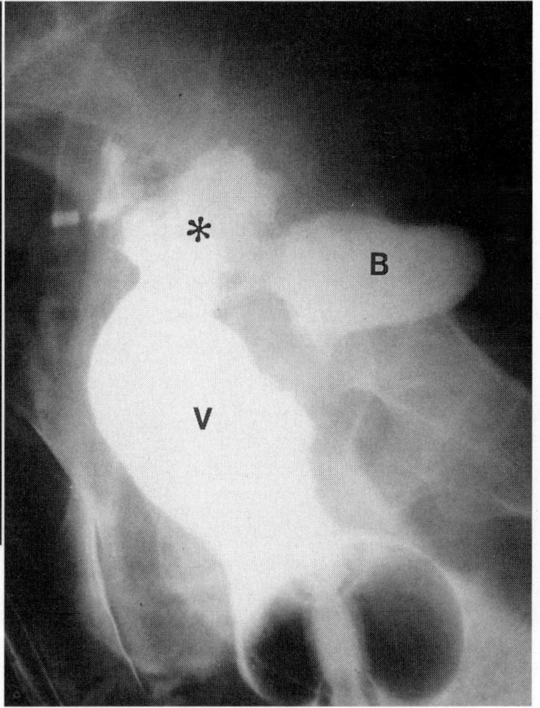

Fig. 5-9 A, Anteroposterior view early during the vaginography shows a very irregular cavity superior to the vagina *(V)*. **B,** A later lateral view of the vaginogram shows an irregular 4-cm cavity (*) connecting the dome of the vagina *(V)* to the posterior bladder *(B)*.

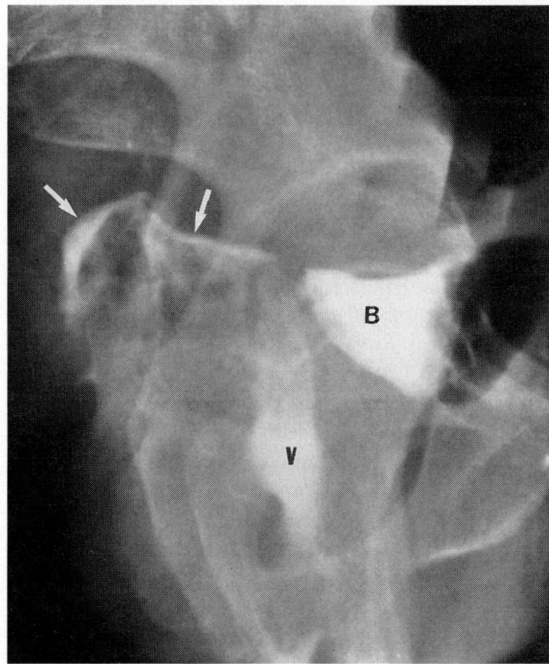

Fig. 5-10 Lateral film shows contrast material spilling from the vagina *(V)* to both the rectum *(arrows)* and, unexpectedly, to the bladder *(B)*.

cerebrovascular accident. Methylene blue dye was placed in her food to assess the laryngeal aspirate for aspiration. Methylene blue was not found in the laryngeal aspirate but was incidentally noticed to be staining the vagina. A vaginogram was then ordered to evaluate the probability of a colovaginal fistula. The vaginogram (Fig. 5-11) shows both the anticipated sigmoidovaginal fistula and an unexpected vesicovaginal fistula. Surgical exploration verified both fistulas and showed them to be the result of diverticulitis.

Case 11 is a 70-year-old patient who underwent an anterior perineal resection as well as radiation therapy 1 year previously because of rectal carcinoma. Three months previously, she had a pelvic abscess and enterocutaneous fistula, which was drained and closed. She now presented with a foul-smelling vaginal discharge. The vaginogram (Fig. 5-12) shows communication with a pelvic abscess.

Case 12 is a 64-year-old patient who was hospitalized because of chest pain. The review of symptoms revealed that she had a yellowish, foul-smelling vaginal discharge of 10 years' duration. Nineteen years before admission the patient had undergone a hysterectomy, bilateral salpingectomy, and right oophorectomy for unknown reasons. Ten years previously, she underwent incision and drainage of a pelvic abscess. The pelvic examination revealed a 4 × 4 cm firm, discrete, nontender mass but no fistula. To evaluate for a possible fistula,

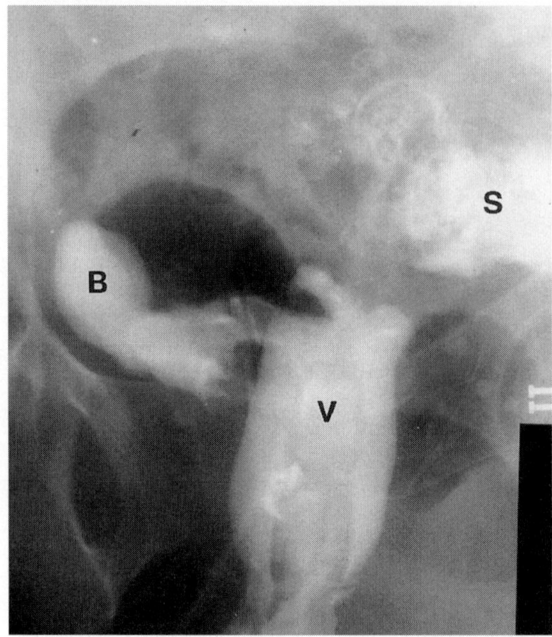

Fig. 5-11 Vaginogram shows communication from the vagina *(V)* to the sigmoid colon *(S)* and, unexpectedly, to the bladder *(B)*.

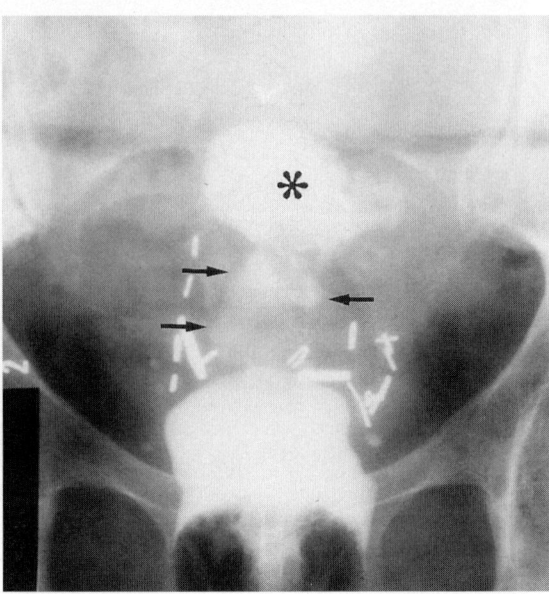

Fig. 5-12 Vaginogram shows a wide track *(arrows)* communicating between the vagina and a 4 x 4 cm pelvic abscess *(*)*.

an IVP and a voiding cystogram were taken. The scout radiograph (Fig. 5-13, *A*) revealed a bilobed, calcified pelvic mass approximately 5 cm in diameter. This was thought to represent the old abscess. Results from the IVP and voiding cystogram were normal. A barium enema was done to search for a fistula, but it showed only a diverticulum and a small polyp. A vaginogram (Fig. 5-13, *B*) revealed a 5-cm track extending from the vaginal cuff to the calcified mass, where slight puddling of contrast material occurred. There were no other fistulas. The patient was diagnosed as having a chronic draining abscess. She refused surgery.

Case 13 is an example of a false-negative vaginogram. This is a 69-year-old patient with a 2-year history of feculent vaginal discharge. A vaginogram (Fig. 5-14, *A*) was unremarkable. A barium enema (Fig. 5-14, *B*) taken the next day shows a very distal rectovaginal fistula of unknown cause.

DISCUSSION

Enterovaginal fistulas may result from diverticulitis,[5-13] rectal cancer,[3] sigmoid cancer,[5,13] vaginal cancer,[13,14] endometrial cancer,[6] radiation,[5,6,13,15-18] abdominal hysterectomy,[6,13] or a combination of these conditions.[6,19] They may also result from unilateral salpingo-oophorectomy for benign ovarian cyst,[6] appendectomy,[20] incision and drainage of pelvic abscess,[6,13] repair of stran-

gulated femoral hernia,[21] Crohn's disease,[5,13,22-24] ulcerative colitis,[6,13] lymphopathia venereum,[13] pelvic tuberculosis,[25] congenital anomaly,[26] ectopic pregnancy,[27] dystocia,[13] or perforation by either a foreign body (chicken bone),[12] a bottle,[13] or the tooth of a dermoid cyst.[28] Periarteritis nodosa[6] and the prolonged use of steroids in the treatment of rheumatoid arthritis[29] have also been suggested as causes of enterovaginal fistulas.

Passage of bowel contents through the vagina is diagnostic of an enterovaginal fistula. However, the site and number of these fistulas must be determined, and it is for this reason that vaginography is more useful than a barium enema or small bowel examination. First, the gastrointestinal study may simply fail to demonstrate contrast material in the vagina, as in cases 1, 4, and 6 and as previously reported.[2,4] Wychulis and Pratt[6] stated that a barium enema examination showed the fistula in only 12 of 35 patients with sigmoidovaginal fistulas. This failure may be due to the fact that contrast material in the gastrointestinal tract can continue to traverse the bowel as a path of least resistance, whereas vaginal contrast material is in a confined space and therefore more likely to enter a fistulous track. Also, although vaginal contrast material may be present, it may be difficult to recognize because of overlapping loops of rectosigmoid, whereas recognition of contrast-stained bowel dur-

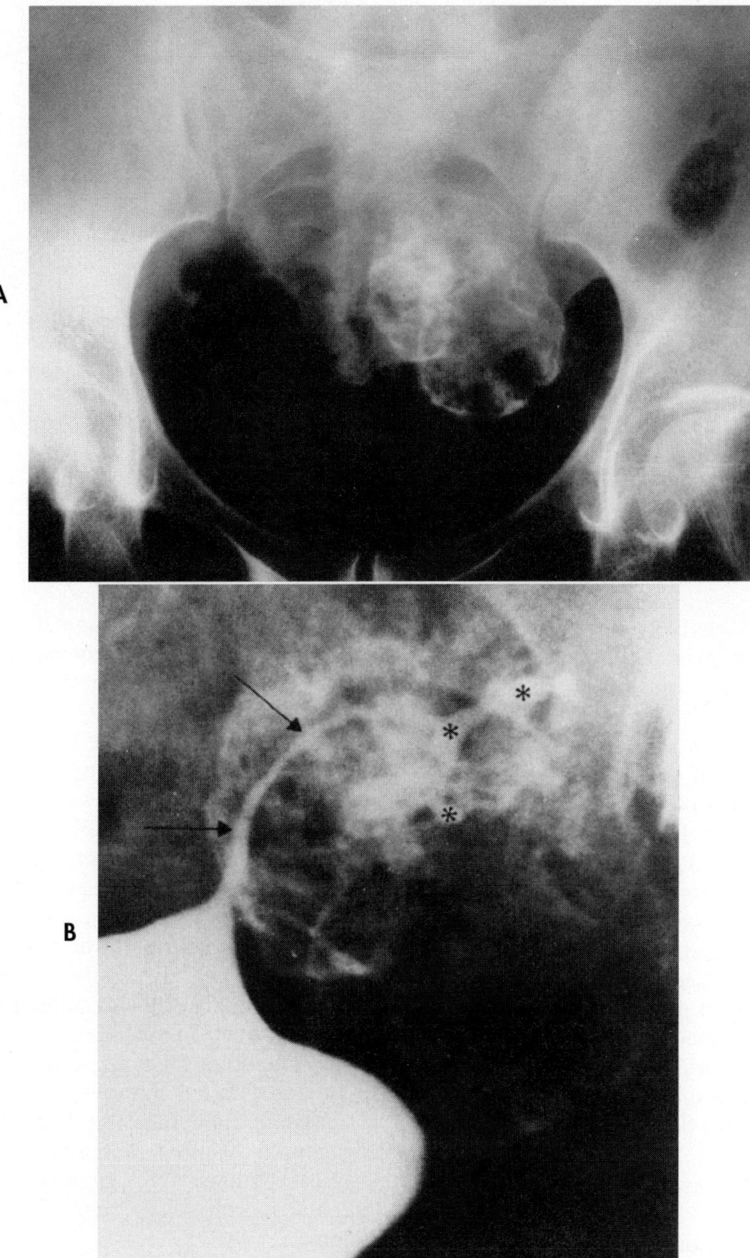

Fig. 5-13 A, Scout film for a cystogram shows a bilobed, calcified pelvic mass compatible with a history of abscess. **B,** Vaginogram reveals a 5-cm fistulous track *(arrows)* from the vaginal cuff to the pelvic calcification, where slight pooling of contrast material occurred (*).

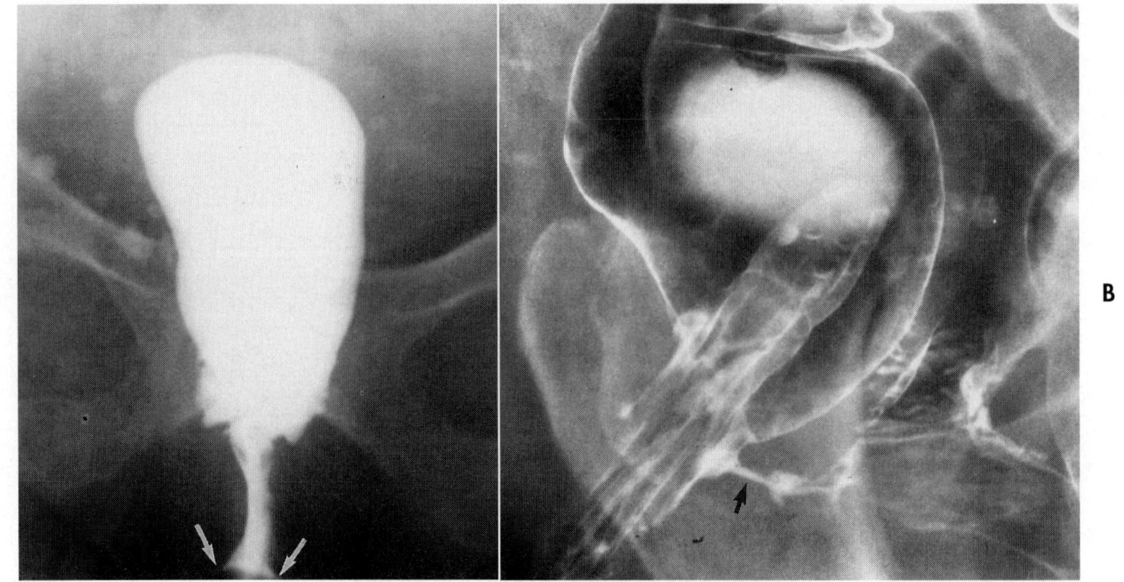

Fig. 5-14 A, This vaginogram shows no evidence of fistula. Note the superior margin *(arrows)* of the intravaginal balloon seen at the bottom of the film. **B,** Coned-down lateral view of a barium enema shows the small, distal rectovaginal fistula *(arrow).*

ing vaginography is relatively simple. Further, although a bowel study may show contrast agent in the vagina, these same overlapping bowel loops may mask the actual track. In addition, the track is often not visualized in small bowel studies because of the difficulty of spot filming.

Although examples of false-negative results from gastrointestinal studies continue, there were many more when vaginography was first performed. However, clinicians now appreciate the value of vaginography, which is often the first and only examination ordered.

Another great advantage of vaginography is that it allows visualization of multiple fistulas (cases 4, 9, and 10) and unsuspected fistulas (cases 5, 9, and 10). Lambie et al[2] reported a case in which a colostomy failed because surgeons were misled by a barium enema study that demonstrated a single sigmoidovaginal fistula. A later vaginogram, however, demonstrated two additional fistulas between the vagina and ileum.

Vaginography allows direct filling of the fistula so that its size can be determined preoperatively. Compare the enormous difference between the scope of the sigmoid vaginal fistulas in cases 2 and 3.

Also, the suspected enterovaginal fistula may be a draining pelvic abscess (cases 11 and 12), which, of course, would not be diagnosed on gastrointestinal studies or by an IVP.

Of the four false-negative examinations, three

were very distal rectovaginal fistulas that were seen only on a barium enema study (case 13) or during clinical examination. In these cases, it is most likely that the intravaginal retention balloon occluded the orifice of the track. One should therefore attempt to repeat a normal vaginogram after deflating the balloon; however, this is not always successful. It is therefore thought that very distal fistulas such as those from grade IV episiotomy tears cannot be reliably detected by vaginography. Indeed, in a patient with just such a tear, there was a normal vaginogram, which was not considered to be a false-negative study because it was beyond the expectations of the examination. Vaginography was performed in such cases to exclude other fistulas. The other false-negative examination was in a patient with a 1-mm vesicovaginal fistula.

Vaginography has also been used to evaluate congenital vaginal abnormalities,[1,30,31] ureteral vaginal fistulas,[3,32,33] vaginal ectopic ureter,[34,35] vaginal morphology,[36] and foreign bodies in the vagina.[37]

In summary, vaginography is a simple, painless, inexpensive fluoroscopic procedure that permits visualization of all types of vaginal fistulas simultaneously without the need to combat the bowel or perform multiple types of examinations.

ACKNOWLEDGMENT

I would like to thank Barbara Medley for her assistance in the preparation of this manuscript.

REFERENCES

1. Coe FO: Vaginography, *AJR* 90:721-722, 1963.
2. Lambie RW, Rubin S, Dann DS: Demonstration of fistulas by vaginography, *AJR* 90:717-720, 1963.
3. Wolfson JJ: Vaginography for demonstration of uretero-vaginal, vesicovaginal, and rectovaginal fistulas, with case reports, *Radiology* 83:438-441, 1964.
4. Cooper RA: Vaginography: a presentation of new cases and subject review, *Radiology* 143:421-425, 1982.
5. Craig O: Intestino-vaginal fistulae, *Br J Radiol* 46:48-53, 1973.
6. Wychulis AR, Pratt JH: Sigmoidovaginal fistulas. A study of 37 cases, *Arch Surg* 92:520-524, 1966.
7. Adachi A, Gold M: Vaginography for enterovaginal fistula, *Am J Obstet Gynecol* 131:227-228, 1978.
8. Carpenter WS, Allaben RD, Kambouris AA: Fistulas complicating diverticulitis of the colon, *Surg Gynecol Obstet* 134:625-628, 1972.
9. Small WP, Smith AN: Fistula and conditions associated with diverticular disease of the colon, *Clin Gastroenterol* 4:171-199, 1975.
10. Walton L, Schwartz M, Photopulos G, Fowler W Jr: Sigmoidovaginal fistulae due to diverticular disease. Two case reports and an update, *Obstet Gynecol* 51:59-61, 1978.
11. Bradford FE: Sigmoidovaginal fistula complicating sigmoidal diverticulitis: report of two cases, *Dis Colon Rectum* 8:44-46, 1965.
12. Rowe RJ, Sullivan ES: Fistulas of the sigmoid flexure, *Dis Colon Rectum* 4:41-49, 1961.
13. Hudson CN: Acquired fistulae between the intestine and the vagina, *Ann R Coll Surg Engl* 46:20-40, 1970.
14. Pride GL, Schultz AE, Chuprevich TW, Buchler DA: Primary invasive squamous carcinoma of the vagina, *Obstet Gynecol* 53:218-225, 1979.
15. Piver MS, Lele S: Enterovaginal and enterocutaneous fistulae in women with gynecologic malignancies, *Obstet Gynecol* 48:560-563, 1976.
16. McIntosh HC: Roentgen differentiation of types of intestinal vaginal fistula, *Am J Obstet Gynecol* 26:231-237, 1933.
17. Alert J, Jimenez J, Beldarrain L, et al: Complications from irradiation of carcinoma of the uterine cervix, *Acta Radiol Oncol Radiat Phys Biol* 19:13-15, 1980.
18. Slot E, Graham J: Rectovaginal fistulas due to radiation, *Neoplasma* 14:313-327, 1967.
19. Zeigerman JH, Stahlgren L, Tulsky EG: Sigmoidovaginal fistulas: review of the literature and report of a case, *Am J Obstet Gynecol* 89:1003-1008, 1964.
20. Bayer L: *Polski Przeg Chir* 29:931, 1957. As cited in Zeigerman JH, Stahlgren L, Tulsky EG: Sigmoidovaginal fistulas, *Am J Obstet Gynecol* 89:1003-1008, 1964.
21. Deshpande PV: Ileovaginal fistula: a complication following repair of a strangulated femoral hernia, *Br J Clin Pract* 18:744-745, 1964.
22. Crohn BB, Yarnis H: *Regional ileitis,* ed 2, New York, 1958, Grune & Stratton, pp 52-60.
23. Colcock BP, Vansant JH: Surgical treatment of regional enteritis, *N Engl J Med* 262:435-439, 1960.
24. Kyle J, Sinclair WY: Ileovaginal fistula complicating regional enteritis, *Br J Surg* 56:474-475, 1969.
25. Chatterjee SK, Talukder BC: Double termination of the alimentary tract in female infants, *J Pediatr Surg* 4:237-243, 1969.
26. Ten Berge BS: *Gynecol Obstet* 49:293, 1950. As cited in Zeigerman JH, Stahlgren L, Tulsky EG: Sigmoidovaginal fistulas, *Am J Obstet Gynecol* 89:1003-1008, 1964.
27. McCammon RE, Geisler HE: Sigmoidovaginal fistula: an unusual complication of ectopic pregnancy, *Obstet Gynecol* 30:414-416, 1967.
28. Lowe GH, Dixon CF, Piper MC: Perforating ovarian cystic teratomas: report of unusual case, *Proc Staff Meet Mayo Clin* 22:117-120, 1947.
29. Tancer ML, Zahiruddin S: Diagnosis of sigmoidovaginal fistula by vaginogram, *Obstet Gynecol* 28:815-819, 1966.
30. Marshall FF, Jeffs RD, Sarafyan WK: Urogenital sinus abnormalities in the female patient, *J Urol* 122:568-572, 1979.
31. Rosenberg HK, Spackman TJ, Chait A: The Dominican Republic conjoined twins: ischiopagus, tetrapus, omphalopagus, *AJR* 130:921-926, 1978.
32. Tramoyeres Celma A, Alonso Gorrea M, Pastor Sempere F, et al: Lesions traumaticas del ureter condicionadas por la cirugia ginecologia. Nuestra experiencia en et tratamiento de 42 casos, *Arch Esp Urol (Spa)* 33:19-50, 1980.
33. Skiba G, Feustal A: Wert der Vaginographie bei der diagnostik postoperativer Ureter-Scheidenfisteln, *Z Aerztl Fortbild (Ger)* 66:679-681, 1972.
34. Katzen P, Trachtman B: Diagnosis of vaginal ectopic ureter by vaginogram, *J Urol* 72:808-811, 1954.
35. Schulman CC: The single ectopic ureter, *Eur Urol* 1:64-69, 1976.
36. Funt MI, Thompson JD, Birch H: Normal vaginal axis, *South Med J* 71:534-535, 1978.
37. Foster A: Vaginal discharge in childhood, *Roentgenblaetter* 28:477-482, 1975.

6   The Cervix

Mitchell D. Schnall

ANATOMY

The uterine cervix is situated at the most caudal portion of the uterus. It is composed of a dense fibromuscular stromal coat that surrounds the endocervical canal. The endocervical canal is thickest in its center, with areas of narrowing of the canal at its junction with the uterine body (internal cervical os) and at its most distal extent (external cervical os) (Fig. 6-1). It is lined by a mucous membrane made up of ciliated columnar epithelium that changes to a squamous epithelium at the external cervical os. There are multiple folds in the mucosa of the cervix that are referred to as arbor vitae uterina. The upper two thirds of the cervix contains deep glandular follicles that secrete an alkaline viscous mucus.[1]

The cervix can be divided into supravaginal and intravaginal components. Paired sacrouterine ligaments originate in the supravaginal cervix and run posteriorly lateral to the rectum to attach to the third and fourth bones of the sacrum. Externally the supravaginal cervix is not covered by peritoneum. In fact, the anterior reflection of the peritoneum onto the bladder can be used as a landmark of the junction between the external surface of the uterine cervix and the uterine body.[1]

SCAN TECHNIQUES

Before a clinical magnetic resonance imaging (MRI) examination, the first decision to be made concerns the coil to be chosen. There are several possibilities to be considered in imaging the cervix. These include the body coil; externally placed surface coils, including multicoil arrays; and endoluminal surface coils, placed in the rectum or vagina. Each of these techniques will be considered in detail.

The most common coil system used to image the cervix is the body coil. This is convenient, since it does not require positioning of surface coils and is available on almost every MRI system. Because of its large size, the body coil is associated with the lowest signal-to-noise ratio (SNR) of any of the coil systems that will be described for cervical imaging; thus, it provides the lowest resolution images. Depending on the size of the patient, the body coil will typically support imaging with a 256 $\times$ 256 matrix over a 28- to 36-cm field of view (FOV), resulting in approximately 1.2 mm in plane resolution. In larger patients the FOV must be increased not only to prevent aliasing artifacts, but also to compensate for the lower SNR that results from the interaction of the larger patients with the body coil.

For imaging the cervix with the body coil, patients can be positioned either supine or prone. The prone position is preferred if tolerated by the patient, since it will result in reduced respiratory artifact.[2] Many patients do not tolerate the prone position well, and attempts to image them in this position usually result in significant motion artifact. These patients can be imaged supine, using a pelvic binder to reduce respiratory effects. An intramuscular injection of 1 mg glucagon helps reduce motion artifacts related to bowel peristalsis. Routine use of bowel preparation for the examination is not required. In most cases the high soft tissue contrast of MRI makes it possible to identify the vagina quite well, rendering the routine use of a vaginal tampon unnecessary. However, if the patient has had extensive surgery, it may be useful to use a vaginal tampon while scanning.

One level of improvement in resolution can be achieved by the use of externally placed surface coils. Best results are obtained when coils are placed both anterior and posterior to the patient[3]; 5-inch diameter circular surface coils provide satisfactory results. The signals from the coils can be combined before digitizing, care being taken to arrange the coils so that the signals from the two coils are in phase. If the coils are positioned so that the signals are out of phase (flipping one coil upside down), the signals from the two coils cancel

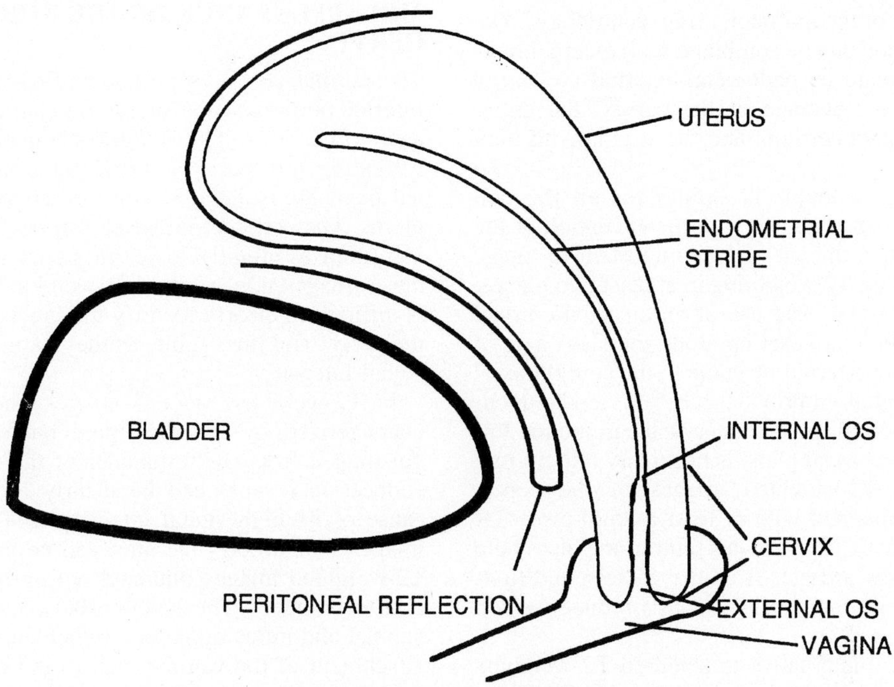

Fig. 6-1 Schematic of the normal uterus and cervix.

and a band of signal void is seen midway between them. The combination of signals can be achieved by the use of a special combiner circuit available from most MRI manufacturers or, in some cases, by a simple T connecter. As in the case of the body coil, positioning the patient prone will help reduce respiratory artifact, but if the patient is uncomfortable in this position, she should be imaged supine. Application of a pelvic binder is particularly important in the case of the external surface coil, where motion artifacts from the anterior and posterior pelvic wall are particularly strong owing to the high signal near the surface coils themselves. It is imperative to image with the frequency encode gradient in the anterior to posterior direction when using external surface coils to image the pelvis. This places the prominent motion artifacts that emanate from tissue near the coils along the anterior and posterior aspects of the pelvis, rather than through the middle of the pelvis.

In addition to the use of an anterior and posterior coil pair as described above, external surface coils can be used as part of a multicoil array.[4,5] This array system provides a means of simultaneously acquiring data from more than one coil. In its current implementation, up to four coils can be sampled at a time. Thus, four separate images are obtained and combined so that only the high SNR part of each image appears in the composite image. This results in the composite image having

the SNR of a signal surface coil and the spatial coverage of up to four surface coils. Although the multicoil array provides increased spatial coverage compared with an anterior and posterior coil pair, it provides only minor advantages when only a small volume in the center of the pelvis is to be imaged.

Maximal resolution of MRI of the cervix can be achieved through the use of intracavitary coils. Both intrarectal and intravaginal coils have been described.[6,7] The endorectal coils appear to offer a larger sensitivity profile and may be better suited to patients with cervical masses that involve the vagina. The actual coil that has been described consists of a 3 × 4 cm square surface coil mounted on a dual cylinder balloon. The balloons serve to expand the coil and prevent the cervix from moving laterally, away from the coil. Endoluminal coils allow pixels with in-plane dimensions of 0.3 to 0.4 mm to be used. As in the case of external surface coils, in order to reduce motion artifacts from the tissue very close to the coil, frequency encoding in the anterior to posterior direction is imperative. When an endorectal coil is used, supine positioning of the patient is preferred to prone positioning, as it reduces patient motion. Glucagon (1 mg IM) is useful to prevent rectal peristalsis.

A major disadvantage of the endorectal coil technique is that it limits the sensitive volume to that very near the cervix. This can be remedied through use of the multicoil array technology.[8] The endorectal coil can be combined with external multicoils to create an endorectal-external coil array that provides coverage of the cervix, the entire uterus, the parametrium, and the vagina with high resolution.

The scan technique is similar for all the coil choices described above, with the exception of the FOV and slice thickness. It is important to image the cervix with T2 weighting in at least two planes, sagittal and axial. The use of an an axial-coronal oblique plane that is set up along the short axis of the cervix is preferred by some to the straight axial plane; they claim it provides a better view to document parametrial spread of cervical carcinoma. Imaging in the coronal plane is necessary only in rare cases. The T2-weighted images of the cervix should be obtained with at least a 2500-msec TR and an 80-msec TE. Vascular saturation pulses help eliminate flow artifacts from the vessels, and first-order moment compensation helps reduce motion artifacts.

A powerful alternative to standard T2-weighted spin echo imaging is the fast spin echo (FSE) sequence. Briefly, this consists of a multiecho spin echo sequence in which each of the echoes collected after a single 90-degree pulse is encoded with a different amount of phase encoding, thus each representing a different line in K space.[9] Typically, 16 echoes can be collected in each echo train, resulting in a 16 times reduction in the time required to collect the image. The long acquisition time of the 16-echo train (usually approximately 320 msec) requires the use of a long TR value, 4 sec, to obtain 12 slices. The long TR also acts to improve image contrast by minimizing T1 effects. Despite the use of this long TR, a stack of twelve 256×256 images can be collected in only 2:26. When applying this technique to the cervix, a TR of 4000 to 5000 is used with an effective TE of 100 to 140 msec. One major difference in the contrast observed in an FSE image relative to a standard spin echo image is the increased signal intensity of fat. This can be reduced by using a fat suppression technique. Either short time inversion recovery or frequency selective presaturation provide adequate results.

The use of Gd-DTPA–enhanced T1-weighted images has been proposed to help evaluate the extent of cervical cancer, particularly in the case of advanced disease.[10] These images can be acquired as either T1-weighted spin echo or spoiled gradient echo images. The use of fat saturation in the post–Gd-DTPA scans has also been suggested to clearly delineate the interface between the high signal–enhancing tissue and the paracervical fat.

MRI APPEARANCE OF THE NORMAL CERVIX

The normal cervix is best identified as the most inferior portion of the uterus on sagittal MR images (Fig. 6-2). On images obtained with T1 weighting, the cervix is of low to intermediate signal intensity, isointense with the remainder of the uterus. The endometrial stripe can occasionally be identified as slightly lower in signal intensity on these images. On sagittal T1-weighted images, it is difficult to clearly identify the junction between the cervix and the vagina, as they exhibit a similar signal intensity.

In T2-weighted sagittal images, the cervix is characterized by its low signal intensity, distinguishing it from the remainder of the uterus. The endocervical canal can be clearly identified because of its high signal intensity in T2-weighted images. The arbor vitae uteri can be identified on T2-weighted images obtained with a high resolution technique.[11] The junction between the supravaginal and intravaginal cervix is identified by the attachment of the vaginal wall to the cervix anteriorly and posteriorly. This is particularly well demonstrated by a higher resolution technique (Fig. 6-2). Fluid within the vaginal vault has high signal on T2-weighted images. The low signal mucosa of the vagina and the intermediate signal muscular wall can occasionally be identified as separate structures.

The axial images best demonstrate the pericervical anatomy. In these images the junction between the cervical stroma and parametrium is well demonstrated. The sacrouterine ligaments are best seen on T1-weighted axial images (Fig. 6-3). On T2-weighted images the endocervical canal is identified by its high signal within the low signal cervical stroma. The canal can be seen to have a very irregular contour, representing the arbor vitae.

CERVICAL CARCINOMA

Cervical carcinoma represents a significant health care issue in women. It is among the more common gynecologic malignancies, and its incidence has been increasing. This is believed to be related to the increasing incidence of papillomavirus and herpesvirus infection, which is considered to be a significant risk factor for the disease. The most common form of cervical cancer is squamous cell carcinoma, representing 90% of all cases.[12] The disease typically begins at the junction of the columnar epithelium of the endocervical canal and the squamous epithelium of the tip of the cervix.[12] The routine use of the Papanicolaou smear to detect early changes of dysplasia and carcinoma in the cervical epithelium, coupled with the aggres-

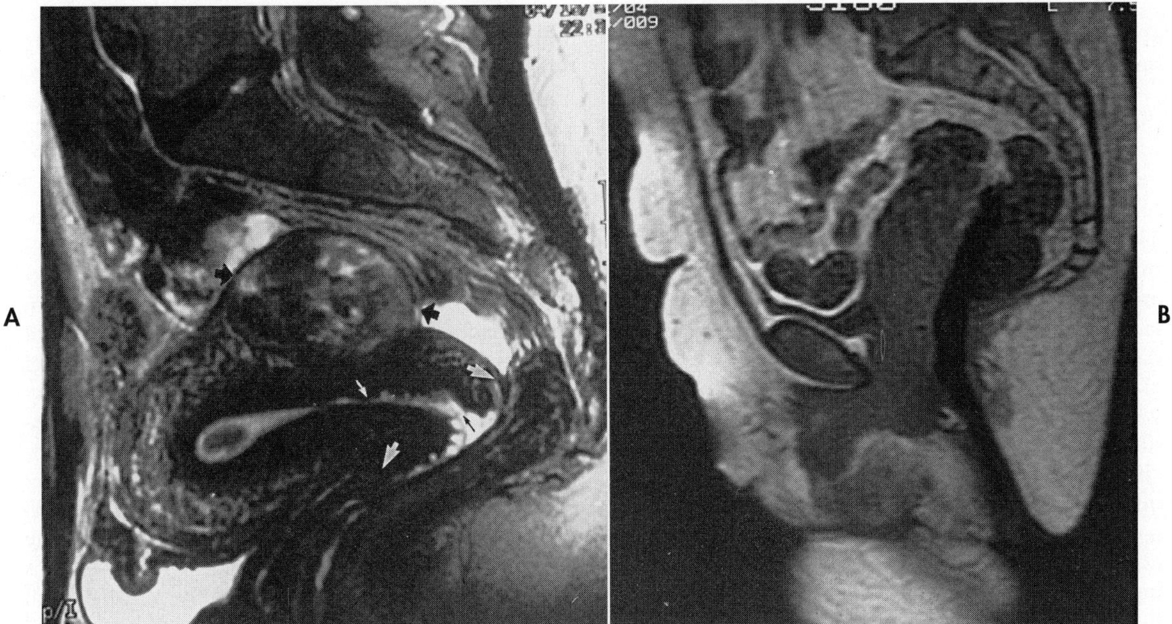

Fig. 6-2 A, Sagittal T2-weighted fast spin echo (FSE) image, obtained with a pelvic multicoil array, demonstrates the normal low signal cervix at the inferior aspect of the uterus. The high signal endocervical canal is demonstrated between the internal os *(small white arrow)* and external os *(small black arrow)*. The anterior and posterior vaginal fornices are also visualized *(larger white arrows)*. Note the large fibroid *(large black arrows)* and the low signal clot within the endometrial canal. **B,** Sagittal T1-weighted body coil image demonstrates the homogeneous low to intermediate signal uterus and cervix. The endometrial and endocervical canal are not seen. The low signal structure in the rectum represents an endorectal surface coil that can be used to obtain high resolution images.

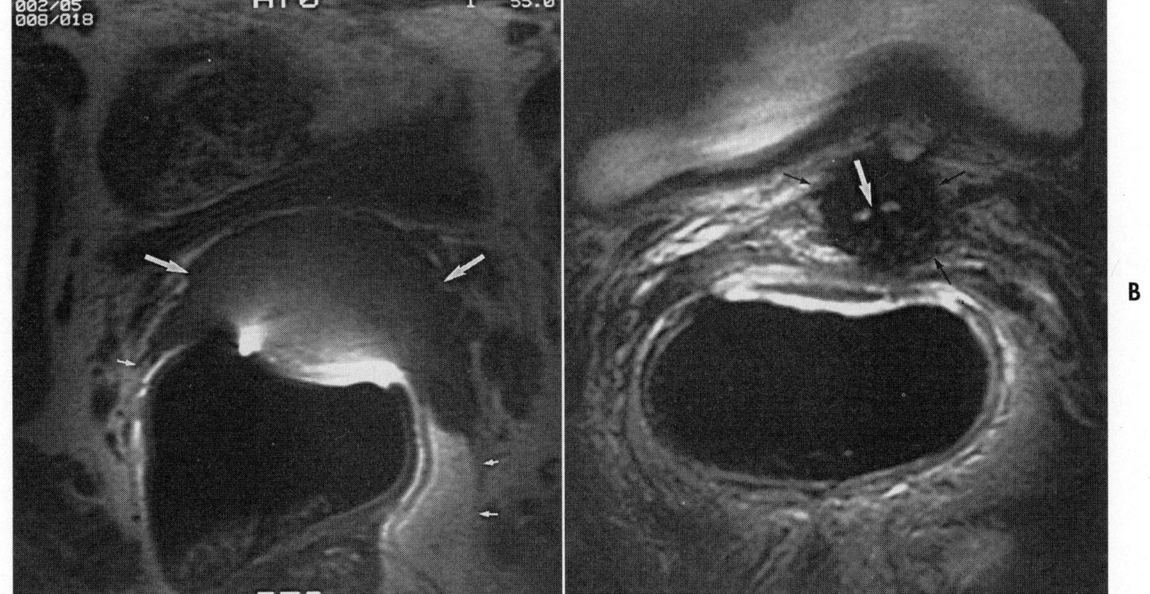

Fig. 6-3 A, T1-weighted axial endorectal surface coil image of the cervix shows a homogeneous low to intermediate structure that represents the cervix and vagina *(large arrows)*. The proximal portions of the sacrouterine ligaments are shown *(small arrows)*. **B,** T2-weighted axial FSE image of a normal cervix demonstrates the low signal cervical stromal ring *(black arrows)* and the high signal endocervical canal *(white arrow)*.

sive use of colposcopic biopsy, has led to earlier detection of the disease where it can be treated successfully with conservative surgical and cryogenic therapies. When the disease becomes invasive, it is often lethal. Invasive cervical carcinoma afflicts approximately 14,000 women each year, and approximately half of its victims die of the disease.[13] Therapy depends critically on the extent of the tumor. The International Federation of Gynecology and Obstetrics (FIGO) staging criteria for cervical carcinoma are shown in the box below (also see Appendix).[14] It is important to understand that this classification is based on clinical criteria combined with specifically determined radiologic examinations (barium enema, intravenous urography, and chest radiography). Although such a clinical staging system does allow for uniform classification of patients across many levels of technology, it does not represent the most accurate means of determining the local extent of cervical cancer. In correlating the FIGO stage with pathologic staging, accuracies of 50% to 75% have been reported.[15] A strong role for MRI in invasive cervical carcinoma is thus to improve the accuracy of preoperative staging of the disease.

MRI of cervical carcinoma

On T1-weighted images, cervical cancer appears as a nodular mass enlarging the normal cervical con-

---

FIGO STAGING OF CERVICAL CARCINOMA

Stage	Definition
0	Carcinoma in situ
I	Carcinoma confined to cervix (extension to corpus disregarded)
IA	Preclinical carcinoma of stage 1 disease
IB	All other cases of stage 1 disease
II	Carcinoma extends beyond cervix without extension to lower third of vagina or to pelvic wall
IIA	No parametrial involvement
IIB	Parametrial involvement
III	Carcinoma extends to pelvic wall and/or lower third of vagina; all cases of hydronephrosis or nonfunctioning kidney (unless due to other cause)
IIIA	No extension to pelvic wall
IIIB	Extension to pelvic wall and/or hydronephrosis or nonfunctioning kidney
IV	Carcinoma extends beyond true pelvis or involves urinary bladder or rectum
IVA	Spread to adjacent organs
IVB	Spread to distant organs

FIGO, International Federation of Gynecology and Obstetrics.

tour. The signal intensity of the lesion is usually identical to that of the normal cervix. When the mass becomes very large, areas of hemorrhagic necrosis can be identified as lakes of high signal within the mass on T1-weighted images. On T2-weighted images, the tumor can be distinguished from the remaining normal cervix by its characteristically higher signal intensity. The signal intensity of the mass can vary from mildly to markedly hyperintense to normal cervix (Fig. 6-4). In the case of large cervical tumors, focal areas of very high signal mark areas of necrosis. In younger women, the mass is characteristically exophytic, while in older women it is often endocervical because of the proximal migration of the squamocolumnar junction (Fig. 6-5).

As indicated above, the primary role of MRI in untreated cervical cancer lies in determining the extent of the lesion. Stage 1A (noninvasive) lesions are difficult to distinguish from the normal high signal of the endocervical canal on T2-weighted images. Stage IB, early invasive cervical cancer, has been reported to be identified in 95% of cases on T2-weighted MR images. Togashi et al suggested that if a macroscopic lesion is identified on body coil MRI examination, the patient has invasive disease.[16] Even with the use of high resolution endorectal surface coil imaging, it has not been possible to identify in situ lesions. Lein et al suggested that the depth of tumor invasion into the cervix can be estimated by measuring the sagittal length of the lesion.[17] They found that one half of the sagittal length provided a reasonable estimate of the amount of invasion.

Findings associated with vaginal wall invasion are thickening and abnormal signal in the vaginal wall on T2-weighted images. This is associated with extension of tumor through the full thickness of the cervical stromal ring in the region of the vaginal attachment.[16,18] Invasion of the anterior and posterior vaginal wall is best demonstrated on sagittal images; invasion of the vaginal fornices is best seen on axial or axial oblique images. If the vaginal wall invasion involves only the proximal third of the vagina, the disease is classified as stage IIa (Figs. 6-6 and 6-7). These are still considered operable lesions. The accuracy of MRI in detecting vaginal wall involvement has been reported as 83% to 93% for body coil imaging.[16,18] No large series has been reported for higher resolution techniques.

Extension of tumor into the parametria elevates it to a stage IIb lesion (Fig. 6-8). This often presents on MRI as tumor extension through the full thickness of the cervical stromal ring in the supravaginal portion of the cervix. This may be associated with nodular soft tissue extending into the

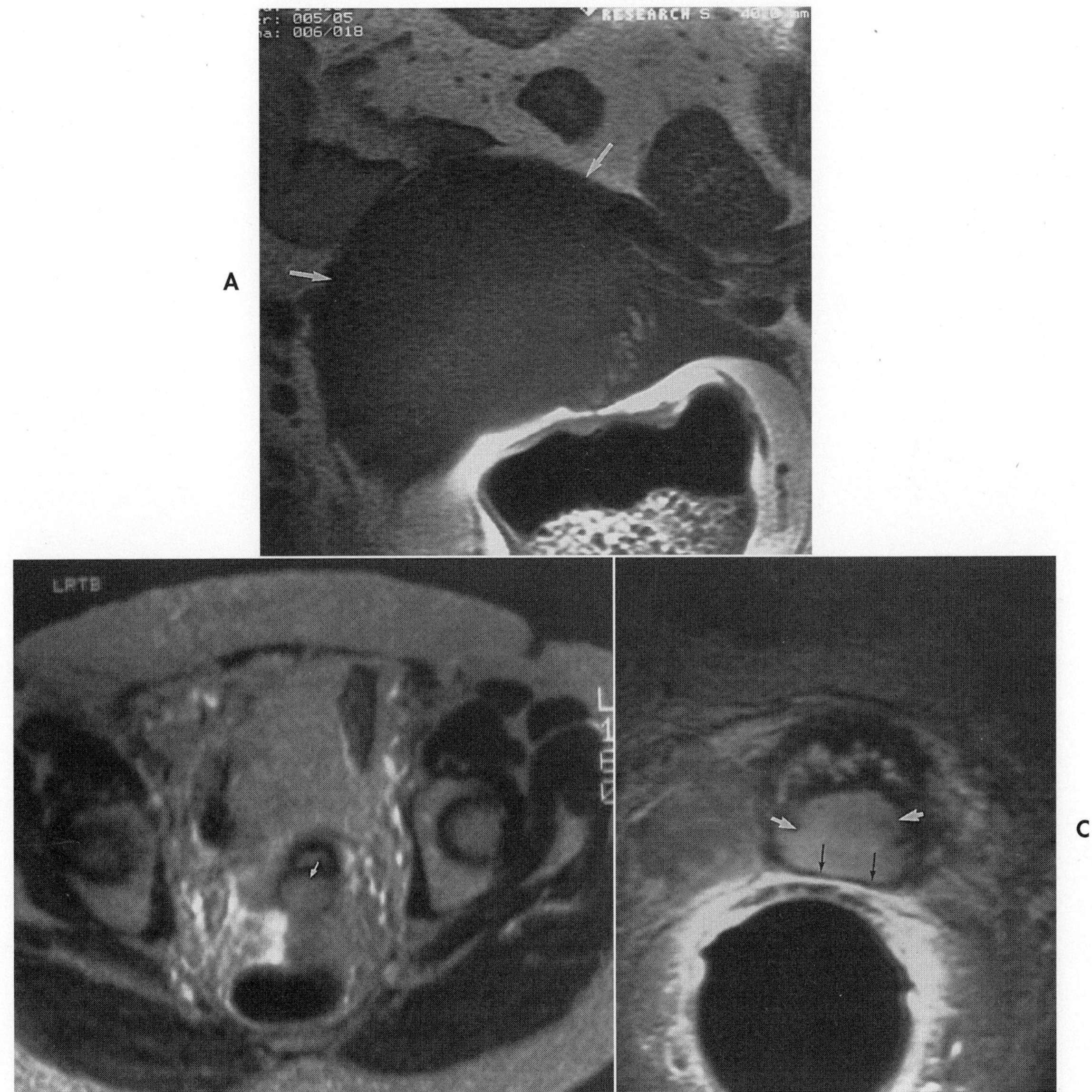

Fig. 6-4 A, T1-weighted axial endorectal surface coil image demonstrates a large soft tissue mass in the region of the cervix, representing cervical carcinoma *(arrows)*. **B,** T2-weighted axial spin echo body coil image shows a high signal mass within the posterior aspect of the cervical stroma that represents carcinoma *(arrow)*. **C,** T2-weighted axial endorectal coil spin echo image demonstrates the same carcinoma *(large arrows),* and clearly shows intact cervical stroma between the mass and the parametrium *(small arrows),* indicating an absence of parametrial invasion.

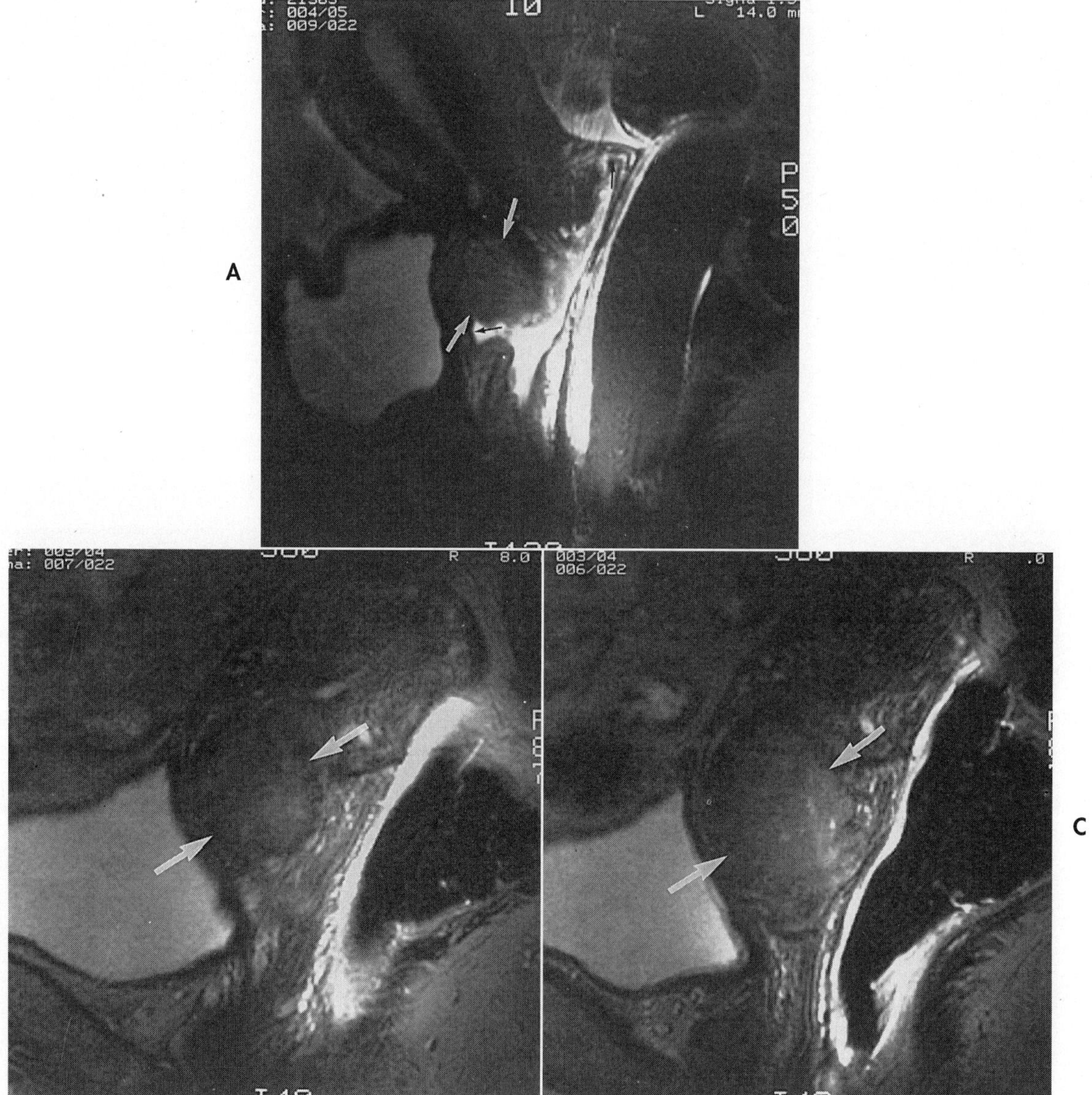

Fig. 6-5 **A,** Sagittal T2-weighted FSE endorectal coil image shows exophytic cervical carcinoma *(white arrows)*. Note the excellent demonstration of the anterior and posterior vaginal fornices *(black arrows)*. **B,** and **C,** Sagittal T2-weighted FSE endorectal coil images show endocervical squamous carcinoma in a postmenopausal woman.

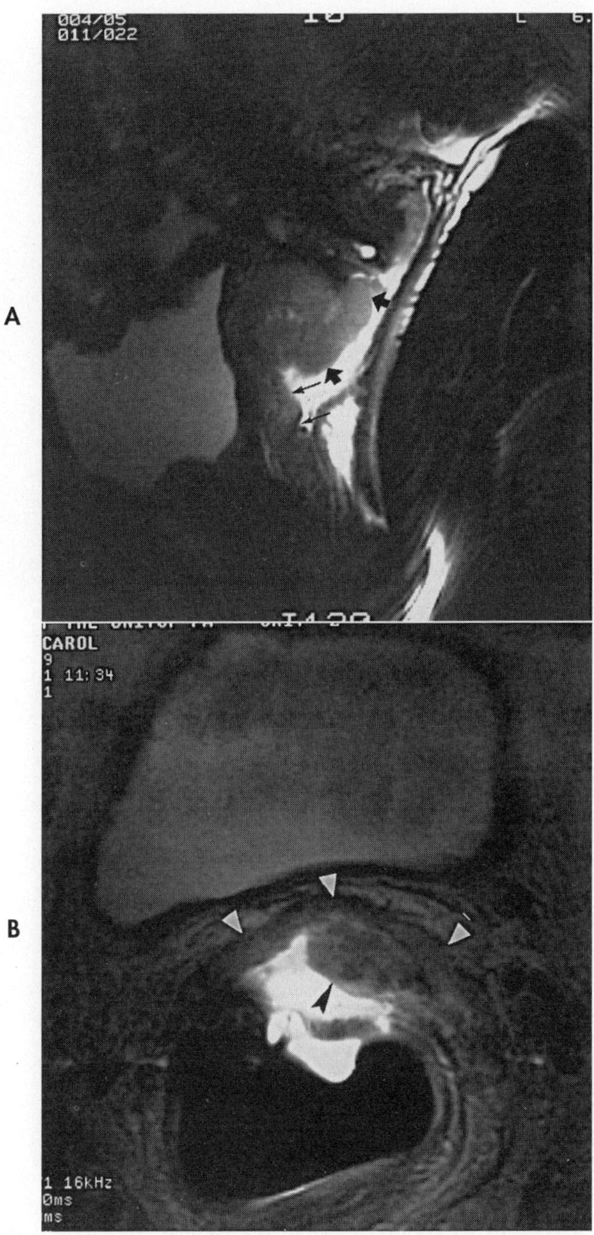

Fig. 6-6 A, Sagittal T2-weighted FSE endorectal coil image demonstrates exophytic cervical cancer *(large arrows)* with associated vaginal wall invasion *(small arrows)*. **B,** Axial image shows vaginal wall invasion. Arrows point to a cervical mass; arrowheads to the thickened vaginal wall.

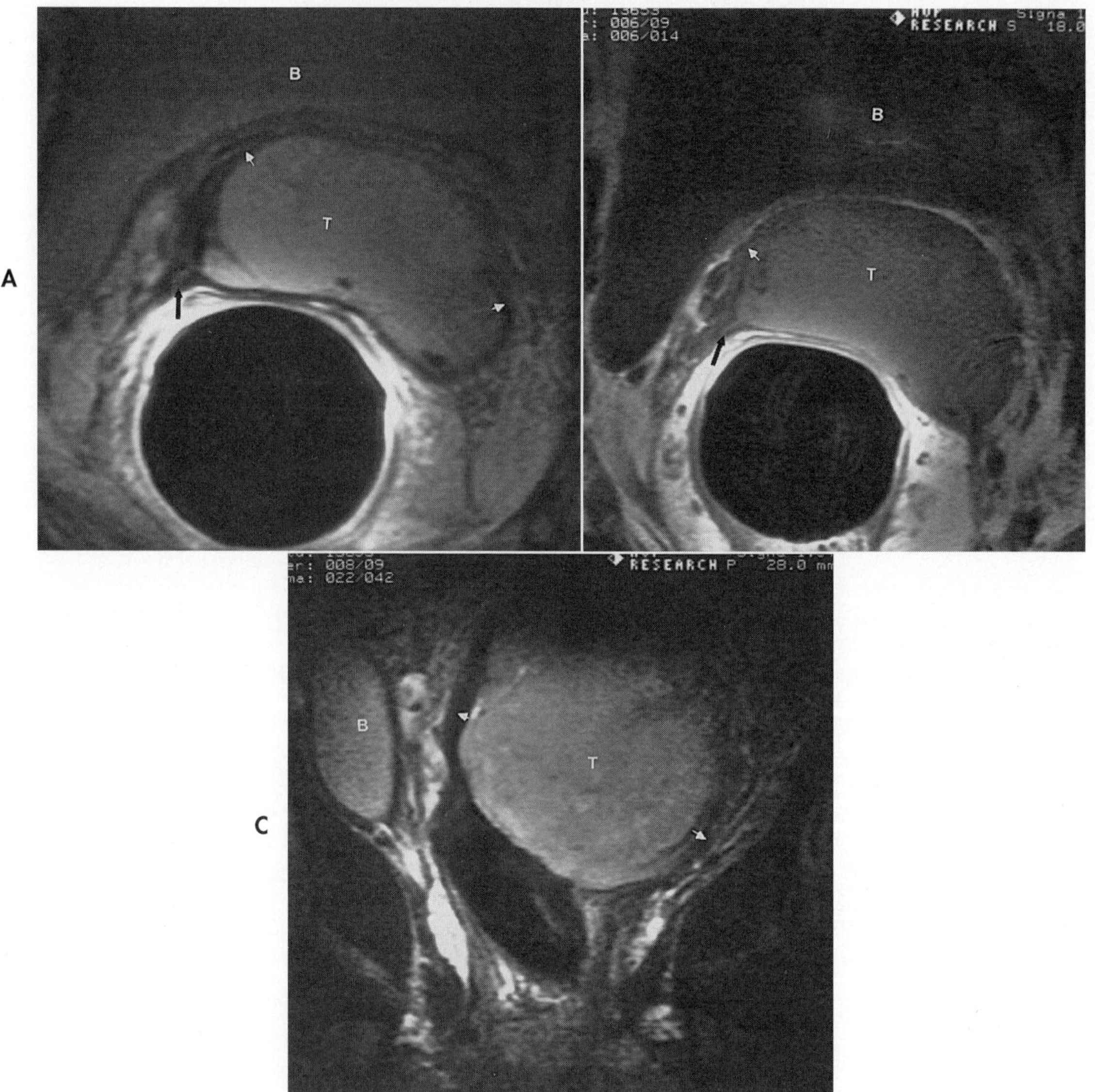

Fig. 6-7 Bulky stage IIa disease: T2-weighted **(A)** and T1-weighted **(B)** axial images obtained with endorectal coil show a large exophytic mass filling the vaginal vault. The left vaginal fornix is effaced, but the right vaginal fornix is well demonstrated *(black arrow)*. A coronal oblique T2-weighted image **(C)** reveals similar findings. *,T, Cervical tumor; b, bladder.

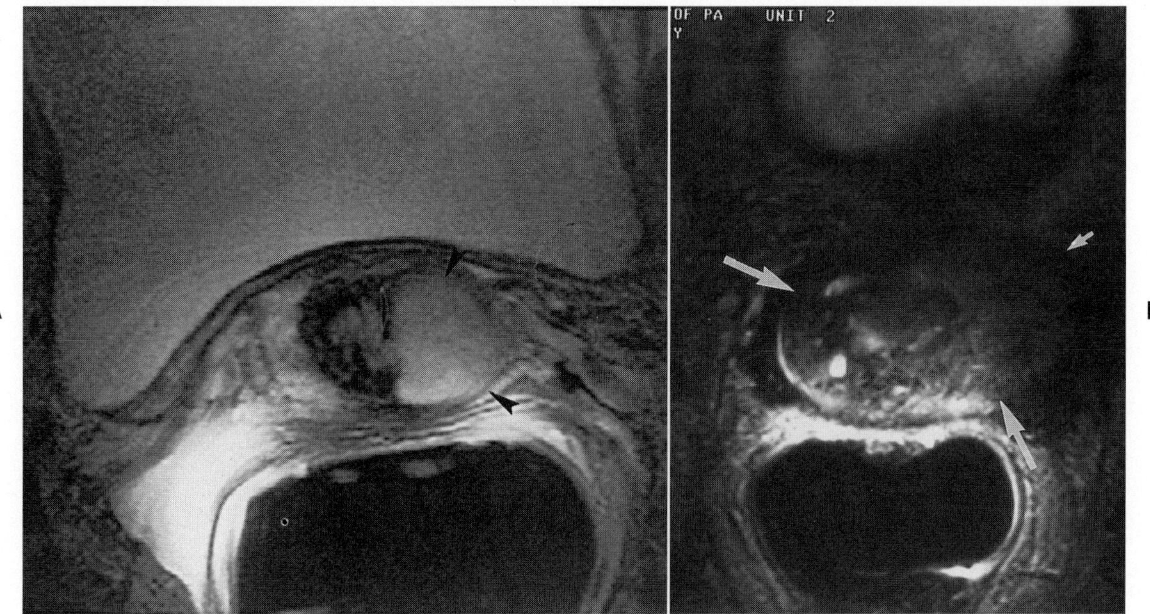

Fig. 6-8 A, Cervical cancer with invasion through the entire cervical stromal ring in the supravaginal cervix, indicating parametrial invasion. **B,** Large, predominantly intravaginal cervical cancer *(large arrow)* with invasion through the vaginal wall into the parametrium *(small arrow).*

parametrium.[16,18-20] Invasion of tumor along the sacrouterine ligaments can present as focal thickening of the cervical attachment of this structure, which may be associated with tethering of the cervix toward the ipsilateral side of tumor invasion.[16] Invasion of tumor into the vaginal and then into the paravaginal tissues is more difficult to identify on MRI because of the poor demarcation of the serosal surface of the vagina, particularly on lower resolution imaging. With high-resolution techniques such as the pelvic multicoil and the endorectal coil, better delineation of this structure is possible, making it easier to detect this type of parametrial invasion. The accuracy of body coil MRI in detecting parametrial invasion has been reported to be 88% to 93%.[16,18]

Pelvic side wall invasion is also well demonstrated on MRI (Fig. 6-9, *A*). On T1-weighted images, there is complete obliteration of the fat plane between the lesion and the pelvic side wall. On T2-weighted images, abnormal signal is demonstrated in the substance of the pelvic side wall musculature. An 86% sensitivity of MRI in detecting pelvic side wall invasion has been reported by Hricak et al.[18]

Cervical carcinoma also invades adjacent structures such as the rectum and bladder (Fig. 6-9, *B*). Invasion of the bladder most often results from anterior extension of tumor along the peritoneal reflection between the bladder and the cervix, which is often referred to as the uterine vesical ligament. It is best identified on T2-weighted sagittal or axial MR images as abnormal high signal extending from the cervix into the normal low signal bladder wall. Tumor may also extend out along the broad ligament to involve the ureter, resulting in hyronephrosis (Fig. 6-9, *C*). On high-resolution MRI, involvement of the ureter is easily detected. Involvement of the rectum with cervical carcinoma may occur through two different routes. Tumor may invade the sacrouterine ligaments and follow these structures posteriorly to involve the rectum. This method of spread also may result in invasion of the presacral space and the sacrum itself. A posteriorly positioned cervical mass may also directly invade the anterior border of the rectum.

Metastatic lymphadenopathy can also be detected with MRI. It is best identified on T1-weighted images as low to intermediate signal structures, contrasted against the high-signal retroperitoneal and pelvic fat. Signal intensity characteristics have not yet proved valuable in separating benign from malignant lymphadenopathy, and therefore the same size criteria used in x-ray computed tomography (CT) apply to MRI. Nodes greater than 1 cm or multiple clusters of nodes are considered pathologic. Thus, as one would expect, the accuracy of MRI in detecting metastatic

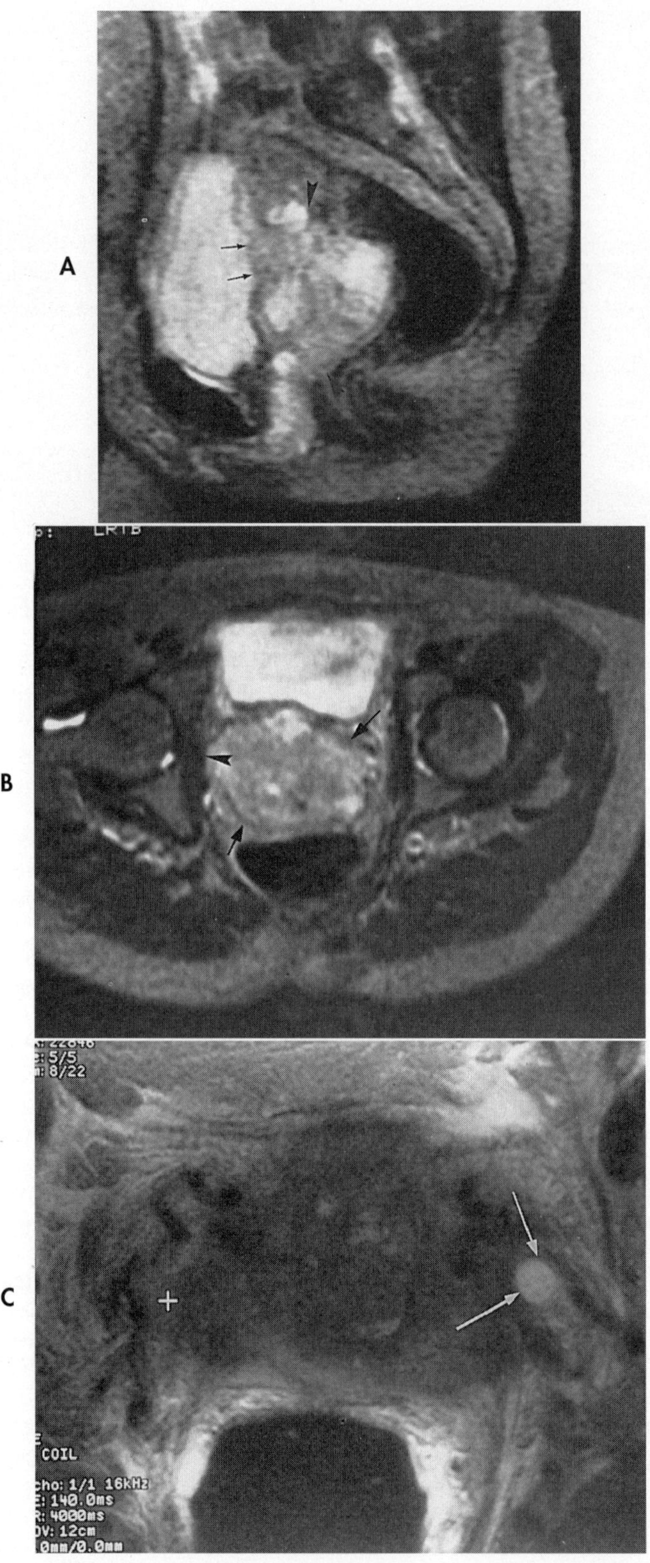

Fig. 6-9 A, Body coil T2-weighted sagittal spin echo image demonstrates a large cervical mass *(arrowheads)* invading the posterior bladder wall *(arrows)*. **B,** Axial body coil T2-weighted spin echo image shows a cervical mass *(arrows)* with associated invasion of the right internal obturator muscle *(arrowheads)*. **C,** Endorectal coil FSE image shows a large intermediate signal intensity mass infiltrating into the parametrium and involving the left ureter *(arrows)*.

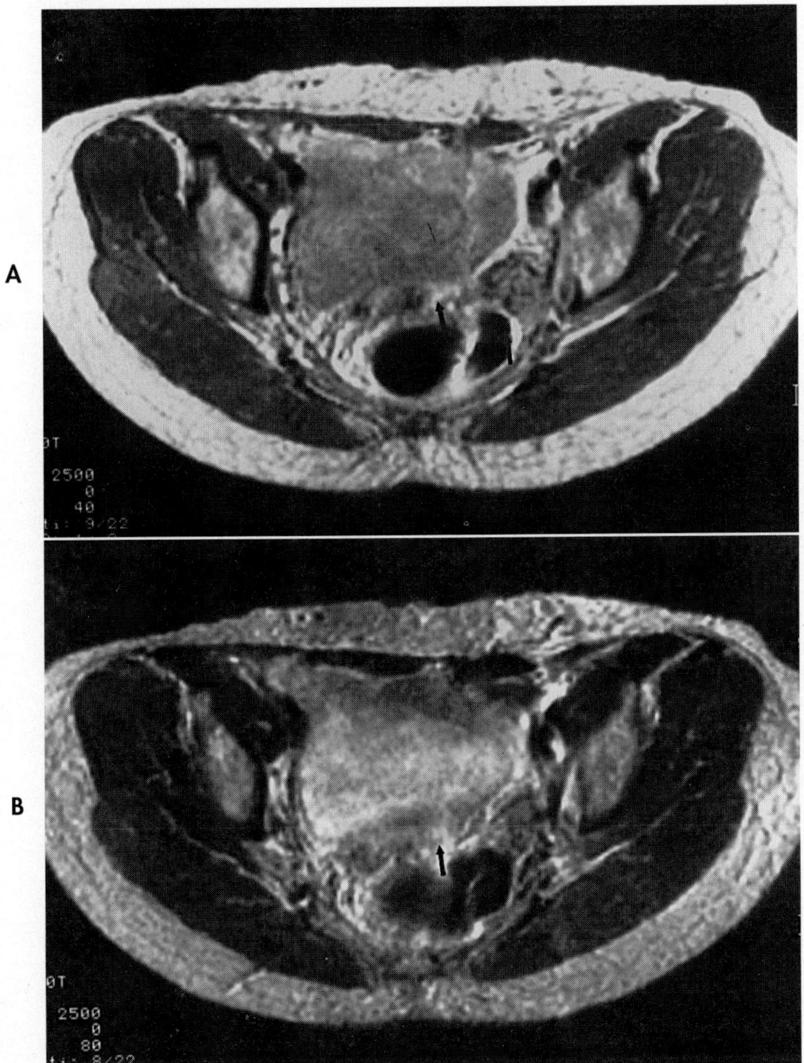

Fig. 6-10 Axial proton density (**A**) and T2-weighted (**B**) standard spin echo images, obtained with the body coil through the region of the vaginal cuff in a patient who has had radical hysterectomy for cervical carcinoma, demonstrate high signal along the left side of the vaginal cuff *(arrow)*. This represents recurrent cervical carcinoma.

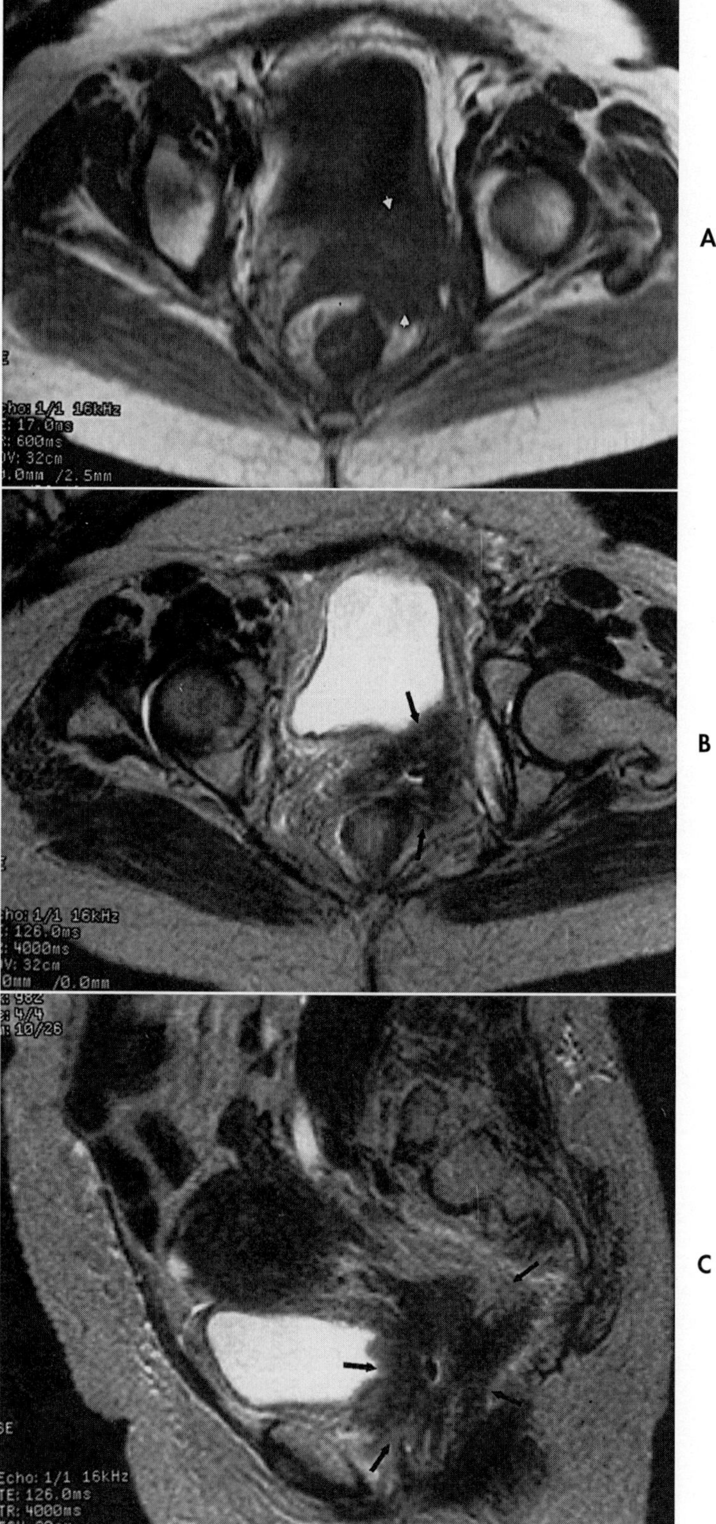

Fig. 6-11 T1-weighted axial image through the region of the vaginal cuff in a patient who underwent radical hysterectomy for cervical cancer (**A**) shows thickening of the vaginal cuff and thickening of the posterior aspect of the bladder *(arrows)*. T2-weighted FSE images obtained in the axial (**B**) and sagittal (**C**) planes demonstrates similar findings. No plane between the vaginal cuff and bladder is noted. The bladder wall appears thickened in its left posterior aspect; this area represents recurrent cervical cancer. Note that the signal characteristics of the recurrent cervical cancer do not appear to be identical between FSE and standard spin echo images.

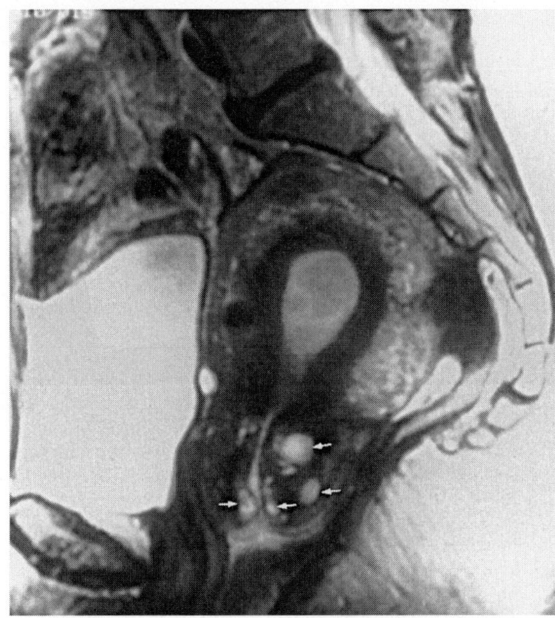

Fig. 6-12 Sagittal T2-weighted FSE image of the uterus demonstrates multiple high signal nabothian cysts *(arrows)* within the cervix.

lymphadenopathy is similar to that of CT. In a large series of prostate cancer patients, the sensitivity of MRI in detecting metastatic lymphadenopathy was 69% and the specificity was 96%.[21] Similar results have been reported in patients with cervical carcinoma.[16-18] One significant advantage of MRI with respect to identifying metastatic lymphadenopathy is that nodes can be easily differentiated from blood vessels because of flow effects. This is particularly valuable in patients in whom intravenous contrast material is contraindicated.

Recurrent cervical carcinoma

MRI is a valuable tool for following patients who have had surgical treatment for cervical cancer. Its advantages in this respect are twofold. First, the multiplanar capability of MRI helps evaluate the distorted and often complicated anatomy of postoperative patients. Second, the soft tissue contrast of MRI makes it possible to distinguish recurrent tumor from mature scar, allowing for earlier detection of recurrent disease.

The most common single site of cervical carcinoma recurrence after radical resection is the vaginal apex (Figs. 6-10 and 6-11) (approximately 20% of cases). The next most common site is along the pelvic side wall. The normal mature scar is low signal on T1- and T2-weighted images, equal to that of muscle. It is important to note that in the first year after surgery the scar will not be mature and often is of higher signal on T2-weighted im-

ages. Ebner et al reported a series of 23 patients in whom the mean signal intensity ratio of mass to muscle on heavily T2-weighted (1.5T; TR, 2500; TE, 80) images was 3.8 ± 1.2 for recurrent tumor, 0.9 ± 0.3 for mature fibrosis, and 2.6 ± 0.8 for early fibrosis. Thus, abnormal high signal within a mature scar on T2-weighted images is indicative of recurrent disease.[22,23]

Benign conditions of the cervix

The most common benign lesion of the cervix is a nabothian cyst. These cysts represent mucous distention of the deep glandular follicles that occupy the upper two thirds of the cervix. They present as 1- to 5-mm mucus-filled nodules on the surface of the cervix. Occasionally, they are larger, up to 1 to 2 cm. The signal intensity of these lesions is variable on T1, but they commonly have high signal on T1-weighted images. This is probably related to the viscosity of the mucus within these cysts. These lesions are high signal on T2-weighted images. They are usually recognized by their very smooth, well-circumscribed borders and their characteristic very high signal on T2-weighted images (Fig. 6-12). If there is any difficulty in distinguishing these lesions from cervical cancer (this occurs rarely), imaging with a very long TE (160 msec) or after gadolinium injection (lack of enhancement for cysts) can be helpful.

The multiplanar capability and high soft tissue contrast combined with improvements in MRI coil design and pulse sequences have made MRI the most powerful pelvic imaging technique. It is now possible to study cervical disease with high resolution and less time than previously possible. The efficacy of MRI in evaluating patients with cervical cancer has already been established and will continue to improve. I believe MRI to be the method of choice for staging primary cervical cancer and for postoperative imaging. It can also be helpful in other aspects of cervical disease.

REFERENCES

1. Gray H: *The classic collectors' edition of Gray's anatomy,* New York, 1977, Bounty Books, pp 1028-1035.
2. Spritzer CE, Kressel HY, Schnall MD: *Magnetic resonance imaging of the female pelvis.* In Kressel HY, editor: *Magnetic resonance annual 1987,* New York, 1987, Raven Press, pp 203-235.
3. Reiman TH, Heiken JP, Totty WG, Lee JK: Clinical MR imaging with a Helmholtz-type surface coil, *Radiology* 169:564-566, 1988.
4. Roemer PB, Edelstein WA, Hayes CE, et al: The NMR phased array, *Magn Reson Med* 16:192-205, 1990.
5. Hayes CE, Hattes N, Roemer PB: Volume imaging with phased arrays, *Magn Reson Med* 18:308-319, 1991.
6. Milestone DN, Schnall MD, Lenkinski RL, Kressel HY: Cervical carcinoma: MR imaging with an endorectal surface coil, *Radiology* 180:91-95, 1991.

7. Baudouin CJ, Soutter WP, Gilderdale DJ, Coutts GA: Magnetic resonance imaging of the uterine cervix using an intravaginal coil, *Magn Reson Med* 24:196-203, 1992.
8. Schnall MD, Connick T, Hayes CE, et al: MR imaging of the pelvis with an endorectal-external multicoil array, *J Magn Reson Imaging* 2:229-232, 1992.
9. Melki PS, Mulkern RV, Panych LP, Jolesz FA: Comparing the FAISE method with conventional dual-echo sequences, *J Magn Reson Imaging* 1:319-326, 1991.
10. Carrington B, Hricak H: *The uterus and vagina in MRI of the pelvis. A text atlas,* In Hricak H, Carrington B, editors: London, 1991, Martin Dunitz, pp 93-184.
11. Smith R, Reinhold C, McCauley TR, et al: Breath-hold T2-weighted imaging in the female pelvis (abstract). SMRM Tenth Annual Scientific Meeting and Exhibition, Book of Abstracts, 1991, vol 2, p 898.
12. Stafl A, Mattingly RF: *Cervical intraepithelial neoplastic invasive carcinoma of the cervix.* In Mattingly RF, Thompson JD, editors: *TeLinde's operative gynecology,* ed 6, Philadelphia, 1985, JB Lippincott, pp 759-844.
13. Silverberg EL: Cancer statisitics: 1986, *CA Cancer J Clin* 36(1):9-25, 1986.
14. American Joint Committee on Cancer, *Manual for staging of cancer,* ed 2, Philadelphia, 1983, JB Lippincott, pp 135-137.
15. Nagell JR, Roddick JW, Lowin DM: The staging of cervical cancer: inevitable discrepancies between clinical staging and pathologic findings, *Am J Obstet Gynecol* 110:973-978, 1971.
16. Togashi K, Nishimura K, Sagoh T, et al: Carcinoma of the cervix: staging with MR imaging, *Radiology* 171:245-251, 1989.
17. Lein HH, Viggo B, Kjorstad K, et al: Clinical stage 1 carcinoma of the cervix: value of MR imaging in determining degree of invasiveness, *AJR* 156:1191-1194, 1991.
18. Hricak H, Lacey C, Sandles LG, et al: Invasive cervical carcinoma: comparison of MR imaging and surgical findings, *Radiology* 166:623-631, 1988.
19. Kim SH, Choi BI, Lee HP, et al: Uterine cervical carcinoma: comparison of CT and MR findings, *Radiology* 175:45-51, 1990.
20. Sironi S, Belloni C, Taccagni GL, Del Maschio A: Carcinoma of the cervix: value of MR imaging in detecting parametrial involvement, *AJR* 156:753-756, 1991.
21. Bezzi M, Kressel HY, Allan KS, et al: Prostatic carcinoma: staging with MR at 15T, *Radiology* 169:339-350, 1988.
22. Ebner F, Kressel HY, Mintz MC, et al: Tumor recurrence vs. fibrosis in the female pelvis: differentiation with MR imaging at 1.5T, *Radiology* 166:333-340, 1988.
23. Williams MP, Husband JE, Heron CW, et al: Magnetic resonance imaging in recurrent carcinoma of the cervix, *Br J Radiol* 62:544-550, 1988.

7   Benign Diseases of the Uterus

Clare M.C. Tempany and Naveed Yousuf

This chapter reviews the imaging of benign conditions of the uterus with particular reference to their appearance on magnetic resonance imaging (MRI). It includes a description of the clinical, pathologic, and surgical issues related to the management of these benign lesions. Specific detail is provided for the evaluation of leiomyomas and adenomyosis, including their diagnostic work-up and the goals of imaging. Newer therapies, including surgical and nonsurgical approaches to leiomyomas, are also discussed.

MAGNETIC RESONANCE IMAGING TECHNIQUES

Imaging of the uterus is fundamental to all MR protocols for the pelvis. The earlier chapter on techniques reviews these in detail. In this chapter the techniques and suggested protocols specifically for benign conditions of the uterus are discussed. As always, the choice of coil type and sequences to be used will depend on the type of scanner and the hardware and software available.

In designing the optimal imaging approach for examining the uterus and its diseases, of which leiomyomas are the preeminent example, the primary goal is not to achieve high spatial resolution but to obtain multiple imaging planes and a wide field of view (FOV), in order to provide three-dimensional analysis and adequate coverage (Fig. 7-1). The images usually cover from the inferior aspect of the pubic symphysis up to at least the

iliac crest. It is always desirable to acquire at least two different imaging planes to allow multiplanar display and a three-dimensional analysis of the uterus (Fig. 7-2).

Thus, the standard transmit/receive external body coil is more than adequate. This will afford a large FOV and allow multiplanar imaging. The newer multicoil phased array arrangements are usually superior, except when one is dealing with a large volume of disease. They are superior inso-

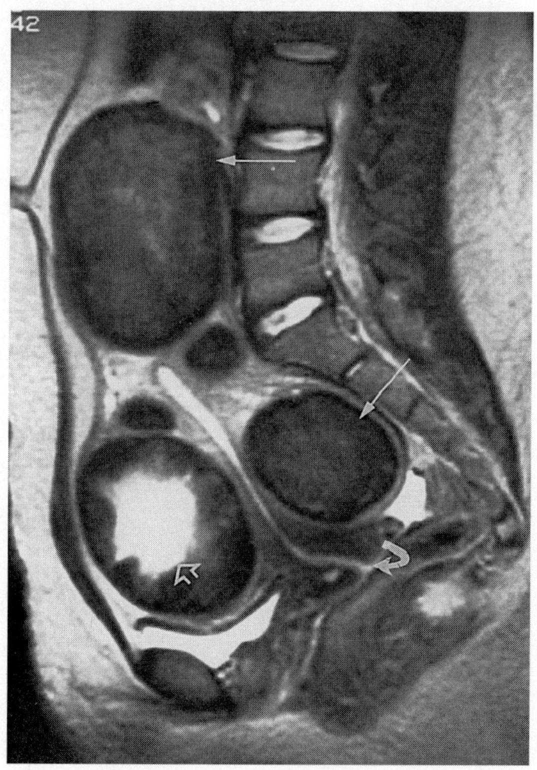

Fig. 7-1 Sagittal T2-weighted image of the uterus shows five intramural leiomyomas. Four of them *(long white arrows)* have the typical T2-weighted appearance of low signal intensity, well-defined masses in the myometrium. The anterior lesion *(open white arrow)* has a high signal center, showing evidence of degeneration. Note the relationship of the two lower leiomyomas to the cervix and its external os *(curved white arrow)*.

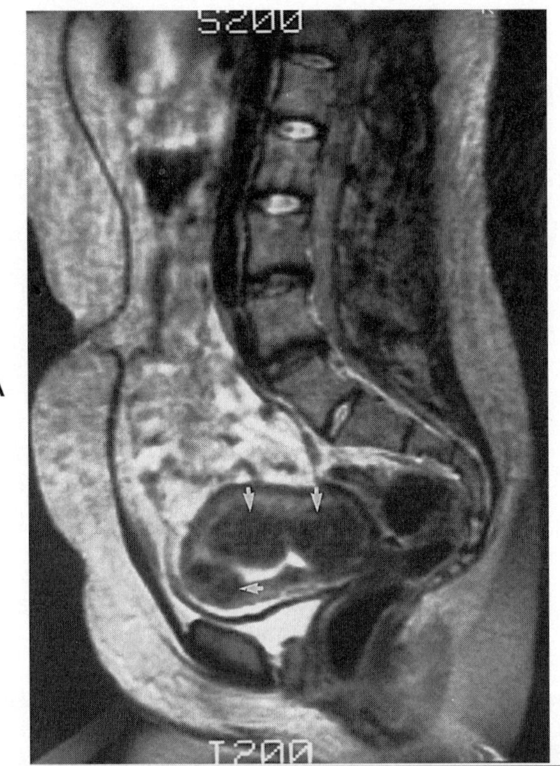

Fig. 7-2 A, Sagittal T2-weighted image of the uterus shows three separate leiomyomas *(short white arrows),* again with a typical T2-weighted appearance. **B,** Axial T2-weighted image of the same patient shows innumerable leiomyomas in submucosal *(curved white arrow),* intramural *(short white arrows),* and subserosal locations *(black arrow).* The endometrial cavity is markedly distorted *(long thin white arrow).*

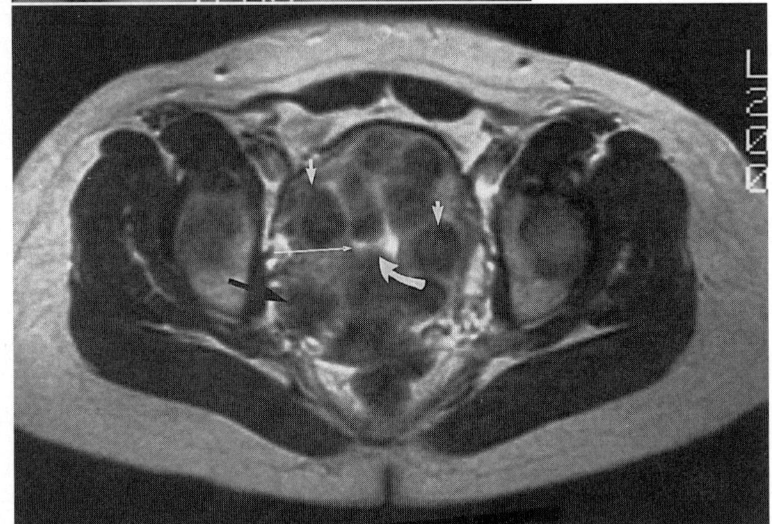

far as the images can be achieved with a smaller FOV and with higher signal-to-noise ratios. The phased array images have their own specific protocols and their own particular artifacts, which are discussed in Chapter 4, on MR techniques. If there is any suspicion that the patient's abnormalities extend up above the iliac crest, it is better to use the body coil and ensure complete coverage (see Fig. 7-1).

Pulse sequence and imaging planes

The position of the uterus in the pelvis is variable and cannot be predicted ahead of time. Thus, it is best to start with a sagittal plane series to display the uterine body and its orientation. This is particularly important if any off-axis planes are planned. The sagittal plane allows for images to be prescribed along the long or short axis of the endometrial cavity, which is particularly important in adenomyosis, for example (Fig. 7-3).

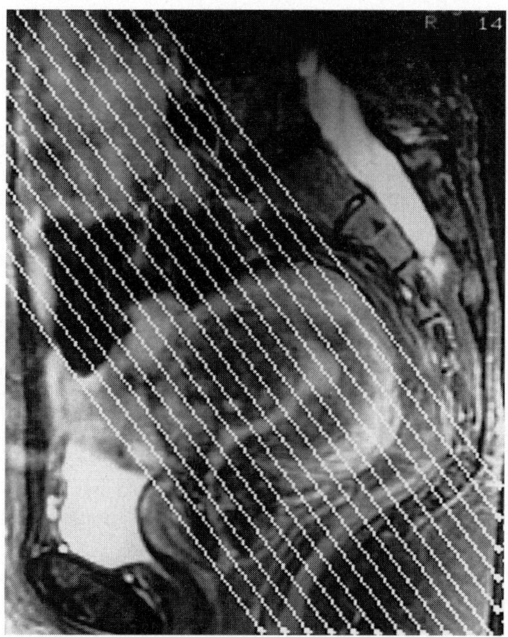

Fig. 7-3 Sagittal T2-weighted image topogram that demonstrates the orientation of the off-axis plane for imaging the short axis of the endometrial cavity in this patient with adenomyosis (see also Fig. 7-34).

Since fast spin echo has become available it is recommended that at least two different planes of T2 weighted (T2W) sequences be acquired. Usually these should be the sagittal and axial, supplemented with a coronal or off-axis sequence, as indicated. For simplicity and for standardized protocols, all three planes can be obtained.

Contrast agents

Intravenous (IV) gadolinium is not essential for imaging benign diseases of the uterus. Unlike malignant neoplasms, benign leiomyomas are most often clearly delineated on T2-weighted images, and there is little to be gained by additional sequences and the expense of gadolinium.[1] On the other hand, oral contrast agents, which have been reviewed previously, may have a potential role to play in the evaluation of leiomyomas, especially in the case of pedunculated degenerated leiomyomas, which can be difficult to separate from adjacent bowel loops and to differentiate from bowel in the first place. Therefore, although these oral agents are not currently in widespread use, there seem to be no compelling reasons to routinely use contrast agents (IV or oral) for evaluating the benign uterus. The main diagnostic information is obtained from T2-weighted sequences, and the examination time can be kept to a minimum by focusing on these high-yield sequences.

DISEASES OF THE ENDOMETRIUM
Normal endometrium

The endometrium of the uterus can be imaged by both ultrasonography and MRI. The normal endometrium is evaluated with specific attention to its thickness and overall texture.

Sonography and MRI can both provide the three imaging planes for evaluation: anteroposterior, craniocaudal (length), and transverse (width). The innermost surface of the endometrium or its interface with the junctional zone (or subendometrial halo in sonography) can be defined. This definition allows both modalities to provide accurate measurements of the endometrial thickness. The zone or stripe actually represents the two layers of endometrium in apposition. It is essential to obtain this measurement in all uterine imaging examinations.

There are established normal measurements available (according to data from Fleischer and colleagues[2]) for both ultrasonography and MRI, usually taken in the anteroposterior dimension (sagittal plane MR) and ideally confirmed on the transverse dimension (axial plane MR). It is important that these images be not oblique in any direction, to ensure accuracy. These measurements are based on data from over 100 patients. The thickness of the endometrium ranges from 4 to 14 mm in premenopausal women during the proliferative and secretory phases. In the proliferative phase the thickness ranges from 4 to 8 mm, and in the secretory phase from 7 to 14 mm. The endometrium is, of course, thinnest during menses (1 to 4 mm). In postmenopausal women the endometrial stripe is 4 to 8 mm.

The clinical history, and in particular the menstrual history, is essential a priori information. It is also important to determine whether the patient is taking exogenous estrogen, as this can cause endometrial stimulation and thus thickening, increasing the normal thickness by 2 to 3 mm. If possible, this information should be available at the time of image interpretation. There are some discrepancies in the ranges of normal, not only between MRI and ultrasonography but also between transabdominal sonography (TAS) and transvaginal sonography (TVS). The compression effect of the full bladder is thought to account for some of the differences in sonographic measurements.

The MR appearance of the endometrium is that of the high signal intensity layer on T2-weighted images (Fig. 7-4). This high signal, as in the ultrasound examination, represents the two layers of endometrium in apposition. Unless the endometrium is bleeding or filled with blood (hematometra), it cannot be distinguished from the other zones of the uterus on T1-weighted images.

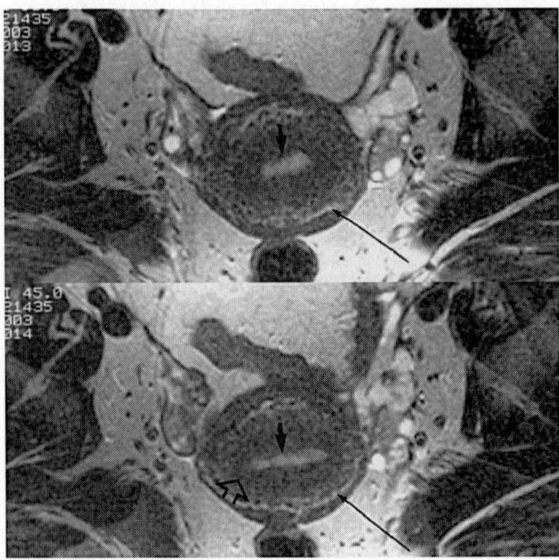

Fig. 7-4 A 45-year-old woman with a normal uterus at subsequent hysterectomy. Two axial T2-weighted images show the normal appearance of the uterus in the secretory phase of the cycle. The normal endometrium *(black arrow)*, junctional zone *(open black arrow)*, and myometrium *(long black arrows)* are all clearly seen. Note the high signal in the myometrium representing the arcuate vessels *(black arrow)*.

The endometrial measurements on MR, although similar to those on sonography, have been found in a study by Mitchell and colleagues to be slightly different.[3] In this study, 20 patients (normal volunteers) all had both transvaginal ultrasound and MR examinations within 24 hours of each other. The average MR endometrial measurements were thinner than the sonography ones in the same patients. The average MR measurement was 6.5 mm versus 7.9 mm on sonography in the proliferative phase and 9.9 mm versus 11.3 in the secretory phase. The authors also found differences in the other zonal measurements. One of the most problematic areas appears to be the exact measurement of the junctional zone on the two modalities. Importantly, the authors do not recommend that their measurements be regarded as normal because of variabilities in the phase of the cycle and differences in the transducers and MR protocols used. However, the study does show that small differences may exist and should not be a cause for concern. The other imaging tools such as computed tomography (CT) and hysterosalpingography (HSG) provide indirect visualization of the endometrium; the latter allows visualization of only the inner surface of the endometrium.

Without doubt, HSG is the only imaging study to provide a view of the surface of the endometrium, and irregularities of the surface such as are noted in hyperplasia or adenomyosis are clearly seen.

Hyperplasia

Benign hyperplasia of the endometrium is usually manifested by a generalized widening or dilatation of the endometrial cavity. Hyperplasia can be seen in patients who are hyperestrogenic or have polycystic ovarian disease, in whom there has been long-term unopposed estrogen stimulation.

Pathology. Hyperplasia of the endometrial glands occurs as a result of estrogen stimulation. If there is no progesterone to regulate it, the endometrium will become hyperplastic. According to Kurman and colleagues, there are two major forms of hyperplasia: invasive and noninvasive.[4] In the past, many different terms have been used to describe hyperplastic states such as adenomatous, atypical, and even carcinoma in situ.

Clinical presentation. Hyperplasia is the most common cause of abnormal uterine bleeding, both before and after menopause. The patient may have menorrhagia (hypermenorrhea), with a normal cycle but excessive bleeding; menses may be prolonged, lasting 5 to 8 days. Alternatively, she may have metrorrhagia, which consists of irregular cycles and irregular quantities of blood, and again prolonged menses.

Diagnostic techniques. The definitive diagnosis is pathologic, usually resulting from examination of the curettage specimens. Prior to pathology the diagnosis can be suspected whenever the endometrial cavity is widened and dilated. This is not a specific finding, but in a young woman it is highly suggestive of hyperplasia.

Ultrasonography. In keeping with the pathology, the sonographic findings consist of prominence and thickening of the echogenic endometrial stripe. The endometrium is the layer of bright central echoes, which normally vary during the menstrual cycle. The echogenic stripe is thickened in hyperplasia: usually a generalized thickening without any associated masses or alteration of the myometrium.

Polyps may be indistinguishable, also causing a thickening of the echogenic layer. Importantly, endometrial carcinoma may have an identical appearance, and thus endometrial thickness of greater than 14 mm in perimenopausal women and 10 mm or greater in postmenopausal women should always be regarded as abnormal.[5] It has been recommended that ultrasonography be used to monitor postmenopausal women before and during estrogen replacement therapy.[6] These patients are at risk not only of hyperplasia, but more important, of carcinoma. Lin and colleagues recommend that all patients with an endometrial thickness of at

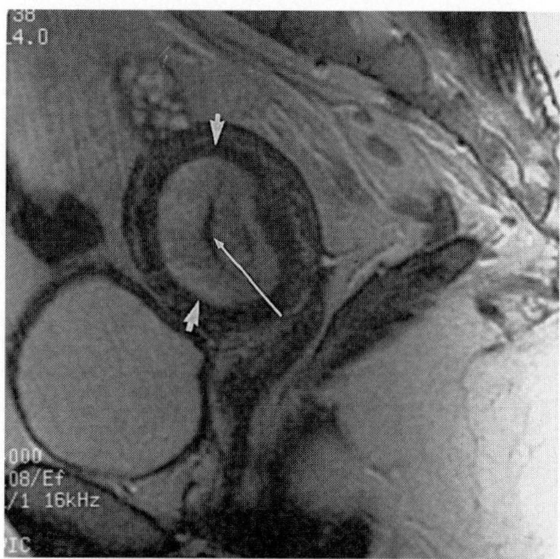

Fig. 7-5 Endometrial hyperplasia and polycystic ovaries in a 25-year-old woman with irregular menses. This sagittal T2-weighted image shows marked endometrial thickening *(white arrows)*. A low signal line is seen centrally *(long white arrow),* which probably represents the interface of both endometrial surfaces.

least 1.5 cm should undergo a biopsy, regardless of symptoms and hormonal status.[6]

Magnetic resonance imaging. The MR appearance of hyperplasia consists of an increase in endometrial thickness on T2-weighted images, beyond the expected normal ranges for the patient's age and hormonal status. The measurements are taken in the sagittal plane, and an endometrium of 10 mm or greater is abnormal (Figs. 7-5 and 7-6). Whenever the endometrium is abnormal, the MR images should also be used to evaluate the other areas of the uterus, specifically the junctional zone and the ovaries. The junctional zone should be carefully examined for completeness, to ensure that it is intact all the way around the endometrium. This may require a set of off-axis images (Fig. 7-7). Evaluation of the junctional zone is critical, as the major differential diagnosis is endometrial carcinoma. When this is suspected, it is the responsibility of the radiologist to stage the "cancer," which necessitates detailed examination of the uterus, pelvic side walls, and retroperitoneum. If there is hyperplasia, the cause may be found on the scan. The ovaries may be abnormal, and in particular there may be polycystic ovary disease (Figs. 7-6 and 7-8). There are thus several possible diagnoses that may be evidenced by endometrial thickening, primary carcinoma, hyperplasia, polyps, pregnancy (Fig. 7-9), and retained fluid. The myometrium and endometrial cavity should be carefully examined if there is a possibility of pregnancy. The cavity may show a gestational sac, and the myometrium will show a significant increase

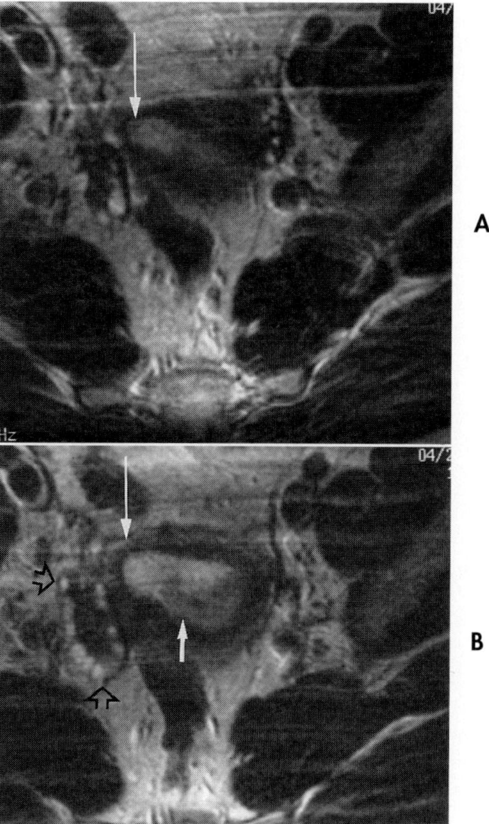

Fig. 7-6 A, B, Axial T2-weighted images (fast spin echo [FSE] TR 4000, TE effective 108, field of view [FOV] 20 cm, slice thickness 4 mm, gap 0.5 mm, and 256 matrix with two signal averages) of the patient in Fig. 7-5. The junctional zone did not appear complete on the right side *(long white arrows).* **B,** Of particular importance in this case is the right ovary, which is abnormal with numerous small peripheral cysts *(open black arrows),* the typical appearance of polycystic ovaries.

in T2 signal, a decidual response (Fig. 7-9).

In the case of retained fluid or mucus, the images should be carefully evaluated for any possible obstruction of the cervix or uterine cavity. Cervical carcinoma or adhesions from radiation therapy are both common causes of cervical os stenosis. If there is no apparent mass or cervical abnormality causing obstruction, careful examination of the T1-weighted images with added IV gadolinium can help differentiate tumor and hyperplasia from fluid; the former will have a higher T1 signal both before and after gadolinium.

Polyps

Pathology. Endometrial polyps are hyperplastic outgrowths of the endometrial tissue containing some glandular, vascular, and stromal elements. They are variable in origin (broad-based or on a

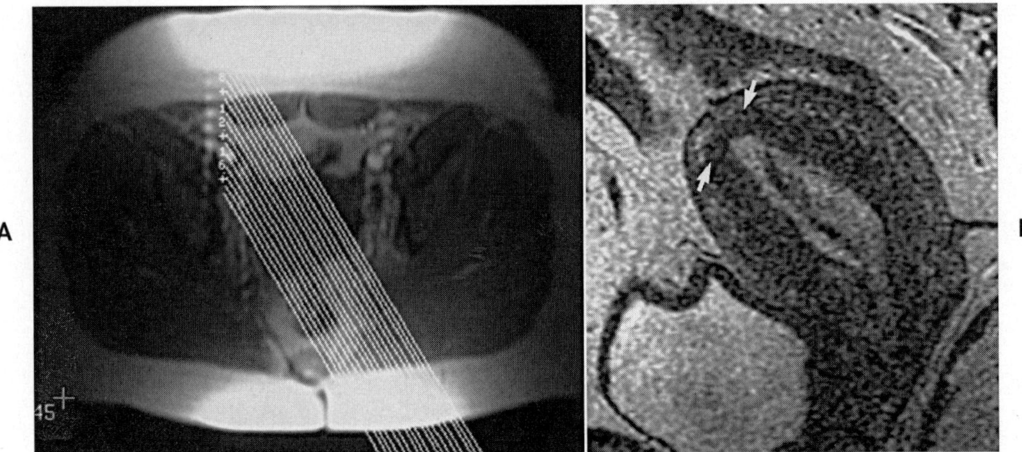

Fig. 7-7 Off-axis images of the uterus (same patient as in Figs. 7-5 and 7-6) are planned from the topogram **(A)** and **(B)**. One of the resulting oblique images shows the junctional zone to be completely intact all around the endometrial cavity *(short white arrows)*. For comparison with Fig. 7-6, this image was obtained with a 16-cm FOV, 3-mm slice thickness, 0.5-mm gap, a matrix of 192, and two signal averages.

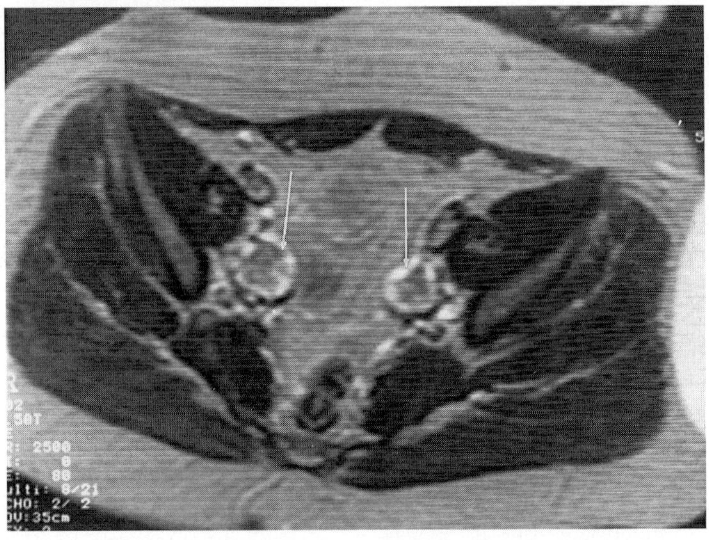

Fig. 7-8 Axial T2-weighted images (0.5T) showing the MR findings of bilateral polycystic ovaries *(long white arrows)*.

stalk) and in size, ranging from a few millimeters to as large as the endometrial cavity itself. They can even prolapse through the endocervical canal. They are most often benign, being either hyperplastic or adenomatous, and rarely develop into carcinoma or carcinosarcoma.

Diagnostic techniques. The diagnosis of endometrial polyps is based on the clinical findings. Hysteroscopy is the most sensitive (100%) and specific (96%) diagnostic procedure.[7]

Ultrasonography. Transabdominal ultrasonography has had limited success in detecting endometrial polyps. The transvaginal approach to sonography of the uterine cavity has allowed more accurate imaging and may help detect polyps, but in many cases this is difficult. If the polyp is on a stalk, it may be mobile, and the detection of motion or alteration in its position may be appreciated during the ultrasound examination.

Magnetic resonance imaging. The MR appear-

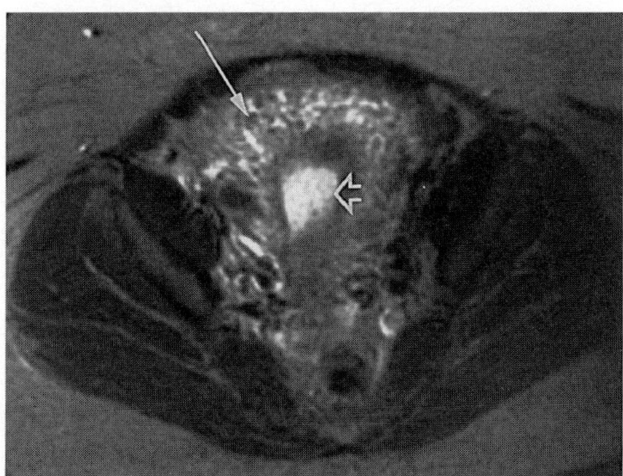

Fig. 7-9 Axial T2-weighted image of a woman with an ectopic pregnancy, showing the endometrial thickening *(open white arrow)* and markedly increased signal in the myometrium *(long white arrow)*, and the vascular engorgement and edema secondary to the hormonal stimulation.

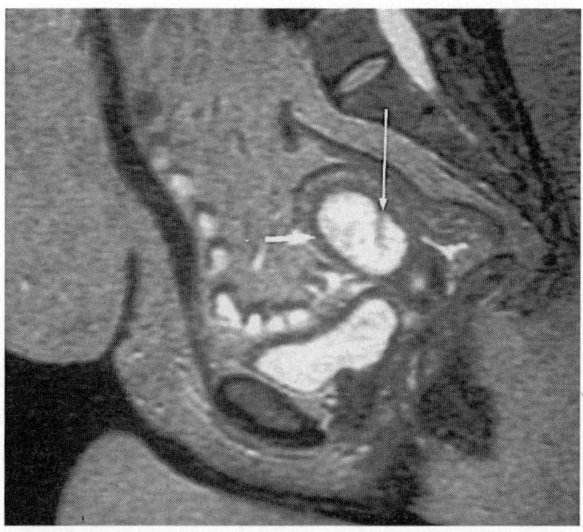

Fig. 7-10 Sagittal T2-weighted images of the uterus in a postmenopausal woman. The endometrial cavity is abnormally widened *(short white arrow)*. At hysterectomy, this patient had a large hyperplastic polyp filling the cavity of the endometrium. The MR findings, although abnormal, were not diagnostic of a polyp. In retrospect, there is a linear low signal intensity area *(long white arrow)*, which may represent the stalk of the polyp. Note the appearance of the normal postmenopausal myometrium, which is thin and homogeneously low in signal intensity.

ance, similar to that of hyperplasia and carcinoma, is again endometrial thickening seen on T2-weighted images (Fig. 7-10). No specific signs or features have been described on unenhanced MR to help differentiate polyps from these two entities. There is some possible advantage to using IV gadolinium. In Hricak and colleagues' study, the detection of polyps was significantly improved by use of gadolinium: 11 of 14 cases were correctly detected on enhanced gadolinium images versus five of 14 on the T2 images alone.[1] This may be one of the very few instances in which IV contrast may be helpful in examination of the benign uterus.

Uterine instrumentation

Injury to the endometrium as a result of instrumentation, most commonly curettage, is known as Asherman's syndrome. It leads to amenorrhea or hypomenorrhea, particularly if there is concurrent endometritis. It can also lead to infertility, and if the patient does become pregnant it may be complicated by premature labor or placenta increta or percreta.

Pathology. Pathologically, the endometrial cavity is narrowed or even obliterated with synechiae or adhesions consisting of fibrous tissue. Usually, there is no significant inflammation. It is believed that the scars result from vigorous curettage.[8]

Diagnostic techniques. Diagnosis is made either by direct visualization on hysteroscopy or by HSG. The patient usually proceeds to hysteroscopy to confirm the diagnosis, and also in an attempt to

remove and lyse as many of these scars as possible. An inflated intrauterine device (IUD) can be placed in the cavity to hold it open and prevent reformation of the adhesions.

Hysterosalpingography. The HSG findings are typically of a small, distorted, and narrowed uterine cavity. The cavity may be partially obliterated, and the contrast may pass around the scars or "islands" with contrast surrounding.[9] The filling defects are sharply demarcated and may be linear or triangular (Fig. 7-11). Multiple linear, transverse filling defects are seen, representing the bands of scar tissue.

Magnetic resonance imaging. MRI is not generally used to image patients with Asherman's syndrome, because it can be diagnosed by a less expensive modality (HSG). The MR findings in one case that was confirmed hysteroscopically have been described by Dykes and colleagues.[10] In this patient the T2-weighted images showed no normal endometrium or junctional zone signals. She was 1 month post partum, putting the uterus at increased risk of injury. The authors postulated that MRI could provide a precise grading of the severity of the scarring process.

The changes of the endometrium as seen on MRI after an uncomplicated dilation and curettage have also been described by Ascher and col-

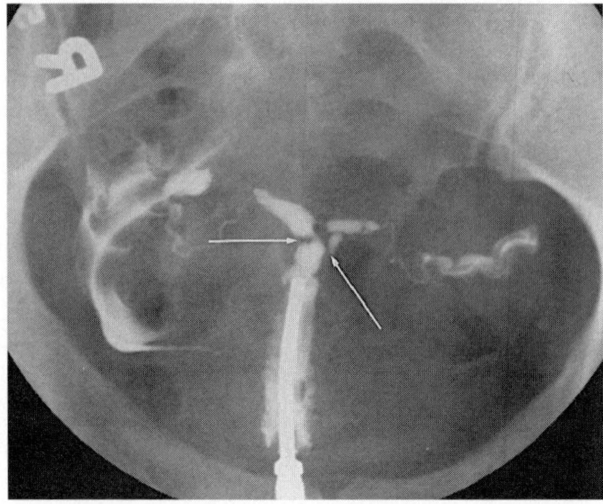

Fig. 7-11 Hysterosalpingogram (HSG) of a 40-year-old woman with Asherman's syndrome. She had a history of two first-trimester spontaneous abortions, followed by dilatation and evacuation. She had undergone resection of multiple synechiae 1 year before this study. The HSG shows multiple filling defects caused by extensive synechiae *(long white arrows),* with resultant marked narrowing of the uterine cavity.

leagues.[11] The most common finding was of curvilinear areas of low signal on T2-weighted images in the endometrial cavity. These were seen early on and either completely resolved or decreased in size on later scans, in all cases. It was thought that the areas most likely represented clot. The endometrial and junctional zone thicknesses were not changed in most cases.

DISEASES OF THE MYOMETRIUM
Normal myometrium

As in the endometrium, two major imaging modalities are used to characterize the myometrium: MRI and ultrasonography. CT has no defined role in myometrial evaluation but has many applications in pelvic imaging in general. The appearance of the uterus and myometrium is similar to that of other soft tissues such as skeletal muscle. The myometrium enhances rapidly after injection of iodinated contrast agents. This allows depiction of the endometrial cavity, which is more obvious when there is fluid within the cavity.

The sonographic appearance of the myometrium does not change with age or menstrual cycle,[12] unlike the MR appearance, which does so change. On sonography the myometrium is homogeneously of low to medium echogenicity.

On MRI the myometrium is best characterized on T2-weighted images (Fig. 7-12), which permit clear delineation of the endometrium, junctional

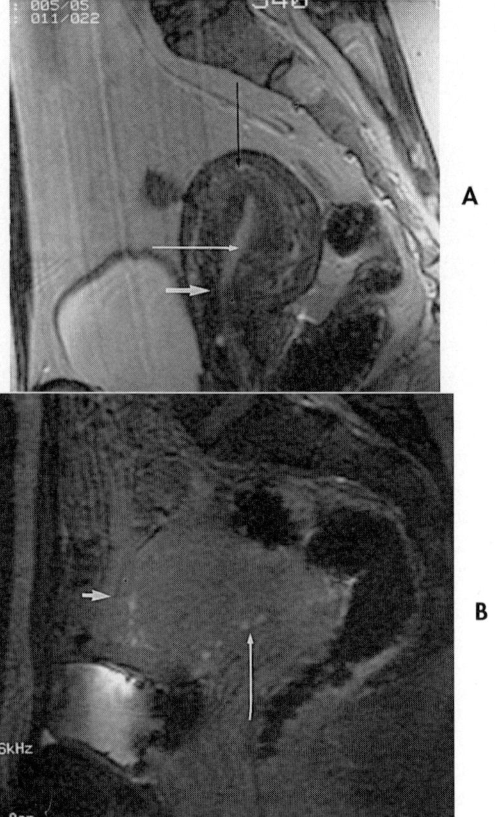

Fig. 7-12 A, The normal myometrium on T2-weighted images acquired with the phased array coil shows three layers: the endometrium centrally *(long white arrow),* junctional zone *(short white arrow),* and myometrium *(long black arrow).* **B,** The arcuate vessels can be identified on this gradient recalled echo in the steady state (GRASS) image in another patient *(long white arrow).* These clearly lie within the myometrium, below the serosal surface *(short white arrow).*

zone, myometrium, and serosal layer. The myometrium is really composed of three layers, starting with the junctional zone and the inner and outer layers of the muscular component beyond the junctional zone. These latter two layers are divided by the arcuate vessels, which can now be routinely visualized (Figs. 7-12 and 7-13). They do not differ in signal intensity at any point, but it is useful to note the location of the arcuate arteries dividing the inner and outer myometrium. These vessels can also be seen as echogenic foci on sonography when they are calcified, as they commonly are in older women. The normal myometrium shows cyclic changes according to the menstrual cycle.

In the proliferative phase the myometrium is of

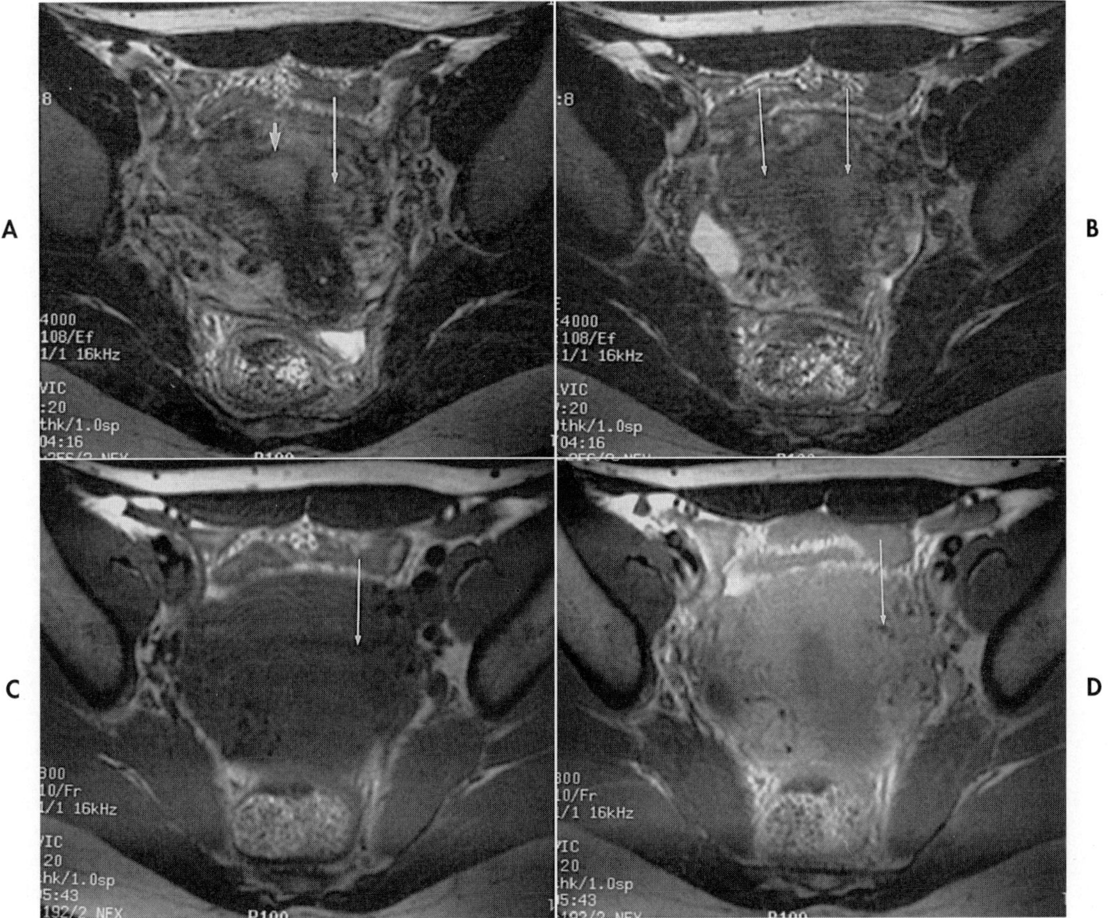

Fig. 7-13 A 31-year-old woman with a normal uterus at subsequent hysterectomy. **A, B,** Axial T2-weighted images of the uterus show a heterogeneous appearance to the myometrium, with focal areas of high signal *(long white arrows),* which are normal, especially with the normal junctional zone *(short white arrow).* This should not be mistaken for adenomyosis. The same areas of high signal are seen before **(C)** and after **(D)** gadolinium administration as nonenhancing branches of the arcuate vessels in the myometrium.

relatively low T2-weighted signal intensity, similar to skeletal muscle. Myometrial contractions may cause problems of interpretation on T2-weighted images, as they resemble leiomyomas or adenomyosis. Since there are usually at least two imaging planes, the contraction, which should be transient, should not be apparent on both sets of images.[13] In the secretory phase the signal rises in response to increasing blood flow, edema, and generalized vascular engorgement. This is even more pronounced in pregnancy (see Fig. 7-9). In postmenopausal women the uterus atrophies and becomes smaller. In the myometrium the signal drops and the zonal differentiation is diminished. As a result of the decreased signal of the myometrium, the junctional zone is no longer seen separately.

Similarly, in the prepubescent uterus, there is no clearly separate uterine junctional zone, and the uterus itself will be small (Fig. 7-14).

Leiomyomas

Leiomyomas are the most common neoplasm of the uterus, occurring in up to 30% of women over 30 years of age. They are rare in women under 18 and in postmenopausal women. They are usually multiple, and the most common site in the uterus is an intramural one. They occur more commonly in black women than in whites. They are hormone sensitive, with a higher ratio of estrogen to progesterone receptors than is normally seen in the myometrium. They are thus hormonally sensitive, becoming larger in women who are pregnant or are

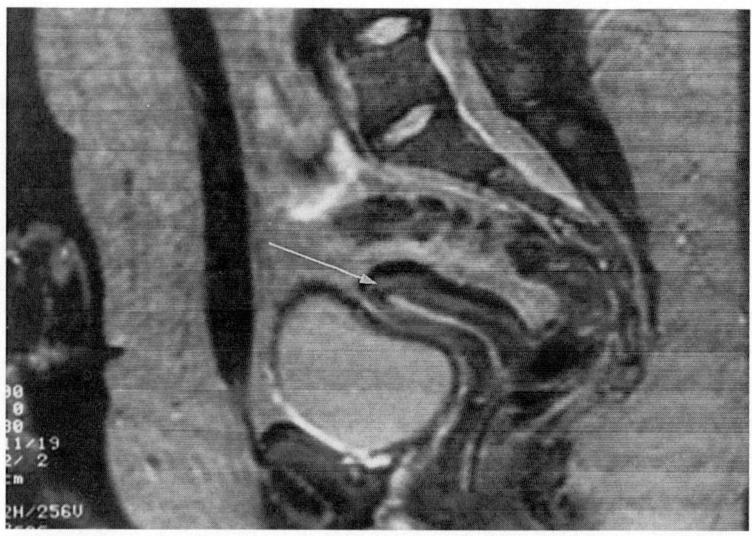

Fig. 7-14 T2-weighted sagittal image (0.5T) of a prepubescent uterus shows no clearly separate uterine junctional zone *(long white arrow),* and the uterus itself is small.

taking estrogen, and smaller after menopause and in women taking luteinizing hormone–releasing hormone agonists.

Clinical presentation. Leiomyomas may have a variety of presenting signs and symptoms, and can also be clinically occult in many women. Most commonly they cause bleeding (hypermenorrhea) and pain, and when very large, compression of adjacent organs (see Fig. 7-1). Thus, when the bladder is compressed, the patient will experience urinary frequency and even ureteral compression, with resultant hydronephrosis. The pelvic vessels may be compressed, leading to venous insufficiency with leg edema. Leiomyomas are also thought to cause infertility, especially when in a submucosal location. It is believed that they can cause an obstruction to implantation of the fertilized ovum. They are also the source of problems when present in the gravid uterus, causing compression of and obstruction to the growing fetus. When very large, they can block the birth canal and may be so obstructive as to necessitate cesarean section.

Location. The most common organ of origin is the uterus, but leiomyomas can occur in the fallopian tubes, broad ligament, cervix, and ovary. Leiomyomas may occur exclusively in the cervix, representing about 8% of all leiomyomas.[14] Within the uterus, leiomyomas essentially may arise anywhere, in a submucosal, subserosal, or intramural location; last-named is the most common. Subserosal lesions may become pedunculated and markedly exophytic. Pedunculated ones most com-

monly arise from the fundus of the uterus. The exact origin of these leiomyomas may often be difficult to determine.

Pathology. Leiomyomas are classified as mesenchymal, smooth muscle tumors. They appear similar to the uterine corpus but may change in appearance as they grow, degenerating and developing areas of necrosis and hemorrhage. Submucosal lesions in particular may become hemorrhagic and ulcerate, leading to uterine bleeding. Hemorrhage, necrosis, myxoid change, and hypercellular foci are all more likely to occur when a woman is pregnant or undergoing high-dose progesterone therapy. Cystic degeneration, with central liquefaction, may also occur. Histologically the most common degenerative changes are hyaline fibrosis (60%) and edema (50%). Hemorrhage is seen in 10% and cystic degeneration and microcalcification in 4% of all leiomyomas at pathologic examination.

Sarcomatous degeneration is rare, occurring in less than 1% of all leiomyomas. It is seen in older women in their fifties, in whom the incidence is 0.67 per 100,000 women. Intramural and cervical leiomyomas are at increased risk of sarcomatous degeneration.[15] Since leiomyomas are so common, leiomyosarcomas account for 25% of all uterine sarcomas.

Diagnostic techniques. Several specific features of leiomyomas require special attention by diagnostic imaging. These are primarily their detection, followed by the size, specific location (s), status (internal features such as degeneration) and

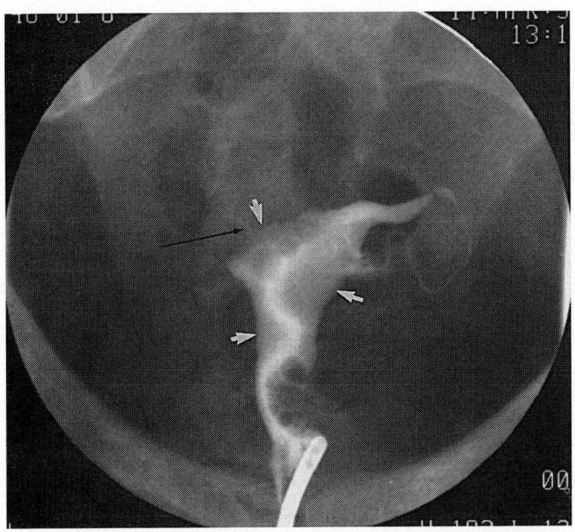

Fig. 7-15 Typical HSG appearance of multiple uterine leiomyomas *(short white arrows)*, causing marked distortion of the endometrial cavity. There is poor filling of the right fallopian tube *(long black arrow)* due to obstruction by the leiomyomas. Note several small air bubbles, which can cause a potential diagnostic dilemma.

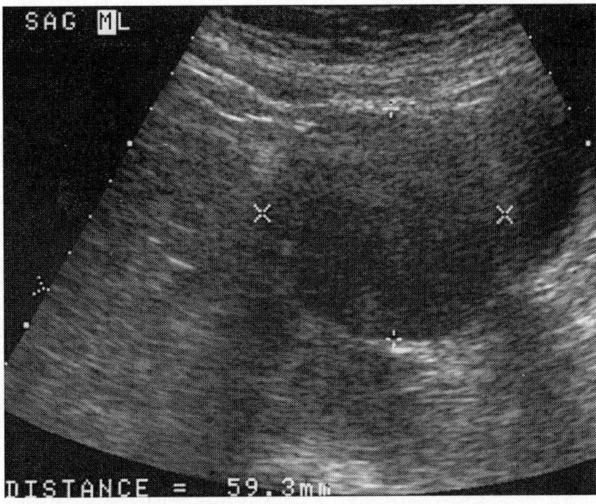

Fig. 7-16 Typical sonographic appearance of a large leiomyoma, which in this case is predominantly hypoechoic, probably because of a large amount of smooth muscle within the lesion.

effects of therapy. Imaging should provide the details for planning surgery (e.g., is the leiomyoma amenable to hys-teroscopic removal?).

Hysterosalpingography. HSG is a common diagnostic imaging modality used in the evaluation of patients with infertility. In view of the increased incidence of infertility due to the presence of leiomyomas, it consequently becomes a common diagnostic study for the detection of leiomyomas. The typical appearance of a leiomyoma is of a smooth, well-defined filling defect that protrudes in the lumen of the endometrial cavity. The appearance relates to the size and location of the lesion. Submucosal lesions cause an impression on the cavity, projecting into it to cause significant mass effect and distortion (Fig. 7-15).

It is important to reduce the possibility of air bubbles entering the cavity. Usually, over multiple films, the air bubbles will move. The leiomyoma may be large enough to cause obstruction to the fallopian tubes (Fig. 7-15). The sensitivity and specificity of HSG relative to MRI for detecting leiomyomas are low. No numerical data are available because there are no prospective studies comparing the two modalities. HSG can perform well when compared with findings at surgery. In a large study of over 800 women in 1969,[16] the preoperative HSG diagnosis was correct in 88% of cases. As would be expected, this study also showed that the diagnostic accuracy rate was highest for submucosal leiomyomas.

Ultrasonography. The classic appearance of leiomyomas on sonography is of large, mild to moderately echogenic, heterogeneous masses (Fig. 7-16). The uterine serosal outline may be distorted, as may the endometrial stripe. The echogenicity of the leiomyoma depends on the ratio of smooth muscle to fibrosis; with more fibrosis, there is increased echogenicity.[12] In some cases, leiomyomas may have a relative cystic appearance, being hypoechoic and only minimally echogenic, but lacking the through transmission and sharp posterior wall of a true cyst. Anechoic areas can be seen if cystic degeneration has occurred, and multiple bright echogenic foci if there is calcification. When there is degeneration, the sonographic features vary, depending on its type and degree.

The diagnosis of leiomyomas on sonography is not usually difficult, but there is a problem in trying to evaluate the number, size, and correct locations of all the lesions, especially when they are multiple. Ultrasound images often show only the tip of the iceberg and just the superior aspect of one of the myomas. Thus, it may be impossible to clearly define the location and number. Evaluation of leiomyomas in the retroflexed uterus can be particularly difficult.

Computed tomography. The most common finding on CT of leiomyomas is an enlarged uterus with a deformed contour.[17] They are usually isodense with the normal myometrium, unless they contain calcium. The latter is a very specific finding in leiomyomas, and its detection usually makes the diagnosis much easier. It often occurs in only a small part of the lesion and may have a circular or whorled shape, conforming to the rings of smooth muscle fibers. Calcification is not thought to be common on pathologic examination, although it was found on CT in 10% of the cases of Casillas and associates.[17] When the lesions degenerate, they develop areas of hyaline and cystic degeneration. Hyaline degeneration tends to liquefy, having a fluid density in the center of the isodense soft tissue mass. Occasionally there may be superimposed infection, with air and debris seen centrally.

Magnetic resonance imaging. The typical appearance of a leiomyoma on T2-weighted images is that of a well-defined uterine mass with a homogeneously low signal intensity, similar to that of muscle (Figs. 7-1, 7-2, and 7-17).[18] T1-weighted images, like CT, most commonly show an enlarged uterus. When there is central hemorrhagic degeneration, foci of high T1 signal blood may be seen. The T2-weighted appearance is so specific that there is little else that looks similar.

MRI has proved superior to sonography and HSG for diagnosing leiomyomas.[19,20] It has proved particularly useful when a leiomyoma presents as a pelvic mass, when the sonographic findings are indeterminate.[21] The difficulty in this situation may lie in determining the site of origin of the mass (Fig. 7-18). If it is pedunculated or subserosal, or in an unusual location such as the fallopian tube (Fig. 7-19), the ovary should be identified separately and may appear normal. If the

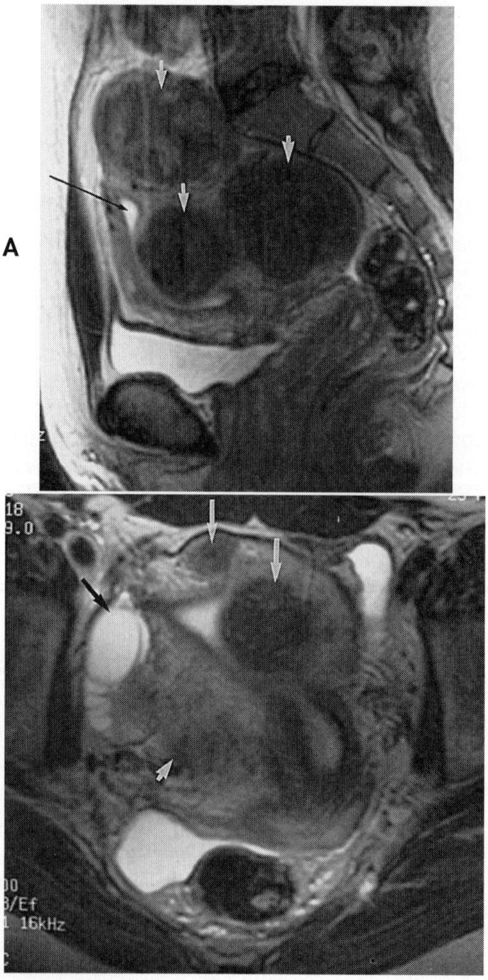

Fig. 7-17 A 29-year-old woman with multiple leiomyomas, showing the typical T2-weighted appearance. **A,** Sagittal T2-weighted image shows at least three leiomyomas *(short white arrows),* all posterior to the endometrial cavity, which is markedly distorted *(long black arrow).* **B,** The same patient in the axial plane shows the submucosal location of the lesion on the left. A simple cyst is seen on the right ovary *(black arrow).*

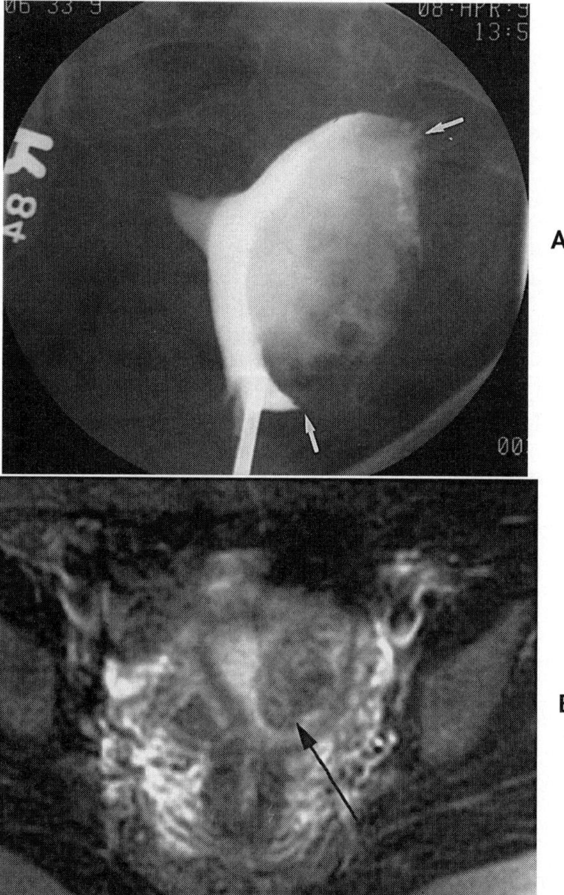

Fig. 7-18 A, HSG showing a large submucosal leiomyoma *(white arrows)* that markedly distorts the cavity. **B,** Axial T2-weighted image of the uterus in the same patient again shows the large submucosal leiomyoma *(long black arrow)* arising from the left lateral myometrium.

mass is in the ovary, it may be either a leiomyoma or a stromal ovarian tumor such as a fibroma or thecoma. HSG and MRI are both helpful for imaging the endocervix and its involvement with leiomyomas (Figs. 7-18 and 7-20).

The advantage of MRI lies in its clear depiction of the leiomyoma and its location. In planning surgery, the volume of submucosal surface involved is important, as well as its depth or extent into the myometrium (Figs. 7-2 and 7-21 to 7-23). This is important if hysteroscopic resection is being considered.

Degenerated leiomyomas may demonstrate a heterogeneous signal, with foci of high T2-weighted signal interspersed within the mass. As the degeneration progresses or the center becomes necrotic, the areas of high signal become confluent and larger in size (Figs. 7-1 and 7-23 to 7-25). Areas of calcification will be seen as areas of low signal. Carneous (red) degeneration will have high spinal or T1 weighted images.

A subgroup of leiomyomas have a high T2-weighted signal and heterogeneous architecture, and are not degenerative. In a study by Yamashita and colleagues, these lesions were found to represent the cellular leiomyomas and also to be edematous.[22] Gadolinium administration was helpful in differentiating these: the cellular lesions showed diffuse enhancement on early dynamic images; the

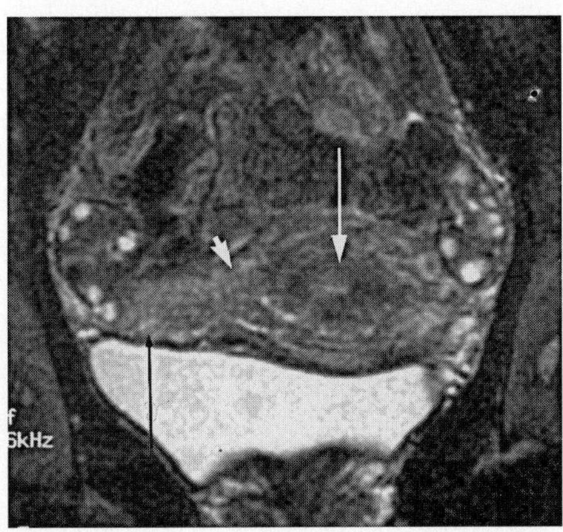

Fig. 7-19 Coronal T2-weighted image of the uterus *(long white arrow)* shows a leiomyoma, with signal similar to that of the myometrium, just to the right of the uterine body, extending along the fallopian tube (between *short white arrow* and *long black arrow*) toward the right ovary.

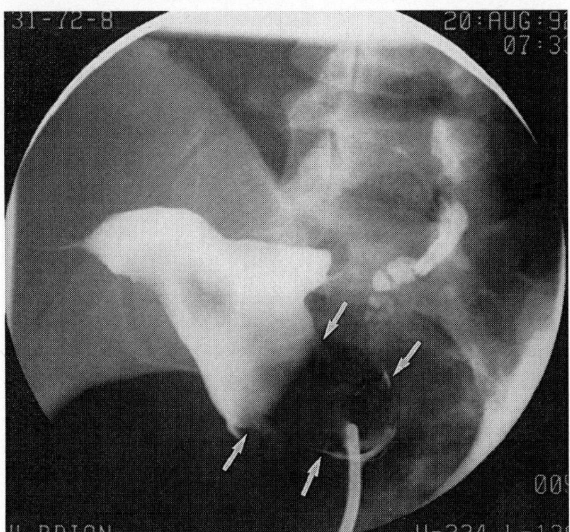

Fig. 7-20 Leiomyoma of the endocervix. HSG shows a large mass just above the catheter tip and the lesion is outlined by a thin layer of contrast material *(white arrows)*.

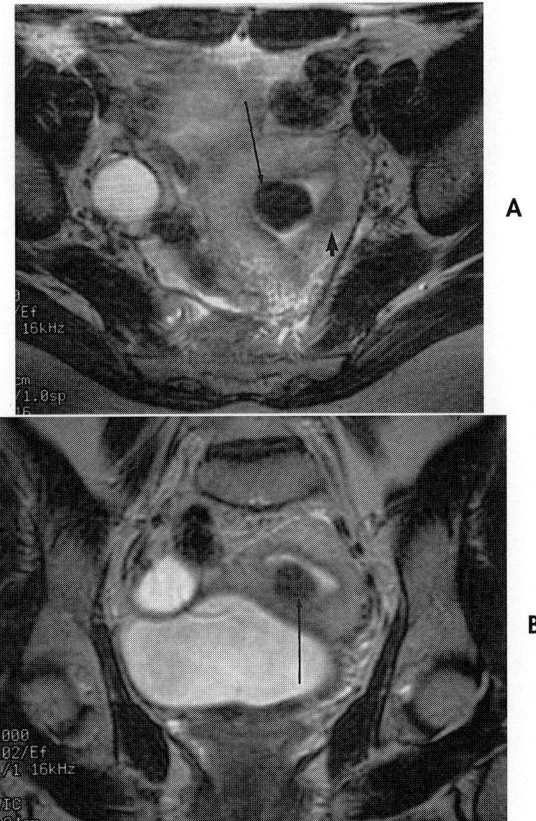

Fig. 7-21 A 33-year-old woman with two small submucosal leiomyomas on T2-weighted axial **(A)** and coronal **(B)** images. The axial image shows how much of the larger lesion *(long black arrow)* extends into the cavity of the uterus. The smaller lesion *(short black arrow)* has no significant mass but is based on the submucosa.

hyperintense degenerative lesions showed irregular delayed enhancement.

Sarcomatous change is very difficult to diagnose on any imaging modality. No specific imaging criteria are available. When a leiomyoma rapidly changes in size or appearance, a sarcoma should be suspected. When there is extensive degeneration, it is also possible (Fig. 7-26), particularly if significant interval growth can be demonstrated. However, it is important to beware of extreme degeneration in a leiomyoma, which may cause

it to appear neoplastic. This may cause confusion, especially when it occurs in a pedunculated leiomyoma, which may be confused with a primary ovarian neoplasm (Fig. 7-27). Even gadolinium is not helpful, as there will be heterogeneous areas of enhancement (Fig. 7-27).

MRI can help assess tumor burden when there are disseminated metastases (Fig. 7-28). When a leiomyoma is frankly malignant, it will be large, infiltrative, and very heterogeneous on T2-weighted images. There may be a very large mass with no clear site of origin (Fig. 7-28).

Treatment. Current therapies for leiomyomas are either surgical, ranging from myomectomy to full hysterectomy, or medical, usually a gonadotropin releasing hormone (GnRH) analog. The choice between the two depends on the symptoms and long-term objectives. If the patient is suffering from severe bleeding and is postmenopausal,

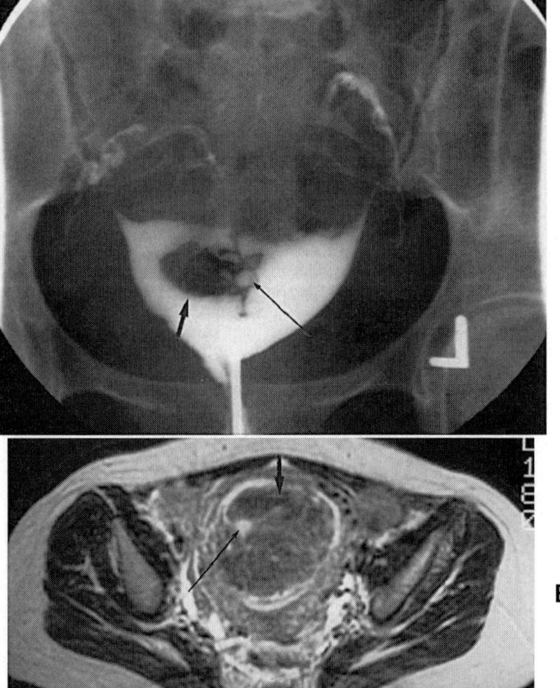

Fig. 7-22 Comparison of sonography and MRI in a 45-year-old woman with multiple leiomyomas. **A,** Transvaginal scan shows at least two leiomyomas *(short white arrows)* that are adjacent to the cervix *(long white arrow).* A third mass *(white arrow)* is outlined by cursors on film. It was unclear whether this represented a third leiomyoma. The bladder is seen anteriorly *(small white arrows)* **B,** Axial T2-weighted FSE image, at the same level as the ultrasound image, shows all three lesions to be typical leiomyomas *(short white arrows).* The cervix *(long white arrow)* is seen in the center with several high signal nabothian cysts. The bladder is seen anteriorly *(small white arrows),* correlating well with the ultrasound scan.

Fig. 7-23 A 40-year-old woman with a large submucosal leiomyoma shown on HSG and MRI. **A,** HSG shows a large intracavitary mass *(black arrow)* that is irregular and contains focal areas of contrast *(long black arrow)* within surface ulcers. **B,** Axial T2-weighted image shows the same mass extending into the cavity *(black arrow).* There are foci of high signal that represent fluid within the mass and on its surface *(long black arrow),* correlating with the HSG areas of ulceration.

a hysterectomy may be indicated. On the other hand, if the patient is younger and infertile, the goal of therapy is to preserve the uterus. More conservative surgical approaches are becoming popular, including hysteroscopic removal of small submucosal lesions. This is done under direct vision, usually by electrocautery. One of the problems with this approach is that the deep or inner margin of the leiomyoma is not visible. MRI can be very helpful in the preoperative planning of such an approach. Other, larger lesions can be removed by either laparoscopy or laparotomy. As the larger lesions can be very vascular, especially if near the uterine artery, an open surgical procedure is often necessary.

The GnRH analogs (e.g., leuprolide acetate [Lu-

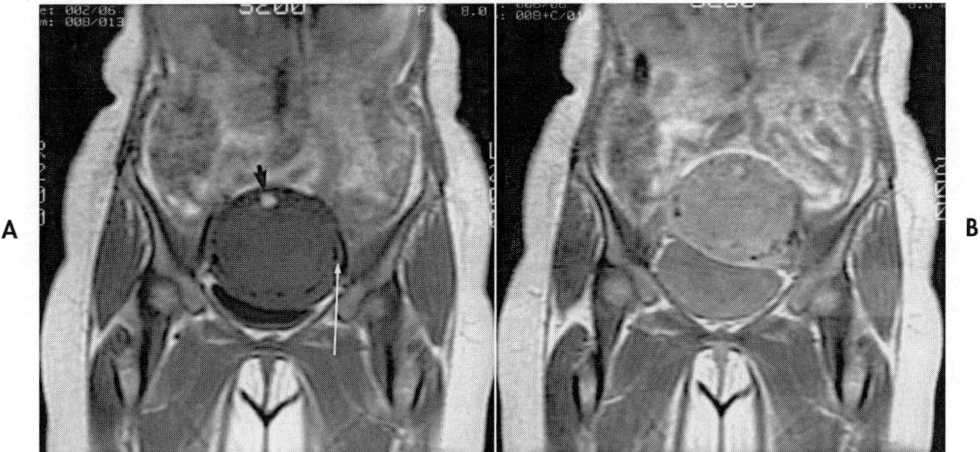

Fig. 7-24 Degenerative leiomyoma in the patient seen in Fig. 7-23. **A,** Coronal T1-weighted image shows a large uterine mass in the midline with a small high signal intensity focus superiorly *(short black arrow)*. As is normally seen with leiomyomas, there are multiple small feeding vessels in the periphery *(long white arrow)*. **B,** After injection of 10 ml IV gadolinium, the leiomyoma enhances, similarly to the myometrium.

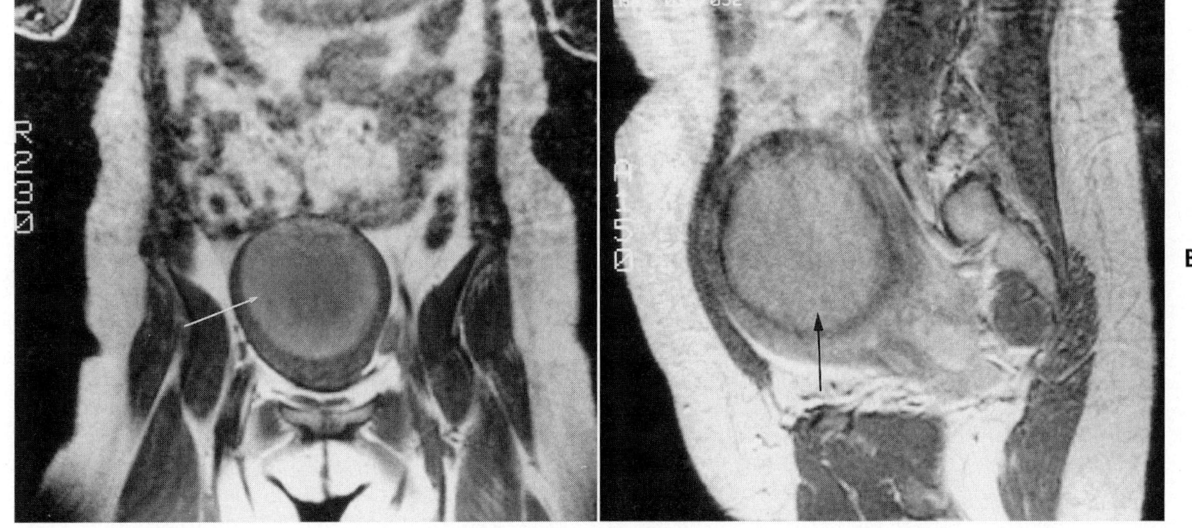

Fig. 7-25 A 29-year-old woman with a large leiomyoma who has been treated with a gonadotropin releasing hormone (GnRH) analog. **A,** Coronal T1-weighted image shows a large high signal intensity mass *(white arrow)* occupying the uterus. **B,** On the sagittal proton density image (TR 2500, TE 20), the leiomyoma *(black arrow)* is almost entirely high signal, compatible with extensive degeneration. This leiomyoma was not shrinking on therapy, and the patient subsequently underwent a myomectomy.

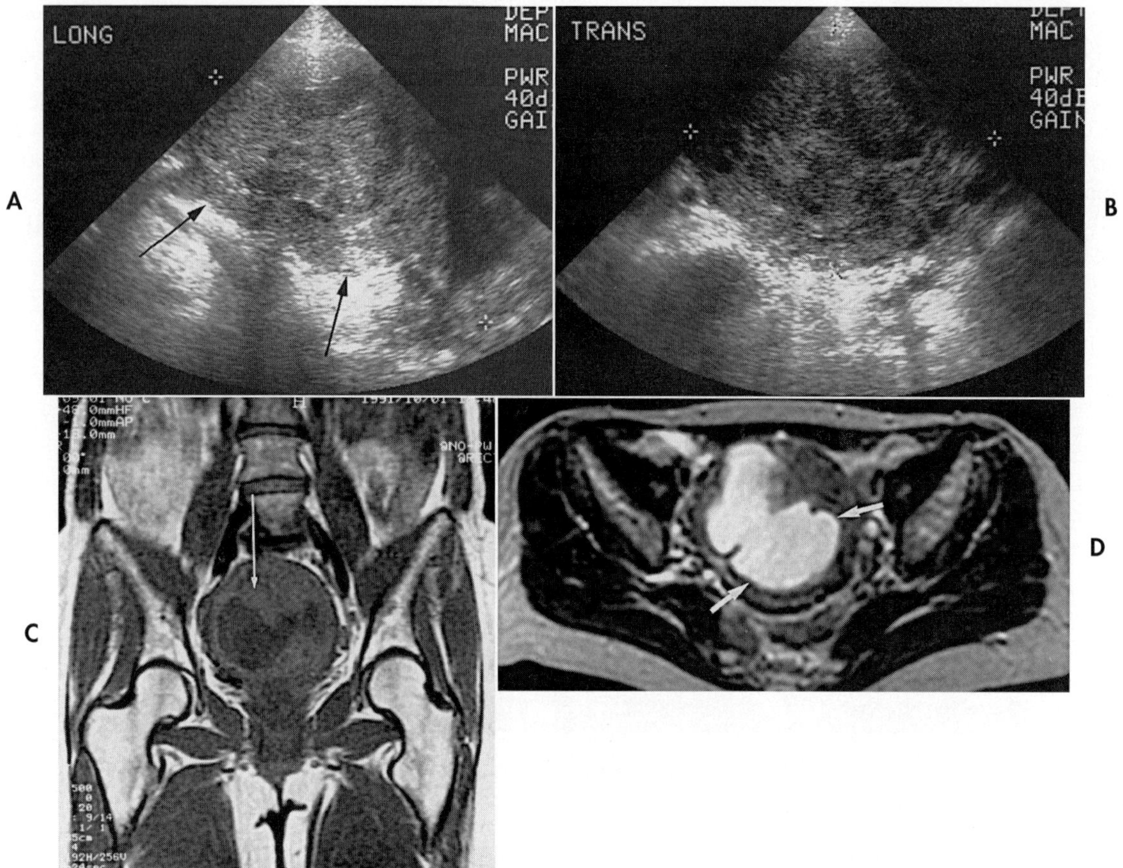

Fig. 7-26 A 48-year-old woman with a uterine sarcoma arising from a previous leiomyoma. **A, B,** Transabdominal (TAS) sonography performed 2 years previously showed a large heterogenous uterus *(black arrows and cursors),* compatible with multiple leiomyomas. **C,** Coronal T1-weighted image at 0.5T shows a large mass in the enlarging uterus, which has a large low signal area centrally. **D,** Axial T2-weighted image shows the uterine mass to be of very high signal, compatible with either a sarcoma or severe necrosis.

pron]) induce a hypoestrogenic state by inhibiting gonadotropins, thus constituting a medical oophorectomy. This hormonal manipulation is successful in reducing the size of leiomyomas and has been used both in infertile women and in symptomatic women who are perimenopausal. In this latter group, the goal of therapy is to avoid hysterectomy by using the medication to control the symptoms until the woman is fully postmenopausal.

Role of imaging in therapy. MRI has been used successfully to monitor the effects of medical therapy on leiomyomas. Zawin and colleagues demonstrated the application of MRI to the monitoring of 19 patients with leiomyomas in a double-blind study of Lupron.[23] The MR images were used to perform a volumetric analysis, which demonstrated a significant reduction of both the overall uterine volume and of the largest individual

leiomyoma in the patients receiving the drug. The authors also noted a decrease in the leiomyomas' gross vascularity as a result of the drug. This may be advantageous in patients who will proceed to surgery, as leiomyoma surgery can be associated with considerable blood loss. It is also important to know that in this same study the authors noted an increased difficulty in identifying the ovaries in patients on GnRH analogs. Ovarian follicular development is suppressed, making it difficult to identify the ovaries on T2-weighted images. On MRI, leiomyomas in patients on these drugs may appear very degenerated (see Figs. 7-24 and 7-26). Yamashita and colleagues showed that the leiomyomas that are markedly degenerated prior to therapy revealed less reduction in size than the cellular leiomyomas.[22]

MRI, because of its superb demonstration of leiomyomas, has great potential in providing a

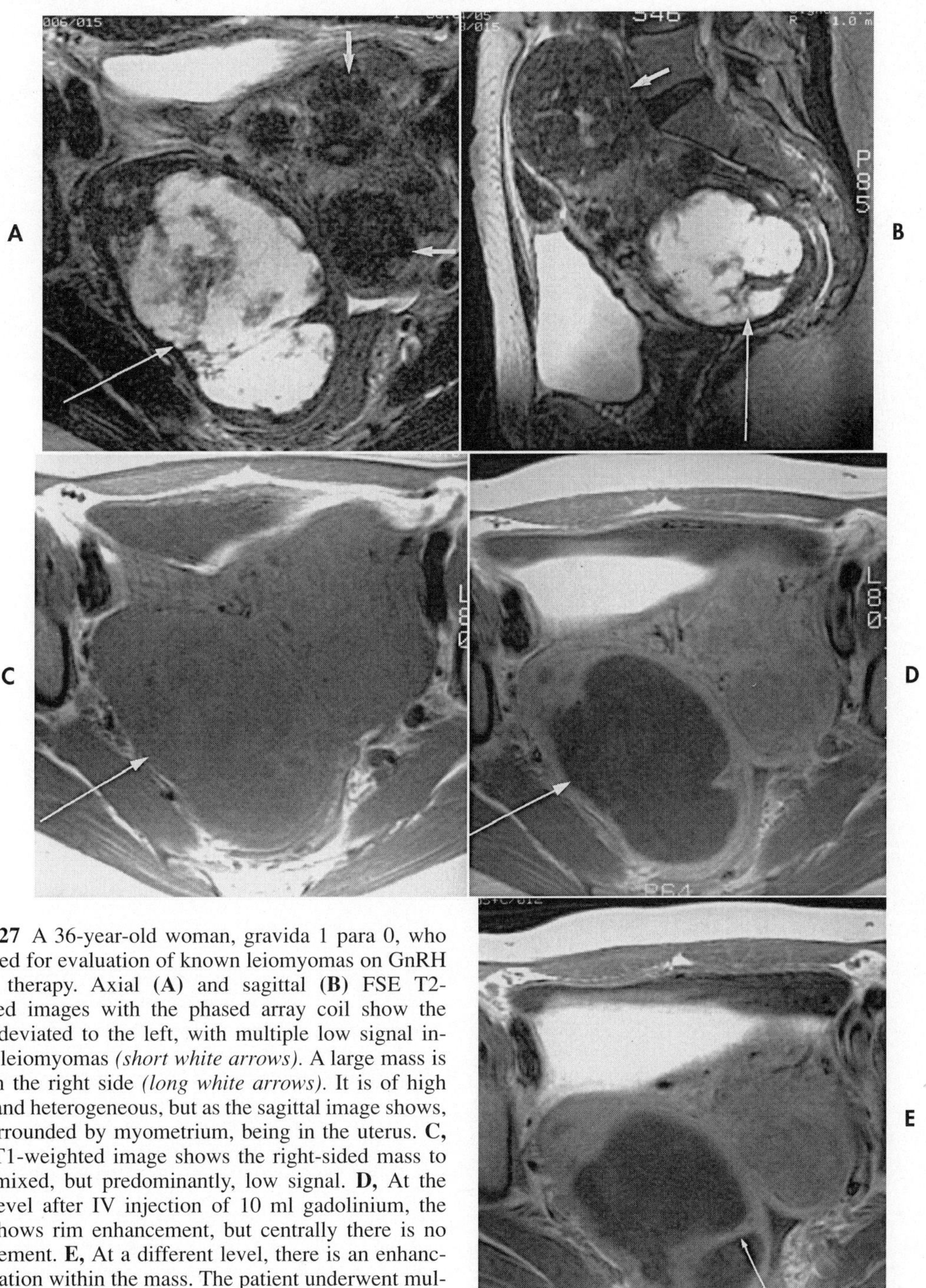

Fig. 7-27 A 36-year-old woman, gravida 1 para 0, who presented for evaluation of known leiomyomas on GnRH analog therapy. Axial (**A**) and sagittal (**B**) FSE T2-weighted images with the phased array coil show the uterus deviated to the left, with multiple low signal intensity leiomyomas *(short white arrows)*. A large mass is seen on the right side *(long white arrows)*. It is of high signal and heterogeneous, but as the sagittal image shows, it is surrounded by myometrium, being in the uterus. **C,** Axial T1-weighted image shows the right-sided mass to be of mixed, but predominantly, low signal. **D,** At the same level after IV injection of 10 ml gadolinium, the mass shows rim enhancement, but centrally there is no enhancement. **E,** At a different level, there is an enhancing sepation within the mass. The patient underwent multiple myomectomies, and the right mass was a large, degenerated leiomyoma.

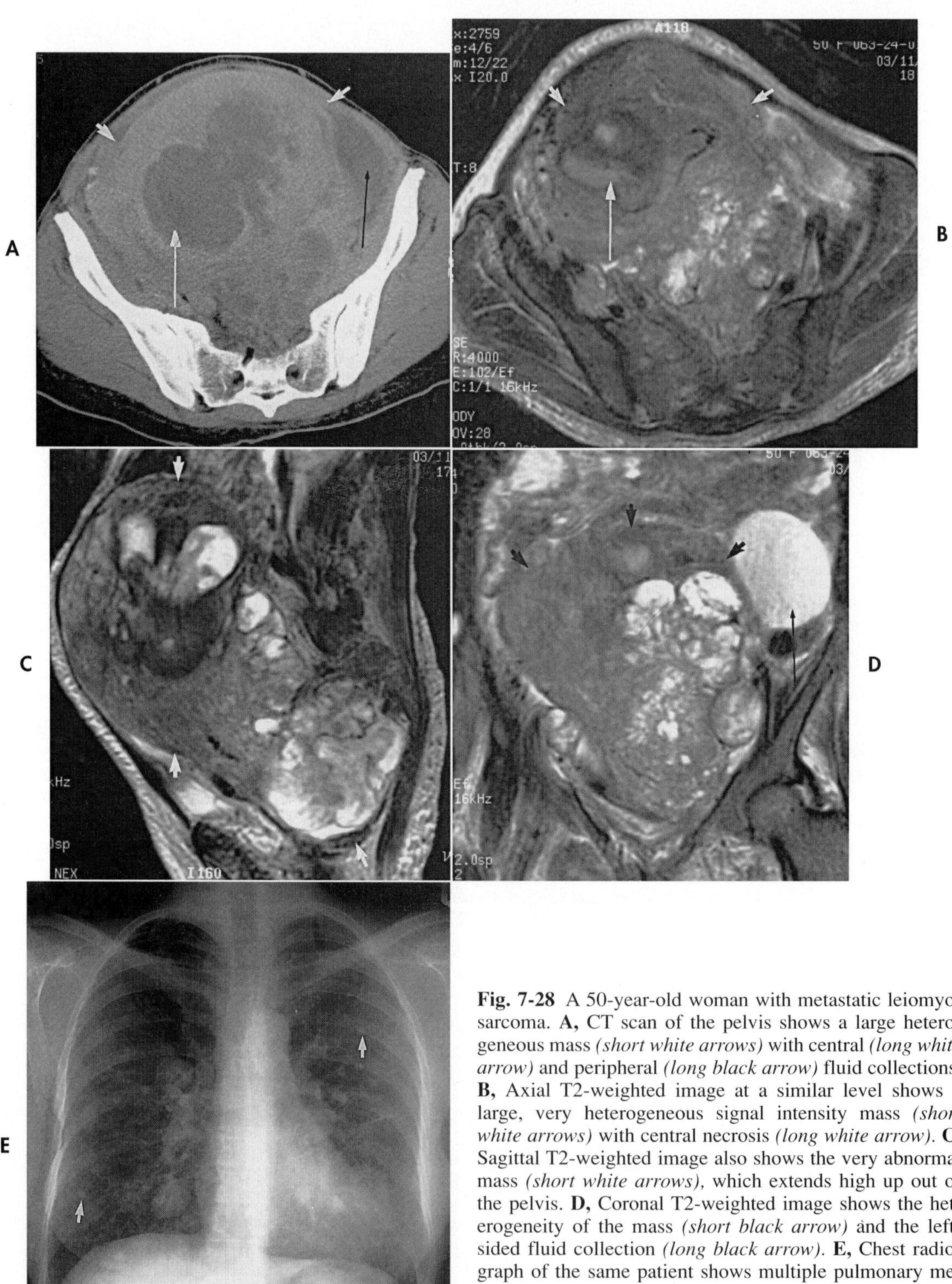

Fig. 7-28 A 50-year-old woman with metastatic leiomyosarcoma. **A,** CT scan of the pelvis shows a large heterogeneous mass *(short white arrows)* with central *(long white arrow)* and peripheral *(long black arrow)* fluid collections. **B,** Axial T2-weighted image at a similar level shows a large, very heterogeneous signal intensity mass *(short white arrows)* with central necrosis *(long white arrow)*. **C,** Sagittal T2-weighted image also shows the very abnormal mass *(short white arrows),* which extends high up out of the pelvis. **D,** Coronal T2-weighted image shows the heterogeneity of the mass *(short black arrow)* and the left-sided fluid collection *(long black arrow)*. **E,** Chest radiograph of the same patient shows multiple pulmonary metastases.

powerful modality for image-guided surgical intervention in treatment of leiomyomas. This is an area of future research and clinical application, as new open MR therapy units become available. For both diagnosis and therapeutic management of leiomyomas, MRI provides the most complete evaluation among the imaging tools available.

Adenomyosis

Adenomyosis is a benign disease of the uterus characterized by the ectopic presence of endometrial glands and stroma within the myometrium, and is associated with myometrial hyperplasia.[24] This is primarily a disease of premenopausal women; 70% to 80% of cases occur in women in their fourth and fifth decades, and 90% of these are parous.

The cause of adenomyosis is unknown. Various pathogenic mechanisms have been proposed, including uterine trauma of childbirth, chronic endometritis, and hyperestrogenemia, but none of these have proved causative.

Epidemiology. The true incidence and prevalence of adenomyosis are unknown. Population-based studies are lacking owing to inability to diagnose the disease preoperatively. The disease has traditionally been diagnosed pathologically from surgical specimens of hysterectomy. The frequency of diagnosis varies with the number of biopsy samples studied in each hysterectomy specimen, the selection criteria of myometrial specimens, and varying histologic criteria for the diagnosis. In view of all these variables, the estimates of frequency of adenomyosis vary widely in various series, from 5% to 70%, with a mean of 20% to 30%.

Pathology. Adenomyosis occurs in two forms: a more common diffuse form, and a less common localized form known as adenomyoma. Traditional pathologic criteria require the presence of endometrial glands within at least one low-power field (4 mm) beneath the endomyometrial junction. The ectopic mucosa in adenomyosis, as opposed to endometriosis, consists of nonfunctional basal endometrial layer, and thus is not altered by the hormonal changes of the menstrual cycle. The posterior myometrial wall is the most common site of involvement.

Clinical presentation. Adenomyosis has been labeled "the elusive disease" owing to lack of reliability of a preoperative clinical diagnosis.[24] The patient may be completely asymptomatic (19%) or may present with menorrhagia (22%), dysmenorrhea (15%), or dyspareunia (7%). Menorrhagia is possibly due to an increased endometrial surface of the hypertrophic uterus accompanied by diffuse intramural fibrosis, creating ineffective hemostasis during the myometrial contractions of menstrua-

tion. Dysmenorrhea may be due to excessive synthesis of prostaglandins by an enlarged endometrial surface, and to propulsive uterine contractions from the presence of endocavitary clots. Physical examination may show an enlarged tender uterus, usually the size seen is less than 12 gestational weeks.

About 60% to 80% of women with adenomyosis have associated pelvic pathology, including leiomyomas (35% to 55%), endometriosis (6% to 20%), endometrial polyps (2% to 3%), and adenocarcinoma of the uterus (1.4%). Adenomyosis is a frequent finding in pregnancy (17.2%), although obstetric or surgical complications are rare.[25]

Diagnostic techniques. Although myometrial biopsy (hysteroscopic or laparoscopic) has been tried for diagnosis of adenomyosis, this procedure is invasive in nature and is fraught with possible complications and sampling errors. The role of biochemical markers such as Ca-125 antigen for the diagnosis of adenomyosis remains to be established. Radiologic imaging remains the mainstay for the diagnostic work-up of adenomyosis.

Hysterosalpingography. HSG may demonstrate multiple marginal irregularities, speculations, or tuft defects in the endometrial cavity (Fig. 7-29). Unfortunately, such findings are not distinguishable from those produced by vascular or lymphatic intravasation. Using HSG, Marshak and Eliasoph were able to diagnose adenomyosis in only 38 of 150 cases (25%).[26] The finding may be very subtle, and it is important to obtain early films before there has been extensive spill into the peritoneum

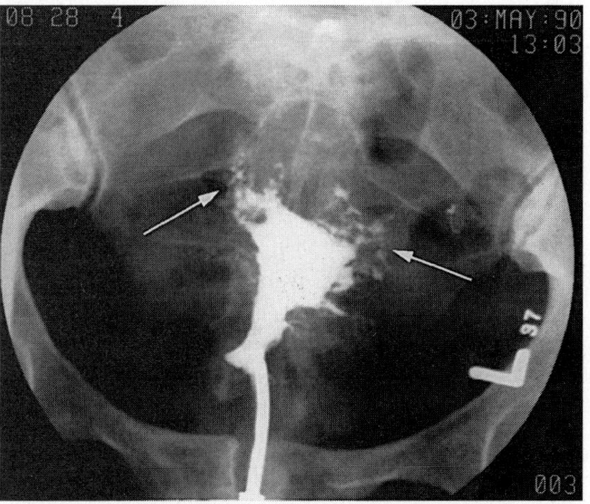

Fig. 7-29 HSG in an infertile 35-year-old woman demonstrates extensive irregularities of the endometrial cavity with multiple diverticular outpouchings *(white arrows)*. Histologic examination of the hysterectomy specimen revealed advanced adenomyosis. (Courtesy of Dr. Harry Z. Mellins.)

(Fig. 7-30). The overall diagnostic accuracy of HSG is so low that it is not currently used to diagnose adenomyosis.

Computed tomography. Although the role of CT in the diagnosis of adenomyosis has not been formally studied, it is presumed not to be of much clinical value because of low resolution of the zonal architecture of the uterus.

Ultrasonography. Ultrasonography is a useful and readily available tool for the diagnosis of adenomyosis. The sonographic picture of adenomyosis consists of thickened myometrium with asymmetry of anterior and posterior uterine walls, and increased echo texture of the myometrium with heterogeneous indistinct areas.

Siedler and colleagues used TAS to study 80 women undergoing hysterectomy, and demonstrated a 63% sensitivity and 97% specificity in distinguishing adenomyosis from leiomyomas.[27] Fedele and colleagues used TVS to study 43 women with suspected adenomyosis.[28] The diagnostic criteria included the presence of nonencapsulated, heterogeneous myometrial areas containing anechoic areas of 1 to 3 mm (Fig. 7-31). This study demonstrated a sensitivity of 80%, specificity of 74%, negative predictive value of 81%, and positive predictive value of 73% in diagnosing adenomyosis. The same group in another study of 405 women tried to distinguish adenomyomas from leiomyomas on the basis of TVS (Fig. 7-32).[29] For adenomyoma, the study resulted in 87% sensitivity, 98% specificity, 74% positive predictive value, and 99% negative predictive value. Overall, the sensitivity and specificity of TVS are far better than those of TAS for the detection of adenomyosis.

Magnetic resonance imaging. MRI has proved superior to TVS for the diagnosis of leiomyomas and is considered the preferred modality for the evaluation of adenomyosis (Fig. 7-33).[30,31] Adenomyosis is often seen as either diffuse or focal widening of the junctional zone (greater than 5 mm) on T2-weighted images, and a myometrial mass with indistinct margins of primarily low signal intensity on all sequences. Sometimes, high signal intensity areas on both T1 and T2-weighted images may occur within these areas, which represent hemorrhage. High signal areas that are seen only on T2-weighted images represent nonbleeding endometrial islands (Figs. 7-3 and 7-34).[32] The adenomyoma is similar in signal to a leiomyoma but appears much less defined, and its borders are indistinct (Fig. 7-35). Mark and associates were the first to report the use of MRI in differentiating adenomyosis from leiomyoma in 21 women.[33] Ten out of 12 leiomyomas and all eight cases of adenomyosis were correctly diagnosed. Togashi and colleagues studied 93 women with uterine enlargement prospectively (71 leiomyomas and 16 adenomyosis).[34] MRI accurately diagnosed the etiology of uterine enlargement in all but one of the cases. Hricak and colleagues used gadopentetate dimeglumine–enhanced T1-weighted MR images to study adenomyosis.[1] Although the widening of the junctional zone was more apparent after contrast administration, T2-weighted images were still superior to contrast-enhanced T1-weighted images in diagnosing adenomyosis.

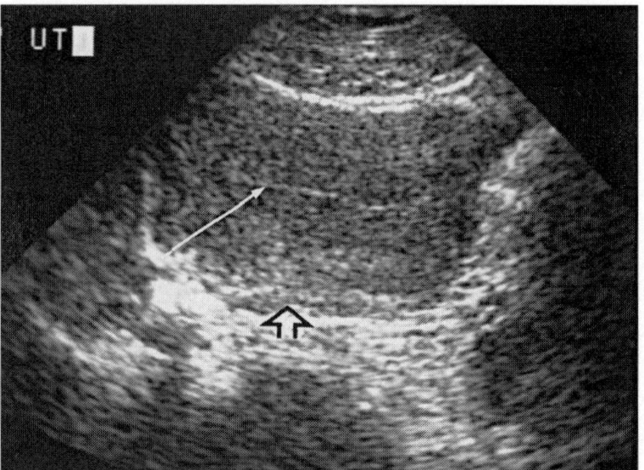

Fig. 7-31 Transverse view of the uterus seen on TAS of the uterus in a 22-year-old woman with a history of spontaneous abortion. There is diffuse asymmetric thickening of the myometrium, which has a heterogeneous echotexture *(open black arrow)*. The endometrium is normal *(long white arrow)*. Uterine leiomyomas were suspected on clinical examination, but the histologic appearance of the hysterectomy specimen revealed adenomyosis.

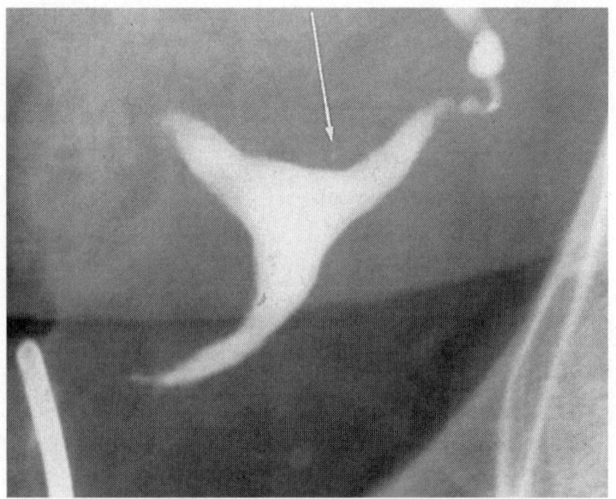

Fig. 7-30 Mild adenomyosis. HSG in a 39-year-old woman with right salpingectomy secondary to an ectopic tubal pregnancy reveals an area of subtle intravasation of contrast, in a small outpouching near the uterine fundus *(long white arrow)*.

After contrast administration the signal enhancement was lower in adenomyosis foci as compared with the normal myometrium in both diffuse and focal forms of the disease, and no rim enhancement was seen. The detection rate with all sequences in this study was 89% (17 of 19 cases), and both proton density and T2-weighted images showed similar sensitivity in detection and characterization of adenomyosis.

MRI can provide a full examination of the pelvis, specifically of the adnexa, in patients with adenomyosis or adenomyomas. It is important to

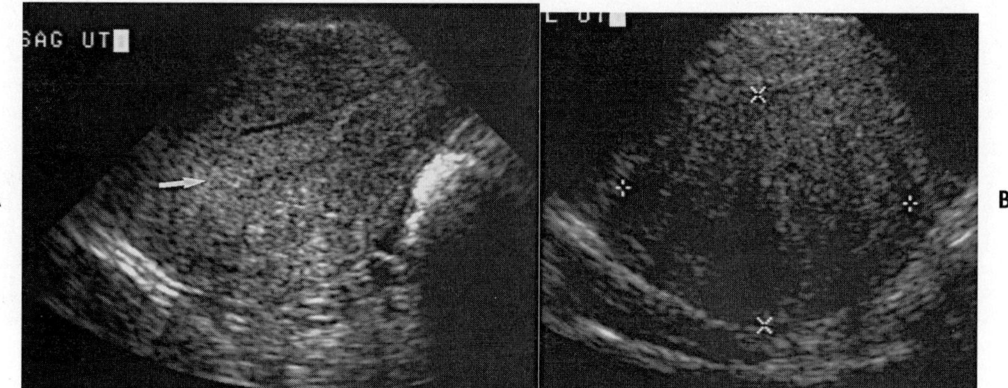

Fig. 7-32 Transvaginal sonogram (TVS) in a 28-year-old woman with a history of fibroid uterus. Sagittal **(A)** and transverse **(B),** images demonstrate nonencapsulated heterogeneous areas involving the posterior myometrium *(white arrow and cursors).* Pathologic examination revealed focal adenomyosis or adenomyoma.

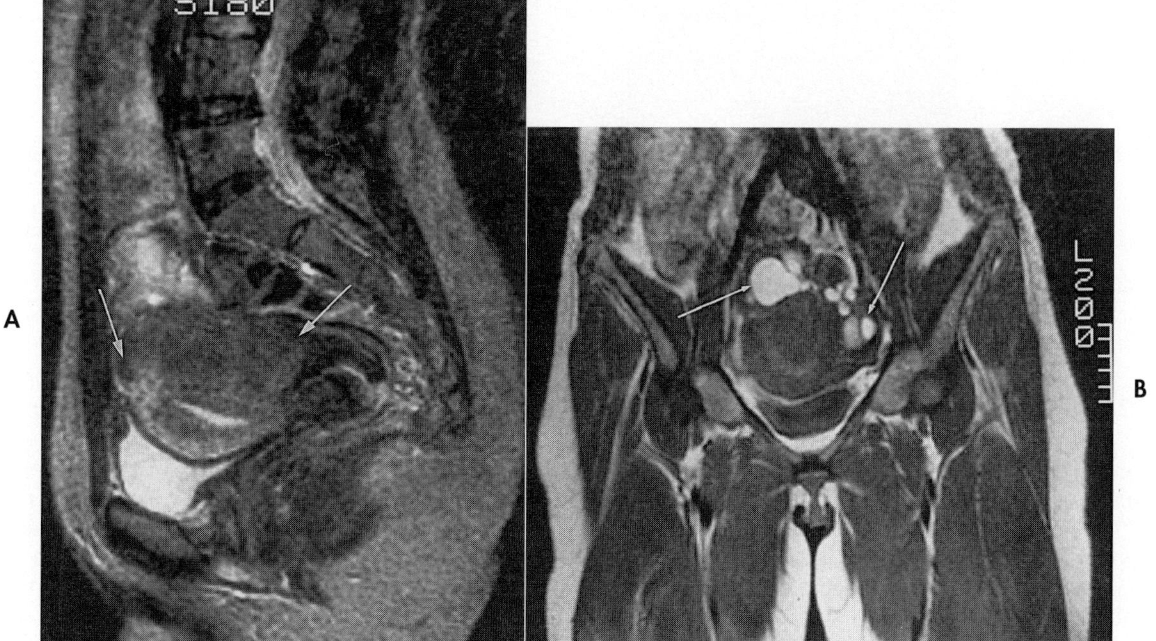

Fig. 7-33 A 30-year-old woman with infertility due to both endometriosis and a large uterine adenomyoma. **A,** Sagittal T2-weighted image shows an ill-defined low signal mass *(white arrows)* involving the posterior wall and fundus of the uterus representing the adenomyoma, and diffuse thickening of the junctional zone. **B,** Coronal T1-weighted MR images demonstrate multiple high T1 signal masses consistent with endometriomas *(long white arrows).*

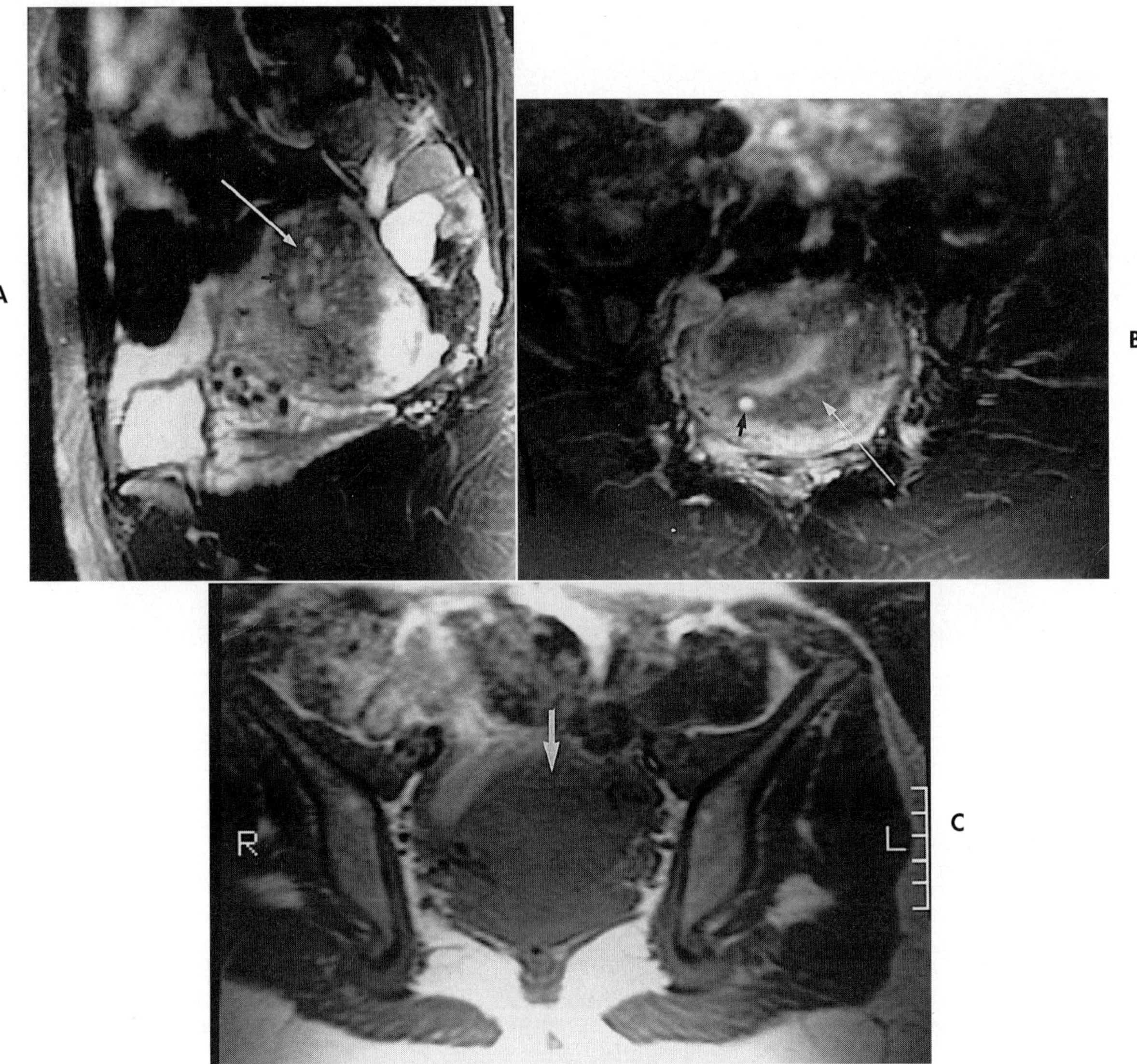

Fig. 7-34 A 45-year-old woman with adenomyosis. T2-weighted sagittal **(A)** and oblique off-axis **(B)** images show the irregularity and widening of the junctional zone of the uterus *(long white arrows),* with areas of high signal intensity in the myometrium *(short black arrows).* **C,** The corresponding oblique T1-weighted image shows the uterus *(white arrow)* (see also Fig. 7-3).

evaluate such women for any associated pathology such as endometriosis (Fig. 7-35).

Although adenomyosis was described as long ago as 1860 by Rokitansky, little is known about the epidemiology and pathogenesis of this potentially debilitating condition. With the current therapeutic approaches, it is critical to differentiate leiomyoma from adenomyosis; the former can be treated by myomectomy, whereas hysterectomy is the definitive treatment for severe forms of adenomyosis. In recent years, hormonal manipulation (GnRH, danazol) has been successfully tried for

medical management of adenomyosis, and reliable noninvasive means for monitoring the effects of such therapies are warranted. TVS and MRI offer such diagnostic means. It is hoped that these modalities will help provide new insights into the etiology and pathogenesis of adenomyosis.

Both ultrasonography and MRI have a major role to play in the evaluation of women with benign disease of the uterus. MRI is particularly advantageous in the work-up of women with infertility as illustrated in this chapter and even more. As illustrated in the Chapter 5 by Fielding and col-

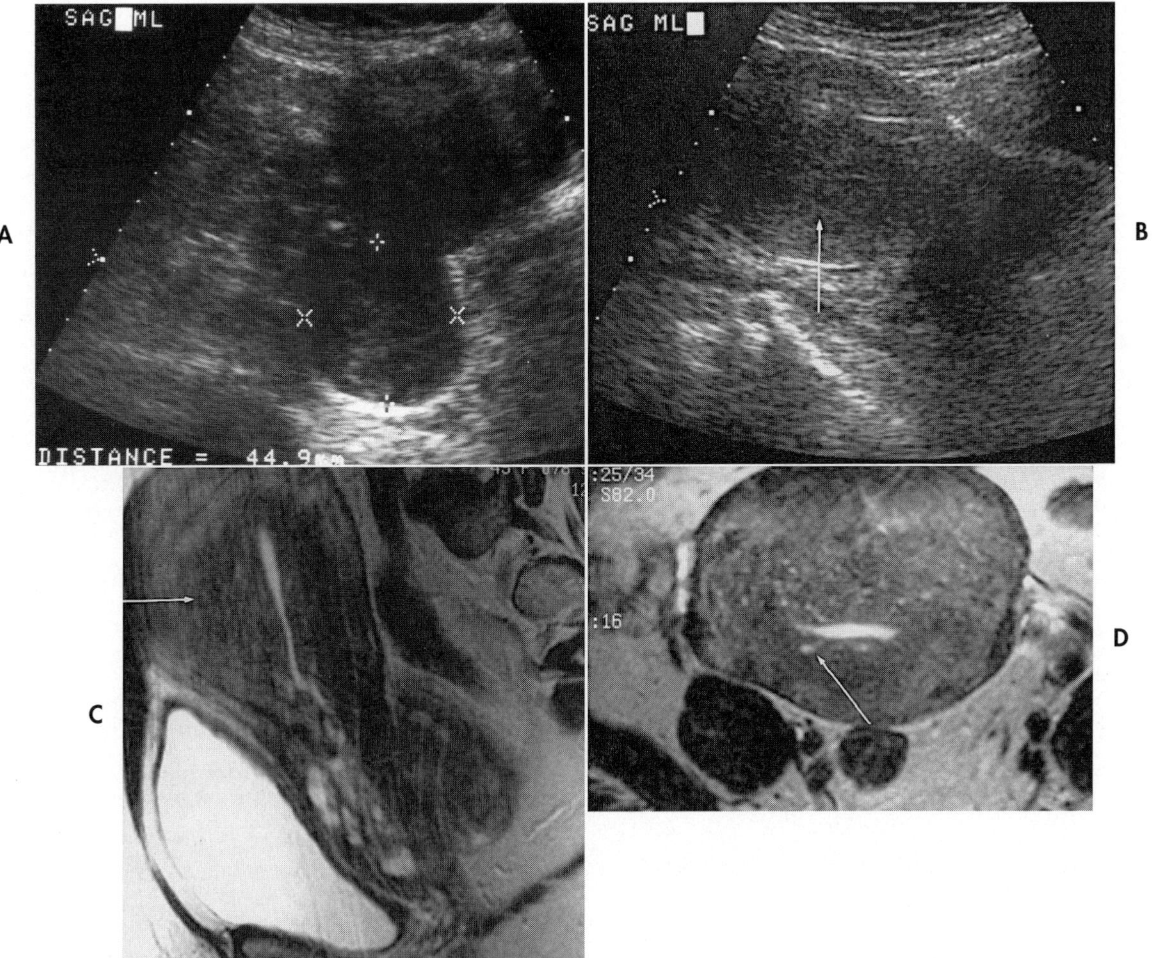

Fig. 7-35 Adenomyosis and multiple leiomyomas in a 45-year-old woman. **A,** Sagittal TAS demonstrates an exophytic mass in the cul-de-sac, with mildly thickened and **(B)** the heterogeneous myometrium *(arrow)*. Sagittal **(C)** and axial **(D)** T2-weighted MRI demonstrates the diffusely thickened junctional zone, with multiple punctate high signal areas within it *(arrows),* most likely representing nonbleeding endometrial islands.

leagues, MRI is excellent for the evaluation of women with congenital anomalies. In a single noninvasive study, many of the common causes of infertility can be assessed.

REFERENCES

1. Hricak H, Fink S, Honda G, Goranson H: MR imaging in the evaluation of benign uterine masses; value of gadopentetate dimeglumine–enhanced T1 weighted images, *AJR* 158:1043-1050, 1992.
2. Fleischer AC, Gordon AN, Entaman SS, Kepple DM: *Transvaginal sonography of the endometrium; current and potential clinical applications.* In Fleischer A, Romero R, Manning F, et al, editors: *The principles and practice of ultrasonography in obstetrics and gynecology,* ed 4, Norwalk, CT/San Mateo, CA 1991. Appleton & Lange, pp 583-595.
3. Mitchell DG, Schonolz L, Hilpert PL, et al: Zones of the uterus: discrepancy between US and MR images, *Radiology* 174:827-831, 1990.
4. Kurman RJ, Norris HJ: *Endometrial hyperplasia and metaplasia.* In Kurmam R, editor: *Blausteins's pathology of the female genital tract,* ed 3, New York, 1978, Springer-Verlag, pp 321-336.
5. Fleischer AC, Gordon AN, Entaman SS, Kepple DM: *Transvaginal sonography of the endometrium; current and potential clinical applications.* In Fleischer A, Romero R, Manning F, et al, editors: *The principles and practice of ultrasonography in obstetrics and gynecology,* ed 4, Norwalk, CT/San Mateo, CA, Appleton & Lange, pp 583-595.
6. Lin MC, Gosink BB, Wolf SI, et al: Endometrial thickness after menopause: effect of hormone replacement, *Radiology* 180:427-432, 1991.
7. Fedele L, Bianchi S, Dorta M, et al: Transvaginal ultrasonography versus hysteroscopy in the diagnosis of uterine submucosal myomas, *Obstet Gynecol* 5:745-748, 1991.
8. Yoder IC: *Hysterosalpingography and pelvic ultrasound.* In Yoder IC, *Imaging in infertility and gynecology,* Boston, 1988, Little, Brown, pp 139-143.
9. Tristant H, Benussa M: *Atlas d'hysterosalpingographie,* Paris, 1981, Masson, pp 119-129.

10. Dykes TA, Isler RJ, McLean AC: MR imaging of Asherman syndrome; total endometrial obliteration, *J Comput Assist Tomogr* 15:858, 1991.

11. Ascher SM, Scoutt LM, McCarthy SM, et al: Uterine changes after dilation and curettage; MR imaging findings, *Radiology* 180:433-435, 1991.

12. Fleischer AC, Entman SS: *Sonographic evaluation of the uterus and related disorders.* In Fleischer A, Romero R, Manning F, et al, editors: *The principles and practice of ultrasonography in obstetrics and gynecology,* ed 4, Norwalk, CT/San Mateo, CA, Appleton & Lange, pp 565-582.

13. Togashi K, Kawakami S, Kimura I, et al: Uterine contractions; possible diagnostic pitfall at MR imaging, *J Magn Reson Imaging* 3(6):889-893, 1993.

14. Fingerland A, Sikl H: Ganglioneuroma of cervix uteri, *J Pathol Bacteriol* 47:631, 1938.

15. Zaloudek C, Norris HJ: *Mesenchymal tumors of the uterus.* In Kurmam R, editor: *Blausteins's pathology of the female genital tract,* ed 3, New York, 1978, Springer-Verlag, pp 373-408.

16. Pietila K: Hysterography in the diagnosis of large submucus uterine fibroids. Acta Obstet. Gynecol. Scandinav. 48, Suppl. 5) 1969.

17. Casillas J, Joseph RC, Guerra JJ: CT appearance of uterine leiomyomas, *RadioGraphics* 10:999-1007, 1990.

18. Hricak H, Tscholakoff D, Heinrichs L, et al: Uterine leiomyoma: correlation of MR, histopathologic findings, and symptoms, *Radiology* 158:386-391, 1986.

19. Dudiak CM, Turner DA, Patel SK, et al: Uterine leiomyomas in the infertile patient; preoperative localization with MR imaging versus US and hysterosalpingography, *Radiology* 167:627-630, 1988.

20. Riccio TJ, Adams HG, Munzing DE, Mattrey RF: Magnetic resonance imaging as a adjunct to sonography in the evaluation of the female pelvis, *Magn Reson Imaging* 8(6):699-704, 1900.

21. Weinreb JC, Barkoff ND, Meigibow A, Demopoulos: The value of MR imaging in distinguishing leiomyomas from other solid pelvic masses when sonography is indeterminate, *AJR* 154:295-299, 1990.

22. Yamashita Y, Torashima M, Takahashi M, et al: Hyperintense uterine leiomyoma at T2-weighted MR imaging: differentiation with dynamic enhanced MR imaging and clinical implications, *Radiology* 189:721-725, 1993.

23. Zawin M, McCarthy SM, Scoutt L, et al: Monitoring therapy with a gonadotrophin-releasing hormone analog; utility of MR imaging, *Radiology* 175:503-506, 1990.

24. Vercellini P, Ragni G, Trespidi L, et al: Adenomyosis: a déjà vu?, *Obstet Gynecol Surv* 48:789-794, 1993.

25. Azizz R: Adenomyosis: current perspectives, *Obstet Gynecol Clin North Am* 16:1, 221, 1989.

26. Marshak RH, Eliasoph J: The roentgen findings in adenomyosis, *Radiology* 64:846, 1955.

27. Siedler D, Laing F, Jeffrey RB Jr, et al: Uterine adenomyosis: a difficult sonographic diagnosis, *J Ultrasound Med* 6:345, 1987.

28. Fedele L, Bianchi S, Dorta M, et al: Transvaginal ultrasonography in the differential diagnosis of adenomyoma versus leiomyoma, *Am J Obstet Gynecol* 167:603, 1992.

29. Fedele L, Bianchi S, Dorta M, et al: Transvaginal ultrasonography in the diagnosis of diffuse adenomyosis, *Fertil Steril* 58:94, 1992.

30. McCarthy SM: MR imaging of the uterus, *Radiology* 171:321, 1989.

31. Olson M, Posniak H, Tempany CM, Dudiak CM: MR imaging of the female pelvic region, *RadioGraphics* 12:445, 1992.

32. Ascher S, Arnold L, Patt R, et al: Adenomyosis: prospective comparison of MR imaging and transvaginal sonography, *Radiology* 190:803, 1994.

33. Mark AS, Hricak LW, Hendrickson MR, et al: Adenomyosis and leiomyoma: differential diagnosis with MR imaging, *Radiology* 171:531, 1987.

34. Togashi K, Ozasa I, Konishi I, et al: Enlarged uterus: differentiation between adenomyosis and leiomyoma with MR imaging, *Radiology* 166:111, 1989.

Harold V. Posniak and *Mary C. Olson*

The advent of diagnostic ultrasonography (US), computed tomography (CT), and magnetic resonance (MR) imaging has allowed direct visualization and evaluation of the normal and pathologic conditions of the uterus. Before this, radiologic evaluation relied on the effect of uterine pathology on adjacent organs as evidenced on barium studies and urography. This chapter discusses the epidemiology, clinical features, and pathology of endometrial carcinoma, uterine sarcoma, and gestational trophoblastic disease. We describe our techniques for US, CT, and MR imaging and illustrate the normal uterus and examples of the different uterine malignancies. The strengths and weaknesses of the different imaging modalities are discussed. Finally, the management of these tumors is briefly addressed.

TECHNIQUE
Ultrasonography

The female pelvis can be examined by US via transabdominal and transvaginal approaches. Transabdominal ultrasonography requires the patient to have a full urinary bladder to provide an acoustic window. Real time examinations are performed and images taken in sagittal and transverse planes; additional images can be taken in oblique planes. The images may be degraded in obese patients; in those who have a large amount of bowel gas, abdominal wounds, and dressings; and in those who are unable to maintain a full bladder. These factors may be overcome by performing transvaginal scans. With this technique, the bladder must be empty; sagittal and coronal images are obtained. By being closer to the uterus, higher-frequency transducers can be used that give better resolution than the transabdominal images. Transvaginal ultrasonography (TVUS) is limited by the restricted view and limited range of visibility. Doppler US may be used to assess blood flow in suspected pathologic processes; this may be facilitated by color flow imaging. A limitation of US is its operator dependence in which excellent image quality is related to the experience and expertise of the sonographer.

Computed tomography

In the management of uterine malignancies, we use CT primarily for evaluating metastatic or recurrent disease. When examining the chest and abdomen for metastases, we take contiguous 1-cm unenhanced images through the chest and liver. These images are reviewed, and if necessary, additional 5-mm thick sections are taken through the hila during rapid infusion of intravenous (IV) contrast material. Contiguous 1-cm enhanced images are then taken through the entire abdomen and pelvis. It is important to stress the need for optimal bowel opacification, particularly in assessing the omentum and peritoneum. We administer 800 ml of oral contrast material 1 to 2 hours before the scan and 400 ml immediately before the examination. Thinner sections, additional contrast, and images in decubitus or prone positions may occasionally be required in difficult cases. When intracranial metastases are suspected, contiguous 1-cm sections without and with IV contrast material are performed.

Magnetic resonance

MR images are obtained with the patient supine during quiet respiration. Partial distention of the bladder is preferred, as this displaces small bowel loops from the pelvis. We administer glucagon, 1 mg intramuscularly or IV, if there is significant artifact caused by bowel peristalsis. We find the routine use of a vaginal tampon to be unnecessary. Occasionally, additional information may be obtained by imaging the patient prone with rectal air insufflation.

A complete examination requires both T1-weighted (short TR, short TE) and T2-weighted (long TR, long TE) pulse sequences. The uterus and cervix are best evaluated sagittally; the ovaries, parametria, and pelvic lymph nodes are best assessed axially. T1-weighted images are useful in detecting tumor extension into the parametria and lymphadenopathy. T2-weighted images delineate the internal anatomy of the uterus and cervix and their relationships to the bladder and rectum.

Imaging in more than one plane is essential. We usually begin with T1-weighted axial and T2-weighted sagittal images, using an image thickness of 5 to 10 mm for T1-weighted images, 3 to 5 mm for T2-weighting, and an interimage gap of 1 to 2 mm. Additional T2-weighted images in axial, coronal, or oblique planes are then obtained to optimally visualize areas of possible myometrial invasion.

ENDOMETRIAL CARCINOMA
Epidemiology

Endometrial carcinoma is the most common gynecologic cancer in the United States, more so than carcinoma of the ovary and cervix combined.[1] It is primarily a disease of postmenopausal women. The median age at the time of diagnosis is 61 years, with the largest number of reported patients between 50 and 59 years.[2] Only 5% of cases develop before the age of 40. When the tumor occurs in younger women, it is commonly a well-differentiated, less aggressive type. Approximately 75% of patients with endometrial carcinoma present with stage I disease.[2]

Associated risk factors include a history of endometrial carcinoma in a first-degree relative; failure of ovulation as evidenced by infertility, dysfunctional bleeding, or amenorrhea; obesity; chronic estrogen intake; and late menopause. An endocrine imbalance with unopposed exposure of endometrial tissue to estrogen may be a predisposing factor.[3] There is an increased incidence in women with the Stein-Leventhal syndrome and in postmenopausal women with feminizing tumors of the ovary. Several studies have indicated an association of hypertension and diabetes with endometrial carcinoma; it is unclear whether this is a casual or a causal relationship. Endometrial carcinoma is more frequent in Jewish women

than in women of other ethnic origins. There is a higher incidence in highly industrialized countries than in developing countries.

Clinical features

The most common presenting symptom is vaginal bleeding. Among all women with postmenopausal bleeding, uterine malignancy is the cause in 15% to 25% of cases. In pre- and perimenopausal women, menorrhagia is frequently observed. Intermenstrual spotting may also occur. Some patients present with an abnormal discharge, which at first is watery but soon becomes bloody. Patients who have obstructing lesions may experience pressure symptoms due to a large hematometra. Pain is not an early symptom and usually indicates widespread disease or involvement of nerve trunks in the lateral pelvis. Endometrial carcinoma is not routinely detected by Papanicolaou (Pap) smears, and endometrial biopsy is necessary for diagnosis. Fractional dilation and curettage (D&C) is the definitive method of diagnosis.

Histologic grade of tumor, stage of disease, and depth of myometrial invasion are the most important prognostic features. These factors directly relate to regional lymph node involvement and tumor recurrence and ultimately to 5-year survival, and are addressed in the revised staging system of the International Federation of Gynecology and Obstetrics (FIGO) (Table 8-1 and see Appendix).[4] Clinical staging, including that based on findings from fractional D&C, is inaccurate in the assessment of the extent of disease in up to 51% of patients.[5,6] In one series, 30.4% of patients with stage I carcinoma were inaccurately staged clinically before surgery.[5]

Pathology

At least 90% of malignant tumors of the uterine corpus are adenocarcinomas. They usually arise within the uterine fundus and are polypoid or infiltrative in nature. The tumors are graded histologically on the basis of differentiation and gland formation. Grade I lesions are highly differentiated with glandular structures that do not appear greatly different from the normal endometrium. In grade III lesions, there is complete loss of architecture and no gland formation. As the grade of the tumor increases, the risk of deep myometrial invasion increases and the chance of survival decreases. Patients with lower uterine segment tumors have a higher incidence of pelvic and periaortic lymph node metastases than those with only fundal disease.[2]

Extension of tumor into the endocervical canal occurs in 10% to 15% of patients.[3] Extension into the vagina is rare and usually involves the anterior

Table 8-1 FIGO staging of endometrial carcinoma (Also see Appendix)

FIGO stage	Criteria
IA G123	Tumor limited to endo-metrium
IB G123	Invasion to less than half of myometrium
IC G123	Invasion more than half of myometrium
IIA G123	Endocervical glandular involvement only
IIB G123	Cervical stromal invasion
IIIA G123	Tumor invades serosa and/or adnexae and/or positive peritoneal cytology
IIIB G123	Vaginal metastases
IIIC G123	Metastases to pelvic and/or para-aortic lymph nodes
IVA G123	Tumor invasion bladder and/or bowel mucosa
IVB	Distant metastases including intra-abdominal and/or inguinal lymph nodes

G, Histologic grade; *FIGO*, International Federation of Gynecology and Obstetrics.

wall. At the time of surgery, approximately 10% of patients with clinical stage I disease have ovarian metastasis.[2] The incidence of ovarian metastasis increases with deep myometrial invasion and involvement of the lower uterine segment or endocervix. Metastases to the omentum and peritoneum, as well as ascites, are uncommon at the time of presentation but are frequent manifestations of recurrent disease.

Histologic variants of adenocarcinoma occur infrequently. Of these, adenosquamous, clear cell, and papillary carcinoma are considered more virulent than adenocarcinoma, while adenoacanthoma is better differentiated and it has a better prognosis.[2]

Imaging

No imaging modality is able to differentiate between endometrial carcinoma and other causes of endometrial widening such as endometrial hyperplasia or blood clot.[7] The diagnosis of endometrial carcinoma needs to be established histologically. We use MR imaging of the pelvis to evaluate the depth of myometrial invasion of tumor and to stage local disease; others have recommended US for this purpose. In assessing extrapelvic spread, we utilize CT.

Ultrasonography. There have been conflicting reports about the usefulness of US in the evalua-

tion of endometrial carcinoma. Using transabdominal US, Fleischer et al were accurate in assessing the depth of tumor invasion within 10% of actual measurements in the gross specimen in 70% of 20 patients.[8] Cacciatore et al found a correlation between endometrial volume and myometrial invasion, correctly predicting the depth of invasion in 80% of 93 patients.[9] However, Thorvinger et al could not reproduce these results and concluded that US was not accurate in defining the local extent of endometrial carcinoma.[10]

In women of child-bearing age, the uterus varies considerably in size. In nulliparous women, it measures approximately 8 cm in length, 5 cm in width, and 4 cm in anteroposterior diameter. In multiparous women, all dimensions increase by approximately 1 cm. In postmenopausal women not on replacement hormonal therapy, the uterus atrophies and ranges from 3.5 to 6.5 cm in length and 1.2 to 1.8 cm in anteroposterior diameter in women over 65 years of age.[11] The uterus in postmenopausal women on replacement hormonal therapy is usually similar in size to that in premenopausal women.

The normal myometrium has a homogeneous, uniform, low to moderate echopattern (Fig. 8-1). Peripheral uterine veins may be seen. The endometrium is composed of functional and basal layers. The normal endometrial echo varies during the

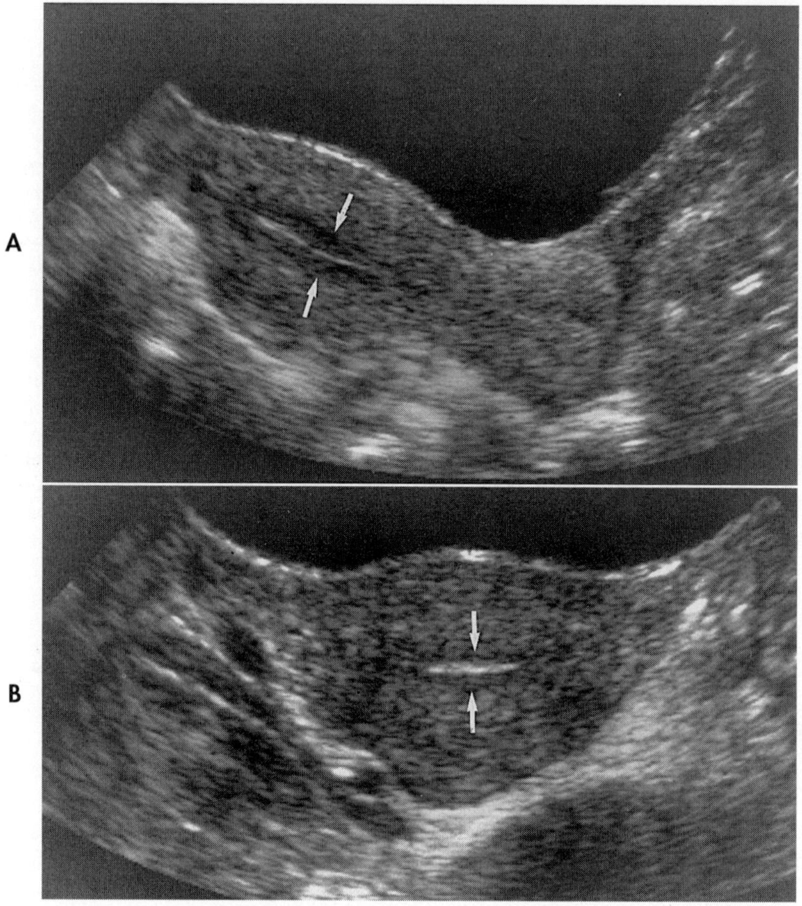

Fig. 8-1 Normal uterus in the proliferative phase. Sagittal **(A)** and axial **(B)** transabdominal ultrasound (US) images demonstrate a thin echogenic line surrounded by a hypoechoic region *(arrows),* which represents the functional layer of the endometrium.

menstrual cycle; in the early proliferative phase, it is seen as a thin echogenic line surrounded by a relatively hypoechoic region that represents the functional layer (Fig. 8-1).[11] This hypoechoic area increases in size and becomes more well defined in the late proliferative phase, with the endometrium measuring 2 to 4 mm in diameter. After ovulation, the endometrium becomes uniformly echogenic and increases to approximately 6 mm in diameter in the late secretory phase. A thin sonolucent layer, known as the subendometrial halo, surrounds the relatively echogenic endometrium; this most likely represents the inner layer of the myometrium.[11]

The endometrium is usually thin in postmenopausal women, measuring 2 to 3 mm. In women receiving hormonal replacement therapy, it may be up to 6 mm thick. It is usually homogeneously echogenic relative to the myometrium, with a well-defined interface between them. The hypoechoic subendometrial halo is usually maintained in these women.

In patients with endometrial carcinoma, the endometrial echoes are usually irregular and the endometrial canal is widened (Fig. 8-2). Most tumors are relatively echogenic. There appears to be a correlation between the echogenicity and the degree of differentiation: better-differentiated tumors are echogenic, and less well differentiated tumors (grades II and III) are heterogeneous or hypoechoic.[8,9] Preservation of the subendometrial halo indicates tumor confined to the endometrium or superficial invasion, whereas absence of a halo has been associated with deep invasion (Fig. 8-3).[8] Low-lying tumors may obstruct the cervical canal, causing hydro- or hematometra. This will manifest as a distended, fluid-filled endometrial cavity (Fig. 8-4). Stage II disease is manifested by extension of the abnormal endometrial echoes into the cervical canal.

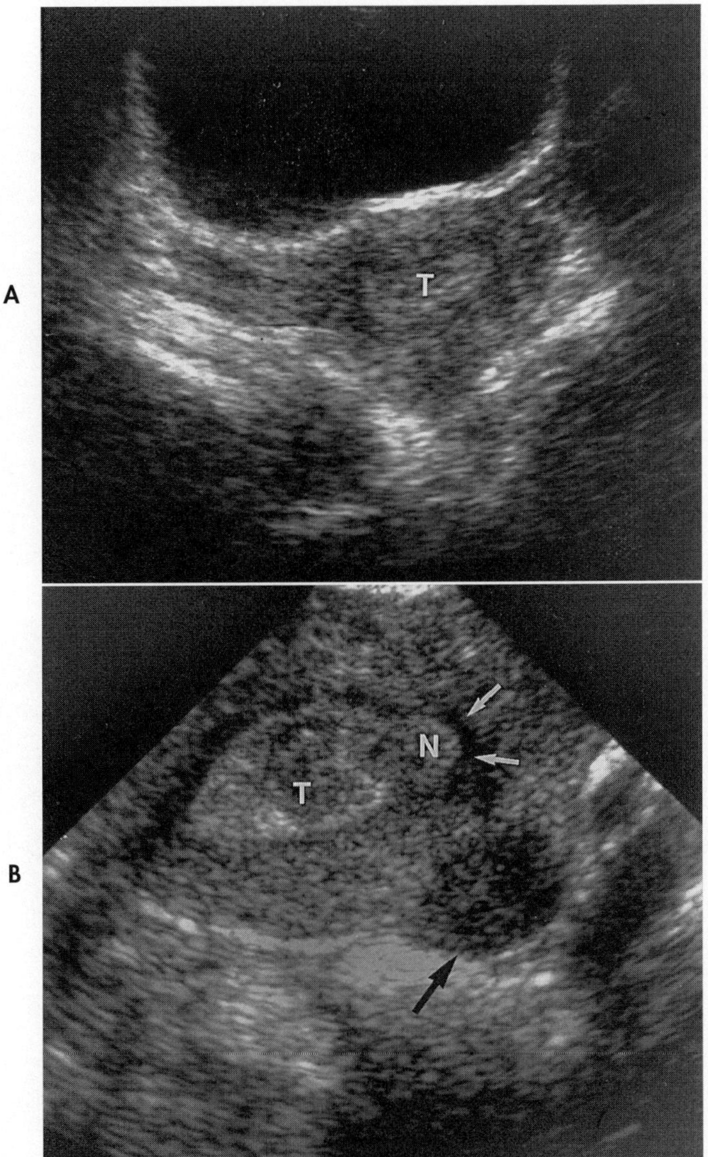

Fig. 8-2 Axial transabdominal **(A)** and transvaginal **(B)** US images of a woman with stage IA endometrial carcinoma. Mixed echogenicity tumor *(T)* distends the endometrial cavity. The subendometrial halo *(white arrows)* in **B** is intact adjacent to a tumor nodule, *(N),* indicating tumor confined to the endometrium. The black arrow points to subserosal leiomyoma.

Initial studies using TVUS suggest that it is more sensitive than transabdominal US in evaluating the depth of invasion and better defines the extent of the tumor (Figs. 8-2 and 8-4). Gordon et al report that TVUS was correct in detecting the depth of invasion (within 15%) in 84% of 25 patients.[12] However, they were able to detect cervical involvement in only one of three patients. Conte et al report 90% accuracy in detecting the depth of invasion in 20 patients.[13] Although these results are encouraging, further studies are necessary to evaluate the role of TVUS in assessing myometrial invasion.

Computed tomography. On unenhanced images the normal uterus is isodense with skeletal muscle. A central area of lower attenuation may sometimes be seen. After administration of IV contrast material the myometrium increases in attenuation and the endometrial cavity is more clearly delineated.[14]

On unenhanced CT in patients with endometrial carcinoma, focal or diffuse enlargement of the uter-

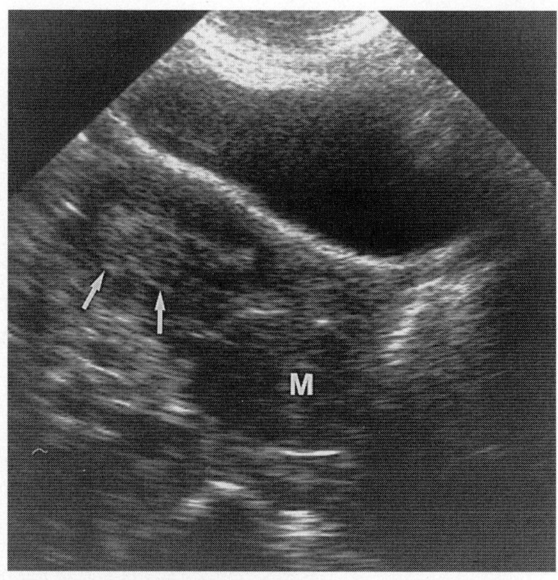

Fig. 8-3 Sagittal transabdominal US image of a woman with stage IC endometrial carcinoma. The endometrial canal is distended with echogenic tumor. There is deep myometrial invasion posteriorly *(arrows)*. *M*, Leiomyoma.

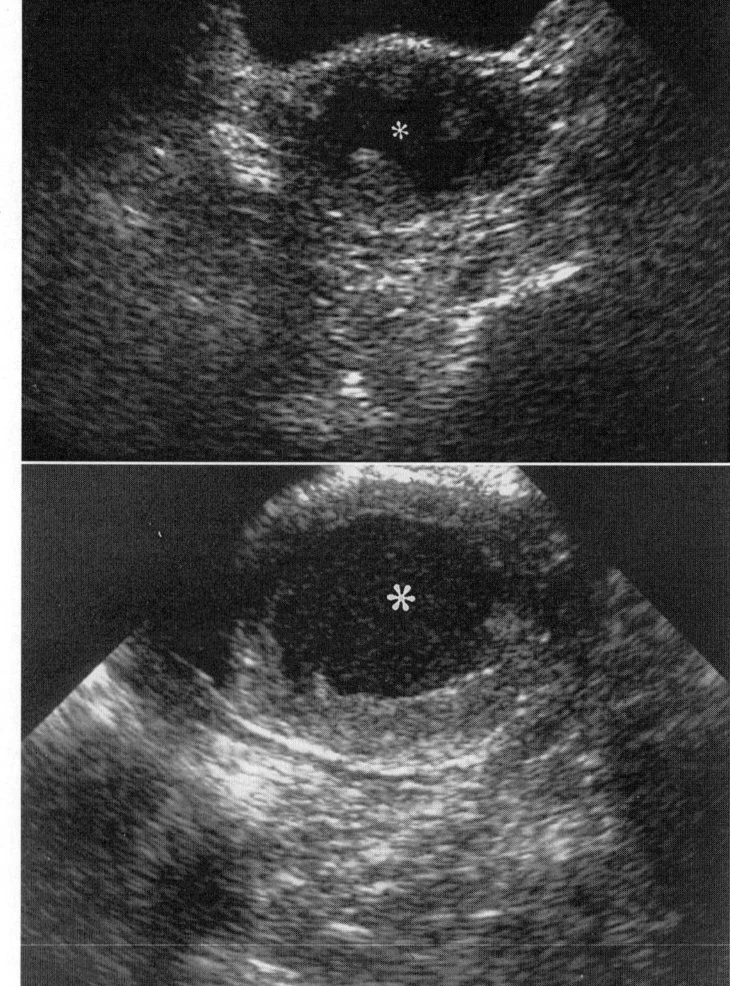

Fig. 8-4 Stage IC low-lying endometrial carcinoma. Axial transabdominal **(A)** and coronal transvaginal **(B)** US images demonstrate hemorrhage *(asterisk)* distending the endometrial cavity. Multiple tumor nodules project into the endometrial cavity.

ine body may be seen. After IV contrast material administration, the neoplasm enhances less than the myometrium but more than nonenhancing uterine secretions (Figs. 8-5 to 8-8).[14] Dore et al evaluated the value of CT in assessing myometrial invasion.[15] Although they reported an overall accuracy of 76%, CT has not been used much in this area.

We use CT in the evaluation of stages III and IV and recurrent disease. Pelvic or retroperitoneal lymph nodes larger than 1 cm in diameter are considered abnormal (Fig. 8-9). Other manifestations include adnexal masses (Fig. 8-10), ascites, and omental or peritoneal masses (Fig. 8-11). The liver is infrequently involved (Fig. 8-11). Differentiation between contiguity and frank invasion between the tumor and bladder or bowel is difficult. Intrathoracic manifestations of stage IV disease include lymphadenopathy and parenchymal masses. Skeletal metastases may be seen (Fig. 8-12). CT-guided biopsy is often used for confirmation of metastatic or recurrent disease (Fig. 8-13).

Magnetic resonance. On T1-weighted images the normal uterus has homogeneous low to me-

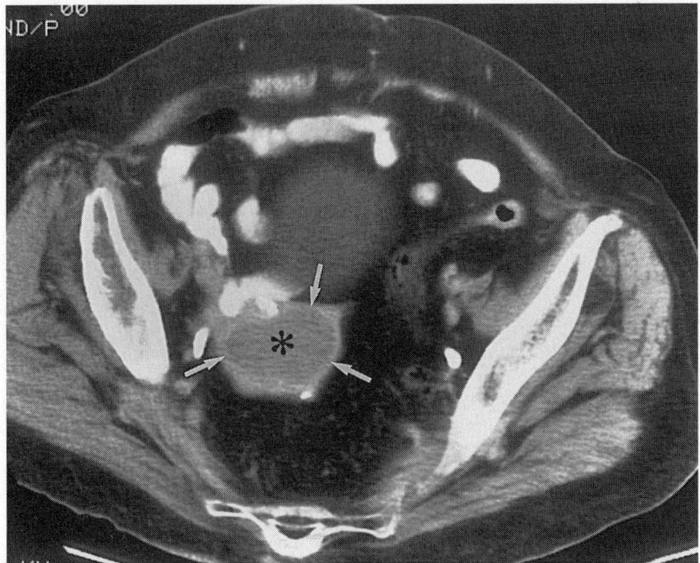

Fig. 8-5 Stage IB endometrial carcinoma. An enhanced computed tomographic (CT) image of a postmenopausal woman demonstrates marked distention of the endometrial cavity by tumor *(asterisk)* and thinning of the myometrium *(arrows)*.

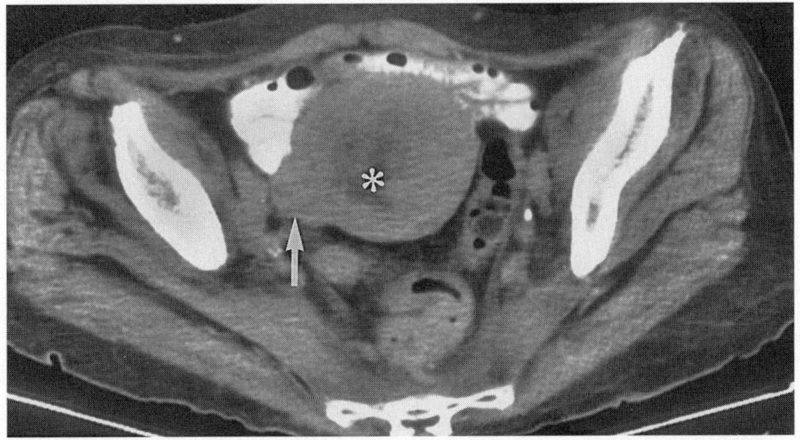

Fig. 8-6 Stage IC endometrial carcinoma. An enhanced CT image in a postmenopausal woman shows enlargement of the uterus with distention and irregularity of the endometrial canal *(asterisk)* by tumor. The arrow points to subserosal leiomyoma.

dium signal intensity (Fig. 8-14, *A*). Uterine zonal anatomy is best appreciated on T2-weighted images. Three zones of different signal intensity may be seen (Fig. 8-14, *B* and *C*).[16-21] The endometrium has high signal intensity, similar to or greater than that of fat. The myometrium has medium signal intensity. Between them is the thin, low signal intensity junctional zone, which is thought to correspond to the innermost portion of the myometrium (Fig. 8-14).[20-22] The junctional zone may not be visible as a distinct structure in premenarchal and postmenopausal women.

The MR appearance of the normal uterus is influenced by the hormonal status of the patient.

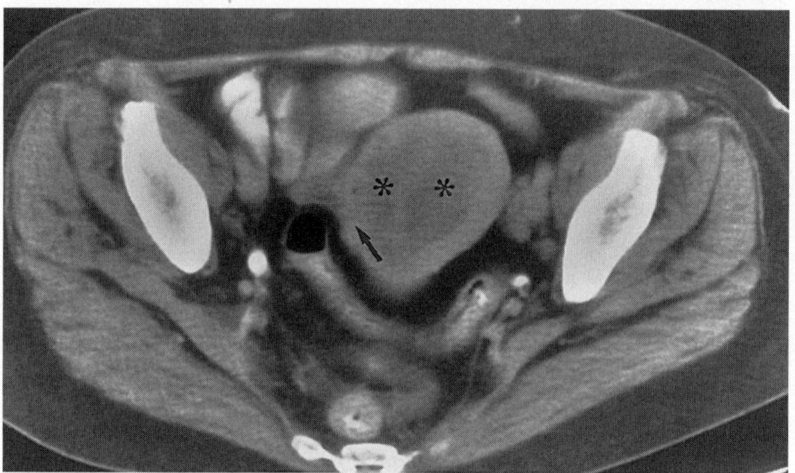

Fig. 8-7 Stage IC endometrial carcinoma. An enhanced CT image demonstrates disruption of the myometrium in the right side of the uterus *(arrow)* due to deep invasion by tumor *(asterisks)* that distends the endometrial cavity.

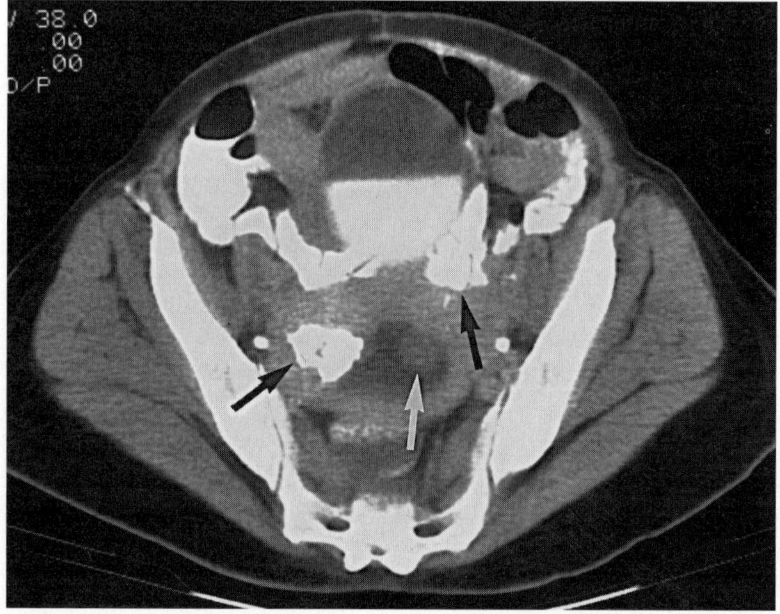

Fig. 8-8 Enhanced CT image of a postmenopausal woman with endometrial carcinoma. The endometrial cavity is widened. An enhancing tumor nodule is present anteriorly *(white arrow)*. The depth of myometrial invasion is difficult to assess. Black arrows point to calcified leiomyomas.

During the reproductive years, there is a distinct temporal variation in uterine appearance in different phases of the menstrual cycle.[16-18] During the proliferative phase, endometrial width is typically 1 to 3 mm. The endometrial zone is widest during the midsecretory phase, when it usually measures 5 to 7 mm but may increase to 10 mm.[16,17,21]

In women taking oral contraceptives, uterine zonal anatomy is less distinct and the endometrial width is usually 4 mm or less.[16,17,21] This appearance is similar to that seen in premenarchal and postmenopausal women. Postmenopausal women taking exogenous estrogen may have an endometrial width greater than 4 mm.

The normal cervix has homogeneous intermediate signal intensity on T1-weighted images. The zonal anatomy of the cervix is appreciated on T2-weighted images (Fig. 8-14). The central zone has high signal intensity similar to that of the endometrium; this is believed to represent cervical epithelium and mucus.[21,23] Surrounding this is the homogeneous, low signal intensity cervical stroma, which is continuous with and similar in appearance to the junctional zone. In some women a third outer

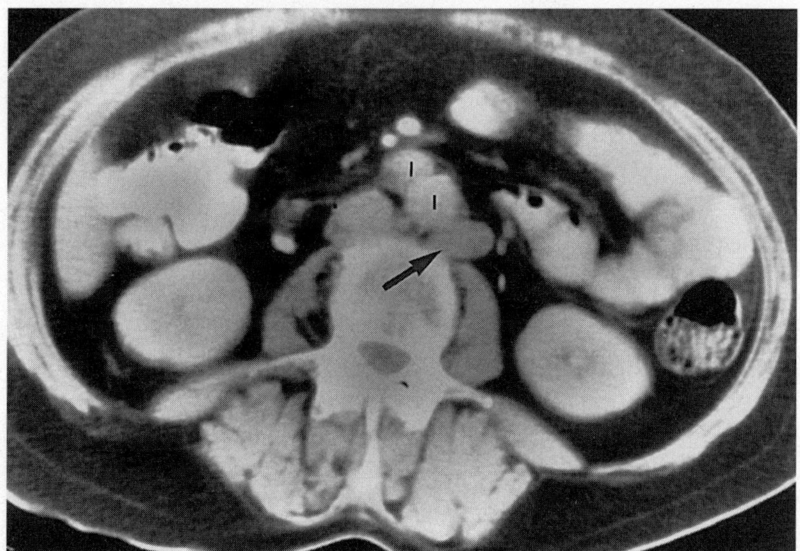

Fig. 8-9 Stage IIIC endometrial carcinoma. An enhanced CT image at the level of the aortic bifurcation demonstrates left common iliac lymphadenopathy *(arrow)*. *I,* Common iliac arteries.

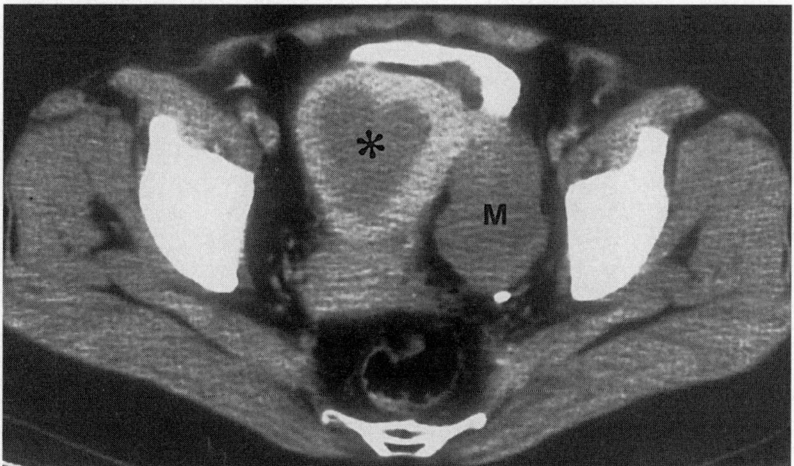

Fig. 8-10 Stage IIIA endometrial carcinoma. An enhanced CT image demonstrates marked distention of the endometrial canal by tumor *(asterisk)*. A large left adnexal metastasis *(M)* is noted.

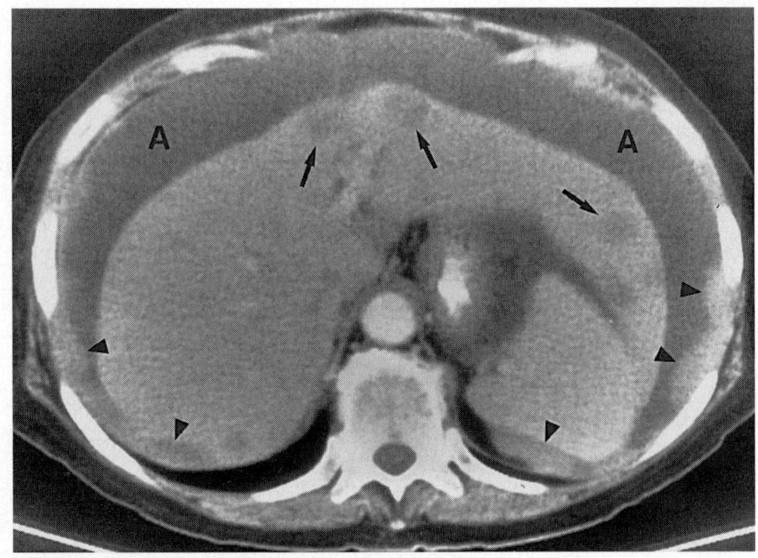

Fig. 8-11 Enhanced CT image of a patient with stage IVB endometrial carcinoma. Arrowheads point to peritoneal metastases, arrows to liver metastases. *A,* Ascites.

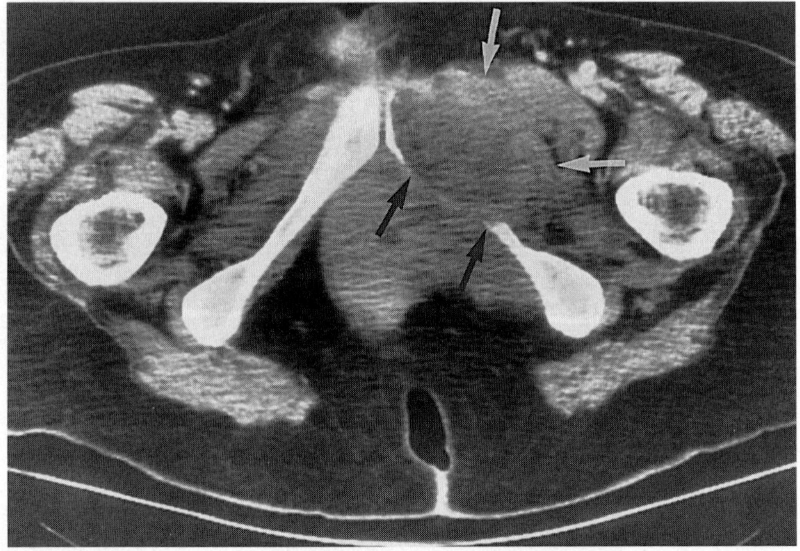

Fig. 8-12 Stage IVB endometrial carcinoma. There is a metastasis with destruction of the left inferior pubic ramus *(black arrows)* and an associated soft tissue mass *(white arrows).*

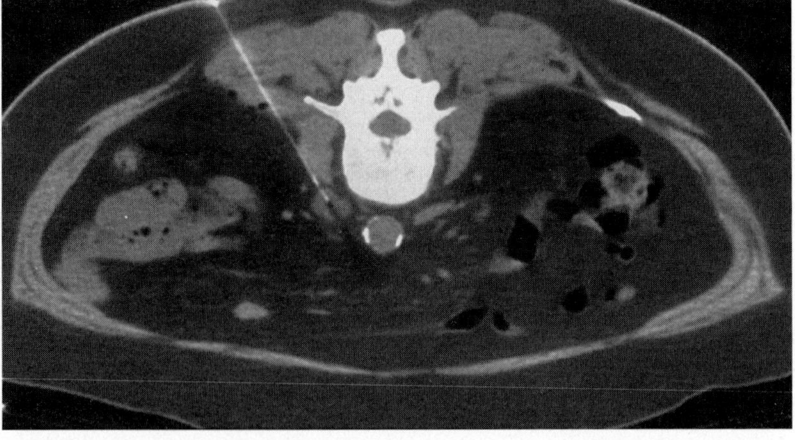

Fig. 8-13 CT-guided biopsy. The tip of the needle is in an enlarged left para-aortic lymph node. Cytologic examination revealed metastatic uterine adenocarcinoma.

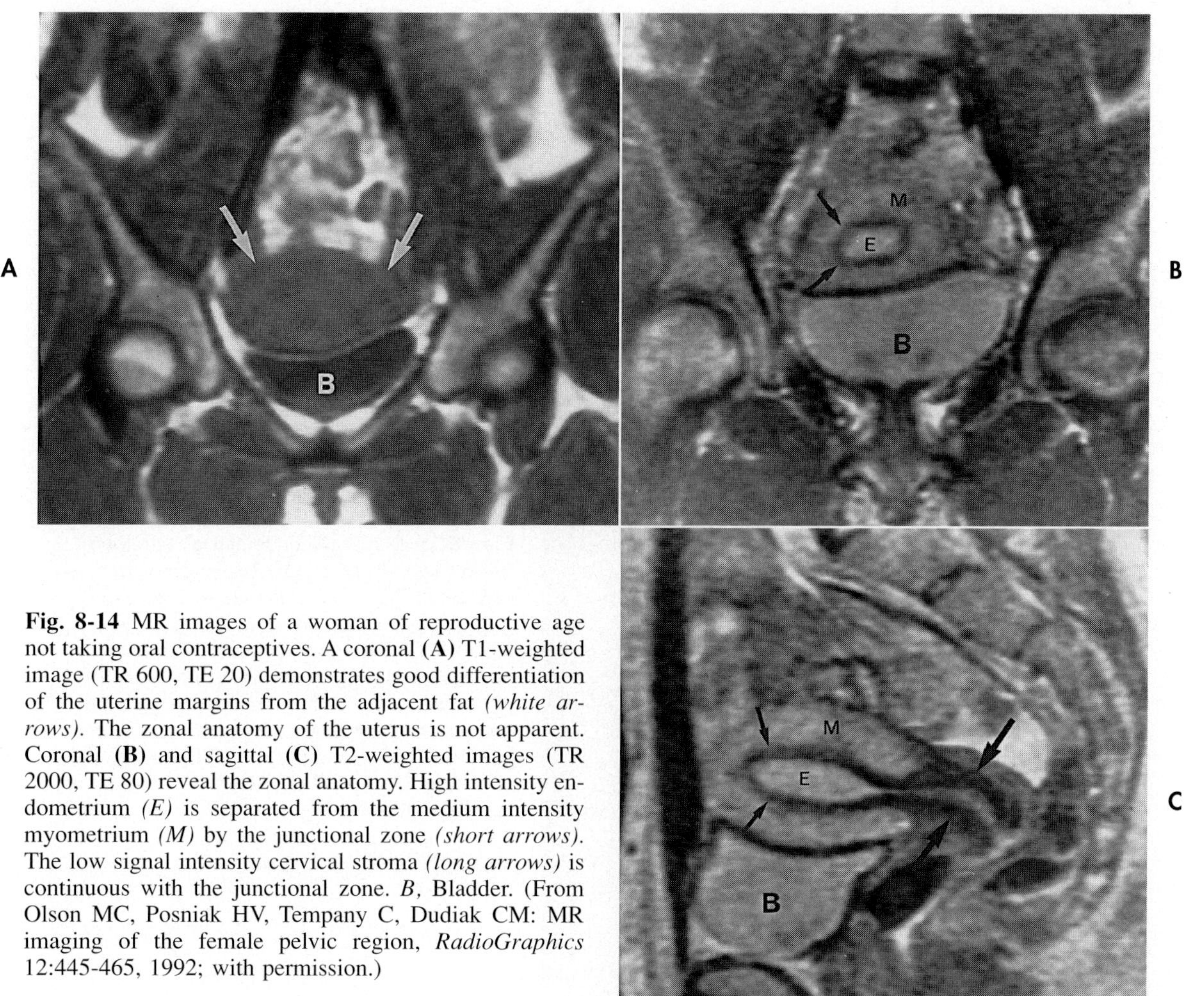

Fig. 8-14 MR images of a woman of reproductive age not taking oral contraceptives. A coronal (**A**) T1-weighted image (TR 600, TE 20) demonstrates good differentiation of the uterine margins from the adjacent fat *(white arrows)*. The zonal anatomy of the uterus is not apparent. Coronal (**B**) and sagittal (**C**) T2-weighted images (TR 2000, TE 80) reveal the zonal anatomy. High intensity endometrium *(E)* is separated from the medium intensity myometrium *(M)* by the junctional zone *(short arrows)*. The low signal intensity cervical stroma *(long arrows)* is continuous with the junctional zone. *B,* Bladder. (From Olson MC, Posniak HV, Tempany C, Dudiak CM: MR imaging of the female pelvic region, *RadioGraphics* 12:445-465, 1992; with permission.)

zone of intermediate signal intensity continuous with the myometrium is seen.[23]

MR has proved effective in evaluating endometrial carcinoma, with overall accuracy rates ranging between 82% and 92% for staging[7,24,25] and between 74% and 87%[7,24-27] for assessing the depth of invasion on nonenhanced examinations. This has important implications in patient management, helping clinicians determine which patients would benefit from preoperative radiotherapy and assisting in planning surgical procedures.

On MR the most frequent manifestation of endometrial carcinoma is widening of the high intensity endometrial canal.[7,25,27-29] This may be focal or diffuse and can be due to the tumor itself, uterine secretions, or both.[28] The endometrium may have an irregular, inhomogeneous signal intensity. Discrete tumor nodules, which may be low or medium intensity relative to the endometrium, may be seen within it.[7,29]

The low intensity junctional zone is important in evaluating myometrial invasion. If this is intact, invasion is essentially excluded. Segmental disruption is a reliable indicator of myometrial invasion.[7,24,28] In the absence of a junctional zone, irregularity of the endometrium-myometrium interface is used as evidence of invasion.[7] Superficial invasion is manifested as extension of the tumor into the inner half of the myometrium (Figs. 8-15 and 8-16); extension into the outer half indicates deep invasion (Figs. 8-17 to 8-20).[4]

The cervix can be involved by direct extension of tumor from the endometrial cavity, or there may be discrete metastases to it.[7] Direct extension of tumor widens the cervical canal (Fig. 8-21) and may invade the cervical stroma.

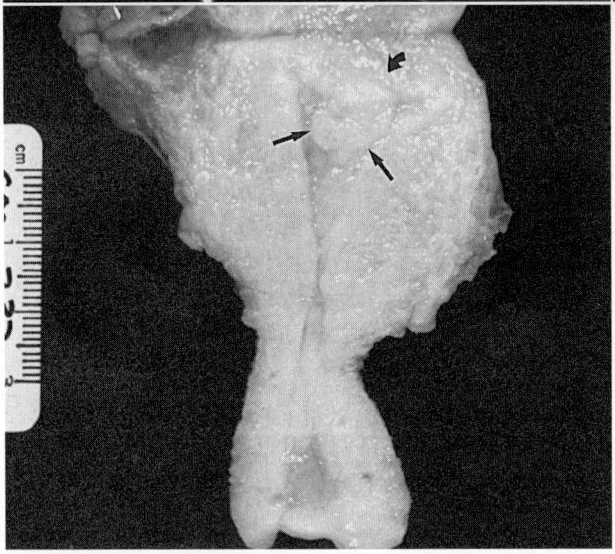

Fig. 8-15 Stage IB endometrial carcinoma. Axial **(A)** and sagittal **(B)** T2-weighted images (TR 2300, TE 70) demonstrate widening of the endometrial canal by tumor *(asterisk)*. *B,* Bladder. **C,** A coronal section of the uterus reveals the tumor *(straight arrows)* near the fundal aspect of an asymmetrically distended endometrial cavity. There is superficial myometrial invasion *(curved arrow)*. (From Posniak HV, Olson MC, Dudiak CM, et al: Imaging of uterine carcinoma: correlation with clinical and pathologic findings, *RadioGraphics* 10:15-27, 1990; with permission.)

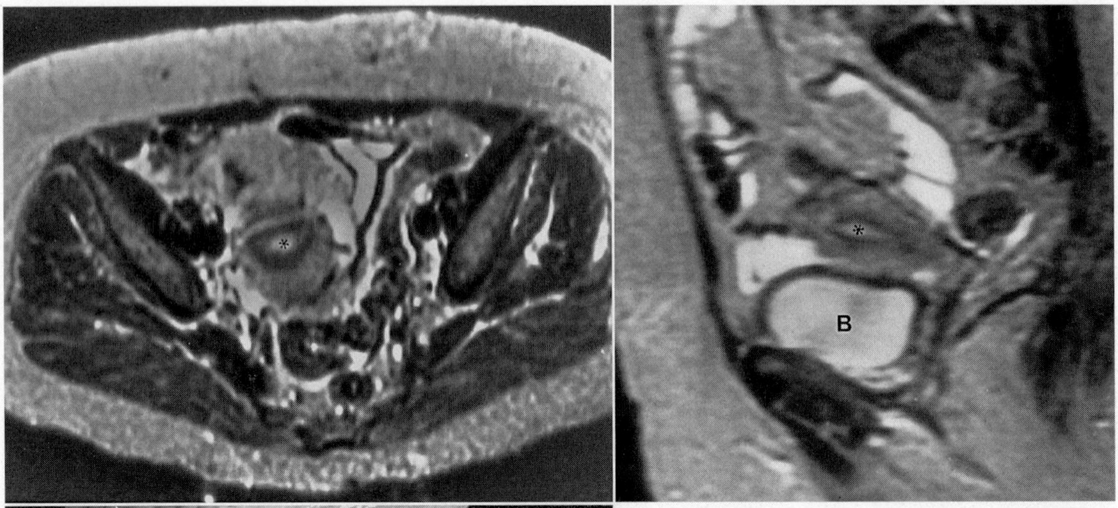

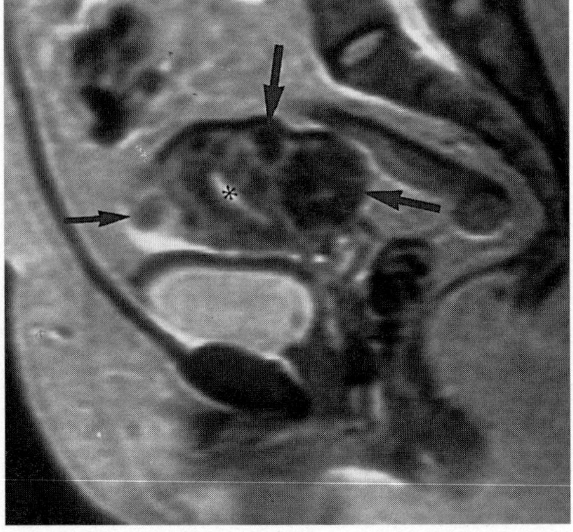

Fig. 8-16 Stage IB endometrial carcinoma. A sagittal T2-weighted image (TR 2200, TE 70) demonstrates minimal widening of the endometrial canal by tumor *(asterisk)*. Multiple uterine leiomyomas *(arrows)* are present.

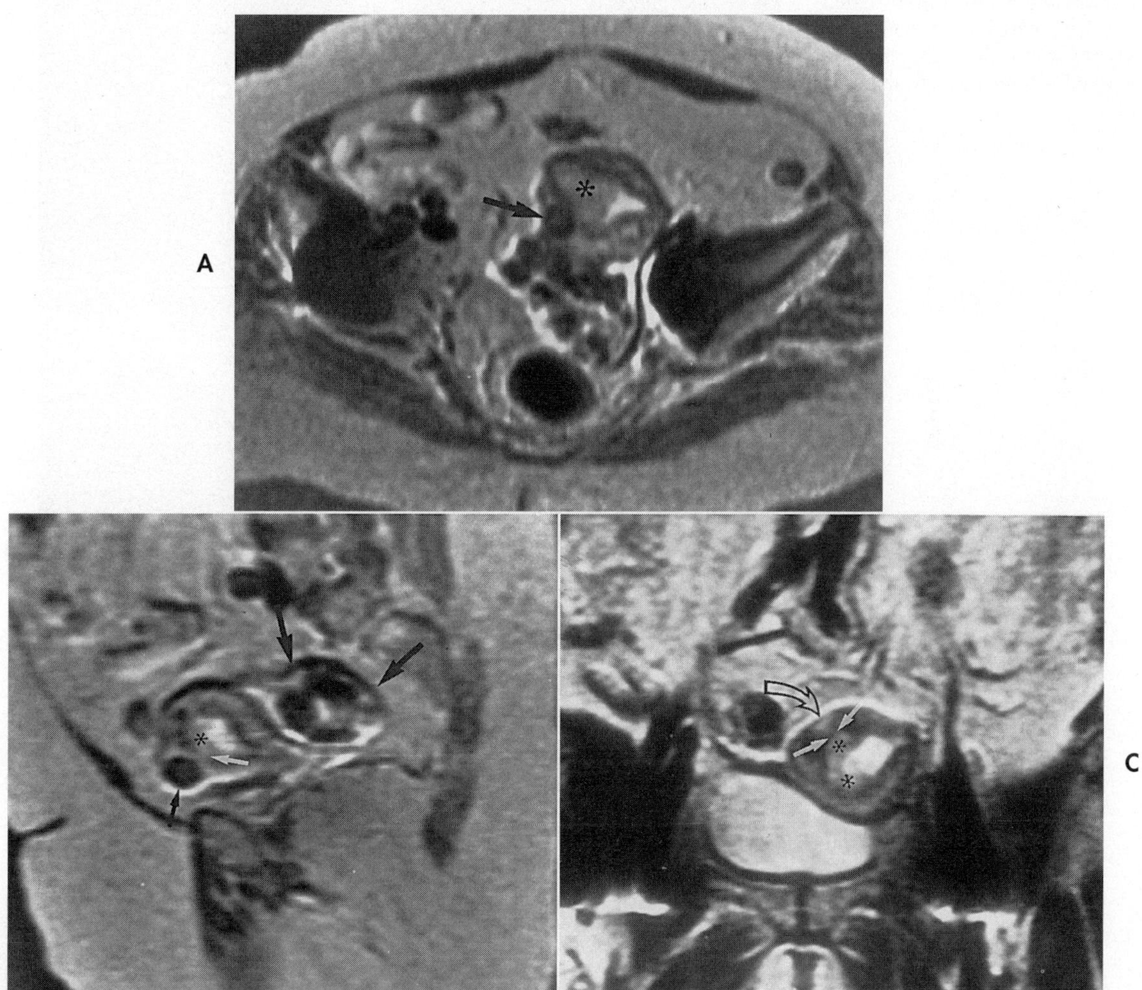

Fig. 8-17 Stage IC endometrial carcinoma. Axial **(A)**, sagittal **(B)**, and coronal **(C)** T2-weighted images (TR 2300, TE 80) show widening of the endometrial canal by tumor *(asterisks)* and higher intensity blood. There is disruption of the junctional zone *(white arrows)* and deep myometrial invasion *(open arrow)*. Black arrows point to leiomyomas. (From Posniak HV, Olson MC, Dudiak CM, et al: Imaging of uterine carcinoma: correlation with clinical and pathologic findings, *Radio-Graphics* 10:15-27, 1990; with permission.)

Fig. 8-18 Stage IC endometrial carcinoma. Sagittal **(A)** and coronal **(B)** T2-weighted images (TR 2300, TE 70) demonstrate widening of the endometrial canal by high signal intensity tumor *(asterisk)* and irregularity of the endometriummyometrium interface. Focal areas of high signal intensity due to tumor extension are noted deep within the myometrium *(straight arrows)*. Curved arrows point to leiomyomas.

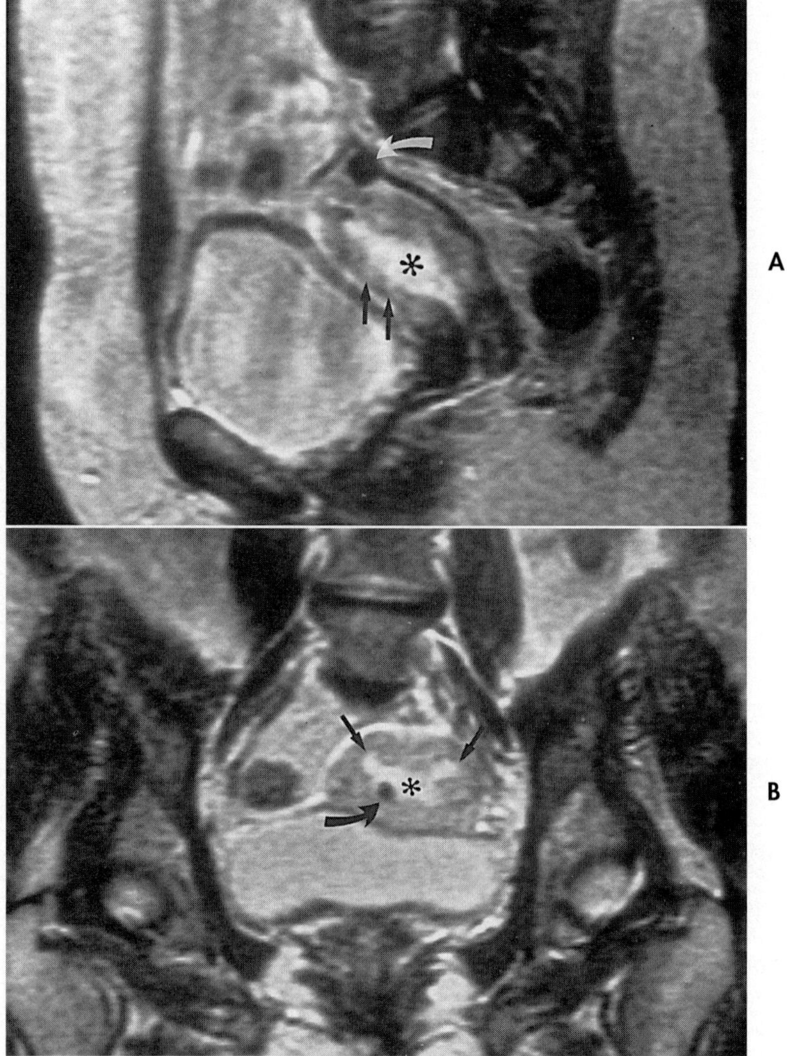

Fig. 8-19 Stage IC endometrial carcinoma. An axial image demonstrates a mixed signal intensity tumor *(T)* distending the endometrial cavity. There is disruption of the junctional zone *(short arrows)* and high signal intensity tumor deep with the myometrium *(long arrow)*. The curved arrow points to a nabothian cyst, which may be confused with a cervical metastasis.

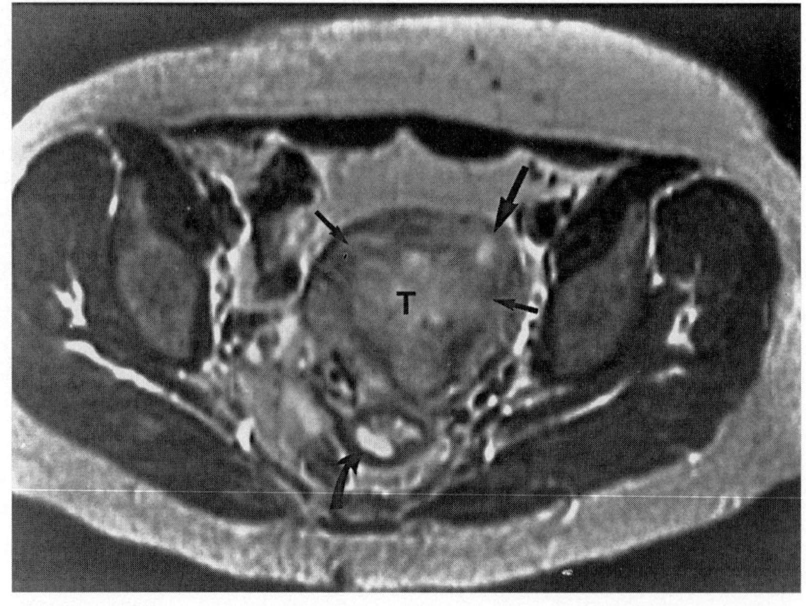

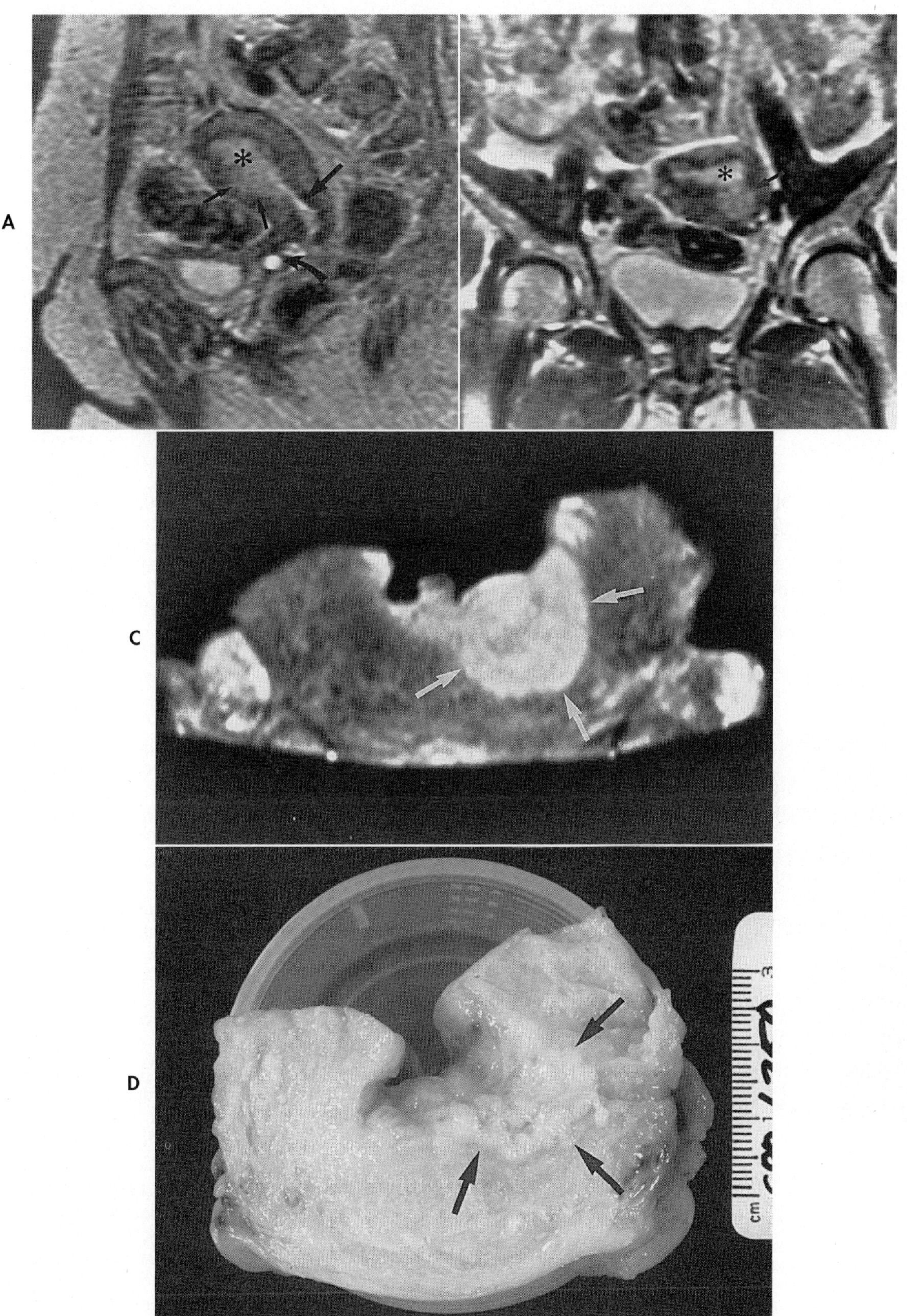

Fig. 8-20 For legend see p. 170.

Continued.

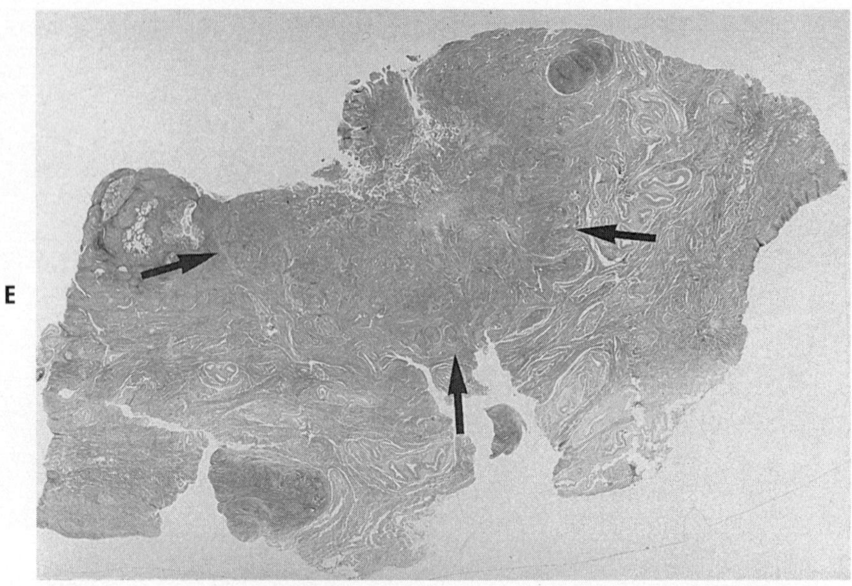

Fig. 8-20 Stage IC endometrial carcinoma. Sagittal **(A)** and coronal **(B)** images (TR 2000, TE 80) show endometrial widening due to tumor *(asterisk)* with extension into the outer half of the myometrium *(short arrows)*. Note the distended cervical canal of higher intensity *(long arrow in* **A**) than that of the tumor, compatible with blood clot. The curved arrow in **A** indicates an incidental nabothian cyst. **C,** Axial MR image of a specimen, opened after surgery, demonstrates deep invasion of tumor *(arrows)*. **D,** Axial section of the uterus reveals tumor *(arrows)* infiltrating deeply into the myometrium. **E,** Transmural section of the anterolateral uterine wall confirms deep tumor invasion *(arrows)*. (From Posniak HV, Olson MC, Dudiak CM, et al: Imaging of uterine carcinoma: correlation with clinical and pathologic findings, *RadioGraphics* 10:15-27, 1990; with permission.)

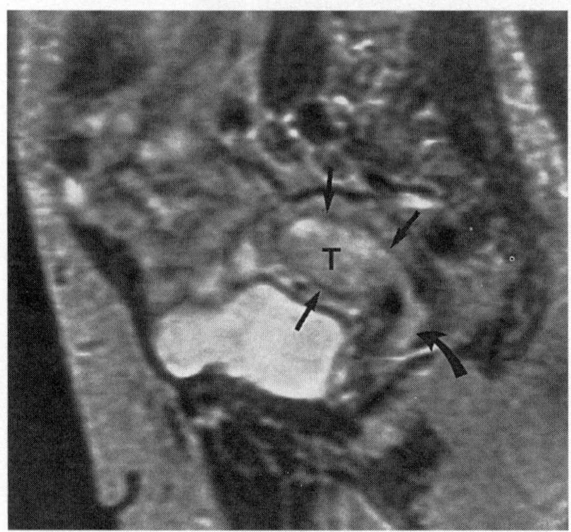

Fig. 8-21 Stage IIA endometrial carcinoma. A sagittal T2-weighted MR image (TR 2200, TE 70) demonstrates the endometrial cavity distended by tumor *(T)* with an intact junctional zone *(straight arrows)*. The cervical canal *(curved arrow)* is widened because of tumor extension. (From Posniak HV, Olson MC, Dudiak CM, et al: Imaging of uterine carcinoma: correlation with clinical and pathologic findings, *RadioGraphics* 10:15-27, 1990; with permission.)

Stage III disease may be manifested on MR as transmyometrial extension of tumor with interruption of the medium signal myometrium, with or without associated serosal masses or parametrial infiltration.[7] The ovaries and adnexae may be involved by direct spread or may have discrete metastases (Fig. 8-22).[7] As with CT, assessment of metastatic lymphadenopathy is based on the size of the nodes (Fig. 8-23). Signal characteristics have not been useful in differentiating metastatic from hyperplastic lymphadenopathy.[30]

As with CT, the role of MR in evaluating invasion of the bladder or rectum in stage IVA disease is unclear. Pelvic manifestations of stage IVB disease include ascites, peritoneal implants, and omental cakes (Fig. 8-24),[7] which are usually readily apparent on MR. MR is also useful for evaluating bone metastases (Fig. 8-25).

The diagnosis of endometrial carcinoma needs to be established histologically, because nonenhanced imaging cannot differentiate between endometrial carcinoma and other causes of endometrial widening such as endometrial hyperplasia or blood clot (Fig. 8-26).

In a 1991 article, Hricak et al indicated that contrast enhancement with gadopentetate dimeglu-

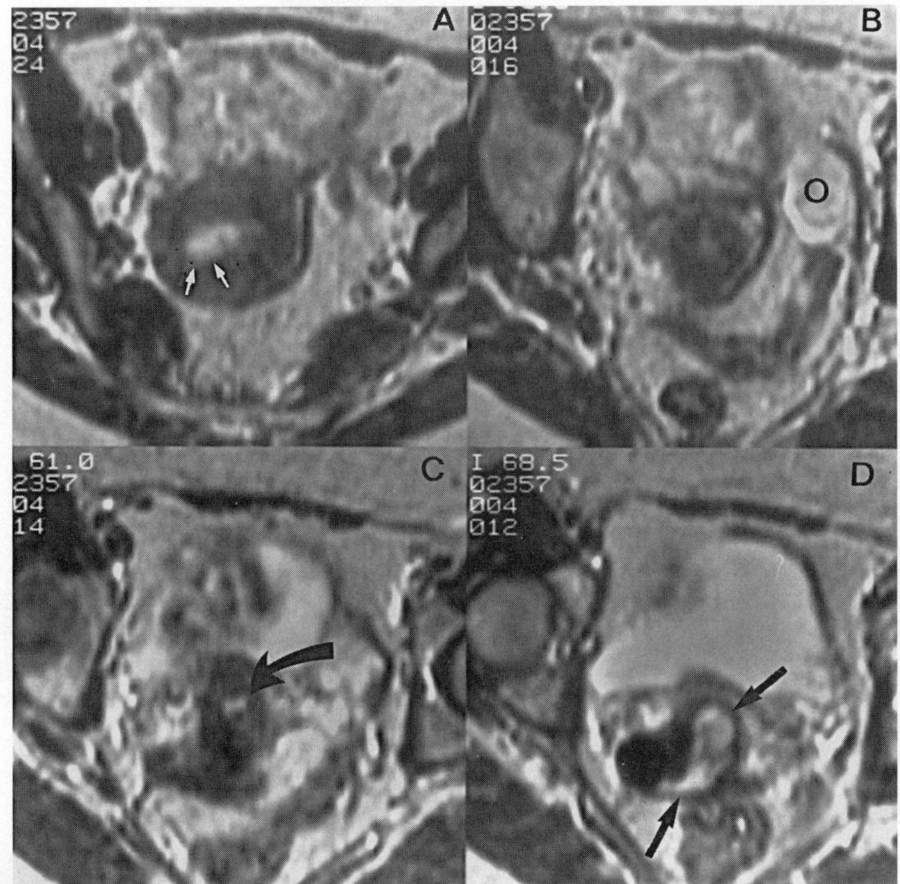

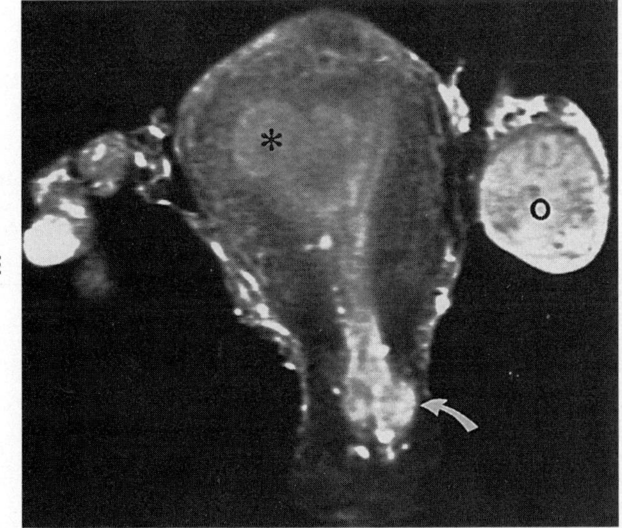

Fig. 8-22 Stage IIIA endometrial carcinoma with metastases to the cervix and left ovary. **A,** Axial T2-weighted images (TR 2000, TE 70) demonstrate a fundal tumor extending into the inner half of the myometrium *(white arrows),* indicating superficial invasion. **B,** The left ovary *(O)* has relatively high intensity but is less intense than the bladder in **D;** this is compatible with a metastasis. **C,** There is no evidence of tumor in the uterine isthmus *(curved arrow).* **D,** A discrete tumor mass *(long arrows)* replaces most of the cervical stroma. **E,** Coronal MR image of a specimen shows superficial invasion of the fundus *(asterisk),* cervical mass *(arrow),* and ovarian metastasis *(O).* (From Olson MC, Posniak HV, Tempany C, Dudiak CM: MR imaging of the female pelvic region, *RadioGraphics* 12:445-465, 1992; and from Posniak HV, Olson MC, Dudiak CM, et al: Imaging of uterine carcinoma: correlation with clinical and pathologic findings, *RadioGraphics* 10:15 27, 1990; with permission.)

Continued.

Fig. 8-22, cont'd F, Coronal section of the uterus reveals tumor filling the fundal portion of the endometrial cavity (*asterisk*) with superficial invasion (*curved arrow*). The uterine isthmus is free of tumor (*open arrow*). **G,** The cervix is distorted by tumor (*asterisks*), with deep stromal invasion (arrows). **H,** The bivalved left ovary reveals replacement by metastasis (*asterisks*).

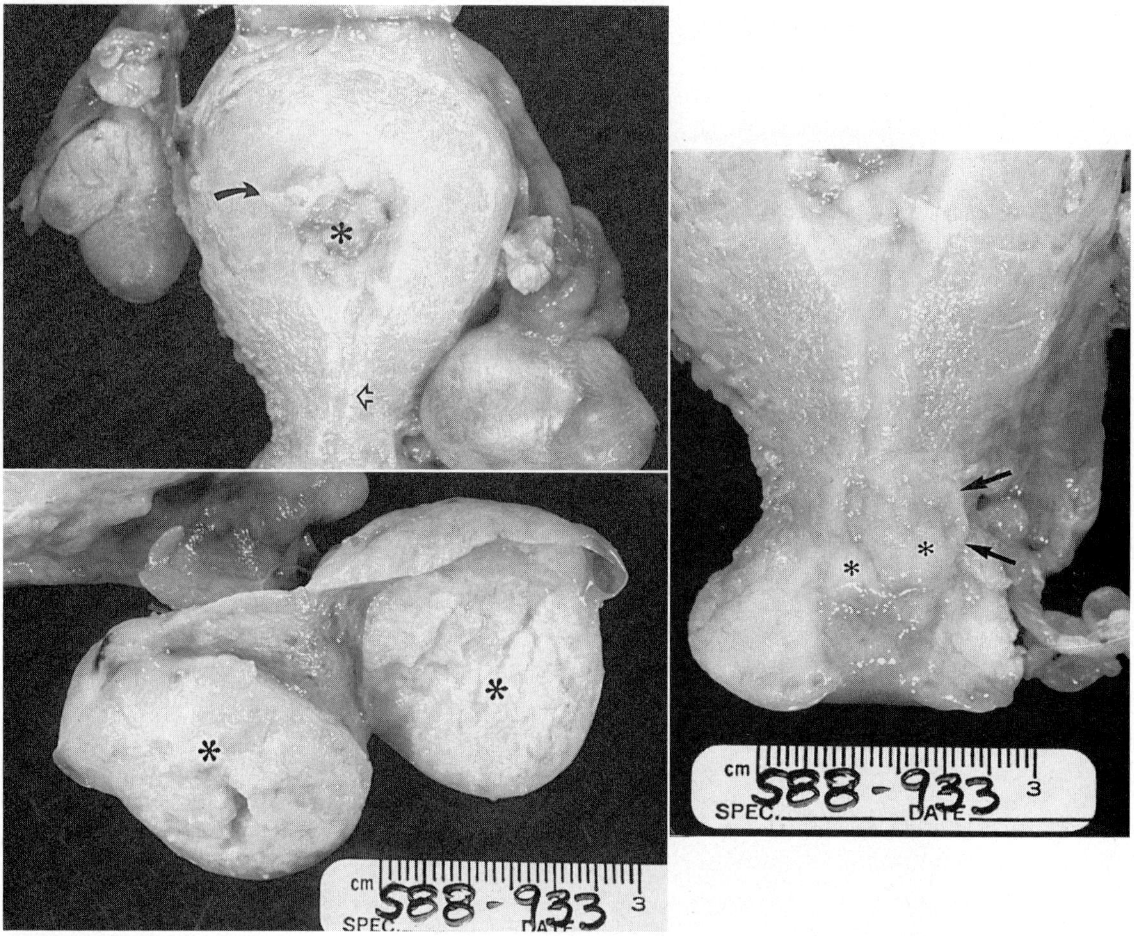

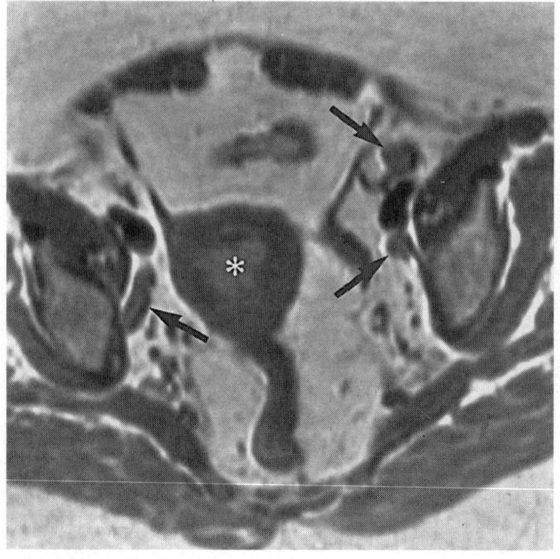

Fig. 8-23 Stage IIIC endometrial carcinoma. There is bilateral iliac lymphadenopathy *(arrows)*. Note the widened endometrial canal *(asterisk)*. (TR 2000, TE 20.) (From Olson MC, Posniak HV, Tempany C, Dudiak CM: MR imaging of the female pelvic region, *RadioGraphics* 12:445-465, 1992; with permission.)

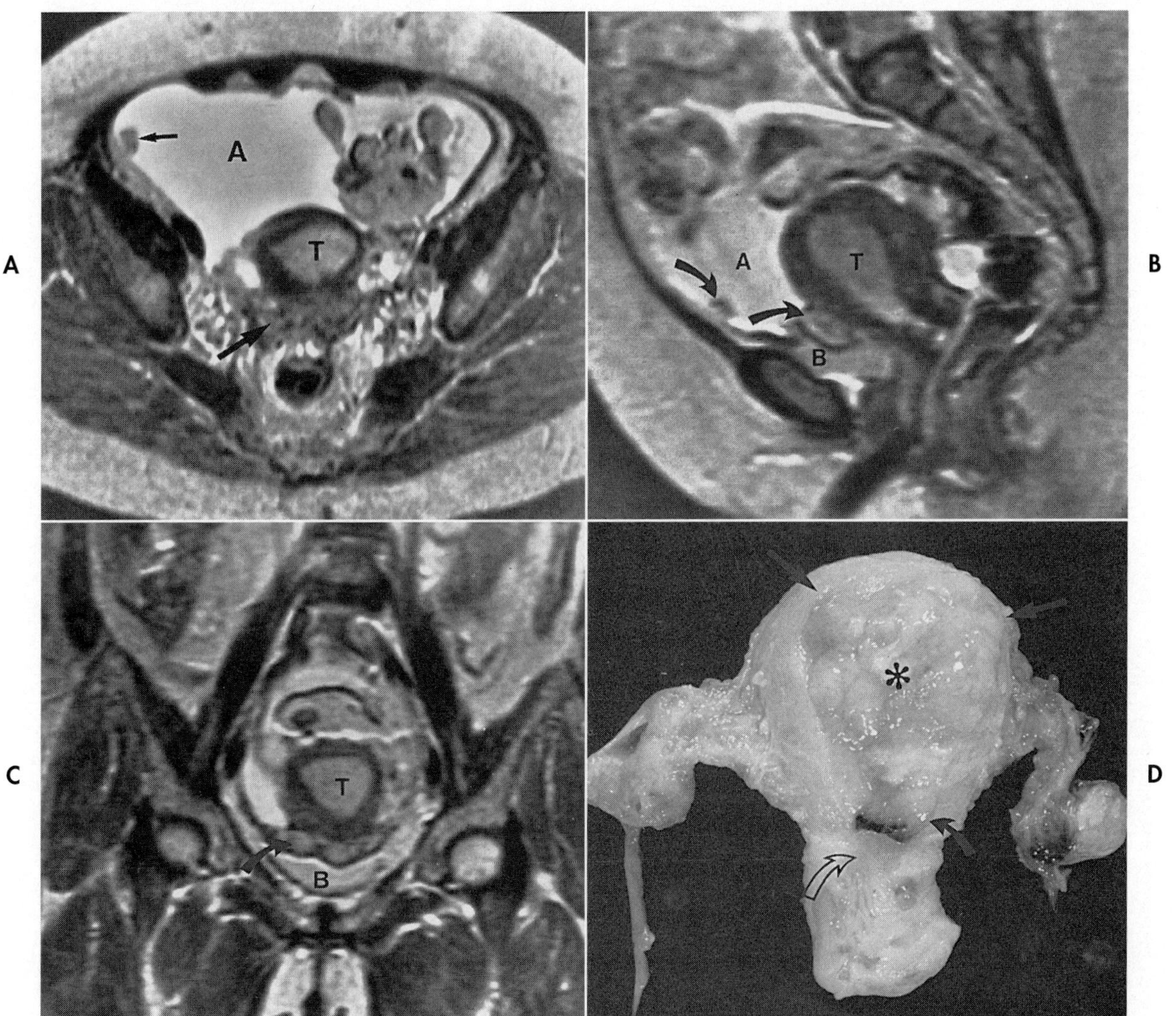

Fig. 8-24 Stage IVB endometrial carcinoma. Axial **(A)**, sagittal **(B)**, and coronal **(C)** T2-weighted MR images (TR 2200, TE 70) demonstrate tumor *(T)* distending the endometrial canal, ascites *(A)*, and peritoneal metastases *(arrows)*. *B*, Bladder. **D,** A coronal section of the uterus reveals a large tumor *(asterisk)* distending the endometrial cavity, with deep myometrial invasion *(straight arrows)*. The curved closed arrow points to the inferior extent of tumor. The open arrow points to a blood clot in the cervical canal. (From Posniak HV, Olson MC, Dudiak CM, et al: Imaging of uterine carcinoma: correlation with clinical and pathologic findings, *RadioGraphics* 10:15-27, 1990; with permission.)

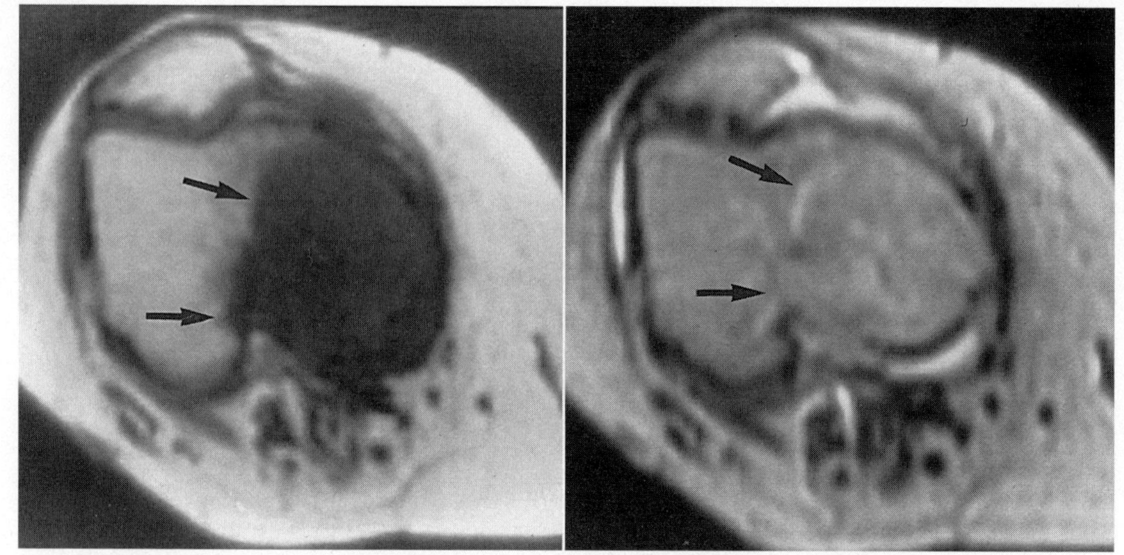

Fig. 8-25 Bone metastasis in a patient with stage IVB endometrial carcinoma. **A,** A T1-weighted image (TR 700, TE20) demonstrates a low signal intensity tumor with a well-defined margin between the tumor *(arrows)* and the normal marrow in the distal femur. **B,** A T2-weighted image (TR 2000, TE 80) shows similar signal intensity of tumor and normal marrow. The tumor margin *(arrows)* is poorly seen on this sequence.

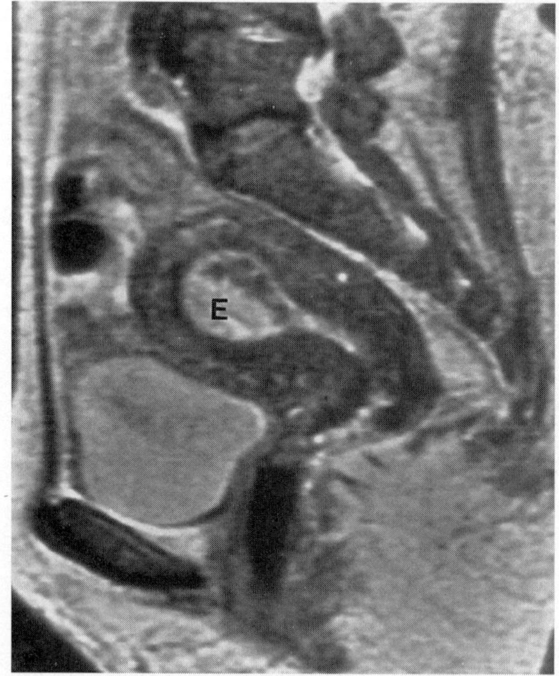

Fig. 8-26 Endometrial hyperplasia. A sagittal T2-weighted image (TR 2200, TE 80) of a postmenopausal woman with distention of the endometrial canal due to endometrial hyperplasia. This case demonstrates the limitations of MR imaging and the need for histologic diagnosis. (From Olson MC, Posniak HV, Tempany CM, Dudiak CM: MR imaging of the female pelvic region, *RadioGraphics* 12:445-465, 1992; with permission.)

mine may have a useful role in evaluating patients with uterine malignancy. They found that the most valuable contribution of contrast enhancement was in differentiating viable tumor from debris.[31] Contrast-enhanced images showed tumors not depicted on nonenhanced images in four of 20 patients.[31] The addition of a contrast medium improved the accuracy of staging and of determination of depth of invasion, but this was not statistically significant.[31]

Management

Total abdominal hysterectomy and bilateral salpingo-oophorectomy are the mainstays of treatment. Adjuvant intracavitary or external beam radiotherapy may be used to prevent vaginal recurrence and sterilize microscopic disease in pelvic lymph nodes and other pelvic structures. Patients with well-differentiated stage I tumors and little or no myometrial invasion have an 85% to 90% survival rate with surgery alone.[3] Those with stage I disease and poorly differentiated tumors or deep myometrial invasion have a 5-year survival rate of 50% or less. Adjuvant radiotherapy is indicated in these cases.

Patients with stage II lesions generally receive combined surgery and radiation therapy. Overall, there is a lower rate of survival than in stage I, which probably relates to increased tumor spread to pelvic and periaortic nodes as well as dissemination to the upper abdomen. With gross cervical involvement, the 5-year survival is 56%.[32]

The 5-year survival rate for stage III is approximately 30%, with a range from 20% to 80%. Patients with tumor limited to the fallopian tubes and ovaries have a better prognosis.[3] Those with stage IV disease receive chemotherapy. The most commonly used systemic therapy is a progestational agent; 30% to 35% of patients respond. Cytotoxic chemotherapy may be used, and 20% to 40% of patients respond to this treatment.[3] Overall 5-year survival rate for stage IV disease is approximately 10%.[32]

UTERINE SARCOMA

Uterine sarcomas are uncommon, accounting for approximately 1% of malignant neoplasms of the female genital tract.[33] Because of this, single institutions have limited experience, and no large studies have been published describing the imaging features.

The first classification scheme for uterine sarcomas was described by Ober in 1959[34] and provided the basis for several other classifications still in use. The Gynecologic Oncology Group has simplified the classification and places uterine sarcomas into one of five groups: mixed mesodermal homologous, mixed mesodermal heterologous, leiomyosarcoma, endometrial stromal sarcoma, and uterine sarcoma type not specified.[33] Mixed mesodermal sarcoma is also known as mixed müllerian sarcoma.

Mixed mesodermal sarcoma and leiomyosarcoma account for 90% of uterine sarcomas.[35] There has been debate in the literature over which of these is more common.

Mixed mesodermal sarcoma is very malignant and contains both carcinomatous and sarcomatous elements. The carcinoma is usually adenocarcinoma but may be undifferentiated or (rarely) squamous cell carcinoma.[36] Stromal sarcoma is the most common sarcomatous element found in these tumors. They are subdivided into homologous and heterologous groups, depending on whether the malignant tissue arises from a cell type common to the uterus or a cell type usually found outside the uterus, such as bone, cartilage, or skeletal muscle.

Mixed mesodermal sarcomas metastasize via vascular and lymphatic routes. Metastases may occur with minimal myometrial invasion. The most important prognostic feature is the extent of tumor at the time of diagnosis, with only rare patient survival when extrauterine disease is demonstrated.

Leiomyosarcoma is often found in association with benign leiomyomas. The prevalence of leiomyosarcoma in patients undergoing surgery for leiomyomas has been reported to be 0.13%.[33] These tumors arise from the myometrium, and most are intramural. Vascular invasion may occur in 10% to 20%[37]; when this occurs, there is a propensity for hematogenous dissemination, with the lungs a common site for metastatic disease. Favorable prognostic features include premenopausal status, confinement within a myoma, low mitotic rate, absence of necrosis, and the presence of hyalinization in the adjacent tissue.

Endometrial stromal sarcoma is less common than mixed mesodermal sarcoma and leiomyosarcoma. Arising from the endometrial stroma, their malignant potential ranges from low grade to very anaplastic, with low-grade lesions predominating. They tend to be locally invasive, but late metastases do occur.

Clinical features

Uterine sarcomas occur most commonly in women over 40. Most patients are postmenopausal, with an average age of 58 years.[36] Stromal tumors tend to occur in younger women between 40 and 50 years of age, and mixed mesodermal tumors occur in the middle to late 60s.[33]

Abnormal uterine bleeding is the most common symptom, and an enlarged, irregular uterus the most common physical finding.[36] Some patients present with abdominal pain and/or abdominal pressure or vaginal discharge. Associated characteristics include obesity, hypertension, and diabetes. In some series, previous pelvic radiation has been an associated finding.

Most patients undergo fractional D&C before hysterectomy. Leiomyosarcoma, owing to its frequent intramural location, is diagnosed by D&C in only 20% to 60% of cases.[33]

No formal staging system is in use for uterine sarcoma, and many physicians use the FIGO staging system for endometrial carcinoma in these patients. Under this staging system, many patients present with Stage I disease, the 5-year survival rate for which is approximately 50%. Survival rates are much lower when the tumor has spread beyond the uterine corpus, with a reported cure rate of 12% or less for stages II to IV combined.[35]

Imaging

The findings of uterine sarcoma on transabdominal US are nonspecific. Transvaginal scanning may be useful in defining the extent of endometrial and myometrial involvement, but, as in endometrial carcinoma, it does not allow a specific diagnosis to be made.

CT has proven value in screening for metastatic disease (Figs. 8-27 and 8-28) and monitoring response to therapy. Its role in staging localized dis-

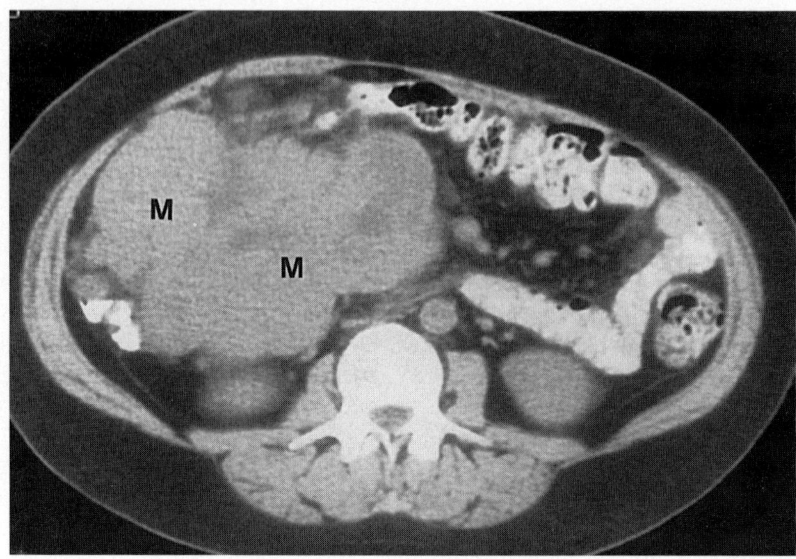

Fig. 8-27 A large mesenteric metastasis *(M)* in a patient with stage IV uterine leiomyosarcoma.

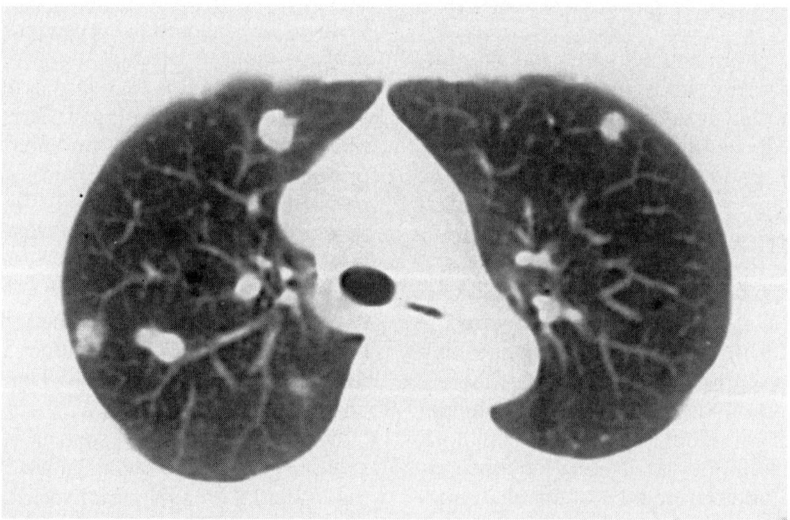

Fig. 8-28 CT of the thorax demonstrates multiple lung metastases in a patient with mixed müllerian uterine sarcoma.

ease has been limited, and there are no specific findings on CT that allow the diagnosis of sarcoma to be made with certainty. It is difficult to distinguish a leiomyoma from a leiomyosarcoma unless metastatic disease is present. Trerotola et al reported the CT features of 14 patients with uterine sarcoma. Eight patients had a large, low-density necrotic mass within the uterine cavity. In seven of these patients, the tumor was larger than 10 cm; in the other six, the mass was smaller and homogeneous, and was either hypodense or isodense with the myometrium. There was no apparent dif-

ference in the CT appearance of the various types of sarcomas.[38]

There have been very few reports of the MR features of uterine sarcoma, and to date, no specific findings have been reported. The reported tumors have been bulky, often distorting the uterine contour. On T1-weighted images the tumors have low signal intensity, becoming hyperintense and often inhomogeneous on T2-weighting (Fig. 8-29).[39] Shapeero and Hricak reported a series of seven patients with mixed müllerian (mesodermal) sarcomas imaged with MR. These patients all had large

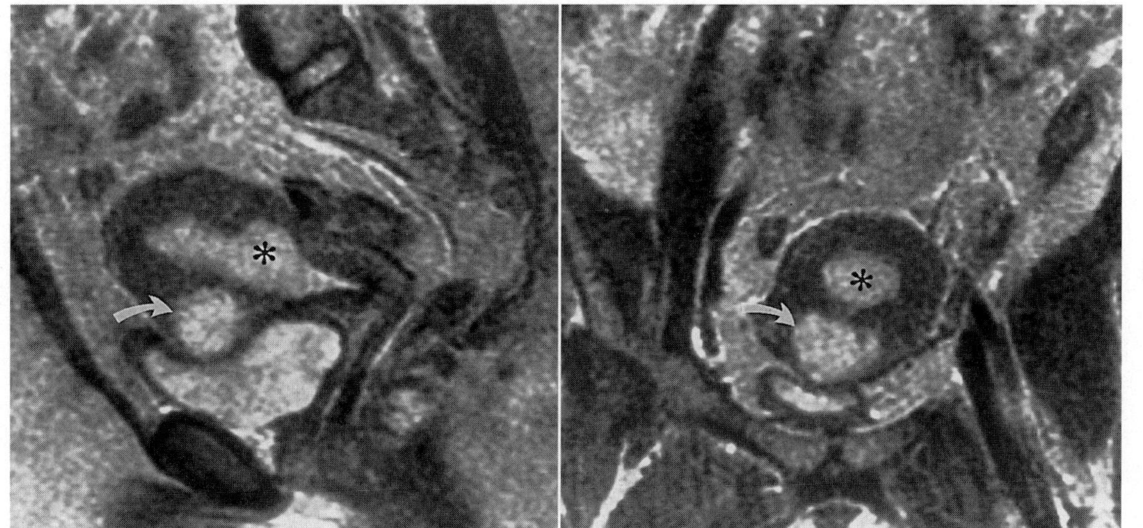

Fig. 8-29 Sagittal (**A**) and coronal (**B**) T2-weighted MR images (TR 2300, TE 70) of a woman with mixed müllerian uterine sarcoma. The endometrial canal is widened by high signal intensity tumor *(asterisk)*. A focal myometrial tumor mass *(arrow)* extends close to the serosal surface. (Courtesy of Dr. Michael Shannon, MacNeal Hospital, Berwyn, IL.)

tumors with deep myometrial invasion. MR was useful in evaluating tumor extent within the myometrium and defining the presence of peritoneal and other pelvic metastases.[40] In this series the MR findings were thought to be nonspecific, simulating those of invasive endometrial carcinoma.

Management

Total abdominal hysterectomy and bilateral salpingo-oophorectomy form the standard treatment for uterine sarcoma. Many physicians advocate pelvic lymph node dissection. Radiation therapy may be helpful in reducing the incidence of pelvic recurrence, but it is uncertain whether or not it improves 5-year survival. The role of chemotherapy has not been adequately defined. Several drugs have proved useful for uterine sarcoma, and there is ongoing evaluation to determine the best regimen. The role of adjuvant chemotherapy is uncertain.

GESTATIONAL TROPHOBLASTIC DISEASE

Gestational trophoblastic neoplasia is a general term for a spectrum of tumors arising from placental villi, including benign hydatidiform mole, invasive mole, and choriocarcinoma. These tumors have a very sensitive serologic marker, the beta subunit of human chorionic gonadotropin (hCG), which is abnormally elevated in the presence of the disease.[41]

Hydatidiform mole is the most common form,

occurring in approximately 1 in 1500 pregnancies in the United States.[42] The incidence is significantly higher in the Far East, where it is reported in as many as 1 in 120 pregnancies.[43] Approximately 80% of patients with hydatidiform mole have a benign course with spontaneous resolution after uterine curettage. About 15% develop locally invasive disease and 5% develop choriocarcinoma.[42] Choriocarcinoma occurs most commonly after a hydatidiform mole but may follow any pregnancy, including normal pregnancy, abortion, and ectopic pregnancy. Malignant trophoblastic disease may occur soon after pregnancy or up to many years later.

Several risk factors have been identified, the most significant being maternal age.[42] Women over 40 and under 15 years old have an increased incidence of trophoblastic disease. Patients who have had molar pregnancies have an increased risk in later conceptions. Nutritional factors may also play a role. It has been suggested that a deficiency of animal fat and carotene may contribute to this disease. Age and parity do not appear to affect the clinical outcome of a patient with hydatidiform mole.[43]

Hydatidiform mole

Pathologically, the chorionic villi become overdistended, forming numerous vesicles. These are derived from both syncytiotrophoblasts and cytotrophoblasts.[44]

Essentially all patients have delayed menses and

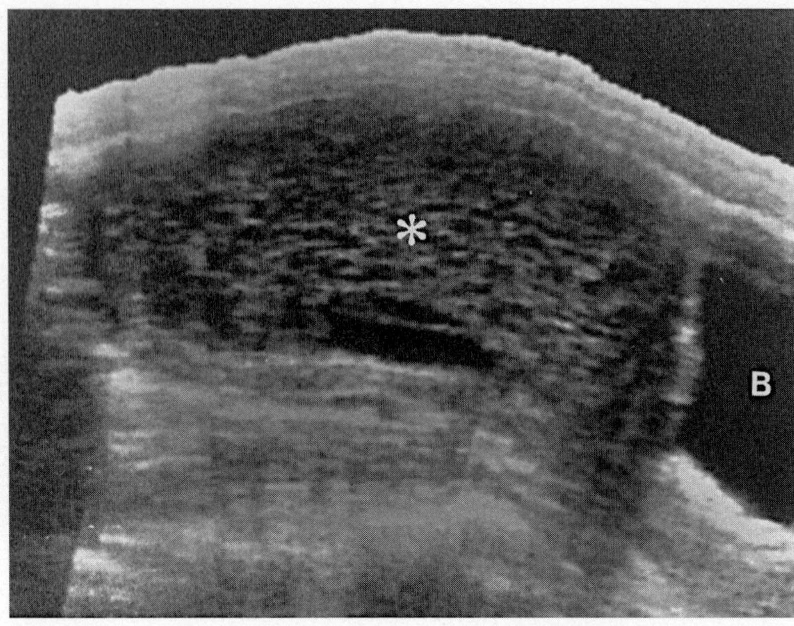

Fig. 8-30 Sagittal transabdominal US image of a woman with a molar pregnancy. The uterus *(asterisk)* is enlarged and filled with echogenic material containing multiple small cystic spaces. *B, Bladder.*

most are considered pregnant. Symptoms and signs include hyperemesis, pain, and vaginal bleeding and/or expulsion of grapelike vesicles. Preeclampsia in the first trimester is virtually pathognomonic. It occurs in approximately 12% of patients. Hyperthyroidism is rare but can precipitate a medical emergency; it is caused by the production of a thyrotropin-like substance by the molar tissue.[43]

Approximately 50% of patients have a uterus that is "large for dates;" 20% have an appropriately sized uterus and 30% have a uterus smaller than expected for the length of gestation.[43] Signs of a normal intrauterine pregnancy are absent. Theca lutein cysts of the ovary are enlarged in approximately 15% of patients, and these are caused by excessive hCG produced by the molar tissue. Patients with enlarged theca lutein cysts have a higher incidence of developing malignant sequelae.[43] Rarely, a fetus may coexist with a mole; the fetus is usually growth retarded and dies in the first trimester. It has a triploid karyotype. Malignant sequelae are much less frequent after a partial mole than after a complete mole.[42]

Diagnosis. Markedly elevated levels of serum hCG suggest the diagnosis. Ultrasonography is the radiologic tool of choice for the initial evaluation of molar pregnancy. If this condition is present, the sonographic appearance varies according to gestational age. Early in the pregnancy, there is diffusely echogenic material in the endometrium represent-

ing multiple tissue-fluid interfaces. Later, multiple cystic spaces become apparent (Fig. 8-30). Coexistent theca lutein cysts manifest as multiloculated cystic ovarian masses (Fig. 8-31). If there is a coexistent fetus, this is readily evident (Fig. 8-32).

The CT and MR findings of hydatidiform mole have been described. On CT images after administration of contrast material, there is enhancement of the endometrial area. There is no extension into the myometrium, and no discrete myometrial lesions are seen.[45] On T1-weighted MR images, there is no distinction between the mole and the myometrium. T2-weighted images demonstrate diffuse high signal in the mole, reflecting fluid in the vesicles. An intact rim of myometrium around the mole indicates that there has been no invasion (Fig. 8-33).[46]

Management. Patients with hydatidiform mole are treated by uterine evacuation and followed with serial measurements of hCG levels. Eighty percent undergo spontaneous regression of any residual trophoblastic disease and resume normal menstrual function. Approximately 15% develop invasive moles, and 5% develop choriocarcinoma.

Malignant gestational trophoblastic disease

The term *invasive mole* applies to moles characterized by abnormal penetrativeness and extensive local invasion, along with excessive trophoblastic proliferation and preservation of the villous pattern

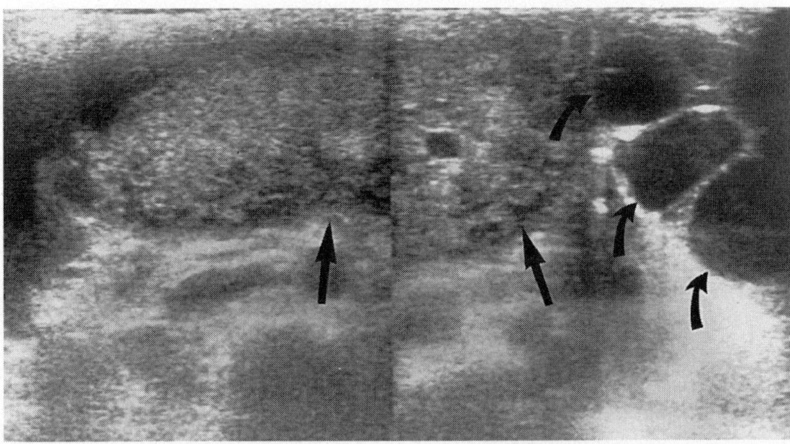

Fig. 8-31 Molar pregnancy with multiple theca lutein cysts. An axial transabdominal US image demonstrates marked distention of the uterus *(straight arrows)* with molar tissue. Theca lutein cysts *(curved arrows)* are noted in the left ovary.

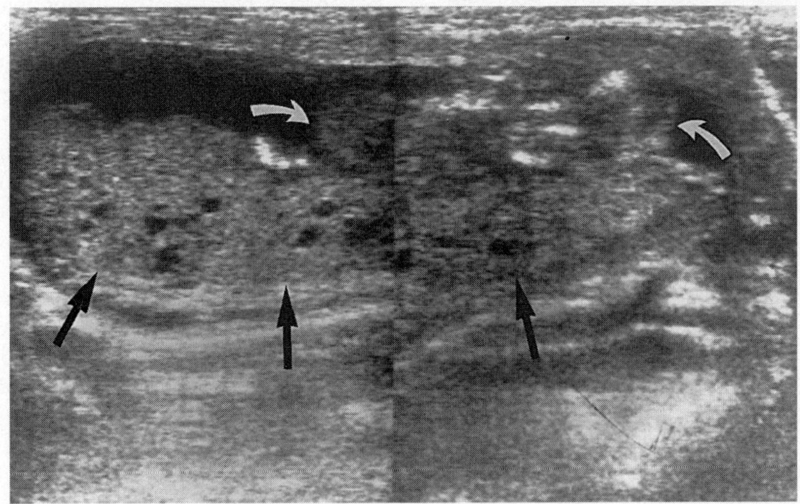

Fig. 8-32 Molar pregnancy with coexistent fetus. A sagittal transabdominal US image demonstrates the fetus anteriorly *(curved arrows)* and molar tissue posteriorly *(black arrows).* The fetus had a triploid karyotype.

seen in benign hydatidiform moles. These proliferative villi may extend locally to invade the parametrium or vaginal wall.[42]

Patients with invasive mole usually present with irregular vaginal bleeding, theca lutein cysts, uterine subinvolution or asymmetric enlargement, and elevated hCG levels. The tumor may erode into uterine vessels, causing vaginal bleeding, or may penetrate the myometrium, producing intraperitoneal hemorrhage. Curettage may be negative if the tumor does not extend to the endometrium.

Choriocarcinoma is characterized microscopically by a disorderly growth of trophoblastic tissue into the myometrium with extensive coagulation necrosis and hemorrhage. It differs from invasive mole in that the villous pattern is absent.[42]

Metastases are frequent with choriocarcinoma, but vaginal bleeding is still the most common presenting complaint. When present, metastases usually appear relatively early and involve the lung, brain, liver, kidney, and bone. On occasion, there may be evidence of metastatic disease without residual intrauterine tumor.

Imaging. An early diagnosis is important to minimize the amount of tumor before therapy. Sonographic findings reflect the wide spectrum of pelvic involvement. The uterus is usually enlarged. The endometrium can be normal or have residual

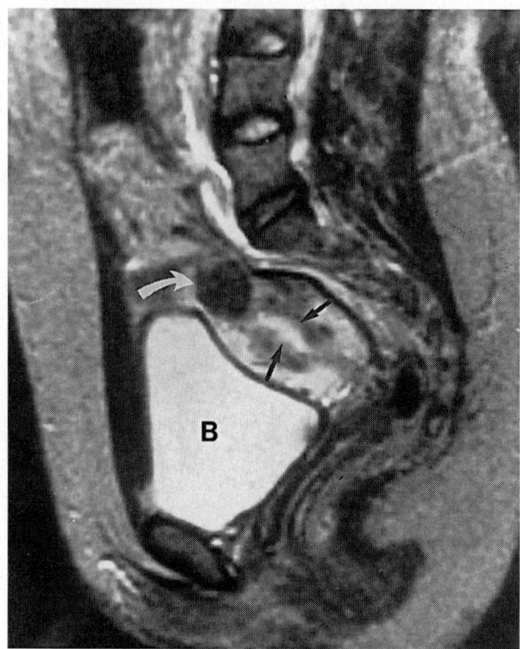

Fig. 8-33 Molar pregnancy. A sagittal T2-weighted MR image (TR 2400, TE 80) in a patient who had a spontaneous incomplete abortion of molar tissue. There is widening of the endometrial canal due to residual high signal intensity molar tissue *(straight arrows)*. Inhomogeneous myometrial signal intensity is of uncertain significance. The curved arrow points to leiomyoma. *B,* Bladder.

tumor, which is echogenic. Higher-grade tumor manifests as a complex echogenic mass with focal sonolucencies.[47,48] Myometrial tumor is also usually echogenic and well defined; it may extend into the parametrium. Large uterine vessels may be seen. Endovaginal US may better delineate the mass and its relationship to the endometrium and surrounding structures.[49]

Doppler US has been reported to be useful in patients with low hCG levels. Long et al[50] found that the pulsatility index in patients with invasive mole or choriocarcinoma was significantly lower than that in normal or pregnant women. The uterine circulation has a characteristic Doppler pattern, suggesting the presence of large, low-resistance blood vessels. Abnormal vascular signals may be elicited from any part of the uterus, even without visualization of enlarged uterine vessels. Color flow imaging may facilitate detection of this abnormal intrauterine blood flow.[52]

CT of the brain, chest, abdomen, and pelvis is used to evaluate patients with persistent gestational trophoblastic disease. The uterus is usually enlarged, with or without focal lobulations; its size does not correlate with hCG levels.[53] The focal masses may enhance on bolus injection of IV contrast material, presumably reflecting their increased vascularity. Hypodense areas following a bolus of contrast material may be due to intra- or peritumoral hemorrhage or necrosis. Local extrauterine extension and dilated uterine arteries may be seen. Bilateral theca lutein cysts were demonstrated in 54% of patients in a series by Kent Davis et al.[53]

The MR findings of malignant trophoblastic disease have been described.[54] On T1-weighted and proton density images the tumors are usually isointense with the uterus. Areas of high intensity consistent with subacute hemorrhage may be seen (Fig. 8-34, *A*). On T2-weighted images there is distortion of the uterine zones, with obliteration of the endometrium-myometrium interface in most patients. The tumors show a heterogeneous pattern of high and low intensity with irregular, indistinct boundaries between the tumor and myometrium. Prominent vessels coursing through the tumor, myometrium, and adnexae are manifested as serpiginous areas of signal void (Fig. 8-34). Tumor extension into the adnexae or vagina is apparent on T2-weighted images, where the tumors have higher intensity than the normal structures. Theca lutein cysts have low or medium intensity on T1-weighted images and high intensity on T2-weighting.

MR is particularly useful in patients in whom the tumor is deep within the myometrium and does not extend to the endometrium, and who may have a negative curettage (Fig. 8-35). MR may also be useful in excluding a uterine source for elevated hCG levels in patients with extrauterine germ cell tumors.

After treatment the return of visible uterine zones, a decrease in adnexal and myometrial vascularity, and the development of intralesional hemorrhage or necrosis usually parallel a decrease in serum hCG.[54]

Management. The treatment of molar pregnancies consists of uterine D&C with follow-up testing of serial serum hCG levels. Persistent hCG elevation or failure to return to normal levels is interpreted as evidence of residual or recurrent disease. Elevated hCG levels occurring many months after D&C may also reflect metastatic disease.

Methotrexate remains the single most effective chemotherapeutic agent for treating gestational trophoblastic neoplasia and local recurrences. Multiple chemotherapeutic agents, with or without adjuvant radiotherapy, may be needed for more aggressive disease. During or after treatment, imaging studies are usually required only when hCG levels plateau or rise unexpectedly.

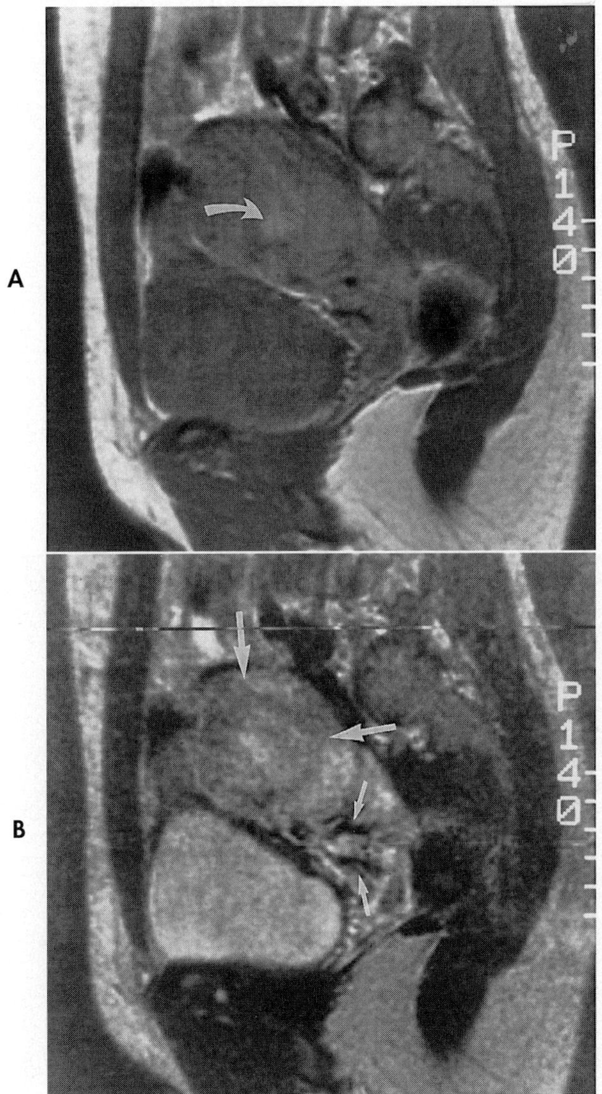

Fig. 8-34 Choriocarcinoma. **A,** A sagittal proton-density image (TR 2500, TE 20) demonstrates an enlarged uterus with a central area of high signal intensity *(curved arrow)* due to hemorrhage. **B,** A T2-weighted image (TR 2500, TE 80) shows an inhomogeneous mass invading the myometrium *(long arrows).* Note the enlarged uterine vessels *(short arrows).*

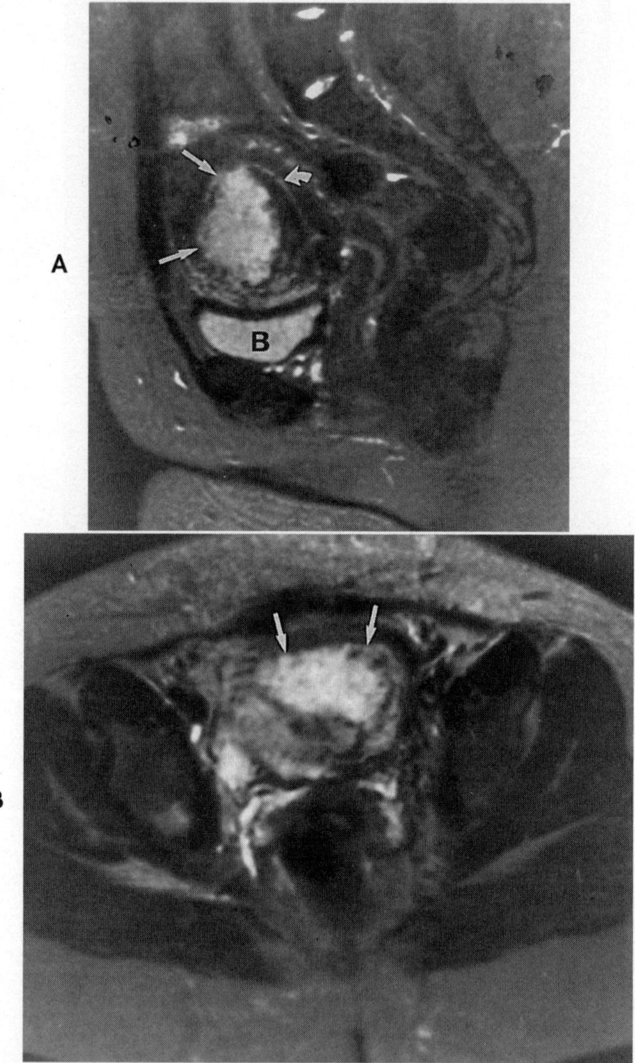

Fig. 8-35 Invasive mole. Sagittal **(A)** and axial **(B)** T2-weighted MR images (TR 3000, TE 80) demonstrate high signal intensity tumor *(arrows)* in the anterior myometrium that does not extend to the endometrial canal. The endometrial canal is displaced posteriorly *(curved arrow)*. *B,* Bladder.

US, CT, and MR may be used to image patients with uterine malignancies. The choice of imaging modality depends on institutional preference, tumor histology, and stage of disease. Patients presenting with abnormal vaginal bleeding often undergo US evaluation of the pelvis. If a molar pregnancy is evident, no additional imaging may be needed. CT, MR, or both are often used for patients with malignant trophoblastic disease. We employ MR to evaluate the depth of myometrial invasion and stage local disease in patients with a known diagnosis of uterine adenocarcinoma. CT is performed to evaluate extrapelvic disease and for routine surveillance of metastatic disease. Uterine sarcomas are uncommon but may be encountered during US, CT, or MR examinations of the pelvis. In a patient with a known diagnosis of uterine sarcoma, we use MR for staging pelvic disease and CT to evaluate extrapelvic and metastatic disease.

REFERENCES

1. *Cancer Facts and Figures, 1989,* New York, 1989, American Cancer Society.
2. DiSaia PF, Creasman WT: *Adenocarcinoma of the uterus.* In *Clinical gynecologic oncology,* St. Louis, 1989, Mosby-Year Book, pp 161-197.
3. Bloomer WD, Howes AE: *Carcinoma of the endometrium.* In Moossa AR, Schimpff SC, Robson ML, editors: *Comprehensive textbook of oncology,* Baltimore, 1991, Williams & Wilkins, pp 1029-1035.
4. Announcements. FIGO stages, 1988 revision, *Gynecol Oncol* 35:125-127, 1989.
5. Cowles TA, Magrina JF, Masterson BF, Capen CV: Comparison of clinical and surgical staging in patients with endometrial carcinoma, *Obstet Gynecol* 66:413-416, 1985.
6. Boronow RC, Morrow CP, Creasman WT, et al: Surgical staging in endometrial cancer: clinical-pathologic findings of a prospective study, *Obstet Gynecol* 63:825-832, 1984.
7. Hricak H, Stern JL, Fisher MR, et al: Endometrial carcinoma staging by MR imaging, *Radiology* 162:297-305, 1987.
8. Fleischer AC, Dudley BS, Entman SS, et al: Myometrial invasion by endometrial carcinoma: sonographic assessment, *Radiology* 162:307-310, 1987.
9. Cacciatore B, Lehtovirta P, Wahlström T, et al: Preoperative sonographic evaluation of endometrial cancer, *Am J Obstet Gynecol* 160:133-137, 1989.
10. Thorvinger B, Gudmundsson T, Horvath G, et al: Staging in local endometrial carcinoma. Assessment of magnetic resonance and ultrasound examinations, *Acta Radiol 30:* 525-529, 1989.
11. Salem S: *The uterus and adnexa.* In Rumack CM, Wilson SR, Charboneau JW, editors: *Diagnostic ultrasound,* St. Louis, 1991, Mosby-Year Book, pp 383-412.
12. Gordon AN, Fleischer AC, Reed GW: Depth of myometrial invasion in endometrial cancer: preoperative assessment by transvaginal ultrasonography, *Gynecol Oncol* 39:321-327, 1990.
13. Conte M, Guariglia L, Panici PB, et al: Transvaginal ultrasound evaluation of myometrial invasion in endometrial carcinoma, *Gynecol Obstet Invest* 29:224-226, 1990.
14. Lee JKT, Marx MV: *Pelvis.* In Lee JKT, Sagel SS, Stanley RJ, editors: *Computed body tomography with MRI correlation,* ed 2, New York, 1989, Raven Press, pp 851-898.
15. Dore R, Moro G, D'Andrea F, et al: CT evaluation of myometrium invasion in endometrial carcinoma, *J Comput Assist Tomogr* 11:282-289, 1987.
16. McCarthy S, Tauber C, Gore J: Female pelvic anatomy: MR assessment of variations during the menstrual cycle and with use of oral contraceptives, *Radiology* 160:119-123, 1986.
17. Demas BE, Hricak H, Jaffee RB: Uterine MR imaging: effects of hormonal stimulation, *Radiology* 159:123-126, 1986.
18. Janus CL, Wiczyk HP, Laufer N: Magnetic resonance imaging of the menstrual cycle, *Magn Res Imaging* 6:669-674, 1988.
19. McCarthy S, Scott G, Majumdar S, et al: Uterine junctional zone: MR study of water content and relaxation properties, *Radiology* 171:241-243, 1989.
20. Brown HK, Stoll BS, Nicosia SV, et al: Uterine junctional zone: correlation between histologic findings and MR imaging, *Radiology* 179:409-413, 1991.
21. McCarthy S: Magnetic resonance imaging in the evaluation of infertile women, *Magn Reson Q* 6:239-249, 1990.
22. Scoutt LM, Flynn SD, Luthringer DJ, et al: Junctional zone of the uterus: correlation of MR imaging and histologic examination of hysterectomy specimens, *Radiology* 179:403-407, 1991.
23. Heiken JP, Lee JKT: MR imaging of the pelvis, *Radiology* 166:11-16, 1988.
24. Yazigi R, Cohen J, Munoz AK, Sandstad J: Magnetic resonance imaging determination of myometrial invasion in endometrial carcinoma, *Gynecol Oncol* 34:94-97, 1989.
25. Hricak H, Rubenstein LV, Gherman GM, Karstaedt N: MR imaging evaluation of endometrial carcinoma: results of an NCI cooperative study, *Radiology* 179:829-832, 1991.
26. Lien HH, Blomlie V, Trope C, et al: Cancer of the endometrium: value of MR imaging in determining depth of invasion into the myometrium, *AJR* 157:1221-1223, 1991.
27. Fishman Javitt MC, Stein HL, Lovecchio JL: MRI in staging of endometrial and cervical carcinoma, *Magn Res Imaging* 5:83-92, 1987.
28. Picus D, Lee JKT: Magnetic resonance imaging of the female pelvis, *Urol Radiol* 8:166-174, 1986.
29. Worthington JL, Balfe DM, Lee JKT, et al: Uterine neoplasms: MR imaging, *Radiology* 159:725-730, 1986.
30. Hricak H: MRI of the female pelvis. A review, *AJR* 146:1115-1122, 1986.
31. Hricak H, Hamm B, Semelka RC, et al: Carcinoma of the uterus: use of gadopentetate dimeglumine in MR imaging, *Radiology* 181:95-106, 1991.
32. Gusberg SB: *Diagnosis and principles of treatment of cancer of the endometrium.* In Gusberg SB, Shingleton MH, Deppe G, editors: *Female genital cancer,* New York, 1988, Churchill Livingstone, pp 337-360.
33. Gordon AN, Kaufman RH: *Sarcoma and lymphoma.* In Gusberg SB, Shingleton MH, Deppe G, editors: *Female genital cancer,* New York, 1988, Churchill Livingstone, pp 459-479.
34. Ober WB: Uterine sarcomas: histogenesis and taxonomy, *Ann NY Acad Sci* 75:568-585, 1959.
35. Thigpen JT: *Cancers of the female genital tract: introduction.* In Moossa AR, Schimpff SC, Robson MC, editors: *Comprehensive textbook of oncology,* vol 2, Baltimore, 1991, Williams & Wilkins, pp 1001-1005.
36. Jones HW: *Sarcoma of the uterus.* In Jones HW, Wentz AC, Burnett LS, editors: *Novak's textbook of gynecology,* ed 11, Baltimore, 1988, Williams & Wilkins, pp 761-772.
37. DiSaia PF, Creasman WT: *Sarcoma of the uterus.* In *Clinical gynecologic oncology,* St. Louis, 1989, Mosby-Year Book, pp 198-213.
38. Trerotola SO, Fishman EK, Kuhlman J: Computed tomography of uterine sarcomas, *Clin Imaging* 13:208-211, 1989.

39. Worthington JL, Balfe DM, Lee JKT, et al: Uterine neoplasms: MR imaging, *Radiology* 159:725-730, 1986.
40. Shapeero LG, Hricak H: Mixed müllerian sarcoma of the uterus: MR imaging findings, *AJR* 153:317-319, 1989.
41. Soper JT, Hammond CB: *Gestational trophoblastic disease and gestational choriocarcinoma.* In Gusberg SB, Shingleton MH, Deppe G, editors: *Female genital cancer,* New York, 1988, Churchill Livingstone, pp 435-458.
42. Jones HW: *Gestational trophoblastic disease.* In Jones HW, Weitz AC, Burnett LS, editors: *Novak's textbook of gynecology,* ed 11, Baltimore, 1988, Williams & Wilkins, pp 863-893.
43. Disaia PF, Creasman WT: *Gestational trophoblastic neoplasia.* In *Clinical gynecologic oncology,* St. Louis, 1989, Mosby-Year Book, pp 214-240.
44. Fishman Javitt MC, Lovecchio JL, Stein HL: *The uterus.* In Fishman Javitt MC, Stein HL, Lovecchio JL, editors: *Imaging of the pelvis. MRI correlations to CT and ultrasound,* Boston, 1990, Little, Brown, pp 77-108.
45. Miyasaka Y, Hachiya J, Furuya Y, et al: CT evaluation of invasive trophoblastic disease, *J Comput Assist Tomogr* 9:459-462, 1985.
46. Powell MC, Buckley J, Worthington BS, Symonds EM: Magnetic resonance imaging and hydatidiform mole, *Br J Radiol* 59:561-564, 1986.
47. Reid MH, McGahan JP, Oi R: Sonographic evaluation of hydatidiform mole and its look-alikes, *AJR* 140:307-311, 1983.
48. Woo JSK, Wong LC, Ma H: Sonographic patterns of pelvic and hepatic lesions in persistent trophoblastic disease, *J Ultrasound Med* 4:189-198, 1985.
49. Schneider DF, Bukovsky I, Weinraub Z, et al: Transvaginal ultrasound diagnosis and treatment follow-up of invasive trophoblastic disease, *J Clin Ultrasound* 18:110-113, 1990.
50. Long MG, Boultbee JE, Begent RHJ, et al: Preliminary Doppler studies on the uterine artery and myometrium in trophoblastic tumours requiring chemotherapy, *Br J Obstet Gynecol* 97:686-689, 1990.
51. Taylor KJW, Schwartz PE, Kohorn EI: Gestational trophoblastic neoplasia: diagnosis with Doppler US, *Radiology* 165:445-448, 1987.
52. Dobkin GR, Berkowitz RS, Goldstein DP, et al: Duplex ultrasonography for persistent gestational trophoblastic tumor, *J Reprod Med* 36:14-16, 1991.
53. Kent Davis W, McCarthy S, Moss AA, Braga C: Computed tomography of gestational trophoblastic disease, *J Comput Assist Tomogr* 8:1136-1139, 1984.
54. Hricak H, Demas BE, Braga CA, et al: Gestational trophoblastic neoplasm of the uterus: MR assessment, *Radiology* 161:11-16, 1986.

9 Ovarian and Adnexal Diseases

Douglas Brown, Stuart G. Silverman, and Clare M.C. Tempany

This chapter deals with a range of neoplastic and non-neoplastic conditions of the ovary and adnexa. The first section reviews the normal anatomy of the ovary and the methods by which it and the adnexa are imaged using sonography, computed tomography (CT), and magnetic resonance imaging (MRI). The middle section briefly reviews the pathology of some of these lesions, and in the final section the appearance of many of these lesions is discussed.

NORMAL ANATOMY

Normal ovaries are ovoid in shape and attached to the body of the uterus by the broad ligament. They lie in the ovarian fossa, which is bounded posteriorly by the internal iliac vessels and ureter, and anteriorly by the obliterated umbilical artery.

They range in size according to the age of the patient. Adult ovaries measure 3.0 to 5.0 cm $\times$ 0.6 to 1.5 cm and weigh on average 5 to 8 g. The ovarian volume is considered to be the most reliable method of measuring their size.[1] The patients in the study of Cohen et al were divided into three groups: menstruating, postmenopausal, and premenarchal. The average volumes for each of these three groups have been found to be 9.8, 5.8, and 3.0 cm^3, respectively. There was a significant difference in the volume between pregnant (11.1 cm^3) and nonpregnant menstruating patients. The volume of the ovary was determined using the formula for a prolate ellipse: 0.523 $\times$ length $\times$ width $\times$ thickness.

Pathologically, on cut section the ovaries have three zones: the outer cortex, inner medulla, and hilus. The superficial cortex consists of the tunica albuginea. Follicular structures (the cystic follicles, corpora lutea, and corpora albicantia) are typically visible in the cortex and the medulla.

The ovary develops from the germinal epithelium, and the primordial ova differentiate from this and migrate into the substance of the ovarian cortex. These primordial follicles decrease in number over the lifetime of the ovary from 7 million at the 30th week of gestation to 450 during the reproductive years, which will mature at ovulation, leaving only a few remaining at menopause.

IMAGING TECHNIQUES

The three major imaging modalities used for imaging the ovaries and adnexae are ultrasonography, CT, and MRI. The ultrasound examination is usually the first performed on the patient suspected of having ovarian or adnexal pathology. Increasingly, however, MRI and CT are being performed to evaluate more complicated cases, often in conjunction with ultrasonography.

Ultrasonography

Sonography usually plays a pivotal role in the evaluation of pelvic masses. It is often the first imaging method employed in women with suspected pelvic masses and is also used in the follow-up of many adnexal masses. This section considers general issues related to the technique of sonography, the gray scale evaluation of adnexal masses, and the newer application of Doppler in evaluating ovarian masses.

Transvaginal sonography (TVS) is usually considered superior to transabdominal sonography (TAS) for evaluating the adenexa, but TAS is far from obsolete. In many cases, TAS provides sufficient evaluation of the uterus and adnexa. It may also supply useful information when an ovary cannot be identified by TVS, when a mass is very

185

large and incompletely evaluable by TVS, or when a patient declines TVS. Attention is devoted here to the technique of TVS because it is a relatively newer technique than TAS, and because there are several issues related to such endocavitary probes that may not be familiar to all readers.

In general, patient acceptance is very good. However, patients should understand that a transducer will be introduced into the vagina, but that it is rarely uncomfortable. We explain to the patient that we generally need to perform TVS because it permits better images of the ovaries or uterus. We also explain that if the examination is too uncomfortable, the transducer will be withdrawn and the examination stopped. It is also important to have two members of the ultrasonography department present during the sonography, one of whom should be female. Although legal charges of assault are very rare, they are not unheard of, and the presence of a "chaperone" helps prevent such occurrences.

If possible, the TVS should be performed in the first 7 to 10 days of the menstrual cycle in premenopausal women. This may not always be feasible, but performing TVS during this part of the cycle helps prevent misinterpretation of the normal corpus luteum as a pathologic condition. A corpus luteum cyst is not uncommon during the latter half of the menstrual cycle. Also, Doppler findings may be misleading during the latter half of the menstrual cycle, when low resistance flow related to the corpus luteum is anticipated (discussed later in this section).

Different transducer designs are available from manufacturers. Some have the transducer element mounted on the end of the transducer; others are on the side or have an angled transducer element. Much depends on personal preference. The most important factor is that one understands the type of transducer orientation for the particular transvaginal probe being used. Various frequencies are used, although most operate at a center frequency between 5 and 7 MHz. The higher frequency of such transducers affords better resolution but at the expense of decreased depth of penetration of the sound beam.

Infection control procedures are also important in transvaginal scanning. Manufacturers' designs may differ slightly, but their guidelines for disinfecting the transvaginal transducer should be followed. In general, this calls for soaking the transducer in a disinfectant solution for a specified period of time between patients. Before use in each patient, the disinfectant solution should be rinsed from the transducer, and a condom or other plastic cover applied. Adequate lubrication of the transducer, both to provide better imaging quality and

to allow easier insertion into the vagina, is important. The ultrasound coupling gel can be used as a lubricant in most patients being evaluated for an adnexal mass.

Patient preparation and positioning is important. The patient should void before the scan, as a distended urinary bladder may place the uterus and ovaries farther from the transducer, compromising image quality. In positioning the patient, there must be room for the transducer handle to be moved in a sufficient range to allow examination of the entire pelvis. We find that the dorsal lithotomy position is the best. This requires a table that can be adjusted to allow this position and has knee rests. Such a table is not mandatory, and another usually acceptable option is to elevate the patient's buttocks with towels or sheets. The patient can then flex both hips and knees.

We usually give the patient the option of inserting the transducer herself. After slow, gentle insertion of the transducer into the vagina, images in the sagittal and coronal planes are obtained by rotating and angling the transducer. As opposed to TAS, in which there is a larger field of view and usually other visible structures providing an easy reference, there is a limited field of view with TVS. Other than perhaps the sagittal images of the uterus, it is often difficult, at least when learning TVS, to know where the image is obtained unless it is accurately labeled or the interpreter is present during the time of the procedure. This is a minor limitation and the increased resolution generally afforded by TVS makes this worthwhile. The entire pelvis should be surveyed as much as possible, by angling the transducer from side to side and rotating it so that the entire uterus is imaged as well as both ovaries and adnexal regions.

In addition to gray scale sonography, color and pulsed Doppler show potential for better characterization of adnexal masses. With color Doppler imaging, color is assigned to pixels in which there is a frequency shift detected, and usual gray scale assignment is made to pixels without a shift. The color assignments of red and blue are interchangeable by most manufacturers and reflect only the vector of flow toward or away from the transducer. Higher velocities or frequency shifts are displayed in lighter shades of each color. Currently, the information available from color Doppler is more qualitative than quantitative. Color Doppler is used as a guide for pulsed Doppler, from which more quantitative information is obtained. Once the pulsed Doppler gate is placed over the area of concern in which color pixels are noted, a uniform waveform is sought and the screen is frozen. Over a cardiac cycle the peak systolic, peak end-diastolic, and mean velocities can be measured.

From these measurements the pulsatility index (PI) and resistive index (RI) can be calculated. The mean velocity used in the PI formula is a mean of the peak velocities and is generally obtained either by manually tracing the envelope over one cardiac cycle or, in the case of some manufacturers, allowing this function to be performed automatically. Pulsatility index is defined by the formula

$$PI = \frac{\text{peak systolic velocity} - \text{peak end diastolic velocity}}{\text{mean velocity}}$$

Resistive index is defined by the formula

$$RI = \frac{\text{peak systolic velocity} - \text{peak end-diastolic velocity}}{\text{peak systolic velocity}}$$

The role of Doppler evaluation is not clear at this point, but there is potential for better characterization of masses. More specifics of Doppler evaluation of ovarian masses are discussed later in this section.

Computed tomography

As with all imaging protocols, the proper technique often depends on the specific clinical indication. Because of the broad applications of abdominal and pelvic CT, ovarian neoplasms may be detected during a general abdominal survey. In this type of examination, practicality and efficiency are almost as important as diagnostic efficacy. The entire abdomen and pelvis is imaged from the diaphragm to the symphysis pubis. The gastrointestinal tract is maximally opacified, using a standard dose of oral contrast medium, generally between 800 and 1000 ml (28 to 35 oz) of dilute barium, or dilute water-soluble iodinated contrast medium. These oral contrast agents need to be administered at least 2 hours before the study; if the goal is to opacify the colon as well, several hours may be required. The CT section thickness and interval prescriptions vary from institution to institution and also depend on the equipment manufacturer. However, to reduce the effects of respiratory misregistration, which results in gaps in the imaging volume, a contiguous study is desirable throughout the abdomen and pelvis using 10-mm sections and 10-mm increments and, if possible, 5-mm sections. Because of the relative stationary position of the pelvic organs, investigators have employed a 5-mm gap in the pelvis and utilized 10-mm sections at 15-mm intervals in the abdomen. The addition of intravenous (IV) contrast material increases the overall sensitivity of abdominal CT and should be used, unless contraindicated, particularly when the liver, pancreas, and kidneys are the regions of primary interest.

Investigators have altered the above survey protocols to enhance the detection and characterization of ovarian neoplasms as well as to stage ovarian cancer more accurately. A variety of specific protocols have been proposed. A study of epithelial neoplasms of the ovary by Buy et al[2] divided the examination into two parts. The first part involved a bolus of 60 ml of contrast medium during which 10-mm contiguous sections were obtained of the pelvis; this was followed by a second bolus during which a full abdominal pelvic CT scan was obtained. Megibow et al[3] altered the conventional approach to gastrointestinal tract opacification and administered an oral cathartic the night before the examination, gave the conventional dose of oral contrast 2 hours before the study (to opacify just the small bowel), and imaged the pelvis in the prone position after air insufflation of the colon. They obtained 10-mm thick sections at 15-mm intervals in the abdomen, and 5-mm thick sections with 10-mm increments in the pelvis. A total of 200 ml iothalamate meglumine (Conray 43) were administered as a 50-ml bolus followed by a rapid infusion of 100 ml, and the abdomen was scanned. The remaining 50 ml of contrast medium was infused while the pelvis was imaged. While these studies demonstrated the ability of CT to detect, characterize, and stage ovarian neoplasms, the relative contributions of each portion of the protocols are not known. What can be concluded, however, is that (1) complete small bowel opacification with oral contrast media, (2) colonic insufflation with air or contrast media, and (3) evaluation of the entire abdomen and pelvis using contiguous 5 to 10-mm thick sections after bolus administration of contrast medium all help maximize diagnostic efficacy. Further study is needed to determine the precise prescription for optimizing abdominal and pelvic CT in patients with ovarian cancer. The advent of spiral volumetric CT allows for the rapid acquisition of CT data during single breath holds. This increased speed should allow data acquisitions during maximal vascular opacification and the elimination of gaps in the image volume, so-called respiratory misregistration. An additional benefit of spiral volumetric CT is that by eliminating respiratory misregistration, more accurate and more consistent tumor size measurements are possible, which allow accurate comparisons of one examination with a previous one. The benefits of spiral CT with respect to detection, mass characterization, and staging all await further study.

Magnetic resonance imaging

As with all MRI examinations, the approach to each case may be slightly different, depending on the clinical history. In the assessment of ovaries and adnexa, the first decision is what coil to use.

Two choices are currently available, depending on the type of MR unit. The commonly used standard body coil works well for the ovaries and pelvis, and allows for easy extension of the imaging up to the upper abdomen, if indicated. The new phased array multicoils allow for smaller fields of view, and thus offer increased spatial resolution and the increased diagnostic accuracy for assessment of the ovaries and adnexal masses (see Chapter 3, the chapter on MR techniques). They are not useful if the mass is very large (greater than 15 cm) or extends beyond the pelvis.

Before the pelvis is scanned, it is recommended that the following preparatory steps be taken. All patients should be NPO status (nothing by mouth) at least 3 hours prior to the scan; this will reduce the amount of peristalsis. They should also have 1 mg of glucagon injected intramuscularly just before imaging. Patients are usually imaged supine, with the abdominal binding used to reduce the anterior abdominal wall motion. If the patient is receiving gadolinium, a long IV line should be placed before she enters the scanner, to allow for the bolus gadolinium-diethylenetetraminepentaacetic acid (Gd-DTPA) to be given dynamically.

The images obtained should be a combination of T1-weighted and T2-weighted, with postgadolinium T1-weighted images in all cases with a mass or adnexal pathology. The T2-weighted images can be obtained with conventional spin echo or fast spin echo (FSE) sequences. The advantage of FSE is that it is much faster and allows time for additional sequences to be obtained as indicated. With the phased array coil, it is possible to obtain high-resolution images with a small field of view (14 to 16 cm), and thin slices can be used (3 to 4 mm with a 1-mm interslice gap). This approach permits visualization of the ovary itself, and it is also usually possible to see the ovarian stroma and the internal matrix of any pathologic mass. This is particularly useful when the assessment of contrast enhancement is performed. Further details on protocol parameters are available in Chapter 3, the chapter on MR techniques.

Oral contrast has recently become available for MR imaging. Although it is still too early to make any definitive statements regarding its value, it is potentially useful in the female pelvis when imaging masses, to determine the relationship to the bowel wall, and especially in ovarian cancer and endometriosis, for detection of bowel implants.

OVARIAN AND ADNEXAL PATHOLOGY
Non-neoplastic lesions

The ovary and fallopian tubes are the common sites of involvement in patients with pelvic inflammatory disease. The organism is commonly sexually acquired, and patients with intrauterine devices (IUDs) are particularly at risk; the risk is three to eight times greater than in those without IUDs. A tubo-ovarian abscess is the typical finding, which can be uni- or bilateral. The common agents of acute infection are *Neisseria gonorrhoeae,* but *Chlamydia trachomatis* and *Mycoplasma hominis* may also be found.[4]

Polycystic ovarian disease, or Stein-Leventhal syndrome, is a condition of abnormal ovaries accompanied by a symptom complex of oligomenorrhea or amenorrhea, hirsutism, and obesity. It is not an uncommon condition, occurring in 3% to 7% of the population.[5] In fact, it may not be a separate clinical entity, but part of the large group of conditions of hyperandrogenism and stromal hyperthecosis. The ovaries are usually both involved, and although they are usually enlarged (two to five times normal), a normal-sized ovary can be seen. When the ovary is examined grossly, multiple small (1-cm) superficial cortical cysts are seen.[6] The central stroma is usually normal.

Vascular lesions

Ovarian hemorrhage can occur when there is an underling cyst that ruptures. The patient will present with an acute abdomen, if there is hemoperitoneum, and this can be very similar clinically to acute appendicitis. Ovarian torsion is likewise an acute condition, also usually occurring in patients with an underlying ovarian lesion, most often benign. The torsion may occur when the ovary is unusually mobile.[7]

Endometriosis is defined as the ectopic implantation of endometrium beyond the uterus. There are many possible sites of involvement, with the ovaries and pelvic peritoneal surfaces being the most common. Distant sites such as the pleura, causing catamenial pneumothorax, and the subarachnoid space are rare. Endometriotic cysts or endometriomas may be bilateral in up to 50% of cases. They are rarely more than 15 cm in diameter and may replace the normal ovary. Grossly, they have a thick fibrous wall and a fluid center that contains blood, the so-called "chocolate cyst." They are frequently surrounded by dense adhesions and may enlarge to produce nodules, cysts, or both. All solid areas or intracystic components must be carefully examined for possible neoplasia. Malignant tumors have been documented in less than 1% of patients with endometriosis.[8] Periodic menstrual changes within the cyst lead to repeated episodes of bleeding, resulting in the presence of blood of different ages in different areas of the cystic mass.[9] Clinically, patients present with repeated episodes of pelvic or abdominal pain, which occurs at menses and is associated with infertility in 30% to 40% of cases. The infertility may be due to tubal adhesions or ovarian dysfunction.

Neoplastic lesions

Ovarian cancer is the most common fatal gynecological malignancy in the United States, with a disturbing increase in cases and in related deaths over the last 10 years. More than one woman in 70 will develop the disease during her lifetime, most frequently between 50 and 70 years of age. Approximately 24,000 new cases are predicted to be diagnosed in 1994, and 13,600 of these women will die of their disease.[10] There is a familial predisposition, which is thought to be inherited as an autosomal dominant trait with variable penetrance. Women with two or more first-degree relatives with ovarian cancer have as much as a 50% chance of developing the disease.[11] Stages I and II tumors have a significantly different 5-year survival rate from stages III and IV. Data from the Surveillance, Epidemiology and End Results (SEER) program show the following 5-year survival rates: stage I, 82%; stage II, 60%; and combined stages III and IV, 17%.[12] The 5-year survival rates for all stages is 26% (SEER data). There are several high-risk groups, including nulliparous or infertile women. Breast cancer will lead to doubling the risk over the normal population, and patients with ovarian cancer have a three to four times increased risk of breast cancer.

The most common malignant ovarian neoplasms in adult women are serous epithelial tumors, constituting 40%; they may be bilateral in up to 50% of cases. There are gross pathologic features that differ between the benign and malignant neoplasms. The malignant tumors are grossly complex solid and cystic masses. Papillary projections may occur on the inner lining, and when these cover the entire surface the tumor is usually frankly malignant. The benign ones are usually large, grossly cystic, unilocular, and filled with clear serous fluid.[13]

Mucinous epithelial tumors occur less commonly and constitute 6% to 10% of all malignant primary neoplasms of the ovary. There is a spectrum of epithelial neoplasms with an intermediate form, the so-called carcinomas of low malignant potential (LMP). These have the capacity to spread, yet are effectively treated by surgery.[14] About 15% of all serous tumors are carcinomas of LMP, and 33% to 60% of these are limited to one ovary.[15] Grossly, these tumors resemble benign serous cystadenomas, except that they have more abundant internal papillary projections. They are associated with a much better prognosis, with a 100% 5-year survival rate.[16]

According to Allen and Hertig (17), the likelihood of malignancy in an ovarian mass is related to its size. There is a 56.2% malignancy rate in masses larger than 15 cm, a 39.9% rate for those in the 5 to 15-cm range, and a 3.9% rate in those smaller than 5 cm.

The Ca-125 is a serologic marker found in approximately 80% of patients with epithelial ovarian cancer. Its level appears to be related to tumor volume, increasing as the disease progresses, and it is elevated in 40% of patients with stage I disease. It is most highly expressed in nonmucinous ovarian cancers.[18] However, it is not specific for ovarian cancer and may be elevated in a number of benign conditions such as endometriosis, pelvic inflammatory disease, and fibroids. Thus, it cannot be used to distinguish benign from malignant masses in premenopausal women.

Ovarian cancer spreads most commonly by contiguous growth and seeding of the peritoneum. Nearly 90% of patients with ovarian carcinoma have peritoneal implants at autopsy, and 60% to 70% have ascites.[19] The presence of metastatic peritoneal implants outside the pelvis is an ominous prognostic feature, defining stage T3 ovarian carcinoma, and defining stage $T3_c$ carcinoma if these implants are greater than 2 cm in diameter. The staging system outlined by the TNM classification is outlined in the appendix. The most common site of metastatic implants is along the surface of the peritoneum. The disease spreads along with the normal flow pattern of ascitic fluid, through the peritoneal pathways; implants occur along the right paracolic gutter, right subphrenic area, and pouch of Douglas preferentially. Eventually, however, they seed and implant throughout the entire peritoneal, omental, and mesenteric surfaces. Implants may also occur in the bowel wall, especially in the rectosigmoid and small intestine.

Management of ovarian cancer

Current management of ovarian carcinoma involves an exploratory laparotomy for the purpose of staging, as well as tumor debulking. The procedure involves a total abdominal hysterectomy, partial omentectomy, peritoneal washings, and debulking of residual disease. The omentum is a particularly susceptible site for metastases, with its network of folds and large surface area.

The surgical treatment of patients with early-stage disease has become more specific. Many can now be spared the toxicities of chemotherapy and have a greater than 90% probability of being cured.[20]

Preoperative knowledge of potential bowel involvement is desirable, because this involves considerable alterations in the surgical technique and preoperative preparation of the patient. Similarly, the presence of bladder wall invasion, although not as common, should be determined. Detection of peritoneal implants at surgery may be difficult and requires careful surveillance of the entire peritoneal cavity. Owing to the extent and occult nature of many of these implants, their complete removal can rarely be accomplished. Unfortunately, 30% to 40% of all cases of ovarian carcinoma are understaged at first surgery. Undetected residual tumor is often left in situ after surgery.[21] This is critical, because the single most important prognostic factor for these patients is the amount of residual tumor left postoperatively prior to initiation of chemotherapy. When the residual tumor masses measure less than 2 cm in diameter, the salvage rates are better.[22]

After initial surgery, most patients with stage III epithelial carcinoma of the ovary will often have no gross residual disease detectable by physical examination or CT scanning. However, many may have persistent elevation of the Ca-125 level, indicating small amounts of residual disease within the peritoneal cavity.

The goal of further postoperative therapy is to eradicate any remaining disease. There are several ways of treating patients postoperatively to accomplish this, the most common being the administration of six cycles of platinum-based chemotherapy. Only 20% to 30% of these patients will be alive 5 years after the diagnosis of advanced cancer, and even then relapses can occur.

In follow-up, a distinction is made between patients who are at high risk (i.e., those who have residual tumor bulk greater than 2 cm at the end of their initial surgery) and those who have a standard risk (i.e., stage T3 disease that has been "maximally" debulked to less than 2 cm). For the high-risk group whose 5-year survival is 5% to 8%, new investigational therapy is justified.

The only way of precisely identifying high-risk patients with residual disease after platinum chemotherapy is by means of "second-look" laparotomy. This involves a second operation and search for persistent tumor. All suspicious areas are resected or biopsied, and washings are taken from multiple sites in the peritoneal cavity. The value of second-look laparotomy is currently under considerable debate, and although it is still performed, it is not widely advocated. It is invasive and has a false-negative rate of 30% to 50% in patients who are deemed to be in complete remission pathologically at the time of the procedure.[23] The literature suggests that second-look surgery does not improve survival and should be reserved for patients enrolled in experimental treatment protocols that require precise detection of residual or recurrent tumor.[24,25]

Patients are followed on a monthly basis during chemotherapy, with physical examinations and testing of Ca-125 levels. CT scans are routinely performed at the end of treatment and at intervals ranging from 3 to 6 months thereafter for up to 1 to 2 years.

For patients failing initial chemotherapy, recent innovative approaches have been proposed and are being tested. Several salvage protocols are ongoing, and phase II trials are being conducted, including high-dose chemotherapy with bone marrow rescue. For a more direct approach to residual disease, intraperitoneal chemotherapy can be used.[26]

DIAGNOSIS

Most patients with adnexal masses undergo surgical resection, especially postmenopausal women or those in a high-risk group (e.g., with a family history of a first- or second-degree relative with ovarian carcinoma). Thus, there is a definite need to increase the predictive value of the imaging studies for the depiction of malignancy prior to surgery. The surgical techniques for the removal of a benign lesion are considerably different from those for complete cytoreductive surgery for malignancy.

Ultrasonography

Gray scale evaluation of ovarian masses. The gray scale appearance of adnexal masses is an important feature in deciding whether surgery is needed. However, many factors must be considered in this decision, such as the patient's age, clinical presentation, and laboratory results. Although some adnexal masses need to be surgically removed when there is little or no concern over malignancy, much effort has been directed toward the sonographic discrimination of benign from malignant ovarian masses.

Gray scale sonographic evaluation of mass morphology is most frequently used to assess the likelihood of malignancy. Qualitative evaluation of masses as well as quantitative scoring systems have been proposed[27-32] in an attempt to predict benignity or malignancy. Regardless of which system is used, the same general sonographic characteristics are sought. A simple cyst has the sonographic characteristics of being anechoic, with smooth imperceptible walls and distal acoustic enhancement. A simple cyst is virtually always benign. Masses with thick septation (generally described as 2 to 3 mm or more), nodularity of the wall or along a septation, or an associated abnormal amount of intraperitoneal fluid are more likely be malignant. Masses that have only thin septations or homogeneous low-level echoes are likely to be benign. A solid mass usually raises concern for malignancy, although many such masses may be benign. Although larger masses are more likely to be malignant, most sonographic testing should be directed toward evaluating morphology. There is evidence that once the morphologic characteristics of an ovarian mass are used to predict malignancy, size does not further improve sensitivity or specificity for malignancy.[32]

Some investigators state that normal ovaries can be identified by TVS in the majority of patients even after menopause,[33,34] but others have been less successful.[35] The normal ovary in a premenopausal woman is ovoid in shape and contains a few small follicles (Fig. 9-1). Since mature-sized follicles can be as large as 2.0 to 2.5 cm in diameter[36,37] a simple cyst less than this approximate size should typically be considered normal in premenopausal women not taking oral contraceptives. In postmenopausal women the ovary is smaller and contains few if any identifiable follicles (Fig. 9-2). Ovarian volume may be calculated, and enlargement has been proposed as a possible screening method for ovarian carcinoma,[38] but the range of ovarian volumes is wider than originally reported.[1] With the improved resolution of TVS, one should be reluctant to report an ovary as abnormal solely based on size when it is well imaged and morphologically normal.

A simple ovarian cyst (Fig. 9-3) is rarely if ever

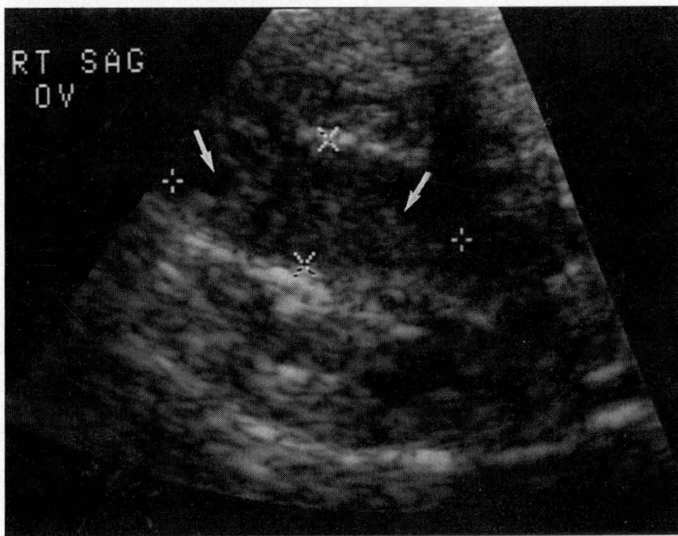

Fig. 9-1 Normal ovary in a premenopausal woman. The premenopausal ovary (marked by cursors) typically has a few small follicles *(arrows)*.

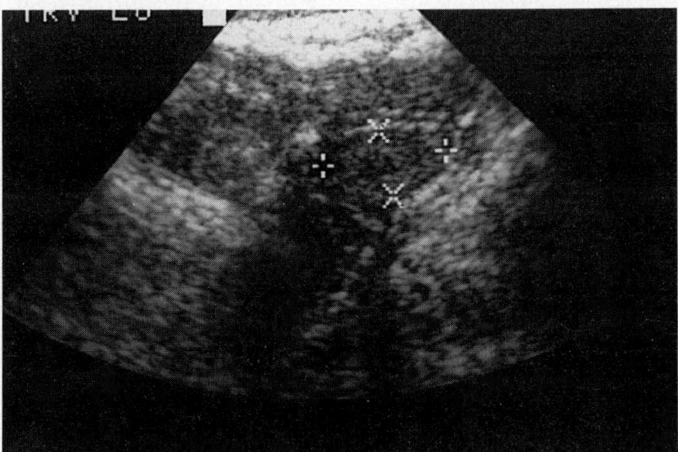

Fig. 9-2 Normal ovary in a postmenopausal woman. Compared with the premenopausal ovary, the postmenopausal ovary (marked by cursors) is smaller and is typically homogeneous, with no identifiable follicles.

malignant[37] and can usually be followed with sonography, unless surgery is needed for other reasons such as pain. Even in postmenopausal women, simple ovarian cysts are more common than originally thought.[39-45] In postmenopausal women, as long as the mass meets the sonographic criteria for a simple cyst (anechoic, smooth walls, distal acoustic enhancement) and is less than 5 cm, the risk of malignancy is so low that the patient can usually be managed conservatively with follow-up sonography. It is important to make sure that the mass is indeed a simple cyst by sonographic criteria; this may require performing both TVS and TAS.

There is overlap in the sonographic appearance of benign and malignant ovarian masses, but there are several sonographic appearances other than simple cysts that are very suggestive of a benign process. When these appearances are present in premenopausal women, benignity should be considered likely. A cyst with homogeneous low-level echoes and/or very fine septations (Fig. 9-4) is typical of a hemorrhagic cyst.[37,46] Endometriomas have a variable sonographic appearance, and may appear as cystic masses and similar to hemorrhagic ovarian cysts.[46] In our experience and that of others,[37] endometriomas often appear as cystic masses with homogeneous low-level echoes (Fig. 9-5). One should not be fooled into thinking that such masses are solid because there are echoes throughout the mass; distal enhancement is a clue to their cystic nature. A cystic mass with a nodular hyperechoic solid component (Fig. 9-6) is very suggestive of a dermoid.[47] Although these are usually removed, the chance of malignancy is low. A cystic mass that is tubular is suggestive of hydrosalpinx.[48] When there is a multiseptated cystic adnexal mass in a patient with gestational trophoblastic disease (Fig. 9-7), theca lutein cysts are the most likely diagnosis. These are typically bilateral and occur in response to elevated levels of human chorionic gonadotrophin.[49] Theca lutein cysts may also occur with ovarian hyperstimulation, a multiple pregnancy, and pregnancy complicated by hydrops.[50,51] In these situations the clinical findings point to the correct diagnosis. Similarly, in a febrile patient with a complex cystic mass, tubo-ovarian abscess (Fig. 9-8) is a likely diagnosis.

When a cystic mass has thick walls, a solid component other than the typical hyperechoic part of a dermoid, or thick septations, the risk of malignancy increases (Fig. 9-9). While such masses, especially in postmenopausal women or when per-

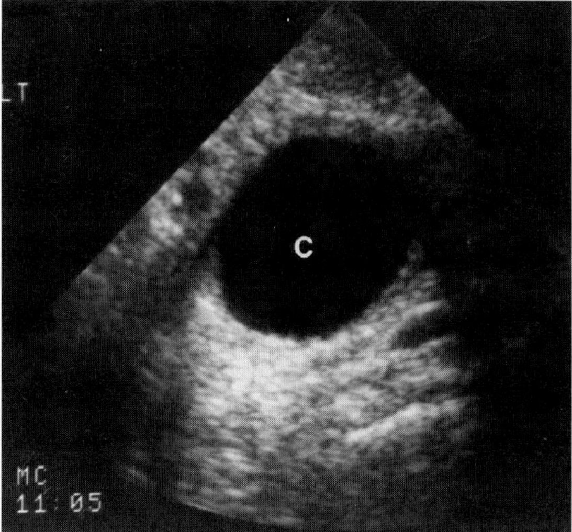

Fig. 9-3 This sonographically simple ovarian cyst *(C)* meets the sonographic criteria for a simple cyst: anechoic, smooth walls, distal acoustic enhancement.

Fig. 9-4 Hemorrhagic cyst. This cystic mass has distal enhancement, low-level echoes, and very fine septations *(arrows)*. Although not specific, this appearance (or that in Fig. 9-5) is typical of many hemorrhagic cysts.

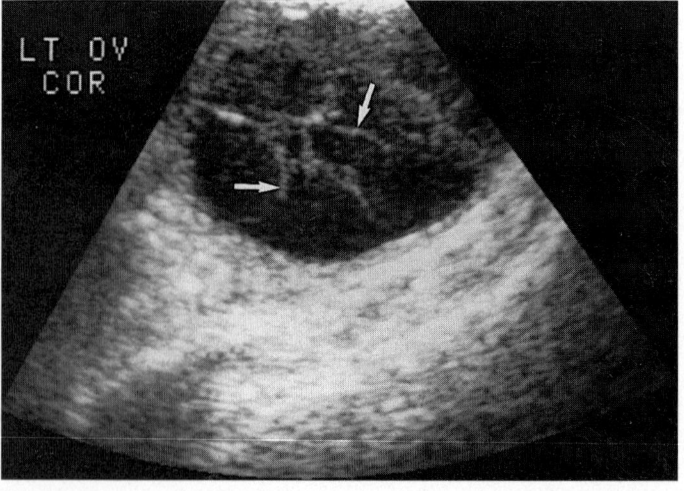

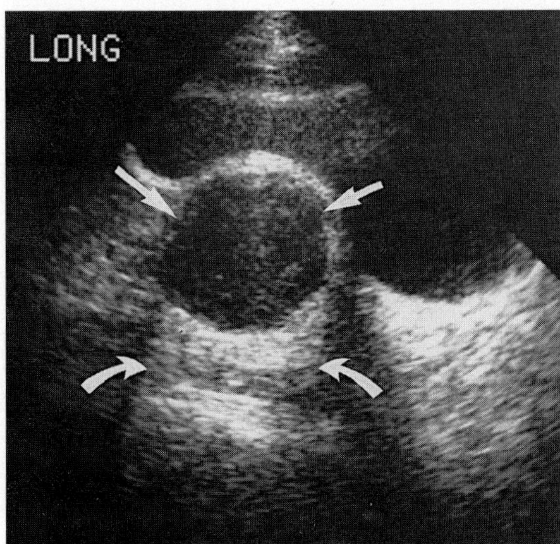

Fig. 9-5 Endometrioma. One should not mistake this mass *(straight arrows)* as solid on the basis of the echoes within it; such echoes are commonly due to blood. Distal enhancement (edges marked by curved arrows) is a clue to its cystic nature.

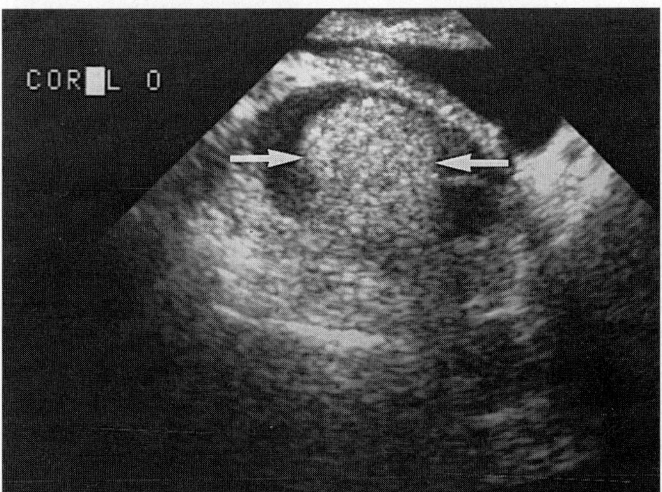

Fig. 9-6 Dermoid. This complex mass has a very hyperechoic nodule *(arrows)*. Such a hyperechoic area is very suggestive of dermoid and corresponds to sebum and hair.

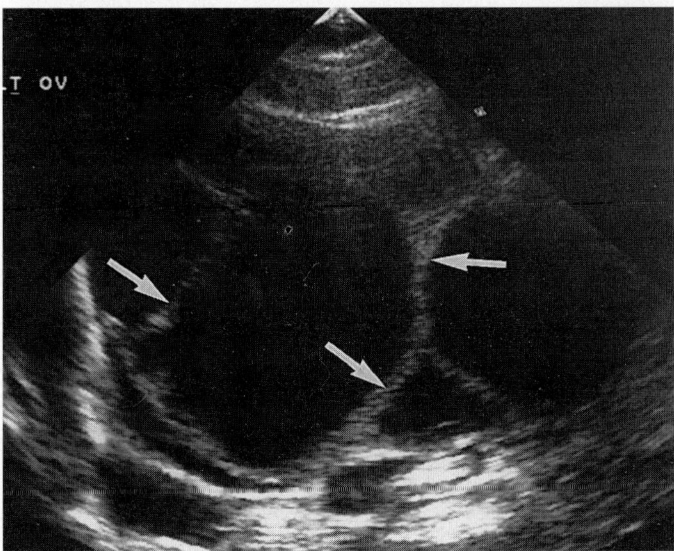

Fig. 9-7 Theca lutein cyst. These cysts are typically multiloculated with several septations *(arrows)*. Clinical settings such as gestational trophoblastic disease, multiple pregnancy, fetal hydrops, or ovarian hyperstimulation help suggest the correct diagnosis.

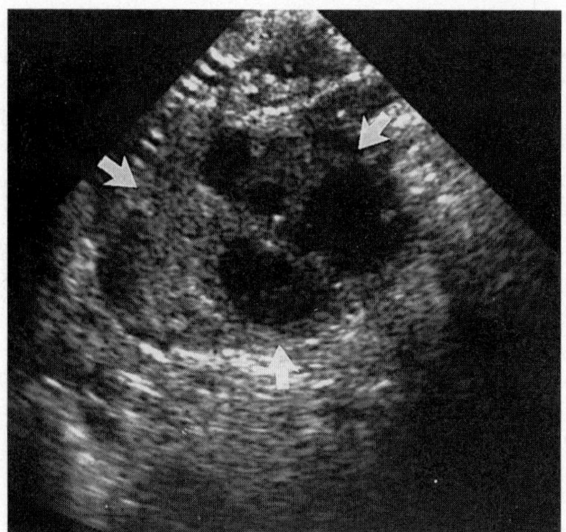

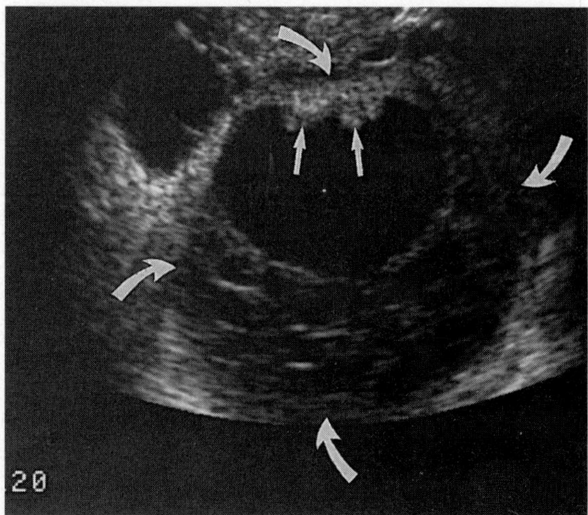

Fig. 9-8 Tubo-ovarian abscess. This complex mass *(arrows)* has both cystic and solid regions. Although indistinguishable from an ovarian neoplasm on the basis of sonographic morphology alone, the clinical presentation often suggests the diagnosis of abscess.

Fig. 9-10 Benign mass with features suggesting malignancy. This complex cystic mass *(curved arrows)* has solid nodular areas *(straight arrows)* that raise concern for malignancy. This is an endometrioma, illustrating how some benign masses appear malignant by sonography.

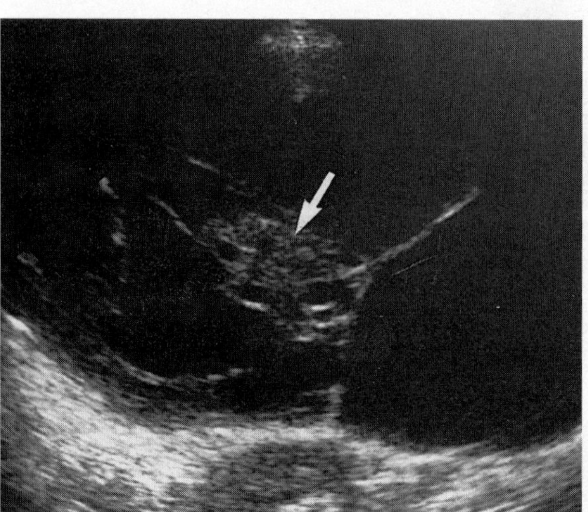

Fig. 9-9 Cystadenocarcinoma of the ovary. Some of the septations in this predominantly cystic mass are relatively thin, but there is a nodular solid area *(arrow)* within the mass that is characteristic of malignancy.

cern about malignancy. Fibroids, however, which are common and typically appear solid, may be pedunculated and simulate a solid ovarian mass. Demonstration of normal ovaries separate from such a mass is the best indication that the mass is not ovarian. Fibroids may occasionally undergo cystic degeneration (Fig. 9-12) and, particularly if pedunculated, be mistaken for an ovarian mass.

Caution should be exercised when a patient is strongly suspected to have an adnexal mass on physical examination, yet no mass is seen on sonography. First, consider that the mass may be relatively superior or lateral in the pelvis. This may occur with pedunculated fibroids and occasionally with ovarian masses. One should attempt to use TAS in these cases, looking superiorly and laterally outside the bladder window. Second, beware of dermoids, which may contain a significant hyperechoic solid component that may be difficult to distinguish from bowel (Fig. 9-13). Strong clinical suspicion of such masses; scanning throughout the pelvis, with firm pressure on the transducer in an attempt to displace bowel; and occasionally CT or MRI can help identify these dermoids.

Doppler evaluation of adnexal masses. In general the sensitivity of sonography, and in particular TVS, for identifying ovarian masses is high. However, most adnexal masses, particularly in premenopausal women, are benign. Research efforts have therefore been directed toward attempts to more reliably discriminate benign from malignant masses. One current method under investigation is

sistent in premenopausal women, are likely to be malignant, the distinction between benign and malignant is not precise. Some masses with a sonographic morphology suggesting malignancy are benign (Fig. 9-10). Cystic masses with septations that are thin (Fig. 9-11) are likely to be benign.

Benign masses, particularly stromal tumors, may appear solid, but solid masses also raise con-

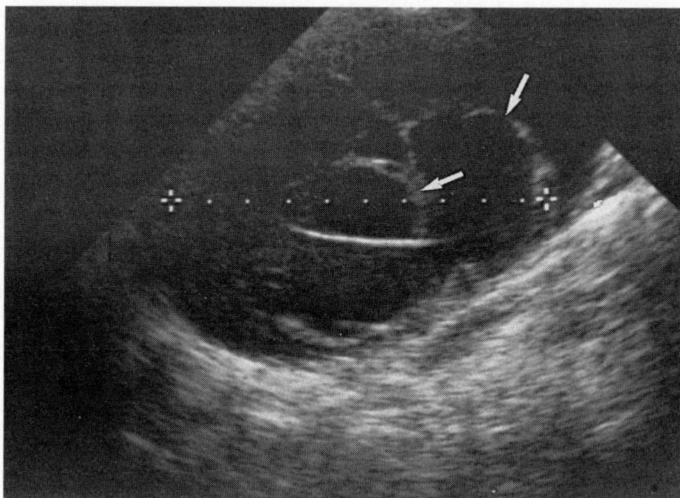

Fig. 9-11 Mucinous cystadenoma. This cystic mass has septations *(arrows)* that are relatively thin (3 mm or less) and without focal thickening. While not diagnostic, thin septations favor a benign etiology.

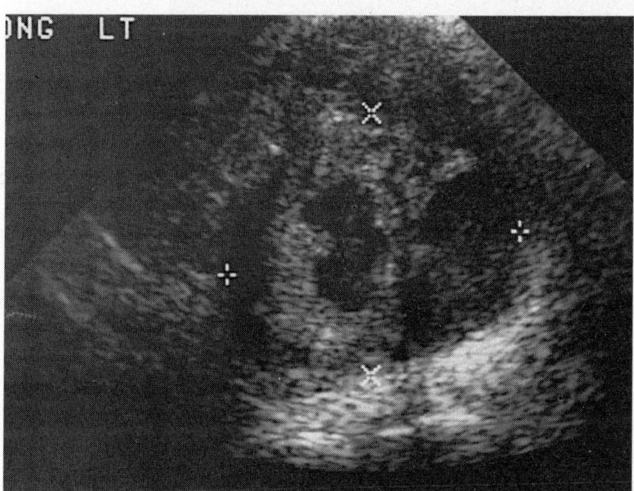

Fig. 9-12 Pedunculated fibroid with cystic degeneration. The adnexal mass (outlined by cursors) has both cystic and solid components. An ovarian mass with this appearance should raise concern for malignancy. However, both ovaries could be identified in this case and were normal. Pedunculated fibroids can occasionally be difficult to distinguish from solid or complex ovarian masses, especially if the ovaries are not identified.

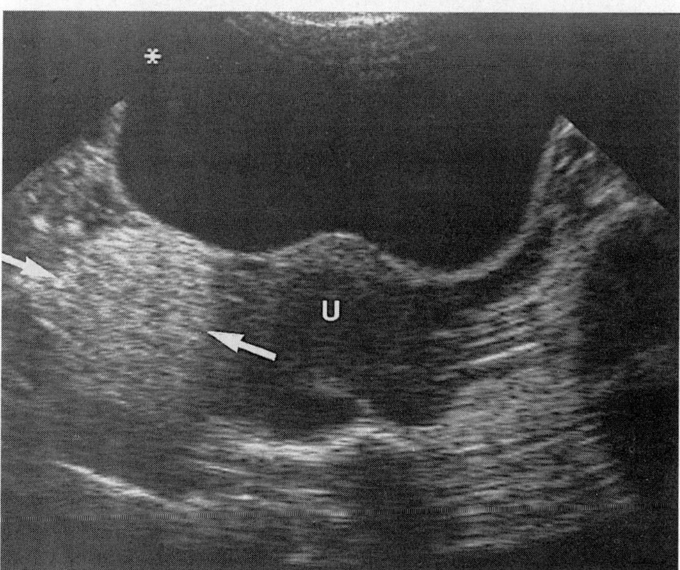

Fig. 9-13 Completely hyperechoic dermoid in a transverse transabdominal image of the pelvis. A dermoid *(arrows)* may have a large hyperechoic component. This one is fairly easily identified, but the hyperechoic appearance can occasionally be obscured by bowel. Awareness of this pitfall and a high index of suspicion help identify such dermoids. *U*, Uterus.

Doppler, which allows noninvasive evaluation of the blood flow characteristics of a mass. Malignant tumors generally have poor muscular support in the arteries,[52] and this produces less vascular resistance. Some malignant tumors also have arteriovenous shunting, which allows for higher flow in the tumor.[53,54] The lower vascular resistance is believed to be reflected in the Doppler waveform by a relatively higher amount of diastolic flow. Lower vascular resistance translates into lower pulsatility and resistive indices. While some studies have reported a mean index, the current trend is to report the lowest PI or RI of each adnexal mass. Although color flow Doppler is not required to obtain the PI or RI, it does permit more rapid evaluation and increased confidence that all areas of the mass have been evaluated. However, color Doppler alone, is not adequate, as a pulsed Doppler image is needed to obtain the velocity measurements.

Initial work in this field suggests that a PI of 1.0 might distinguish between benign and malignant masses, with PI lower than this indicating malignancy. Bourne et al found that all of eight malignant masses and only two of four benign masses had a PI of 1.0 or less.[55] Subsequent investigators found similar, though slightly more variable, results (Figs. 9-14 to 9-16). [56,57] Fleischer et al[53]

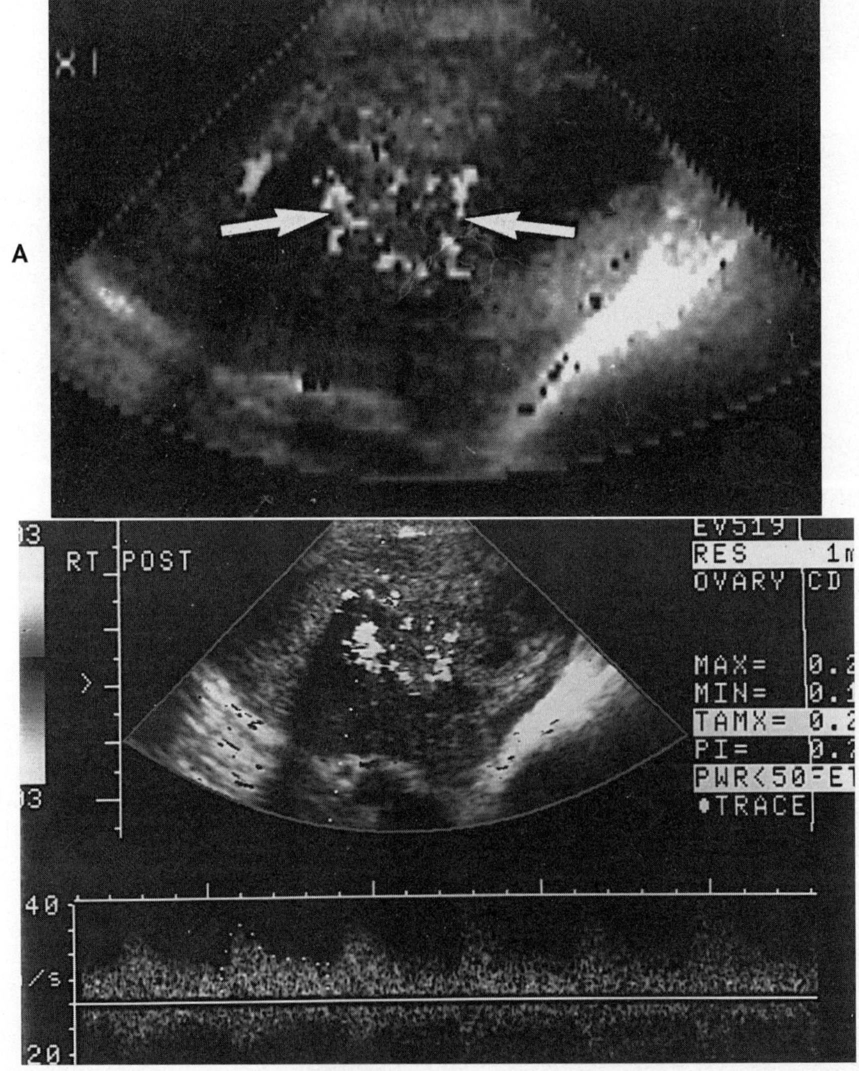

Fig. 9-14 Doppler image of a malignant mass with low vascular resistance. **A,** Transvaginal color Doppler image of a complex cystic ovarian mass. Flow was easily detected in a solid portion *(arrows)*. **B,** Pulsed Doppler image of this area of the tumor shows relatively low resistance flow. The pulsatility index (PI) of this waveform was 0.76 and the resistive index (RI) 0.40. This mass was a mixed cystadenoma of borderline malignancy.

found a similar trend but a wider overlap between the PI of benign and malignant masses. The RI has also been evaluated, and an RI of less than 0.4 has been proposed as a discriminatory value by Kurjak et al.[58] With further experience, more conflicting data are being reported.[59-62] Tekay and Joup-pila[59] found no significant difference in the PI and RI of benign and malignant ovarian masses. Timor-Tritsch et al[60] and Brown et al[61] did find a significantly lower PI and RI in malignant as opposed to benign tumors, but the overlap precluded a single cutoff value for either index that would always dis-

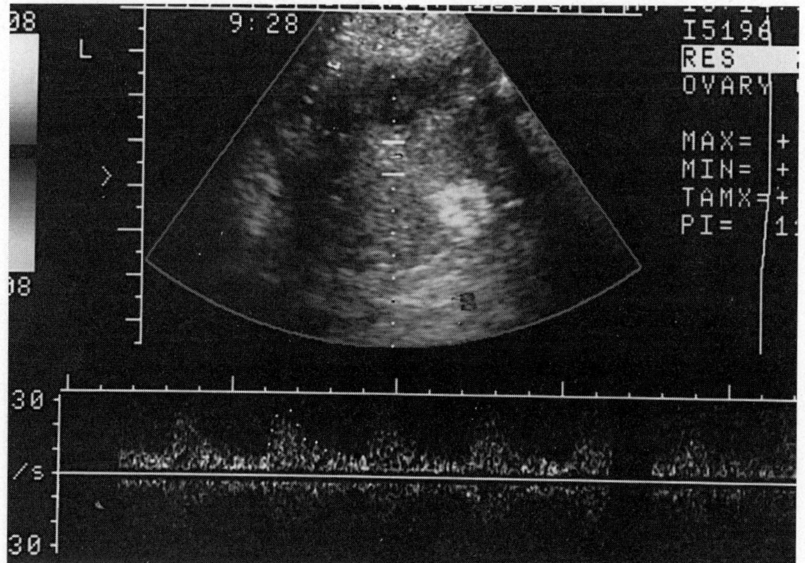

Fig. 9-15 Doppler image of a benign mass with high vascular resistance. A black-and-white representation of a color and pulsed Doppler image from the mass seen in Fig. 9-8, a tubo-ovarian abscess. There is relatively high resistance flow with a PI of 1.1 and RI of 0.67.

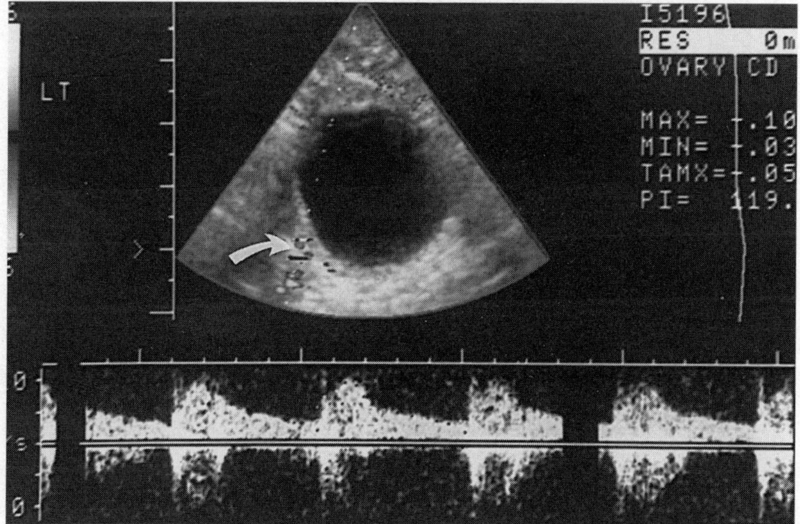

Fig. 9-16 Doppler image of a benign mass with high vascular resistance. A black-and-white representation of a color and pulsed Doppler image from the same mass seen in Fig. 9-3, a simple cyst. There is relatively high resistance flow with a PI of 1.19 and RI of 0.66. This image also illustrates the occasional difficulty in interpreting the location of the vessel interrogated. It is difficult to be sure if the vessel in the sample gate *(curved arrow)* is part of the cyst or if is just close to it but does not supply flow to it.

criminate benign from malignant masses (Figs. 9-17 and 9-18). In our experience, benign ovarian masses often have a relatively low PI or RI, although malignant masses rarely have a high PI or RI.[61,63] Ideally, Doppler evaluation of the ovary or an adnexal mass should not be made during the luteal phase of the menstrual cycle; the corpus luteum normally has low resistance flow that will appear similar to that expected with malignancy (Fig. 9-19). The presence of a notch in the diastolic part of the waveform may also prove useful in excluding malignancy,[53,54] although further experience with this finding is needed. The best cutoff value, if any, and whether the PI or RI is a better predic-

tor of a malignancy, have yet to be determined. It is likely that Doppler parameters will be only another component to factor into the prediction of malignancy. It may be that we can define a PI or RI level above which the chance of malignancy is extremely low, accepting that benign masses may also have a PI or RI below that level. Additionally, the lack of detectable flow by color Doppler does not exclude malignancy. Most malignant masses have detectable flow,[53,60,64] but occasionally no flow is identifiable in an ovarian carcinoma.[56,57,59,61,65,66] The detection of flow by Doppler, however, depends on several imaging parameters, not just on the vascularity of the mass.[59,63]

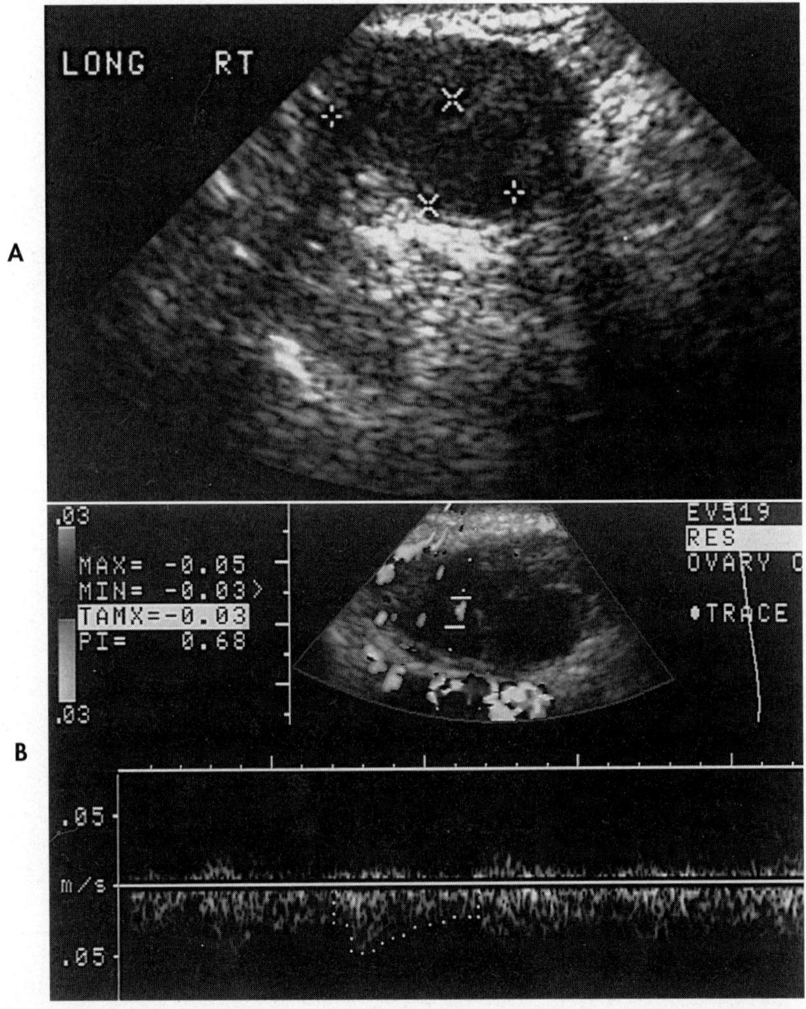

Fig. 9-17 Doppler image of a benign mass with a low PI. **A,** Transvaginal sonogram shows a complex hypoechoic mass (outlined by cursors) in the ovary of a postmenopausal woman. Echoes are present in this mass, with some distal enhancement. **B,** Color and pulsed Doppler image reveals low resistance flow with a PI of 0.68 and RI of 0.40 in this waveform. Despite the gray scale and Doppler findings that both suggested malignancy, this is a benign mass consisting of both cystadenofibroma and endometrioma.

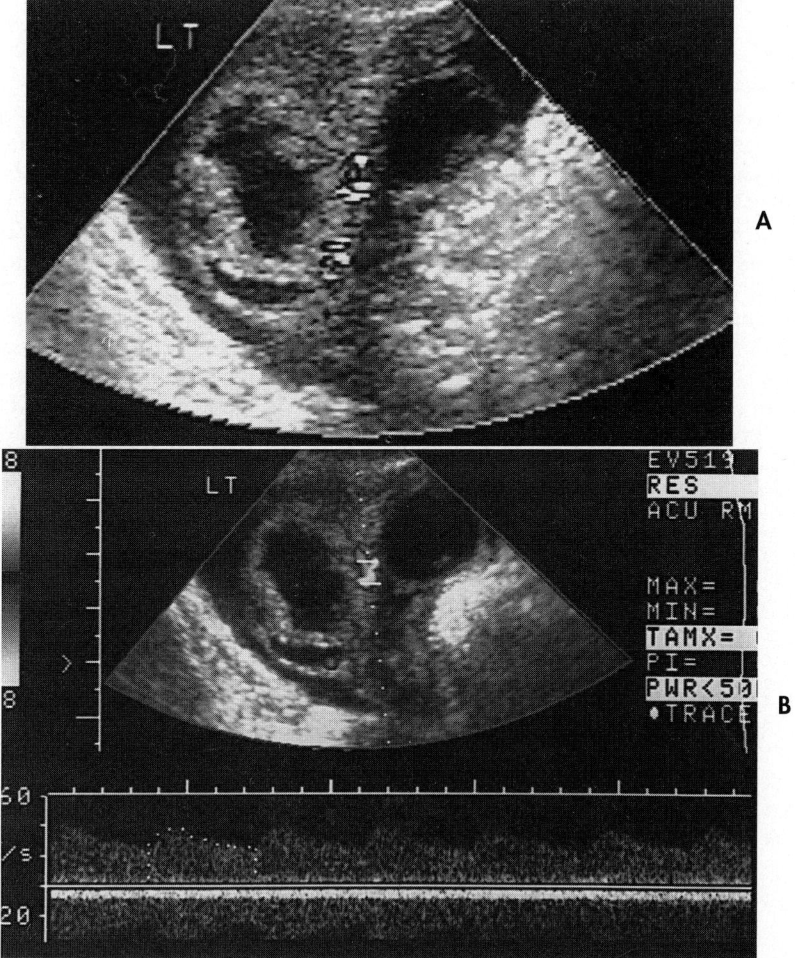

Fig. 9-18 Doppler image of a benign mass with a low PI. **A,** Color Doppler image shows flow in the thick wall of a cystic mass. **B,** Black-and-white representation of a color and pulsed Doppler image in the same area of the mass shows low resistance flow with a PI of 0.42 and RI of 0.34. This mass had resolved on a follow-up sonogram and was presumably a hemorrhagic cyst.

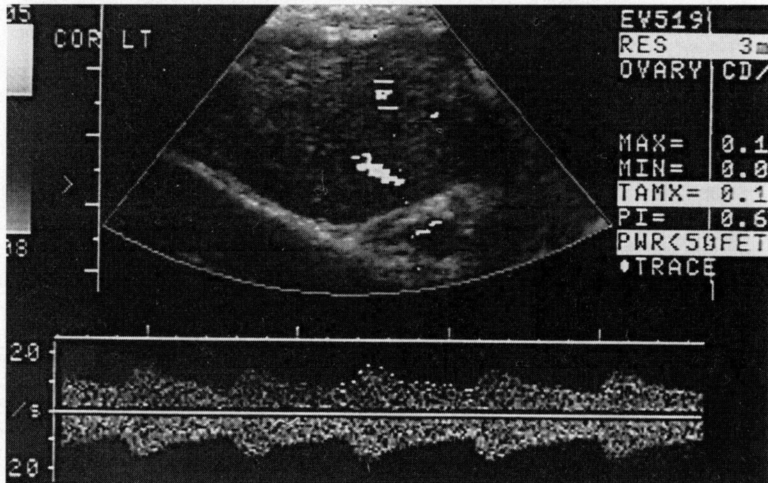

Fig. 9-19 Transvaginal color Doppler image reveals flow around the corpus luteum on cycle day 19. This relatively low resistance flow (PI of 0.65 and RI of 0.50 on this waveform) is similar to what may be seen with malignancy, illustrating the need to perform Doppler studies only during the follicular phase.

The frequency of detectable flow by color Doppler in benign ovarian masses is more variable.[53,56,57]

Because of its relative ease of performance and comparatively lower cost, sonography will likely continue to have an important role in evaluating patients with adnexal masses. Gray scale evaluation of morphology, while sometimes imprecise, still provides useful information in patient management. Doppler findings are not likely to replace gray scale findings, although they may provide another piece of useful information. There is preliminary evidence that a combination of gray scale and Doppler parameters may lead to better characterization of adnexal masses.[60,66]

Computed tomography

Ultrasonography is often the initial imaging modality of choice in the evaluation of pelvic masses and is generally considered superior to CT for determining the adnexal origin of the pelvic mass. Because of the increased resolution of CT and its ability to distinguish subtle differences in x-ray density, the etiology of some tumors may be strongly suggested. Primary ovarian tumors containing fat (dermoid), calcification (psammomatous or dental calcification), cystic or solid nodules, or septation can be identified. The native density of the tumor, as well as the presence of contrast enhancement, are helpful in determining the solid nature of an ovarian mass. Identification of a

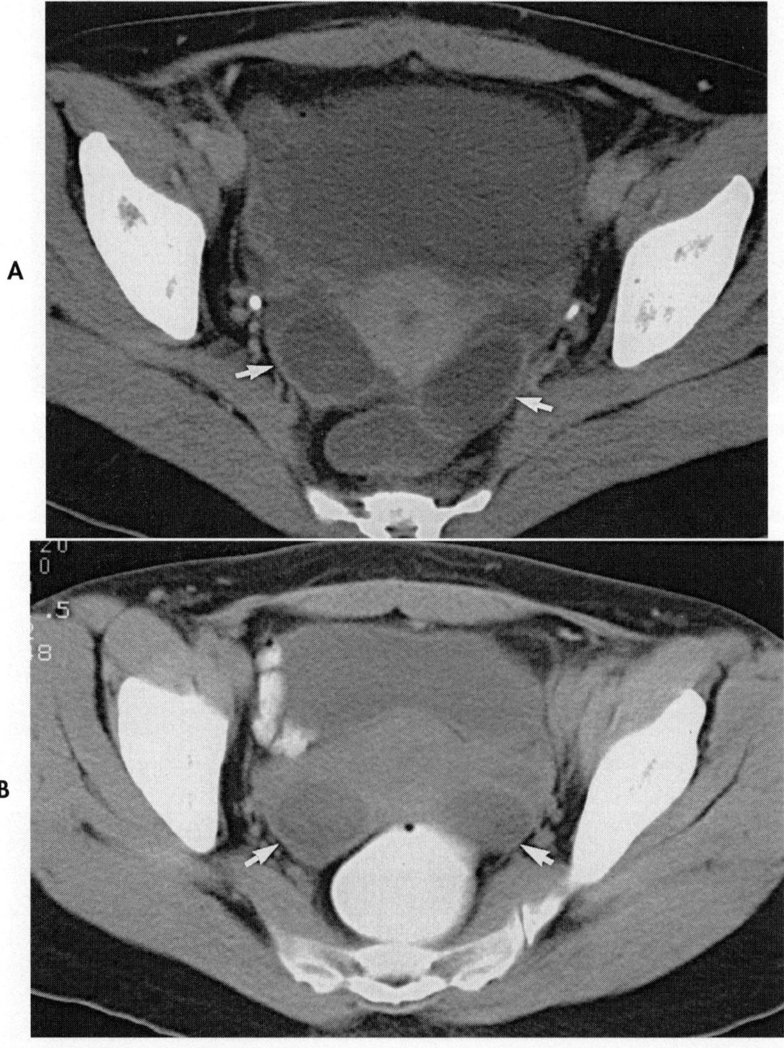

Fig. 9-20 Value of bowel contrast media on computed tomography (CT). **A,** Without bowel contrast media the round, low-attenuation structures behind the uterus *(arrows)* might be mistaken for large intestinal loops. **B,** After rectal contrast medium instillation, bilateral cystic adnexal masses are revealed *(arrows).*

solid component within a mass is predictive of malignant change, although some cases of benign tumors of the ovary demonstrate solid components. This was suggested by a retrospective review of 138 histologically proven ovarian masses. Only five of 104 benign lesions demonstrated solid components such as thickened walls, thickened septa, and papillary projections and could not be differentiated from malignant tumors.[67] Of the Krukenberg tumors, the solid component occupied more than one half the mass. The same authors also suggested that if an ovarian mass is purely cystic and demonstrates no solid components, it can be considered reliably benign. Others argue that most benign ovarian masses have a variable appearance that is often nonspecific, and biopsy may be necessary to exclude malignancy.[68]

Some masslike conditions that can be found in the adnexal region on pelvic CT can mimic an ovarian neoplasm. First and foremost, an unopacified bowel loop should be considered (Fig. 9-20). Uterine masses such as subserosal leiomyomas may be positioned in the adnexa and mimic an ovarian mass. When they degenerate, they can mimic a cystic ovarian neoplasm (Fig. 9-21). As with ultrasonography and MR, identifying a normal ovary separate from the mass is the most helpful clue that the lesion is not ovarian. Identification of a morphologically normal ovary is more easily accomplished with ultrasound examination. A benign ovarian cyst appears as a well-marginated, low-attenuation, nonenhancing structure with an imperceptible or thin wall. Follicular cysts cannot be differentiated from corpus luteum cysts on CT.

Cystic teratomas are benign masses that may contain specific features. Many, but not all, dermoid cysts demonstrate a combination of fat and/or calcification that allows an accurate preoperative diagnosis.[67,69,70] A predominantly fatty mass with a dense or dependent element of globular calcification, bone, or teeth in a solid protuberance into the cyst cavity enables a confident diagnosis of cystic teratoma (Figs. 9-22 and 9-23).[69] These lesions have been classified into three types on the basis of their contents. One type shows layering debris within the tumor.[71] A nodular mural projection and a fat-fluid level have both been described on ultrasound examination.[72] Intracystic fat balls have been noted on both CT and MR.[70] The characteristic finding of a fat-containing mass with a dependent element whose CT numbers are greater than fat, and calcification in a solid prominence that projects from the cyst wall, is highly suggestive. Since a hyperechoic portion of a mass is not specific for fat, ultrasonography can only suggest the diagnosis of fatty tumors. CT allows a specific diagnosis of fat-containing tumors and is superior to sonography for delineating bone and tooth fragments.[69] The presence of thyroid tissue in a cystic ovarian teratoma, so-called struma ovarii, is often asymptomatic. The CT and MR features are not specific enough to permit a preoperative diagnosis based on imaging features.[73]

There is little or no role for CT in the evalua-

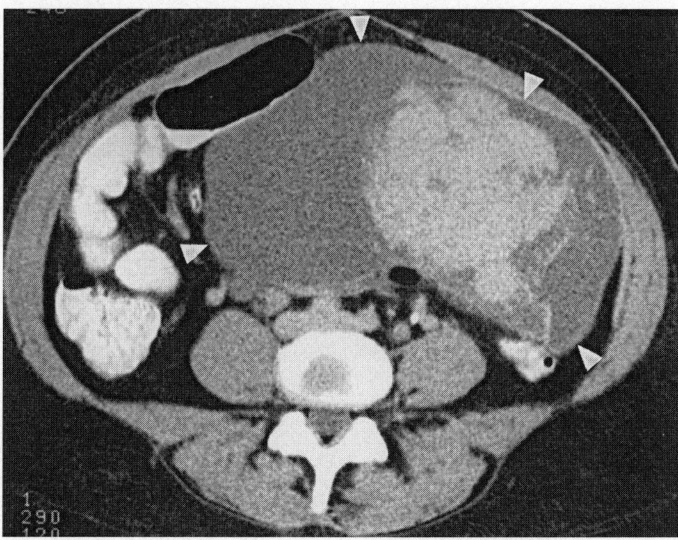

Fig. 9-21 Spiral CT demonstrates a large adnexal mass with solid and cystic components *(arrowheads),* which raised suspicion of a cystic ovarian neoplasm but was shown on pathologic study to be a large, degenerated uterine leiomyoma.

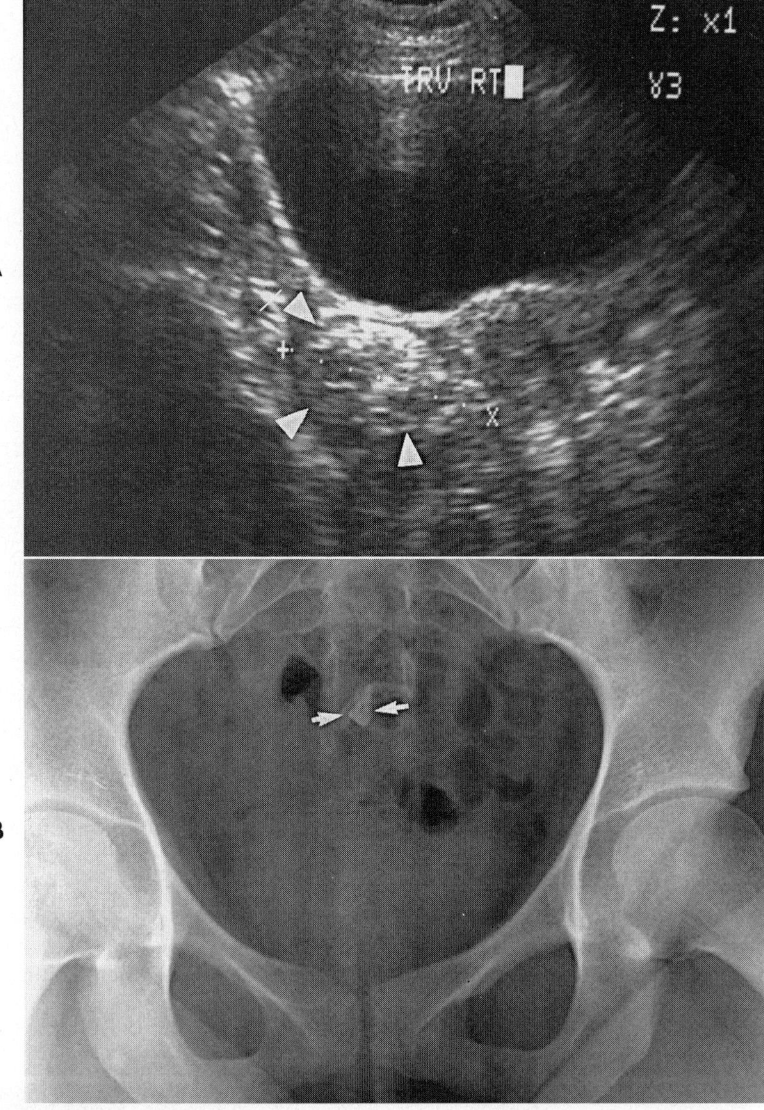

Fig. 9-22 A, A hyperechoic mass *(arrowheads)* in a young woman is suggestive of an ovarian teratoma but should be confirmed with another test. **B,** A plain radiograph in the same patient demonstrates the tooth *(arrows)* and confirms the diagnosis.

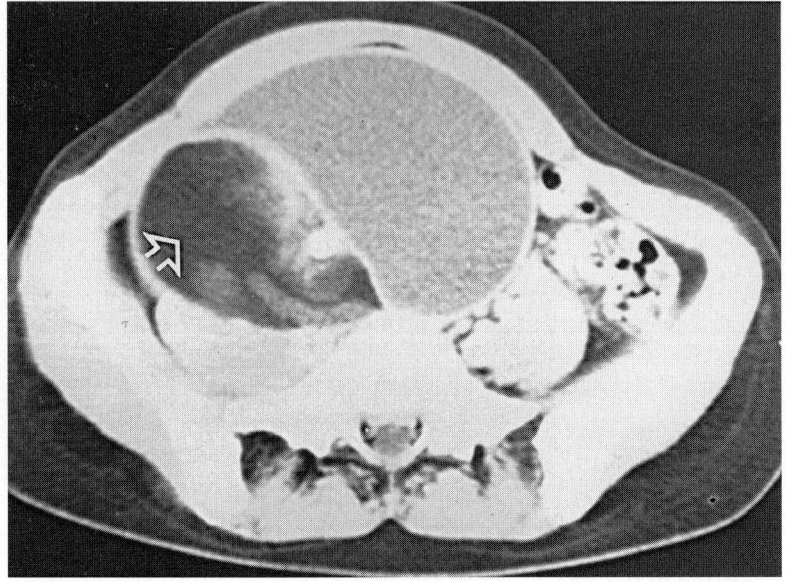

Fig. 9-23 Ovarian teratoma. A CT scan can be highly suggestive alone by demonstrating calcifications as well as fat *(open arrow)*.

tion of patients with suspected endometriosis compared with ultrasonography and MRI. Endometriomas may present as a solid adnexal mass, as a fluid collection with solid and cystic components, or as thick-walled cysts (Fig. 9-24).[74] A high-attenuation component to an adnexal mass is evidence of hemorrhage and may represent an endometrioma or a hemorrhagic cyst. Pelvic inflammatory disease also can present as an adnexal mass, such as a tubo-ovarian abscess or hydrosalpinx (Fig. 9-25).

Metastatic disease to the ovary constitutes 10% of all ovarian tumors.[75] Adenocarcinoma of the endometrium is the most common tumor to metasta-size to the ovary, while the most common extragenital sites are the gastrointestinal tract and the breast. Of the tumors arising in the gastrointestinal tract, the stomach is the primary source in over 90% of cases. In the strictest sense, Krukenberg tumors refer to those tumors containing mucin-secreting signet ring cells. These present as large, lobulated, multicystic masses with soft tissue components that are indistinguishable from primary ovarian cancer.[76,77] The colon may be a more common cause of metastatic disease to the ovary.[77] As many as 3% to 8% of patients with colon cancer develop metastatic disease to the ovaries.[77]

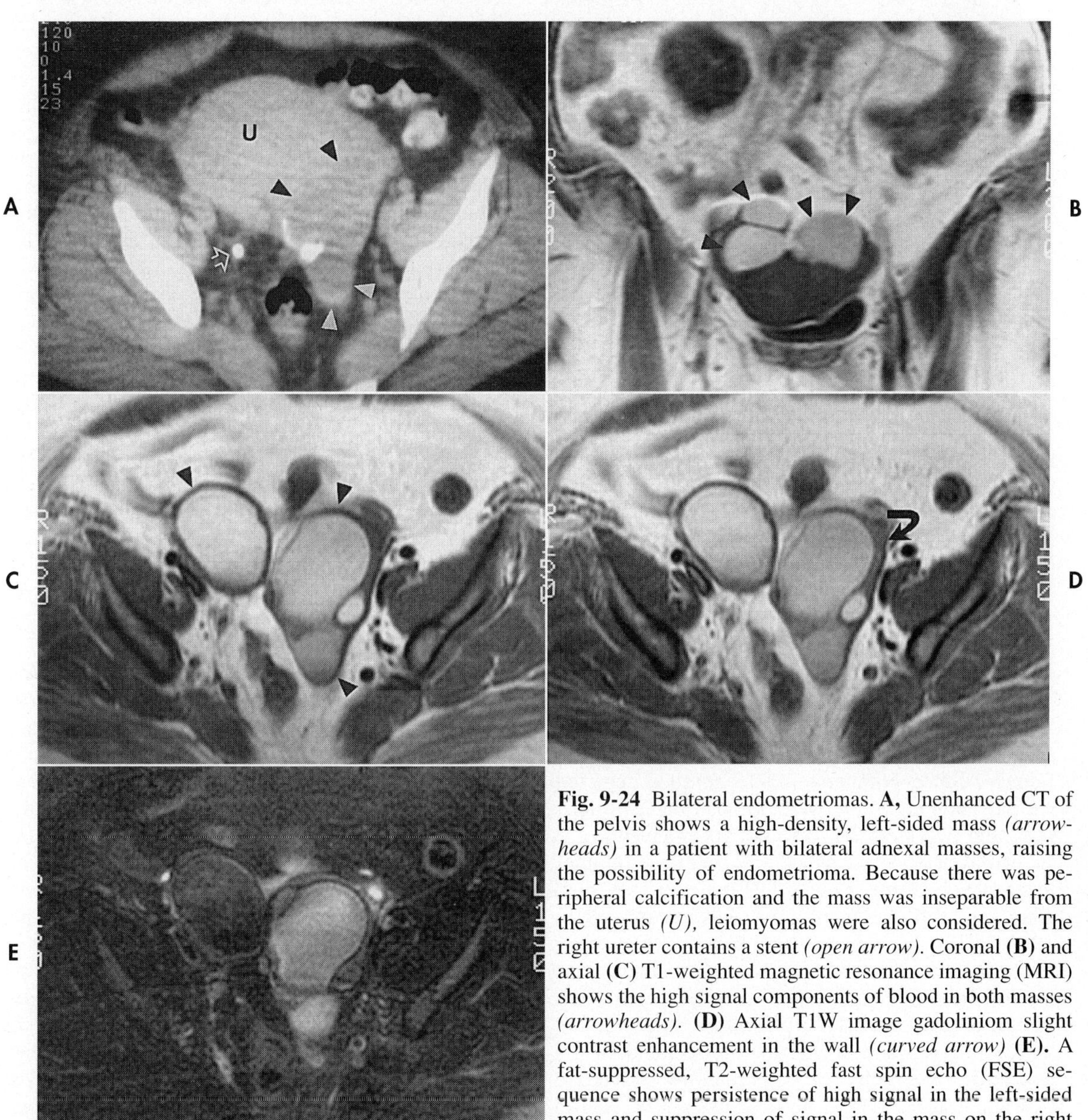

Fig. 9-24 Bilateral endometriomas. **A,** Unenhanced CT of the pelvis shows a high-density, left-sided mass *(arrowheads)* in a patient with bilateral adnexal masses, raising the possibility of endometrioma. Because there was peripheral calcification and the mass was inseparable from the uterus *(U),* leiomyomas were also considered. The right ureter contains a stent *(open arrow).* Coronal **(B)** and axial **(C)** T1-weighted magnetic resonance imaging (MRI) shows the high signal components of blood in both masses *(arrowheads).* **(D)** Axial T1W image gadoliniom slight contrast enhancement in the wall *(curved arrow)* **(E).** A fat-suppressed, T2-weighted fast spin echo (FSE) sequence shows persistence of high signal in the left-sided mass and suppression of signal in the mass on the right side, indicating a mixture of chronic and subacute hemorrhage.

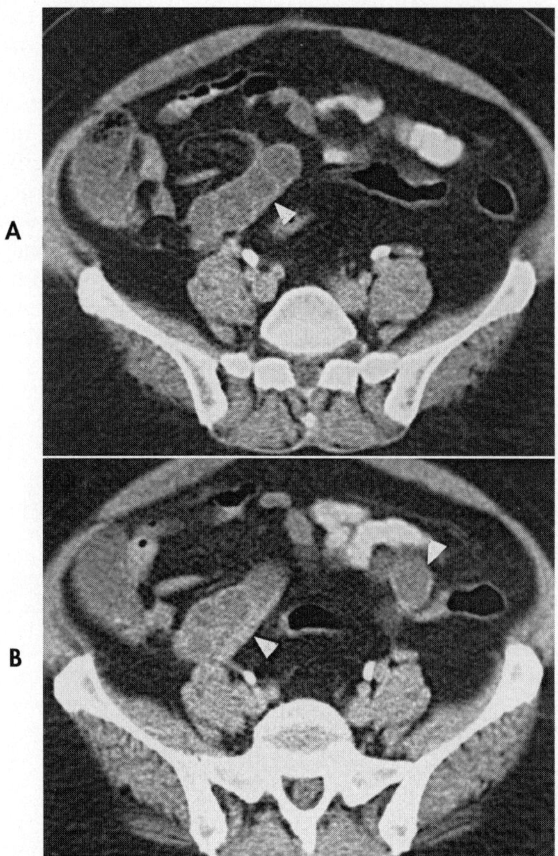

Fig. 9-25 Bilateral hydrosalpinx. **A** and **B,** Conventional CT of the pelvis shows tubular structures *(arrowheads)* that can be mistaken for unopacified bowel. The fold-like walls, shape, lack of change with time, and unopacified appearance are suggestive of dilated fallopian tubes. Only a portion of the dilated left tube is shown.

Both ultrasonography and CT have been used in the preoperative evaluation of pelvic masses, and their utility has been compared and debated. A prospective evaluation of 24 consecutive patients with suspected pelvic masses yielded no significant difference. Since both imaging techniques depicted similar pathology and used similar diagnostic criteria, the two methods were not complementary.[78] A second prospective study of 74 patients thought to have pelvic masses and 110 patients with possible recurrent pelvic tumors was conducted in 1983, and again there was no difference in the ability of the two modalities to identify masses or to predict the extent of disease.[79] A more recent study of 130 patients with 170 epithelial ovarian tumors was conducted to evaluate the ability of both CT and ultrasonography to detect and characterize ovarian masses. These authors assigned specific histologic types to tumors with specific features. A serous cystadenoma was diagnosed on the basis

of a unilocular or bilocular cystic mass with homogeneous water attenuation, containing thin, regular walls or septa without nodularity or vegetations. A mucinous cystadenoma was diagnosed in patients with a multilocular cystic mass containing fluids of different attenuations or echogenicities and without vegetations. A borderline, or malignant, tumor was diagnosed if irregular septa and walls were present, or if either endo- or exocystic vegetations containing contrast enhancement were noted. Evidence of pelvic extension or peritoneal spread was also considered suggestive of cancer. Using these criteria, benign serous cystadenomas were correctly characterized with a sensitivity of 69% on CT and 70% on ultrasonography. Benign mucinous cystadenomas were correctly characterized with a sensitivity of 62% on CT and 50% on ultrasonography. Malignancy was correctly suggested in 64% of patients with borderline tumors on CT, and in 36% of patients with borderline tumors on ultrasound examination. The overall accuracy of characterization of benign versus malignant tumors was 94% with CT and 80% with ultrasonography. The authors concluded that CT was more sensitive than ultrasonography but that there was no difference in specificity. Also, although CT correctly diagnosed serous cystadenomas in 69% of cases, all the falsely characterized serous cystadenomas were found to be benign. This again suggests that purely cystic ovarian carcinoma is indeed rare.[2] Conversely, there are reports of clear pelvic cysts on ultrasound examination that were diagnosed as borderline malignant tumors.[2] Also, borderline and malignant mucinous tumors may present the same findings as a benign mucinous cystadenoma. The poorer performance of ultrasonography in identifying malignant mucinous tumors in this series was attributed to the fact that hyperechoic loculi resembled vegetations on ultrasound, whereas these portions were correctly identified as fluid on CT since they did not enhance with contrast media. The overall high accuracy (94%) of characterization of benign versus malignant disease with dynamic CT was attributed to the demonstration of tumor vessels represented by the accumulation of contrast medium. This finding was absent in all the cases of benign tumors. These authors concluded that when the findings are typical for serous cystadenoma on CT, the mass is virtually always a benign cystic mass that can be treated safely by means of aspiration or at laparoscopy. However, if there are fluids of different attenuation or echogenicities, borderline or malignant (serous or mucinous) tumors are possible. An additional study found that the accuracy for discriminating between benign and malignant ovarian tumors was 86% with MRI and 92% with CT.[80]

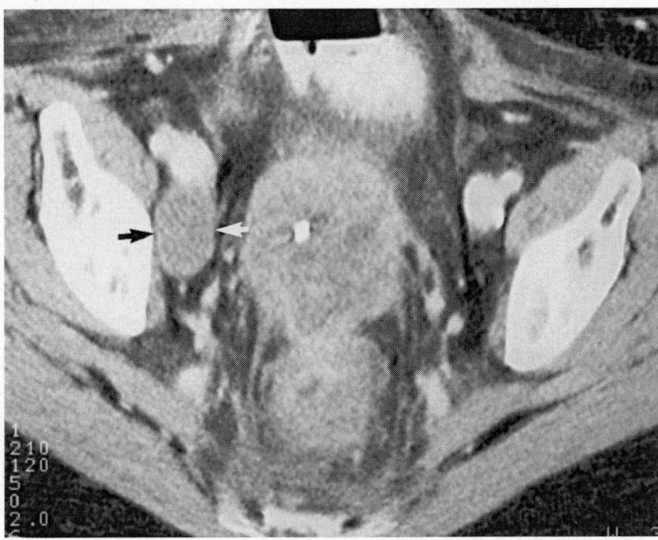

Fig. 9-26 Lymphadenopathy from ovarian cancer. Contrast-enhanced spiral CT of the pelvis (5 mm/sec table feed, reconstructed with 5-mm sections and 5-mm intervals) delineates an enlarged lymph node *(arrows)* posterior to the iliac vessels, which were optimally enhanced, because scanning was rapid and began in the pelvis in a cephalad direction.

In recent years, interventional radiologists have employed image-guided needle biopsy to establish the diagnosis of pelvic masses and obviate the need for surgical exploration. In patients with ovarian cancer, percutaneous biopsy of abnormal areas can eliminate the need for a second-look operation.[75] The indications for fine-needle aspiration and biopsy of ovarian masses have yet to be defined, in large part because of the perceived risk of disseminating tumor throughout the peritoneum and along the needle track. On the basis of this predominantly theoretical concern, surgical excision continues to be the preferred initial approach to any newly diagnosed adnexal mass that may be malignant. However, studies have shown that there is a very low risk of ultrasound-guided needle puncture in nongynecologic lesions.[81,82] Furthermore, laparotomy itself has the potential for spreading tumor cells.[83] A more compelling reason to be cautious in the biopsy of an ovarian mass lies in the risk of false-negative results. Many mucinous ovarian tumors contain predominantly benign tissue with only scattered, small focal areas of high-grade neoplasia. Nevertheless, aspiration of benign-appearing ovarian cysts, with sclerosis in some cases, has been advocated as a means of alleviating symptoms attributed to these mass lesions, particularly in patients with a high surgical risk.[84]

Computed tomography in the staging of ovarian carcinoma. An additional useful role for CT has been in the staging of ovarian cancer. Compared with ultrasonography, CT is superior in delineating the relationship of the mass to surrounding structures and in assessing lymphadenopathy (Fig. 9-26).[77,78] Some investigators believe that CT should be performed preoperatively in all cases of malignant pelvic disease.[85]

Identification of patients with metastatic ovarian cancer includes a search for enlarged lymph nodes, tumor nodules within the abdominal organs, and evidence of spread to the contiguous pelvic structures (Fig. 9-27), peritoneum, and greater omentum (Fig. 9-28). Peritoneal involvement is common and may be subtle. On contrast-enhanced CT the most common finding of peritoneal carcinomatosis is ascites, which may be loculated. A careful search for peritoneal thickening, particularly when nodular, is extremely important in these patients (Fig. 9-29). The three most commonly involved sites are the right subphrenic region, the greater omentum, and the pouch of Douglas, as shown in a study of metastatic peritoneal implants assessed preoperatively with CT.[86] This study, using 10-mm contiguous sections supplemented with 2-mm thick sections in regions suspected of harboring implants, showed that CT allowed the detection of metastatic peritoneal implants in 74% of patients.[86] The major limitation of CT has been its inability to reliably and consistently depict implants on the peritoneal and liver surfaces that are smaller than 2 cm, and those located in certain sites such as the greater omentum.[86] This study also showed that the presence or absence of ascites is a very important factor; it may be the only sign of a

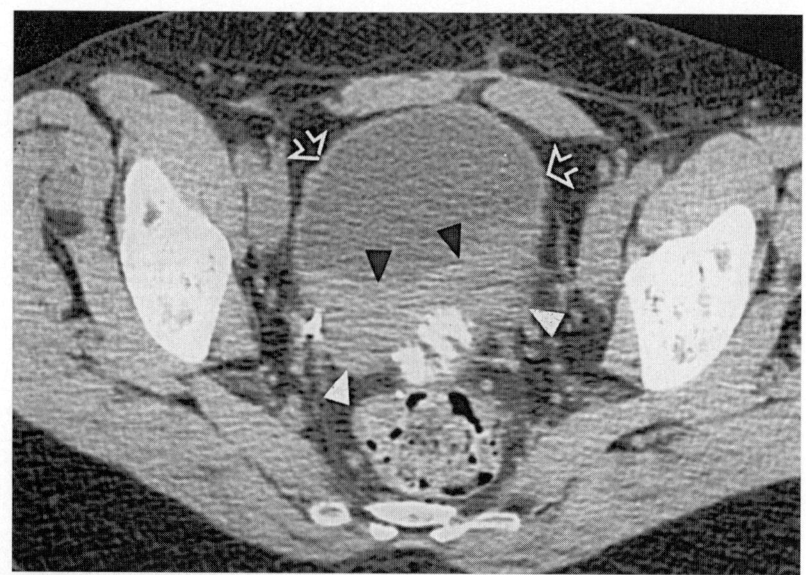

Fig. 9-27 CT shows ovarian cancer involvement of the wall *(arrowheads)* of the base of the bladder *(open arrows)*.

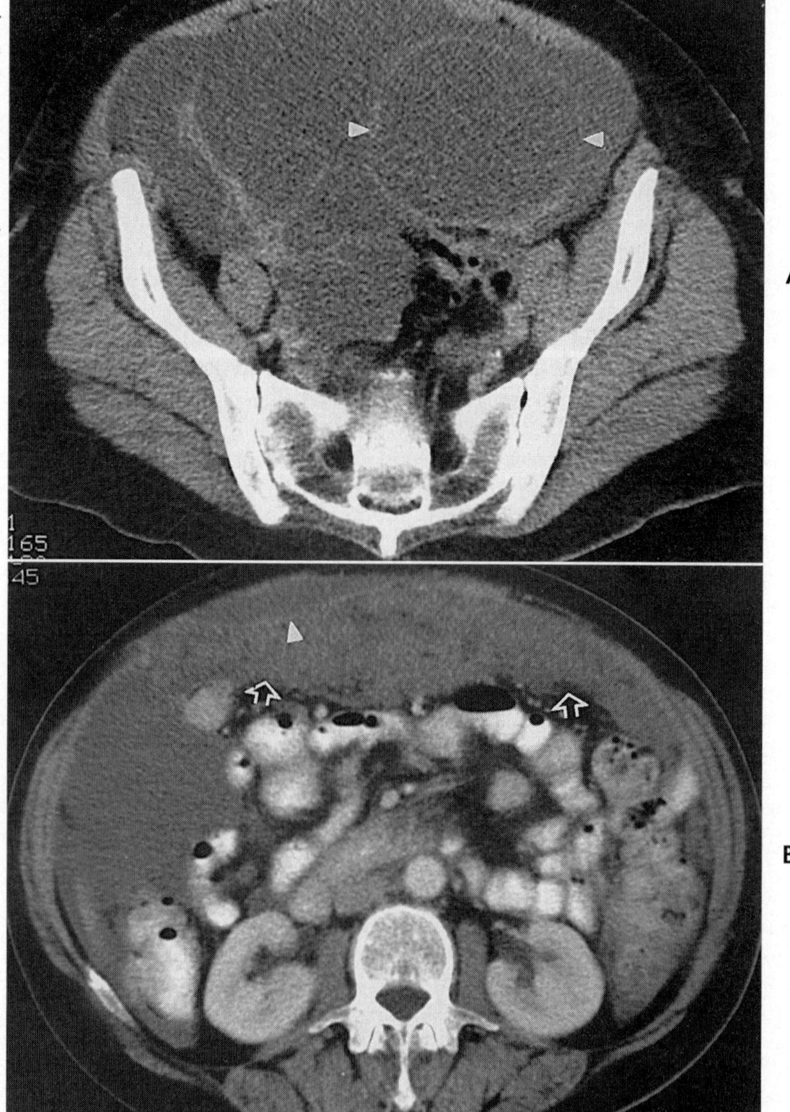

Fig. 9-28 Peritoneal and greater omental metastases from ovarian cancer. **A,** Contrast-enhanced spiral CT (5 mm/sec table feed, reconstructed with 5-mm sections and 5-mm intervals) in the pelvis shows a cystic ovarian cancer *(arrowheads)* surrounded by ascites. **B,** In the abdomen the greater omentum contains tumor *(open arrows)* adjacent to loculated ascites *(arrowhead)*.

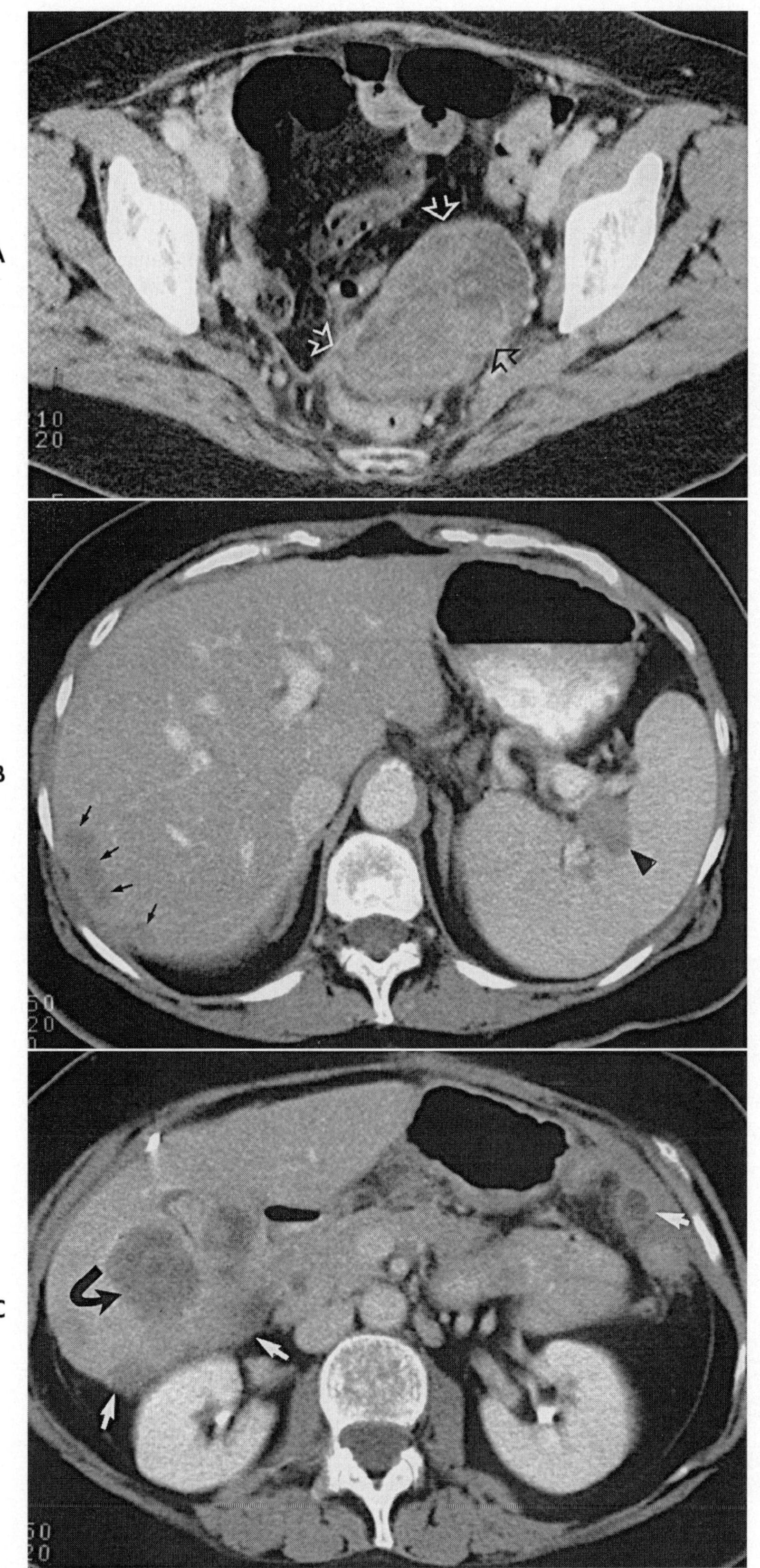

Fig. 9-29 Ovarian cancer, metastatic to multiple sites. Contrast-enhanced spiral CT of the pelvis (5 mm/sec table feed, reconstructed with 5-mm sections and 5-mm intervals) in the pelvis, followed by 8-mm sections every 10 mm using conventional CT technique in the abdomen, shows recurrent tumor in the pelvis *(open arrows)* **(A),** but also shows spread to the right subdiaphragmatic peritoneum *(small arrows),* the perisplenic region *(arrowhead)* **(B),** additional peritoneal sites *(arrows),* and the liver *(curved arrow)* **(C).**

metastasis to the peritoneum that is only 2 to 3 mm in size. However, peritoneal fluid may not always be adjacent to a peritoneal metastasis.

The incidence of peritoneal implants at autopsy has been reported to be as high as 90%.[87] CT may detect peritoneal carcinomatosis. In a series of 60 patients with peritoneal tumor, 35% of whom had metastatic ovarian cancer, the most common CT finding was ascites (74% of patients). Approximately 50% of the patients demonstrated some loculation, and in a small percentage of patients,

absence of cul-de-sac fluid in the presence of generalized ascites was considered by the authors to be suggestive of peritoneal carcinomatosis.[88] A review of a small number of patients with pathologically proved stage III or IV disease revealed that six of 15 patients had calcified peritoneal implants, five of six had perihepatic calcification, and one had a nonenlarged calcified lymph node.[89] Thus, focal peritoneal calcification may be a sign of metastatic disease to the peritoneum even in the absence of ascites (Figs. 9-30 and 9-31). This is

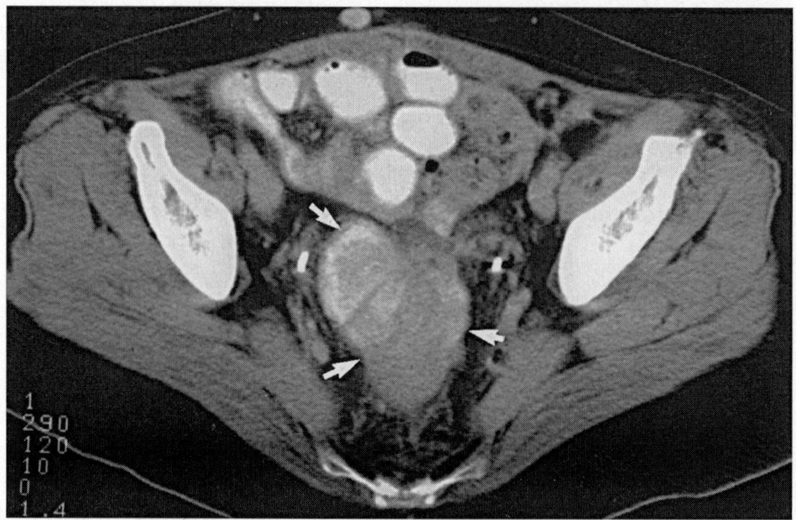

Fig. 9-30 Calcified metastatic ovarian cancer in the pelvis. Metastatic disease may present as a calcified mass *(arrows)*.

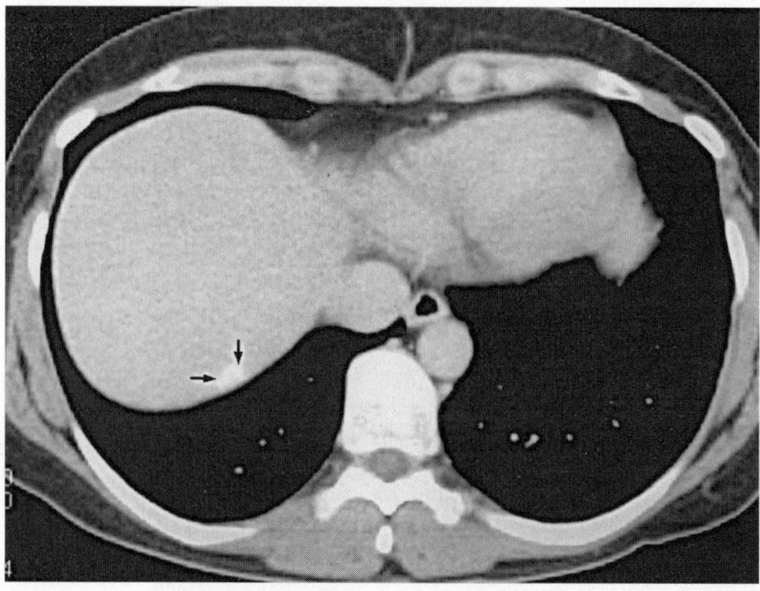

Fig. 9-31 Calcified metastatic ovarian cancer to the peritoneum. CT shows a focal peritoneal calcification *(arrows),* which was the only manifestation of tumor at this site.

explained by the fact that the most common type of ovarian carcinoma, serous cystadenocarcinoma, contains histologic calcification in approximately 30% of cases.[89]

CT as a definitive staging procedure for ovarian carcinoma has been investigated as an alternative to second-look laparotomy, but the results have been disappointing.[3,90-92] These studies show that peritoneal implants are often too small to be detected by CT. In one study,[92] only 7% of tumor nodules 1 cm or less in diameter were detected. To improve the low negative predictive value of CT, Megibow et al suggested employing faster scanners and therefore better contrast enhancement, and routine use of thin sections for the pelvis (5-mm thick, 10-mm table increments) and air contrast colonic opacification.[3] The most common location of recurrent disease is along the pelvic floor, round ligament, infundibulopelvic ligament and cul-de sac.[3] For this reason, careful scanning on high-resolution equipment using thin sections in the pelvis is recommended.

To improve the accuracy of CT in staging ovarian cancer, intraperitoneal injection of contrast media has been employed and shown to demonstrate metastatic disease.[93] This technique was found to be superior to standard CT in the detection of peritoneal metastasis.[94] However, the sensitivity and specificity of CT with intraperitoneal contrast material is not sufficiently better than conventional CT to warrant its routine use.[95]

In summary, therefore, a CT scan before second-look staging laparotomy may obviate the need for surgery by finding unsuspected disease. Although the specificity of CT is relatively high,[92] the findings can be confirmed by percutaneous CT-guided biopsy. However, a negative CT scan does not exclude tiny foci of residual disease, and so a second-look laparotomy may still be warranted.

Magnetic resonance imaging

MRI is often used in the assessment of adnexal masses. Because of its intrinsic "natural" tissue contrast abilities, it has proved useful in the diagnosis of several benign entities such as simple and hemorrhagic cysts, endometriomas, and teratomas. Other lesions such as serosal or pedunculated leiomyomas can also be reliably characterized.[96] With a combination of T1, T2, and fat-suppression and flow-sensitive pulse sequences, accurate tissue characterization can be obtained. MRI with FSE and multicoil techniques depicts the normal ovary as having a low-signal-intensity central stroma with numerous high-signal-intensity follicular cysts (Fig. 9-32). These follicles are more evident on the high-resolution long TR/TE FSE images, with the phased array coils than on conventional

body coil spin echo images. This is due to the high resolution and contrast provided by heavily T2-weighted FSE sequences. Postmenopausal ovaries demonstrate fewer, smaller cysts or an absence of cysts. The added resolution achievable with multicoil and FSE imaging can aid in the localization and detection of ovarian abnormalities. Lesions within the ovary can be recognized by the expansion of the ovarian stroma and displacement of the small follicular cysts to the periphery. Para-ovarian processes displace the ovary while maintaining its internal morphology. Depiction of small morphologic features such as papillae or septa is improved with these techniques.

On MRI, simple cysts have the same characteristics as on sonography and CT: they are smooth walled, homogeneous, with no internal matrix or debris (Figs. 9-33 and 9-34). Hemorrhagic cysts have the typical appearance of blood products on T1- and T2-weighted images (Fig. 9-35). T1-weighted images of hemorrhagic cysts and teratomas can be similar: both appear as masses of high signal intensity. However, owing to the appearance of the hemorrhage, T1-weighted images may have a central area of lower signal typical of subacute blood. Most hemorrhagic cysts of the ovary are

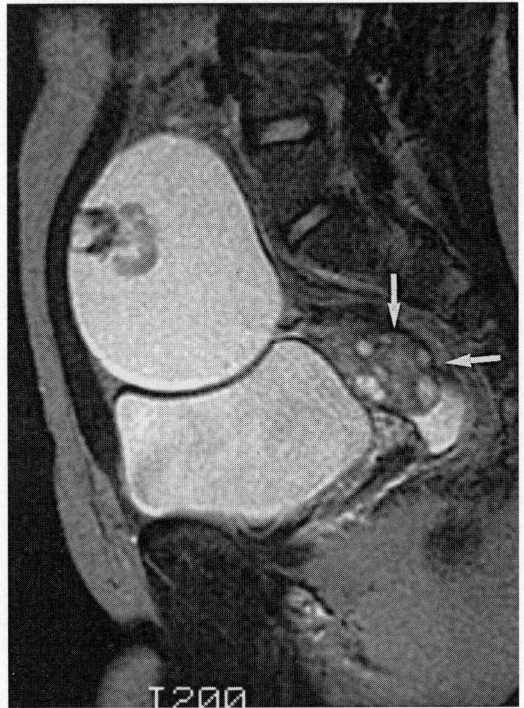

Fig. 9-32 Normal MR appearance of the ovary. A sagittal FSE image with the pelvic phased array coil shows the normal ovary *(white arrows)* in the posterior aspect of the pelvis in this patient with a contralateral teratoma (patient seen in Fig. 9-36).

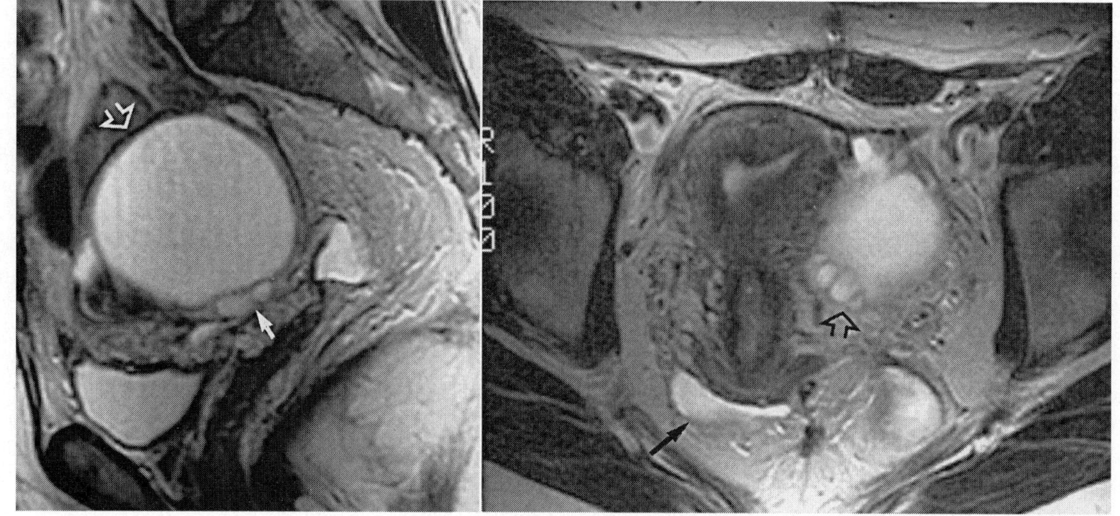

Fig. 9-33 A 26-year-old woman with a simple ovarian cyst **A,** Sagittal FSE image (TR 4000, TE effective 102) shows the cyst *(open white arrows),* with the typical high T2 signal of fluid surrounded by a smooth wall and, again typical of a cyst, the homogeneous internal signal. **B,** Axial FSE image at the inferior margin of the cyst shows several follicles *(open black arrow)* in the rest of the ovary on the left side. Note the small amount of free fluid in the cul-de-sac *(black arrow).*

seen in the subacute or chronic stages. Thus, the T1 signal is usually high, and the signal drops centrally, as the T2 signal decays. Thus, on proton density images, the signal is higher than on the longer echo T2 images (Fig. 9-35). In chronic cases a hemosiderin rim may be seen that has low signal on all pulse sequences (Fig. 9-35). There may be more heterogeneity in the teratomas, as their signal depends on their chemical composition (fat-water mix). Occasionally, they may be difficult to differentiate from each other.

Endometriomas are complex lesions containing multiple hemorrhagic cysts that have blood products of different ages within them. The repetitive cyclic bleeding and rupture leads to the multilocular cystic masses and heterogeneity of blood signal on MRI. Thus the MR appearances of endometriomas are typically multilocular masses, uni- or bilateral, with high signal on T1-weighted images, and hereogeneous high and central low signal or shading on T2-weighted and proton density images (see Fig. 9-24).[97] Chronic hematomas exhibit high signal on both T1- and T2-weighted images, but Togashi et al have suggested that the viscosity and protein content of an endometrioma accounts for the central shading or lower signal seen on T2-weighted images.[97] These authors use the diagnostic criteria of an entirely hyperintense lesion on T1-weighted images and hypointense signal (usually heterogeneous) on T2-weighted or when the lesion consists of multiple hyperintense

lesions on T1-weighted images regardless of the T2-weighted signal.[97] The same authors used their criteria in a study of 374 patients and achieved an accuracy of 96% for the preoperative diagnosis of endometriomas. As these lesions bleed intermittently, there may be associated adhesions and fibrosis seen with fixation of adjacent bowel loops. With fat- and water-suppression techniques, endometriomas can be reliably distinguished from dermoid lesions.[98] Care must be taken when using nonspecific suppression techniques such as short tau inversion recovery (STIR) sequences, as the blood products may in fact have the same T1 relaxation time as fat and may suppress equally (see Fig. 9-24). The specific fat- and water-suppression sequences described by Kier et al are more reliable.

Teratomas have several typical features that can be used by MR and other imaging modalities to define them. As previously discussed, these include the presence of fat, fat-fluid levels, the so-called dermoid "nipple" (Fig. 9-36) or mural nodule, and intracystic fat balls. The fat-fluid level can be identified and due to the dense nature of the fluid not be in the dependent portion of the lesion (Fig. 9-37). Fat-suppression sequences such as frequency-selective presaturation or STIR may be used to specifically demonstrate the fat nature of the lesion. The nipple can have a variable appearance, depending on its histologic make-up (see Fig. 9-36). While MRI is not sensitive for the detec-

Text continued on p. 217.

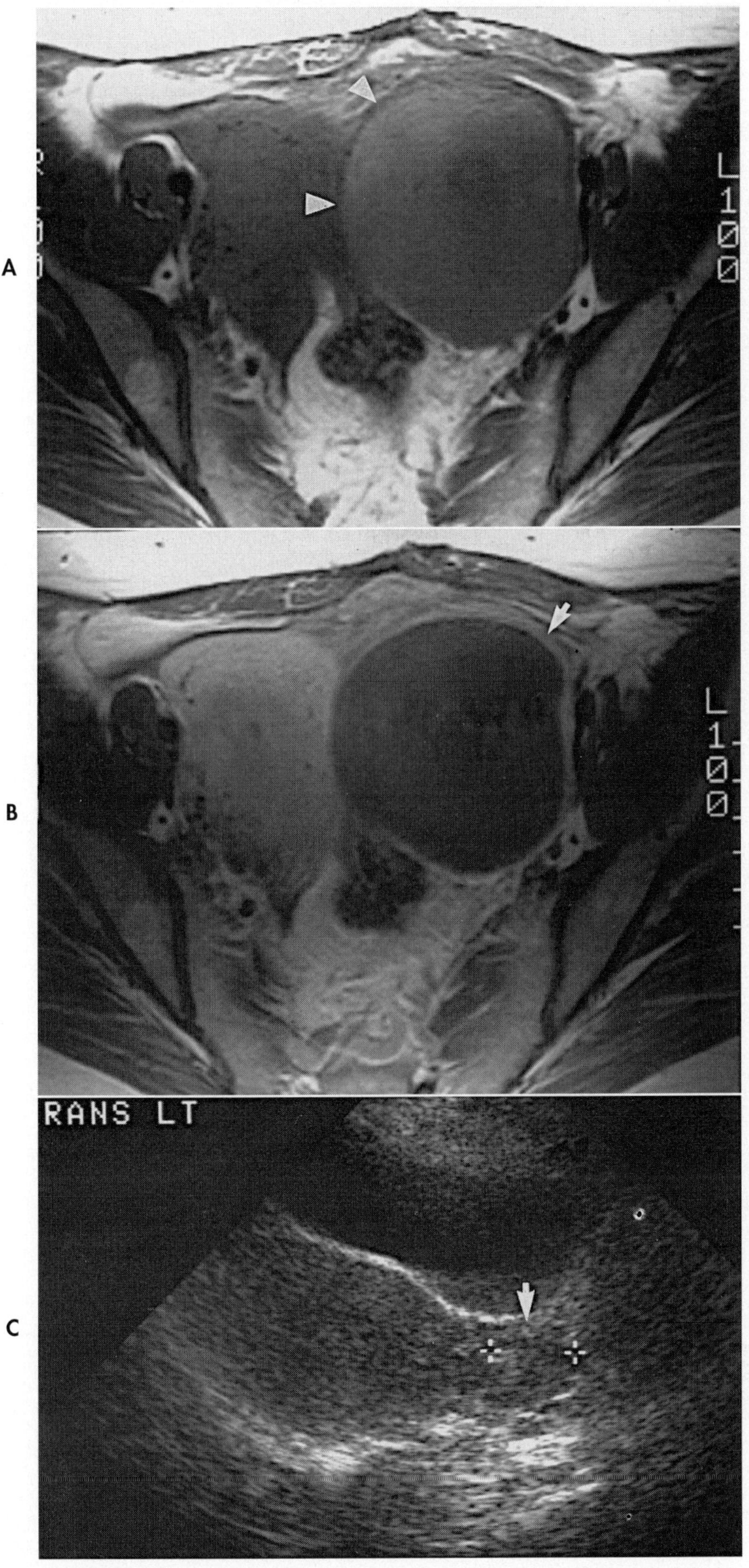

Fig. 9-34 Simple, nonenhancing ovarian cyst. **A,** Axial T1-weighted image before gadolinium administration shows a well-defined left adnexal mass that appears internally homogeneous with a relatively thin wall *(white arrowheads)*. **B,** After injection of 10 ml of intravenous gadolinium the mass shows no evidence of enhancement, with only minimal rim enhancement seen anteriorly *(white arrow)*. This was thought to represent a portion of the normal ovary. **C,** A follow-up ultrasound examination performed 1 month later shows internal disappearance of the mass and a normal-appearing left ovary *(white arrow)*.

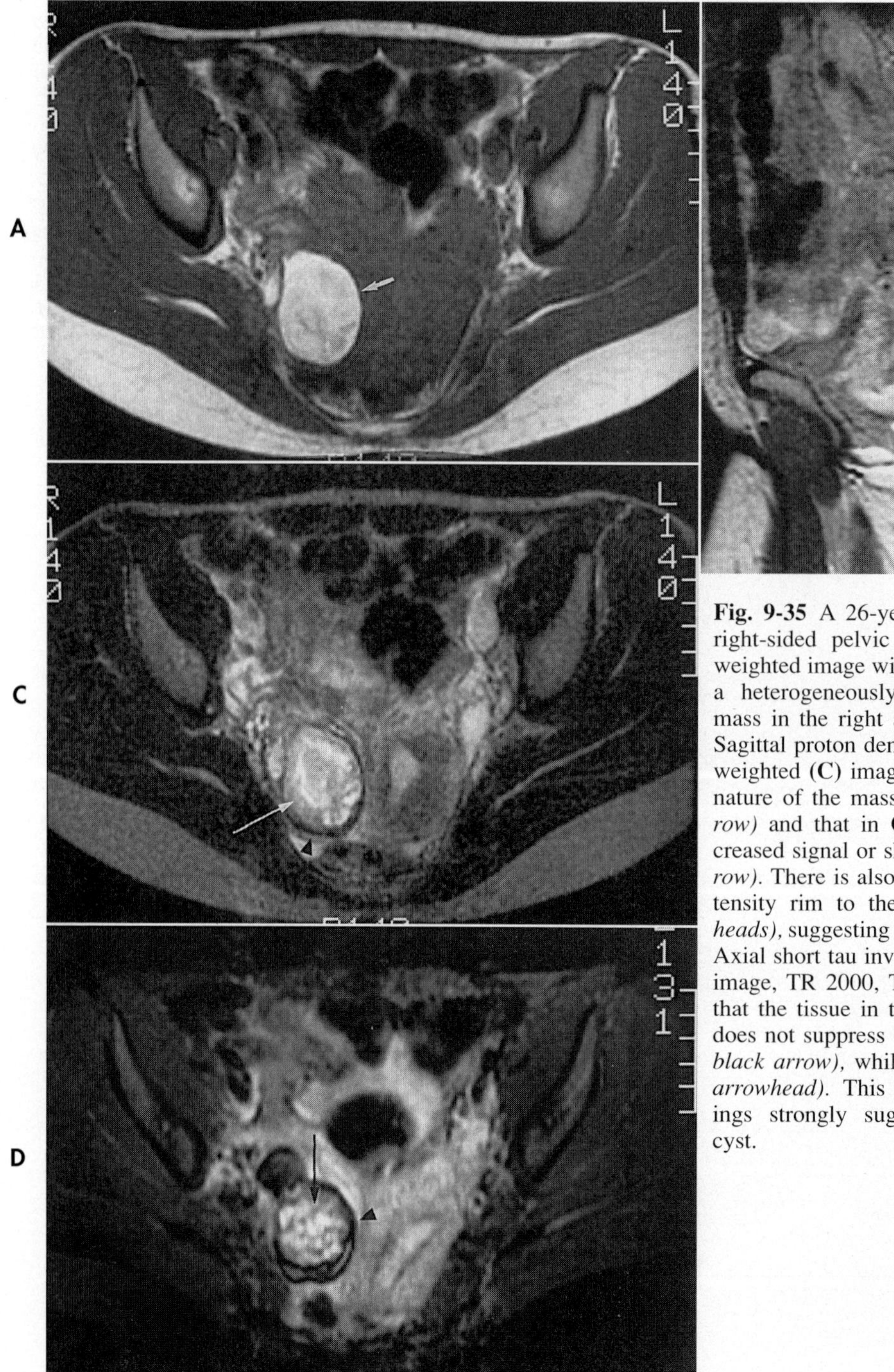

Fig. 9-35 A 26-year-old woman with a right-sided pelvic mass. **A,** Axial T1-weighted image with the body coil shows a heterogeneously high-signal-intensity mass in the right adnexa *(white arrow)*. Sagittal proton density **(B)** and axial T2-weighted **(C)** images show that the fluid nature of the mass is evident *(black arrow)* and that in **C** there is central decreased signal or shading *(long white arrow)*. There is also a thick low signal intensity rim to the mass *(black arrowheads),* suggesting a hemosiderin wall. **D,** Axial short tau inversion recovery (STIR image, TR 2000, TI 160, TE 43) shows that the tissue in the center of the mass does not suppress (as the fat does) *(long black arrow),* while the rim does *(black arrowhead).* This combination of findings strongly suggests a hemorrhagic cyst.

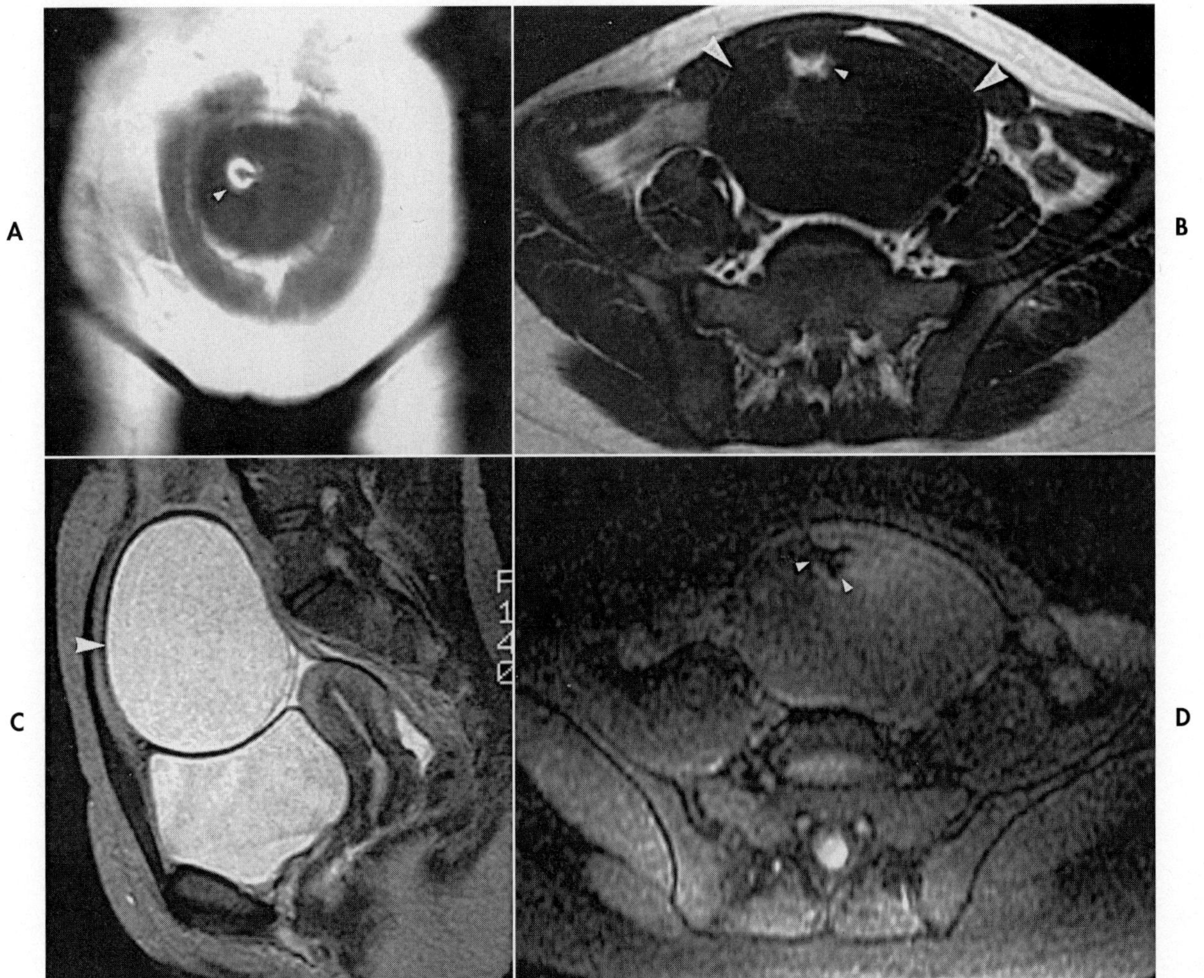

Fig. 9-36 Cystic teratoma in a 31-year-old woman with a large pelvic mass. **A,** Coronal T1-weighted image shows the "nipple" *(small white arrowhead)* in the anteriormost aspect of the mass. On this T1-weighted image the nipple is predominantly fat with a small-low signal center. **B,** Axial T1-weighted image shows the size of the mass *(large white arrowheads)*, which appears predominantly cystic, again with the anterior fat-containing nipple *(small white arrowhead)*. **C,** Sagittal T2-weighted image shows the mass *(white arrowhead)* in relationship to the uterus and bladder. **D,** Axial chemical shift image shows the suppression of the signal in the nipple *(small white arrowheads)*, confirming its fat content.

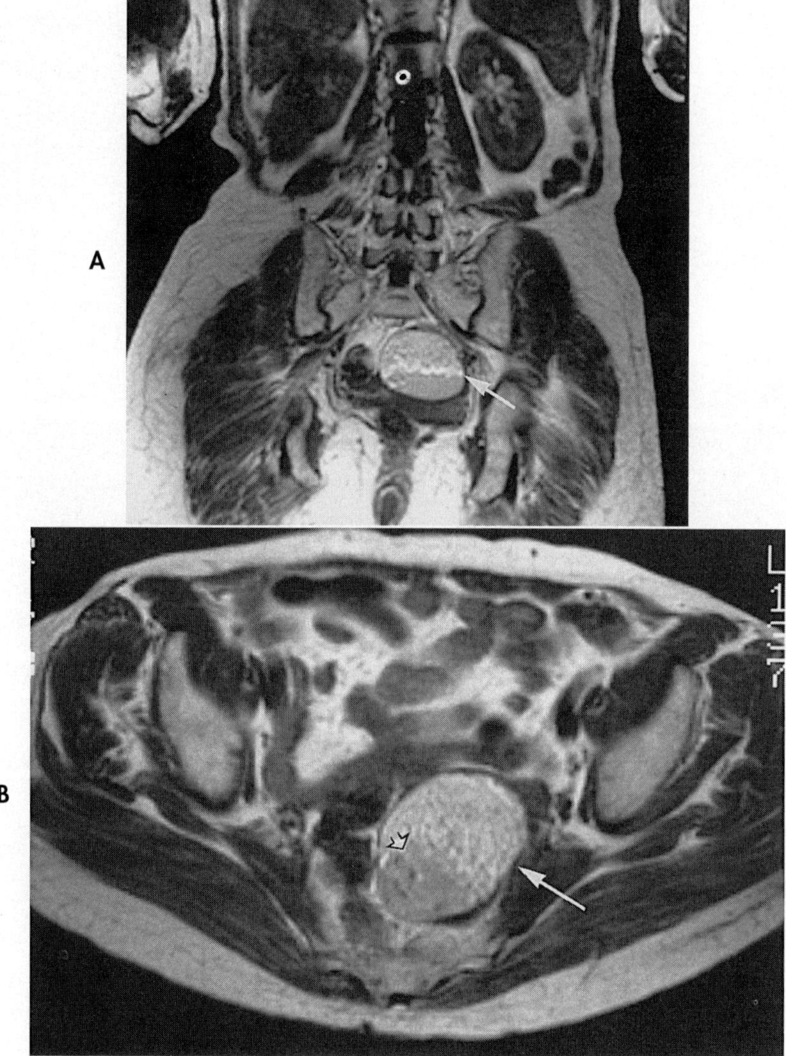

Fig. 9-37 A 73-year-old woman with a left mature cystic teratoma. **A** and **B,** Coronal and axial T1-weighted images show a high signal intensity mass *(white arrows)* with internal heterogeneity *(open black arrow).*   *Continued.*

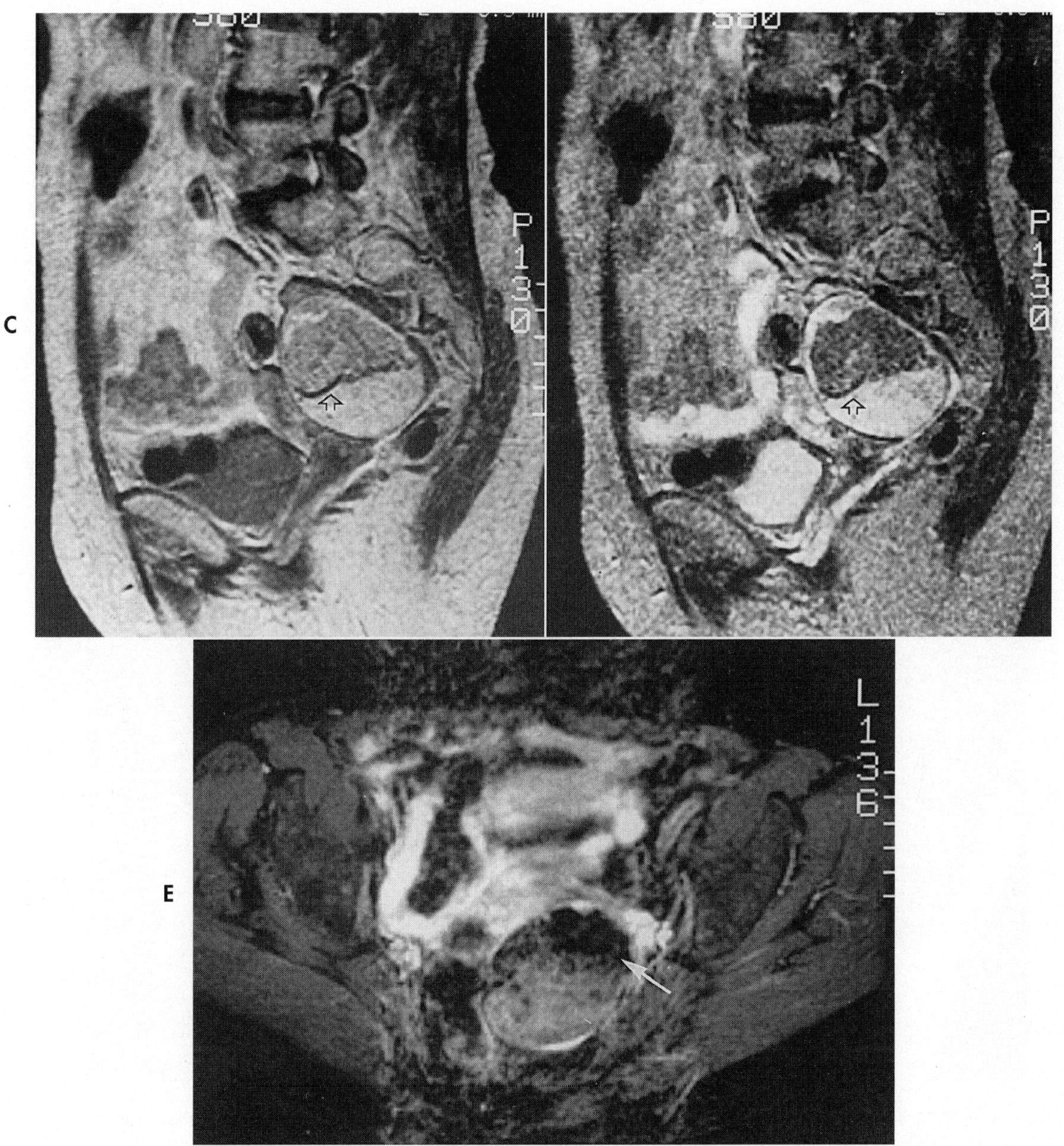

Fig. 9-37, cont'd Sagittal proton density **(C)** and T2-weighted **(D)** images show the internal fat-fluid level *(open black arrows)*. Note that this is not in a dependent position, suggesting that the lesion contains very viscous fat and serous fluid. **E,** Axial STIR (TR 2000, TE 43, TI 160) image shows the superior fat *(white arrow)* to suppress with signal remaining in the dependent viscous fluid.

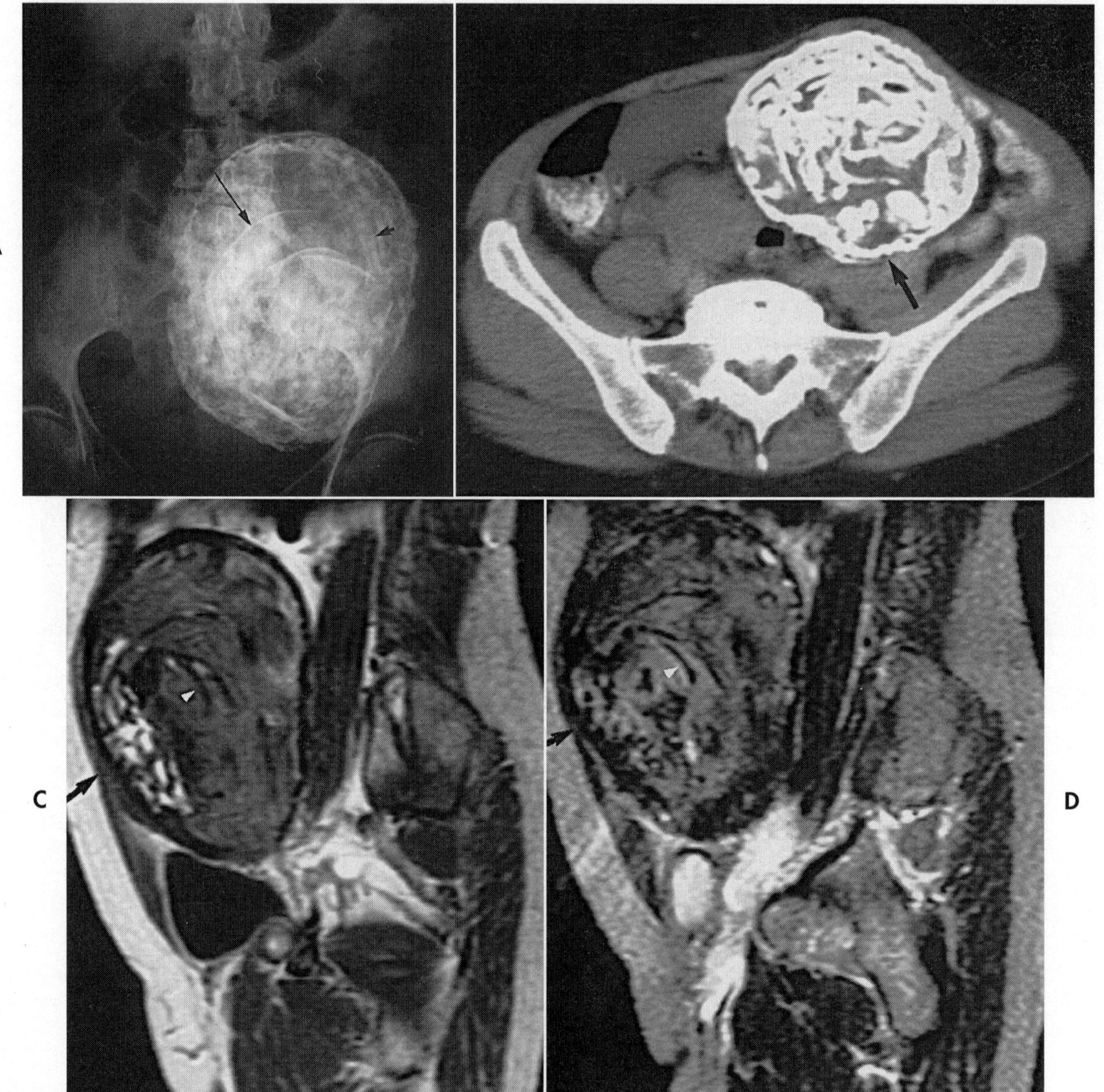

Fig. 9-38 Lithopedion in a 70-year-old woman with a long history of a pelvic mass. **A,** Plain film of the abdomen shows a large, densely calcified and part-ossified mass in the left lower abdomen. The ossification shows some limb formations *(short black arrows),* and portions of the skull bones *(long black arrow)* are seen. **B,** A CT scan of the same mass *(black arrow)* shows the dense ossification and calcification. **C,** Sagittal T1-weighted image shows the mass *(black arrows)* superior to the bladder with linear areas of low signal intensity *(small white arrowhead).* remain low in signal, representing the ossified limbs. **D,** Sagittal T2-weighted image. (Courtesy of Alex Chako, MD, Norfolk, VA.)

tion of small amounts of calcium or bone, when present in large amounts, it will have a low signal on all pulse sequences (Fig. 9-38). The MRI appearance of a heavily calcified mass such as a leiomyoma or the rare lithopedion-containing osseous structures may be easily apparent when these are in abundance (Fig. 9-38). The discrete focal low signal on all sequences is typical.

MRI has been used to evaluate patient with suspected polycystic ovaries. The MR features of polycystic ovarian disease have been described by Mitchell et al[99] and consist of multiple small cysts all located around the periphery of the ovary. The central portion of the ovary in Fig. 9-39 contains a low T2-weighted signal stromal area. This is usually bilateral, and the ovaries may be normal in size (Fig. 9-40). In patients with amenorrhea the uterus is small and shows the typical appearance of a prepubertal uterus (Fig. 9-40). In Mitchell et al's study of seven patients, six had multiple cysts seen on MRI and only one patient had more than two cysts seen on sonography.[99]

Solid lesions of the ovary can be benign or malignant, and in some cases can be differentiated to a degree by MRI. Serosal or pedunculated uterine or ovarian leiomyomas can be readily diagnosed by MRI when they have the typical MR appearance (Fig. 9-41). These are discussed further in Chapter 7, the chapter on benign diseases of the uterus. Other lesions such as fibrothecomas typically appear as solid lesions, uniformly low in signal on T2-weighted images (Fig. 9-43). However, these may become necrotic centrally as they outgrow their blood supply, and may have a hetero-geneous appearance (Fig. 9-43). The normal appearance of the remaining ovary can also be suggestive of the benign nature of the lesion (Fig. 9-44). Primary malignancies of the colon may have significant extraluminal involvement, so that these should be included in the differential diagnosis of a pelvic mass, especially when there is extensive bowel involvement (Fig. 9-45). Other less common nonovarian neoplasms can be found in the pelvis. The MR appearance of pheochromocytomas of the adrenal glands is typically described as "light bulb" bright on T2-weighted images. The extra-adrenal bladder pheochromocytoma in Fig. 9-46 has a high signal, with a central "light bulb."

Malignant lesions of the ovary, the common adenocarcinomas, are typically large, complex masses with extension beyond the pelvis (Fig. 9-47). The literature also supports a role for MRI combined with gadolinium enhancement for the assessment of adnexal lesions (Figs. 9-42 and 9-48).[100,101] The addition of gadolinium has reportedly increased diagnostic accuracies from 56% to 78% when combined with a feature analysis approach. The features used include a large mass (greater than 5 cm), complex internal nodules, thick internal septations (greater than 2 mm), thick wall (greater than 3 mm), and central necrosis.[100] The solid components and the nodules usually demonstrate enhancement with gadolinium, indicating their solid nature (Figs. 9-47 and 9-48). However, there may be overlap in these features when they are used to differentiate benign from malignant lesions.

Text continued on p. 223.

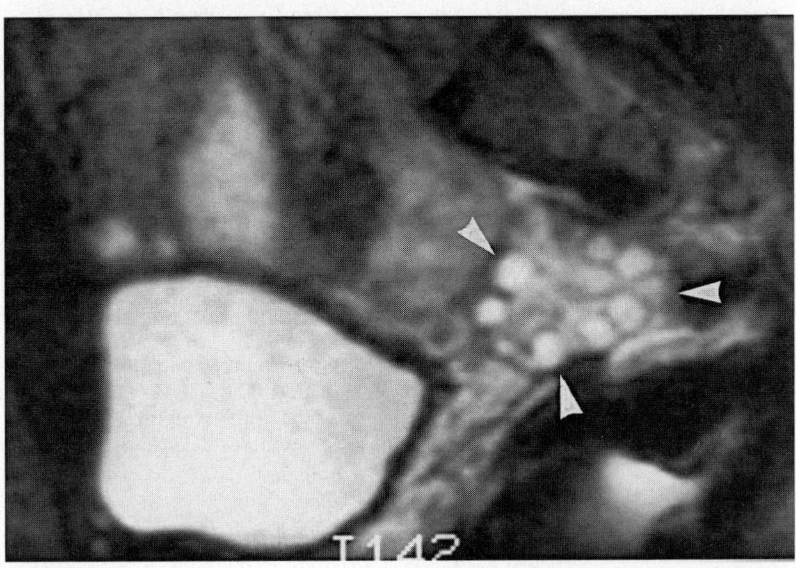

Fig. 9-39 Sagittal FSE image with the body coil shows a polycystic ovary with multiple small peripheral cysts of similar size *(white arrows).*

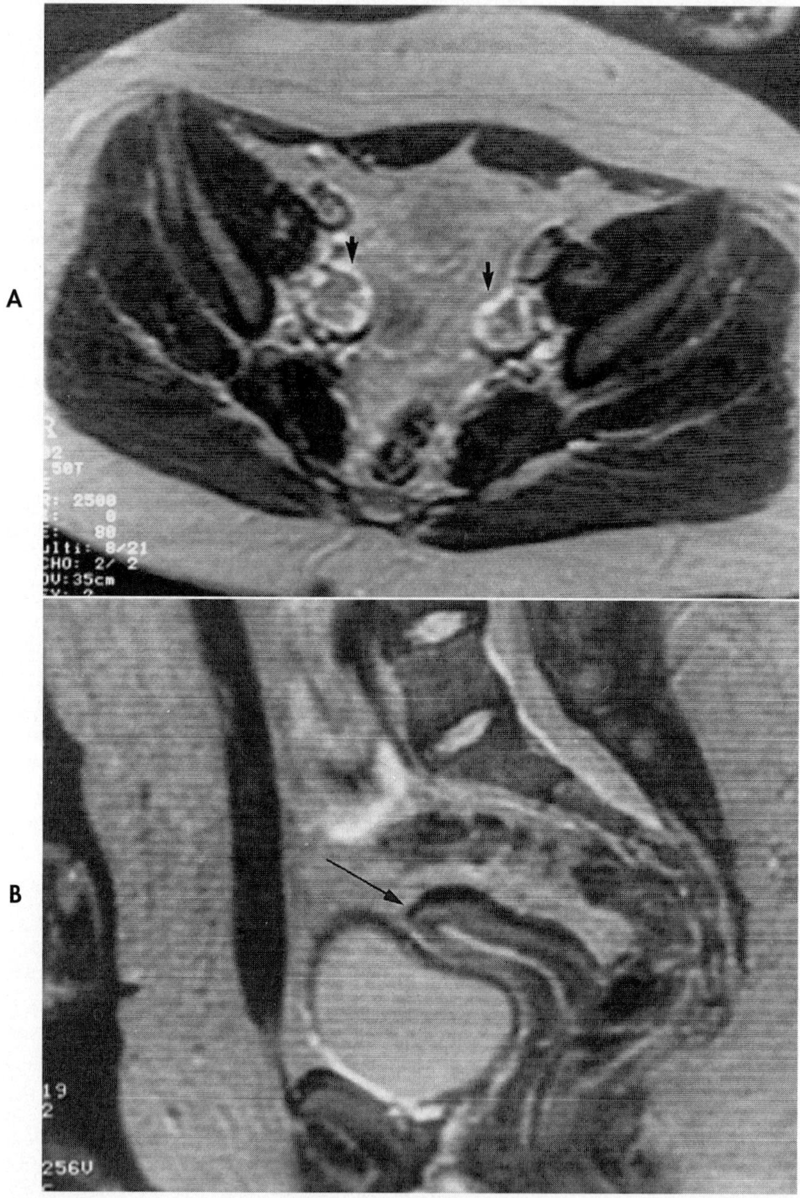

Fig. 9-40 Polycystic ovaries in a 22-year-old woman with primary amenorrhea and an elevated testosterone level. These images were obtained on a 0.5T unit. **B,** Axial T2-weighted image shows the ovaries *(black arrows)* with a thin hyperintense rim bilaterally, which represents the multiple small cysts. **B,** Sagittal T2-weighted image shows a small prepubescent-appearing uterus *(long black arrow)*.

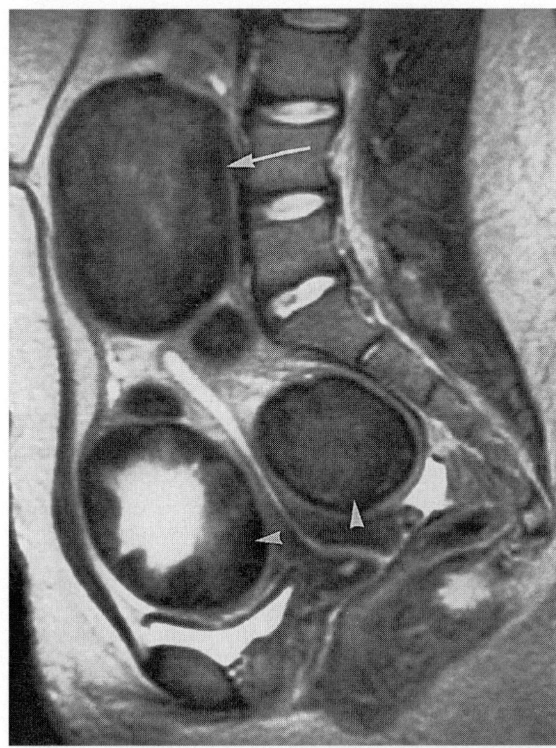

Fig. 9-41 Multiple leiomyomas. Sagittal T2-weighted image shows the typical appearance of uterine leiomyomas *(white arrowheads)*. These can be very large and subserosal *(white arrow)*.

Fig. 9-42 Benign fibroma of the ovary in a 16-year-old girl with a large palpable mass on physical examination. **A,** Sagittal FSE image using the body coil shows a very large multilobular mass of predominantly low signal intensity *(white arrowheads)* superior to the uterus *(long white arrow)*. Axial T1-weighted images before **(B)** and after **(C)** gadolinium administration show a fairly diffuse enhancement pattern *(white arrows)*. In view of the low T2 signal and the patient's young age, the likely diagnosis is a benign tumor of the ovary.

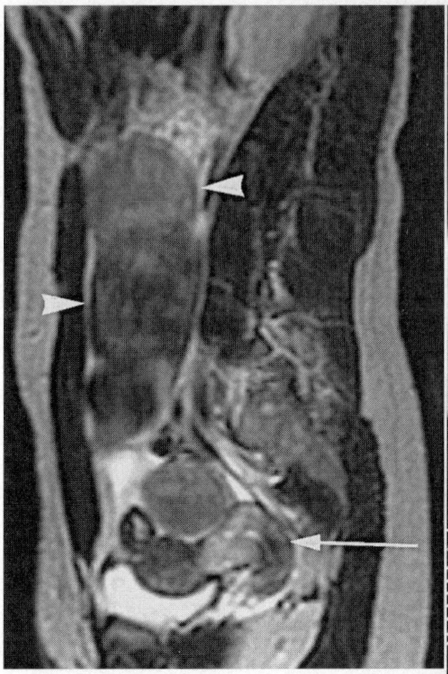

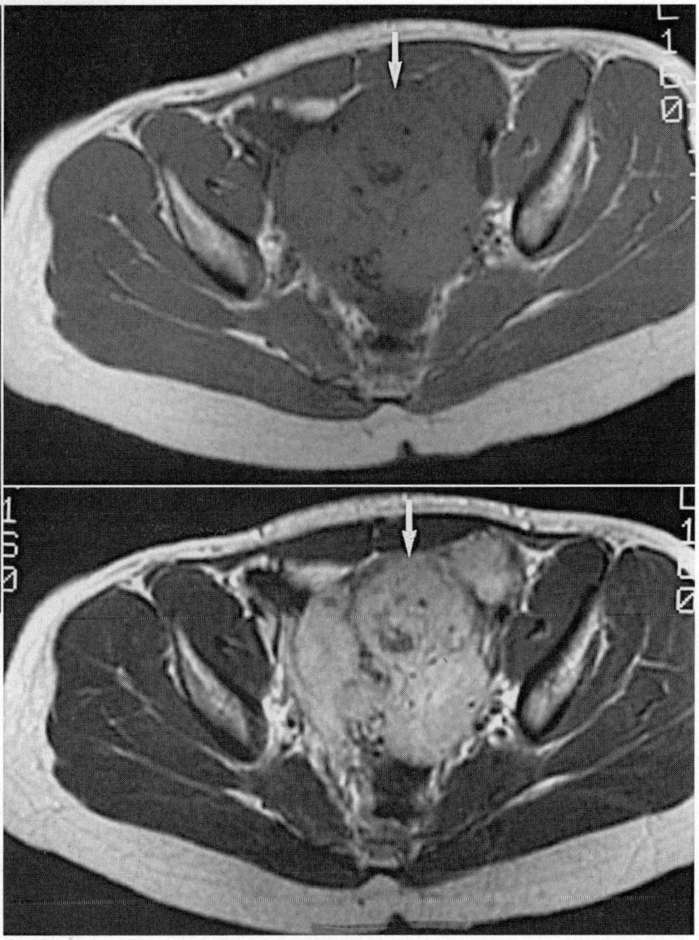

Fig. 9-43 Ovarian fibrothecoma in the patient seen in Fig. 9-38. **A,** CT scan of the pelvis after injection of intravenous contrast material shows a large mass *(white arrowhead)* that is solid and contains some central area of lower attenuation *(small black arrow),* suggestive of fluid. **B,** Axial T1-weighted MR image shows the large mass with low signal intensity *(black arrow).* **C,** Axial T2-weighted image (TR 2400, TE 80) shows the predominantly low signal mass *(white arrows)* to have several focal areas of high signal, similar to the low-attenuation areas on CT, representing fluid or cystic necrosis. (Courtesy of Alex Chako MD, Norfolf, Va.)

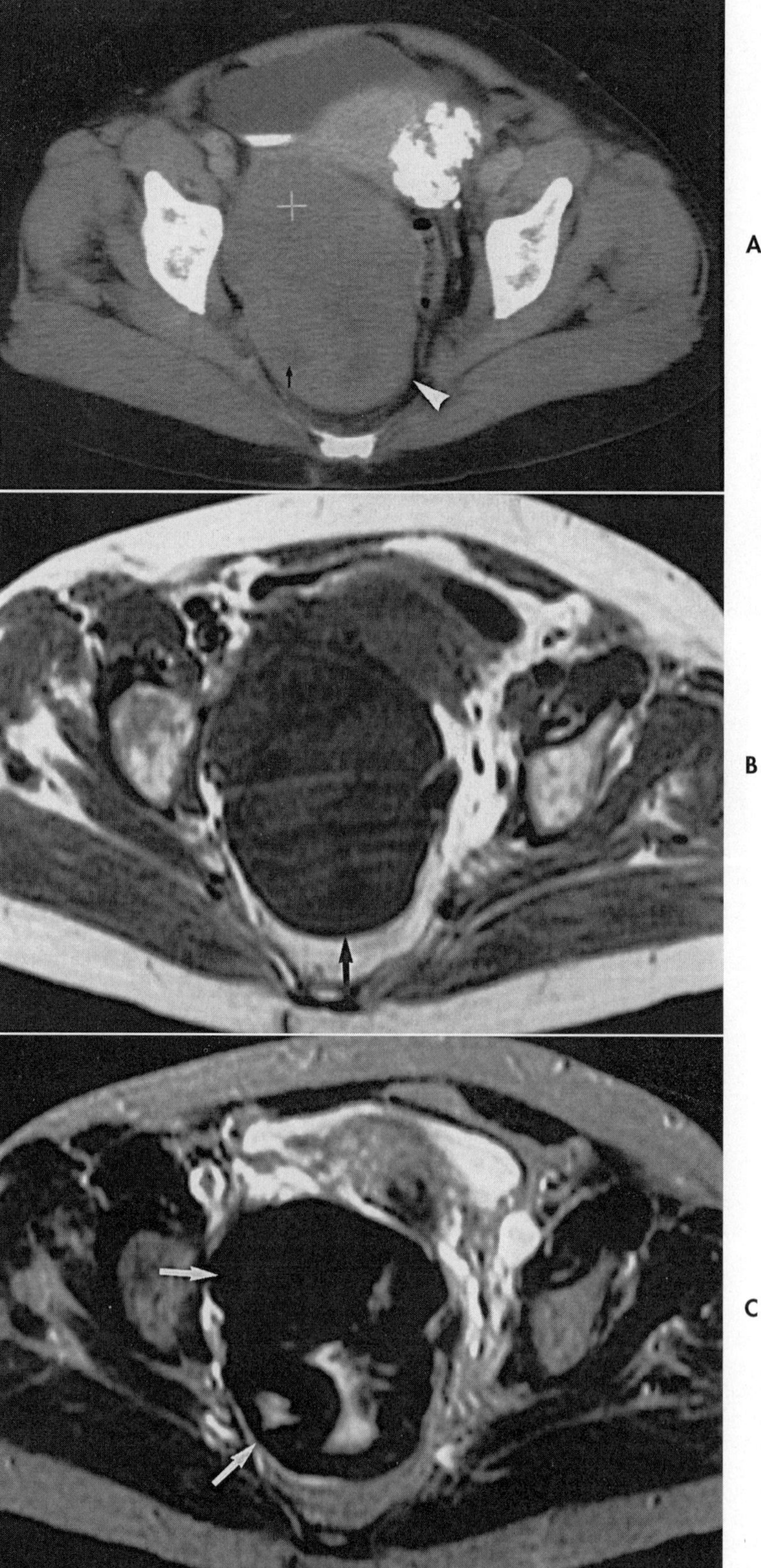

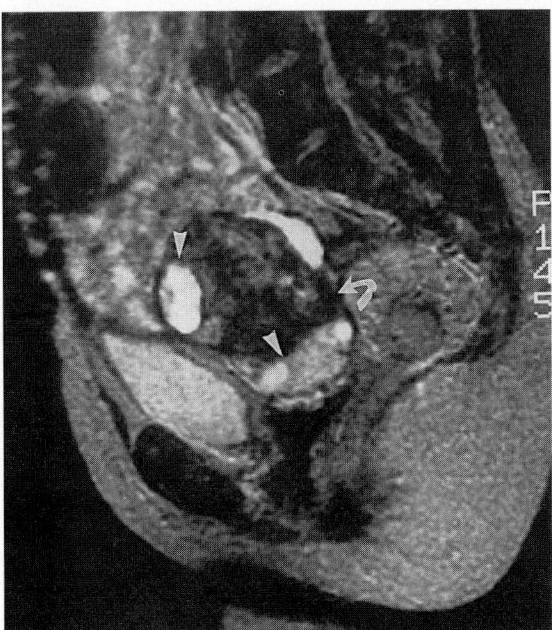

Fig. 9-44 Calcified fibrothecoma in a 64-year-old woman with a mass seen on sonography and CT. This sagittal T2-weighted image shows a mass *(curved white arrow)* arising from the central stroma of the ovary, which has predominantly low signal intensity, with some area of very low signal (likely the calcified component). There are several small cortical ovarian cysts *(white arrowheads)* surrounding the central mass.

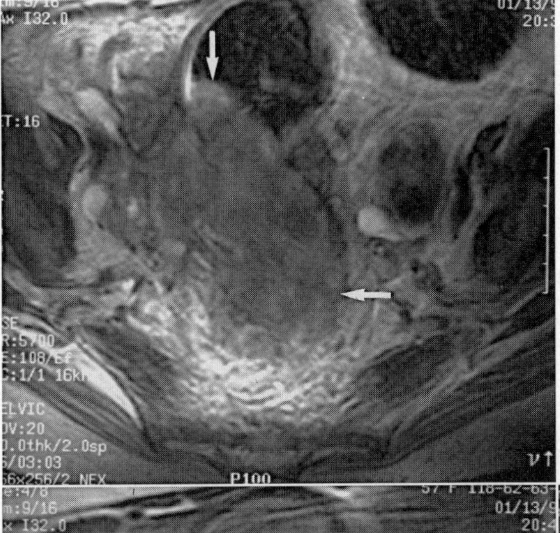

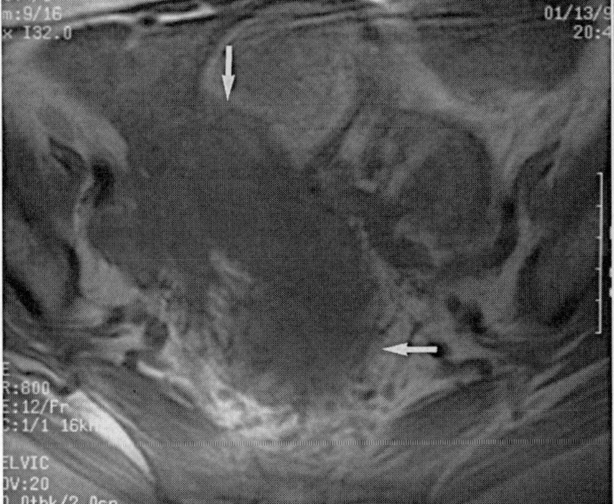

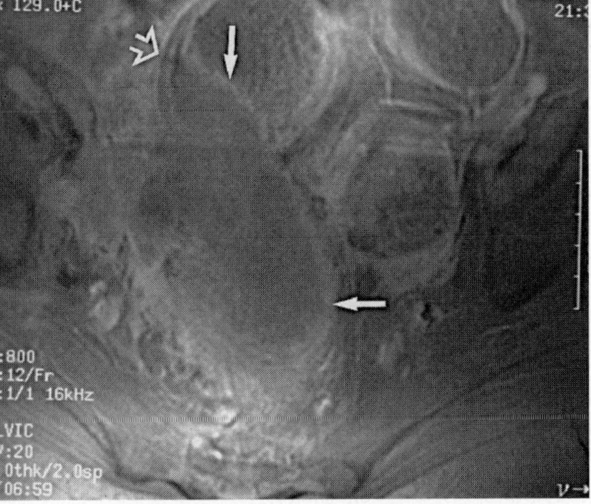

Fig. 9-45 Sigmoid adenocarcinoma in a 57-year-old woman who presented with a long history of altered bowel habits. **A,** Axial FSE image (TR 5700, TE 108), shows a large right-sided pelvic mass *(white arrows)* arising from the lateral aspect of the sigmoid colon. Axial T1-weighted images before **(B)** and after **(C)** 10 ml of gadolinium show the mass *(white arrows)* causing considerable bowel obstruction, and after contrast administration the bowel wall *(open white arrow)* enhances normally, with the rim of the mass outlined (white arrows).

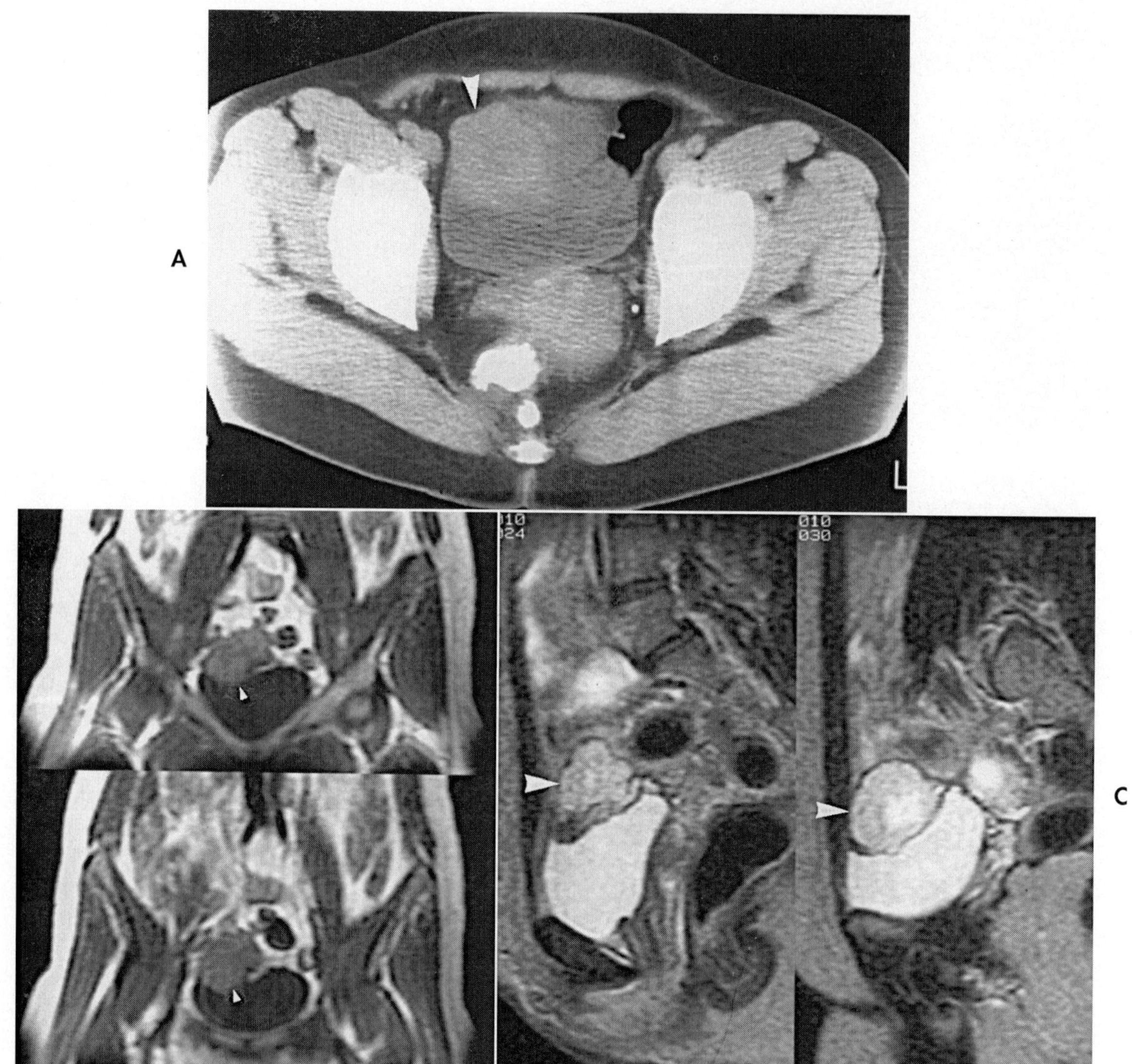

Fig. 9-46 Bladder pheochromocytoma in a 32-year-old woman who presented with a history of recent hypertensive crisis while undergoing pelvic surgery. **A,** CT scan shows a poorly defined mass *(white arrowhead)* on the right lateral dome of the bladder. **B,** Coronal T1-weighted images show the mass *(small white arrowheads)* to be outside the bladder, adherent to its wall. **C,** Sagittal T2-weighted images show the mass *(white arrowhead)* to be superior to the bladder, of high signal with a very high signal center.

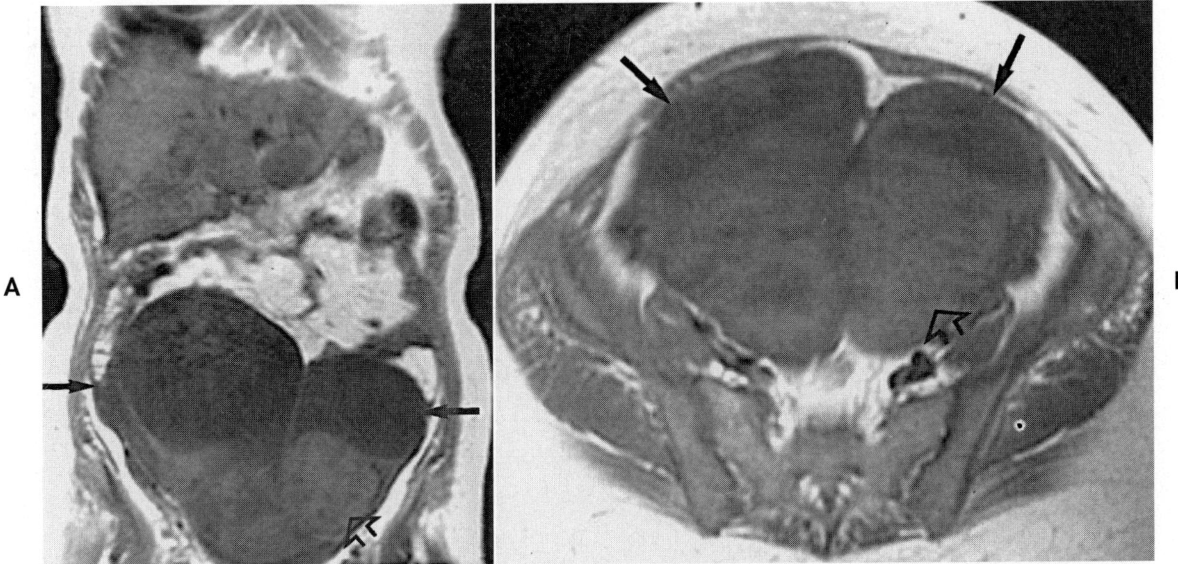

Fig. 9-47 Ovarian cystadenocarcinoma in a 36-year-old woman who presented with a large pelvic mass. Coronal (**A**) and axial (**B**) T1-weighted images show a very large mass extending up out of the pelvic containing cystic *(black arrows)* and solid *(open black arrows)* components.

Magnetic resonance imaging in the staging of ovarian cancer. MRI has a potential role in staging patients with ovarian malignancies. Its diagnostic accuracy is currently being evaluated in a multicenter trial comparing the relative accuracies of MR and CT in staging the pelvic and extrapelvic extent of disease in patients with suspected ovarian cancer. MRI has the advantage of inherent tissue contrast with the multiplanar capability that allows visualization of the entire abdomen and pelvis. It is especially useful for imaging the diaphragm and subphrenic spaces. In the as yet small number of published studies of MRI in staging ovarian cancer, the accuracy rates range from 60% to 83%.[100,102,103]

Like CT, MRI can detect ascites, implants, and lymph nodes. Ascitic fluid is usually clearly apparent on T2-weighted images (Fig. 9-48), and when simple, the fluid has a homogeneous high signal, similar to that of urine. Complex ascites, which is often seen in metastatic ovarian cancer, has a heterogeneous signal and may often be loculated, containing thick-walled septations.

Detection of implants is difficult, especially when they are small and microscopic. They may hard to detect on any imaging modality, including CT, and are often missed at surgery. Larger implants (usually over 2 cm) can be detected by MRI (Fig. 9-49), and more may be picked up with IV gadolinium, even without bowel contrast (Fig. 9-49). The gadolinium signal may be more conspicuous if used with fat-suppressed T1-weighted images. Very small implants, as occur in peritoneal carcinomatosis, can be detected by the presence of complex ascites containing small nodules, best seen on T2-weighted images (Fig. 9-50). It is important to detect peritoneal implants, and the means of detection may improve in the future, possibly with use of monoclonal antibodies for labeled imaging.

The detection of lymph nodes by MRI has been documented and shown to be equal to that by CT. In patients with contrast allergies or other contraindications to iodinated contrast, MRI may be more desirable. The signal void of flow allows for relatively easy differentiation of vessels from lymph nodes (Fig. 9-51). This is particularly helpful in the iliac chains, especially the internal iliacs, where the tortuosity of the vessels may make the detection of small nodes difficult. All nodes greater than 1 cm in length are regarded as abnormal in the female pelvis.

Recurrent or residual disease in the postoperative pelvis and beyond can be detected by MRI. The local recurrence will be similar to the original tumor and have high signal intensity (Figs. 9-52 to 9-54). The effects of local tumor recurrence, such as hydronephrosis, can also be detected on MRI (Fig. 9-54). The detection of residual or recurrent tumor by MRI has been evaluated in patients with lymphoma and found to be useful.[104] The detection of high signal intensity may be re-

Text continued on p. 231.

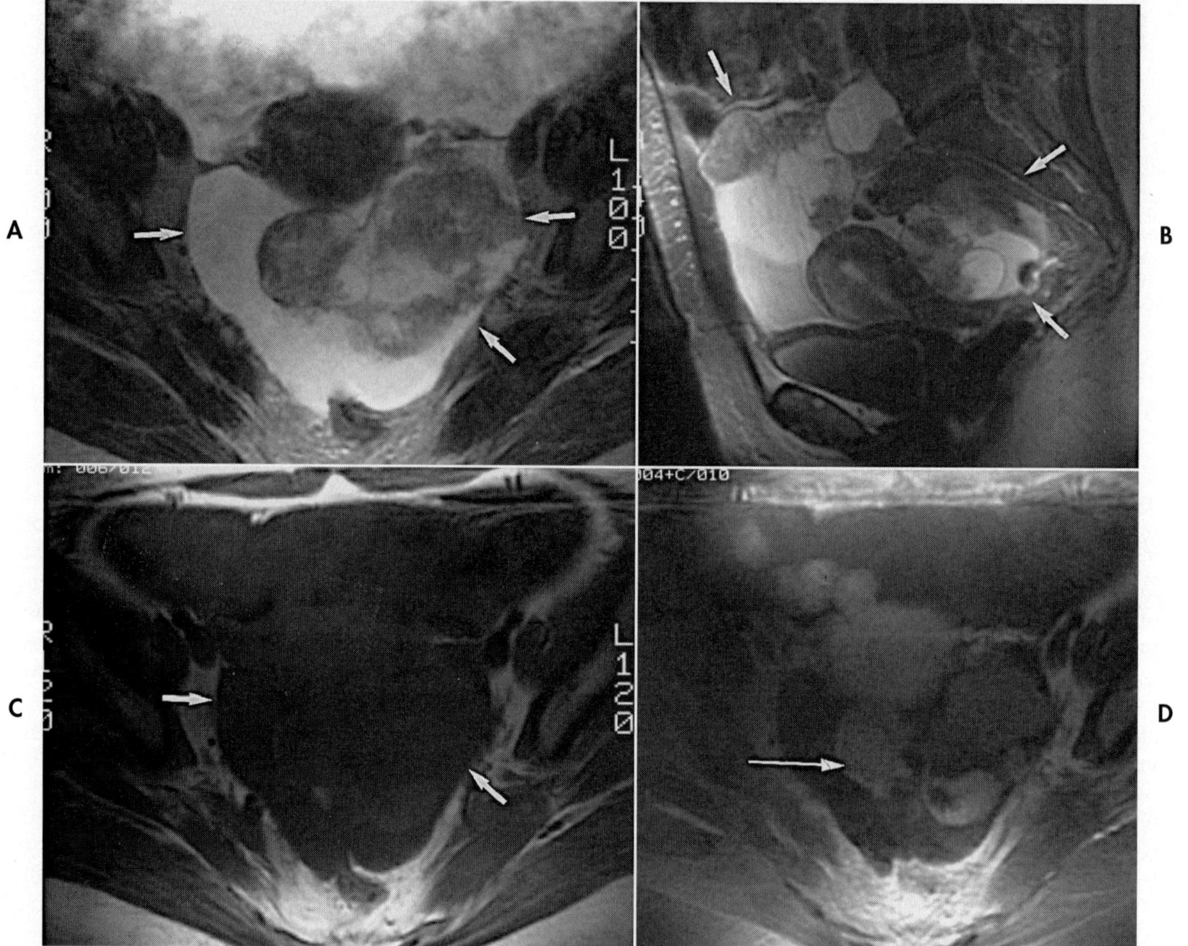

Fig. 9-48 A 45-year-old woman with a large mass in the right adnexa. Axial (**A**) and sagittal (**B**) FSE images with the phased array coil show a very large heterogeneous mass *(white arrows)* with solid and cystic area. **C,** T1-weighted image shows the mass *(white arrows)* to be featureless. **D,** Postgadolinium T1-weighted image with fat suppression shows enhancement in the solid parts of the mass *(long white arrow).* This is an ovarian papillary serous cystadenocarcinoma, grade 3/3.

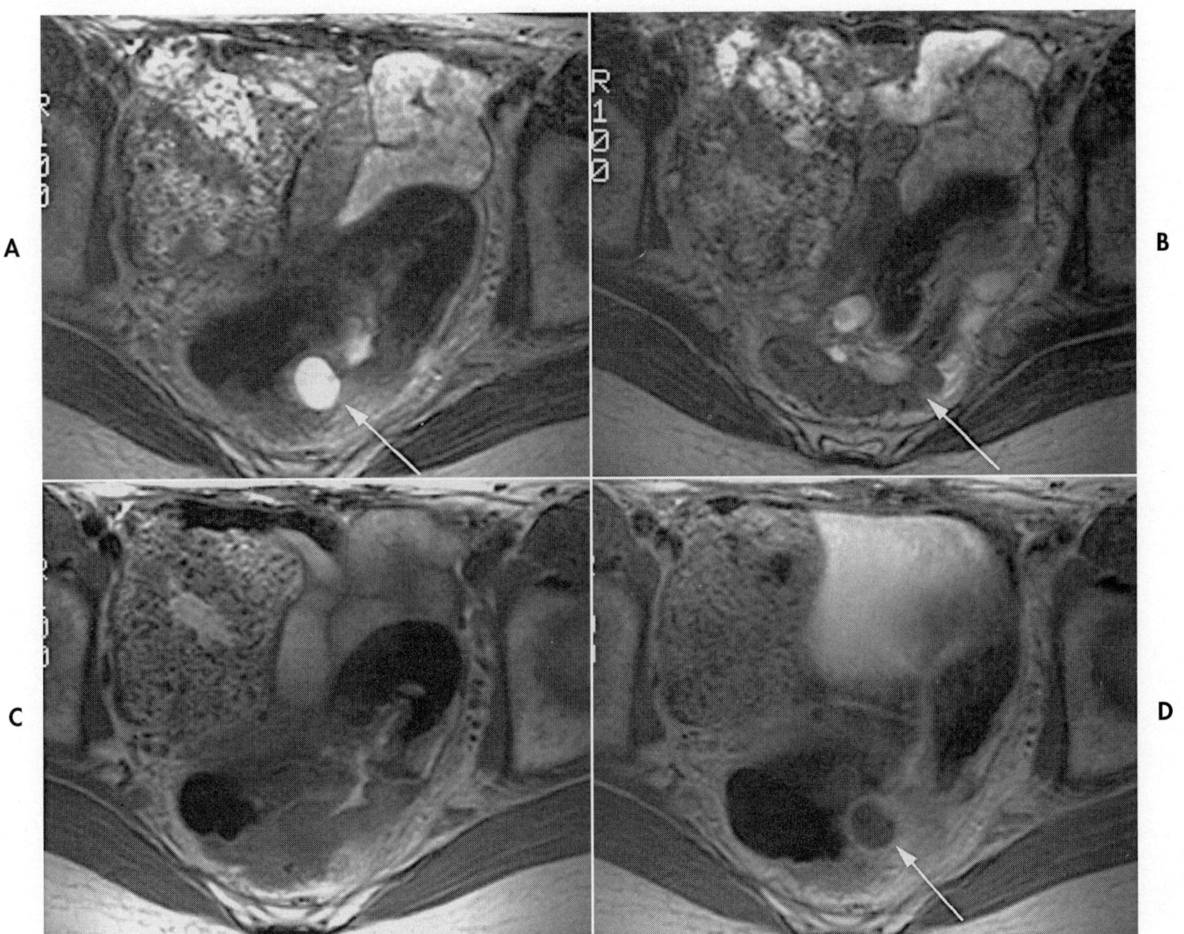

Fig. 9-49 Metastatic ovarian carcinoma implants in a 49-year-old woman with a 3-year history of a poorly differentiated adenocarcinoma of the ovary, stage III. She had had a radical hysterectomy and bilateral oophorectomy. **A** and **B,** Axial FSE images (TR 5700, TE 108) showed several small nodules in the cul-de-sac *(long white arrows),* one of which appeared to have implanted on the wall of the sigmoid colon. Before **(C)** and after **(D)** gadolinium images at the same level again show the bowel implant, which after contrast administration is cystic with rim enhancement *(long white arrow).*

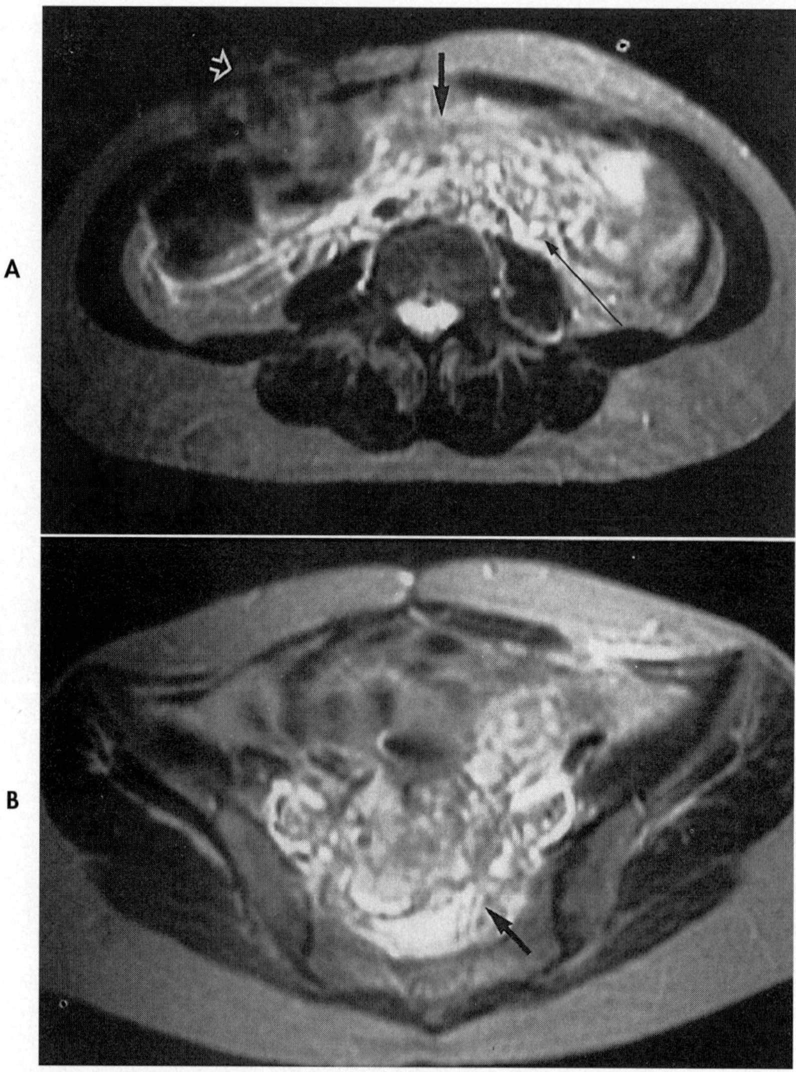

Fig. 9-50 Peritoneal carcinomatosis. **A** and **B** Axial T2-weighted images show a diffuse high-signal-intensity infiltrative process *(short black arrows)* in the peritoneum, with some small nodules *(long black arrow)*. The patient has had a previous ileostomy *(open white arrows)*.

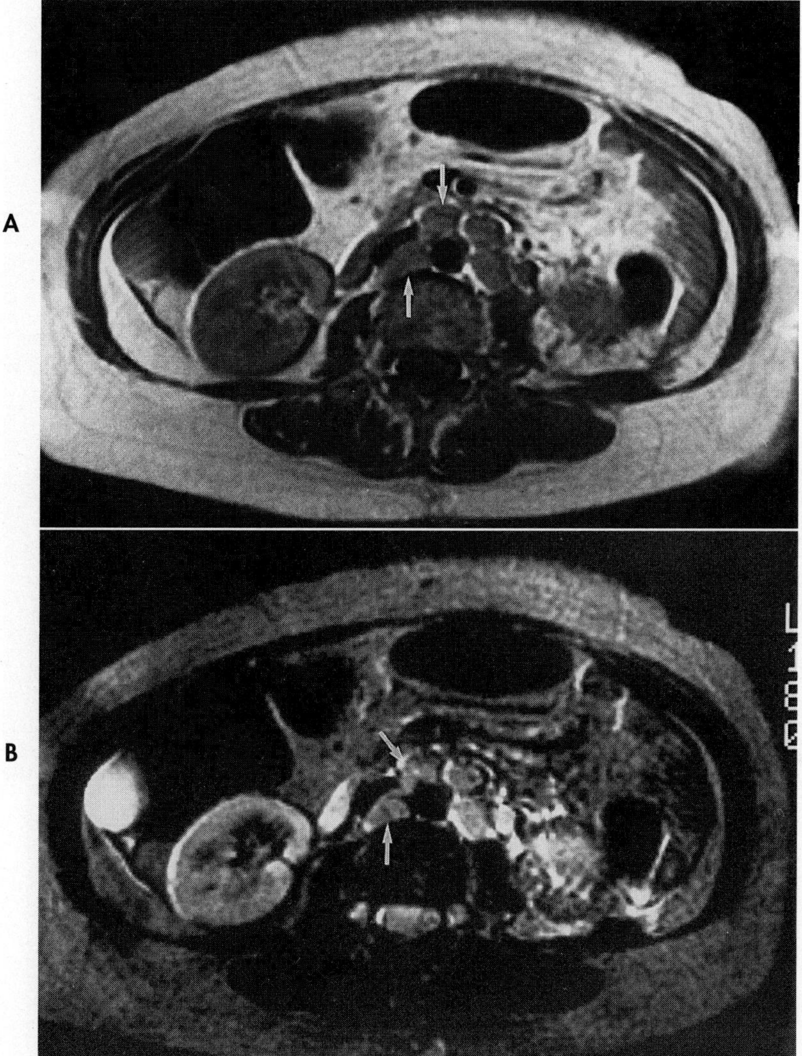

Fig. 9-51 Metastatic lymph nodes. Axial proton density **(A)** and T2-weighted **(B)** images show multiple enlarged retroperitoneal lymph nodes *(white arrows)* in this patient with known ovarian carcinoma.

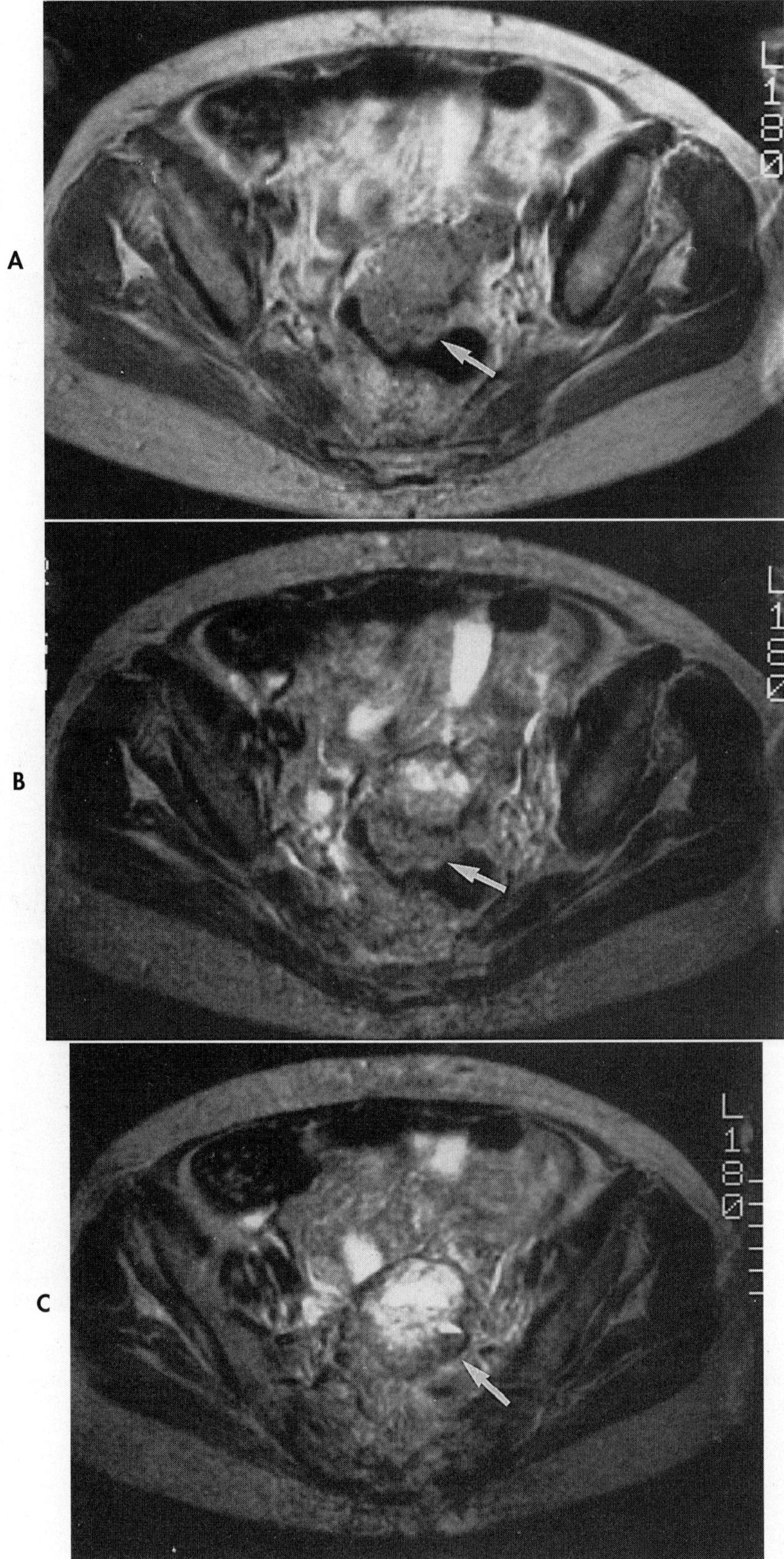

Fig. 9-52 Recurrent ovarian carcinoma. Axial proton density **(A)** and T2-weighted **(B)** and **(C)** images show a large mass *(white arrows)* in the pelvis that has implanted on the surface of the sigmoid colon, in the cul-de-sac. The signal intensity of the mass is very high on the T2-weighted images, typical of a malignant neoplasm.

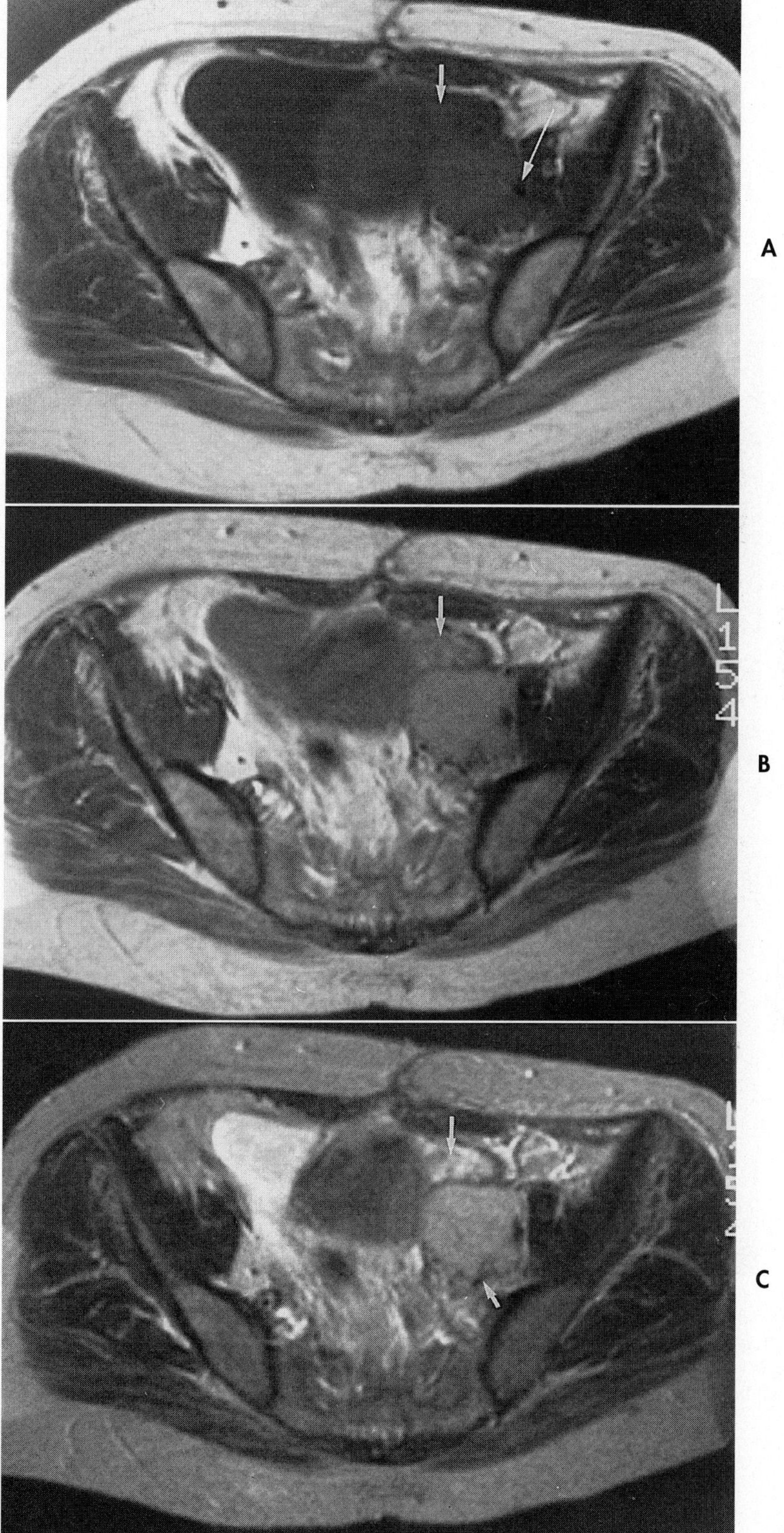

Fig. 9-53 Recurrent tumor with venous thrombosis in a 53-year-old woman with a history of adenocarcinoma of Gartner's duct. **A,** Axial T1-weighted image shows a low signal intensity mass *(short white arrow)* in the left pelvis with a focal signal void *(long white arrow),* representing the left external iliac artery. Axial proton density **(B)** and T2-weighted **(C)** images show the mass *(white arrows)* of increasing signal intensity, compatible with tumor. *Continued.*

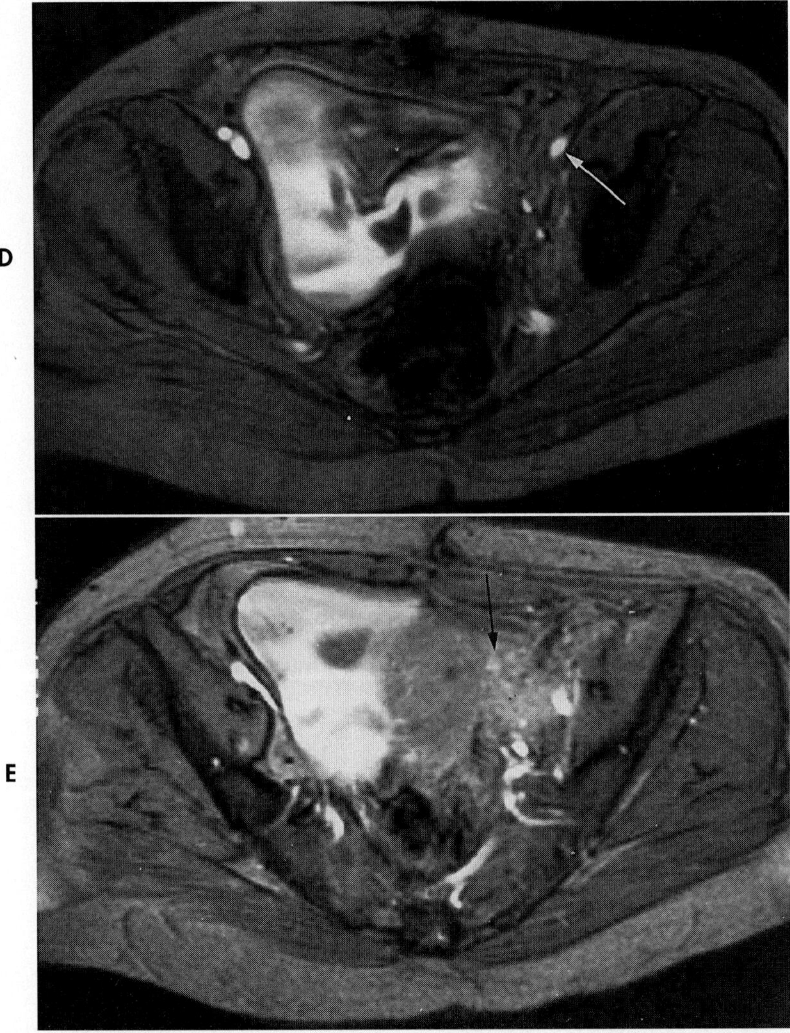

Fig. 9-53, cont'd D, Axial gradient echo (gradient recalled acquisition in the steady state [GRASS] image) shows the patent external iliac artery *(white arrow)* passing through the mass, but the external iliac vein is not visualized. **E,** Axial GRASS image more cephalad shows the small neovascular vessels *(long black arrow)* within the tumor itself.

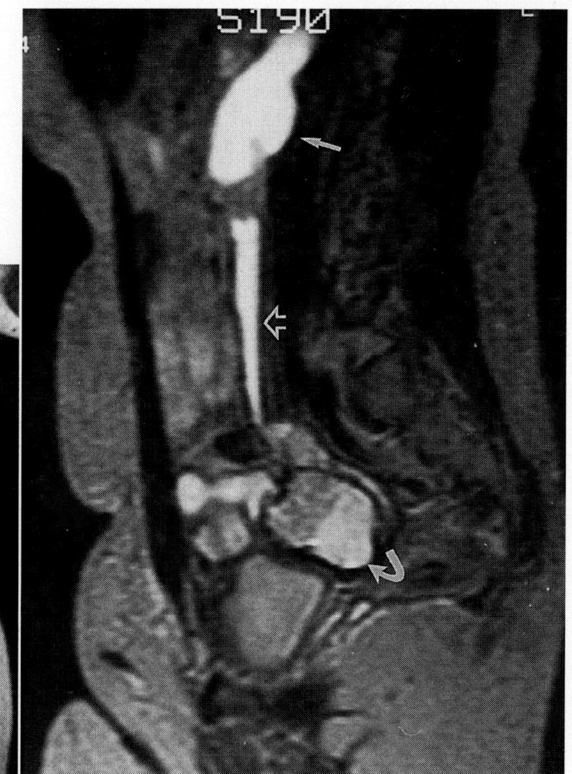

Fig. 9-54 Recurrent tumor with chronic hydronephrosis in a 45-year-old woman with a history of left oophorectomy, hysterectomy, chemotherapy and radiation therapy for ovarian carcinoma. **A,** Coronal T1-weighted image shows the marked chronic hydronephrosis of the left kidney, with only a shell of cortex remaining *(long black arrow)*. The calyces are filled with high T1 signal fluid, due to high protein content, possibly due to pyonephrosis. **B,** Sagittal T2-weighted image shows left hydronephrosis *(short white arrow)* and hydroureter *(open white arrow)* leading down to a large tumor mass *(curved white arrow)* in the pelvis.

lated to tumor activity. It is important to understand that radiation changes can cause a nonspecific increased signal in the pelvis.

The three imaging modalities used in examination of the ovaries and adnexa have been reviewed, and their techniques and applications have been illustrated. Many possible imaging algorithms can be applied according to the clinical presentation, the age of the patient, and the expected management regimen. The relative roles of sonography, CT, and MRI in patients with suspected ovarian neoplasms are currently under investigation by the radiology diagnostic oncology group. In general, for the evaluation of pelvic masses, de novo sonography should be the first examination and either MRI or CT a second examination when indicated.

REFERENCES

1. Cohen HL, Tice HM, Mandel FS: Ovarian volumes measured by US: bigger than we think, *Radiology* 177:189-192, 1990.

2. Buy J, Ghossain MA, Sciot C, et al: Epithelial tumors of the ovary: CT findings and correlation with US, *Radiology* 178:811-818, 1991.

3. Megibow AJ, Bosniak MA, Ho AG, et al: Accuracy of CT in detection of persistent or recurrent ovarian carcinoma: correlation with second-look laparotomy, *Radiology* 166:341-345, 1988.

4. Clement PB: *Nonneoplastic lesions of the ovary.* In Kurman Rj, editor: *Blaustein's pathology of the female genital tract,* ed 3, New York, 1987, Springer-Vérlag p 473.

5. Futterweit W: *Polycystic ovarian disease.* In *Clinical perspectives in obstetrics and gynecology,* New York, 1985, Springer-Verlag.

6. Clement PB: *Nonneoplastic lesions of the ovary.* In Kurman RJ, editor: *Blaustein's pathology of the female genital tract,* ed 3, New York, 1987, Springer-Vérlag p. 486.

7. Clement PB: *Nonneoplastic lesions of the ovary.* In Kurman RJ, editor: *Blaustein's pathology of the female genital tract,* ed 3, New York, 1987, Springer-Vérlag p 502.

8. Scully RE, Richardson GS, Barlow JF: The development of malignancy in endometriosis, *Clin Obstet Gynecol* 9:384-411, 1966.

9. Clement PB: *Endometriosis, lesions of the secondary Müllerian system, and pelvic mesothelial proliferations.* In *Kurman RJ, editor: Blaustein's pathology of the female genital tract,* ed 3, New York, 1987, Springer-Vérlag p 516.

10. Boring CC, Squires TS, Tong T, Montgomery S: Cancer statistics 1994, *CA Cancer J Clin* 44:7-26, 1994.

11. Piver SM, Baker TR, Mettlin C, et al: The Gilda Radner Familial Ovarian Cancer Registry Newsletter, 1990.

12. Westhoff C, Randall MC: Ovarian cancer screening potential effect on mortality, *Am J Obstet Gynecol* 165:502-505, 1991.

13. Czernogilsky B: *Common epithelial tumors of the ovary.* In Blaustein, editor: *Pathology of the female genital tract,* New York, 1987, Springer-Verlag, pp 560-606.

14. Chambers JT, Merino MJ, Kohorn EI, Schwartz PE: Borderline ovarian tumors, *Am J Obstet Gynecol* 159:1088, 1988.

15. Russell P. The pathological assessment of ovarian neoplasms. Introduction to the corinium "epithelial" tumors an analysis of benign "epithelial tumors", *Pathology* 11:5, 1979.

16. Fisher ER, Krieger JS, Skirpan PJ: Ovarian cystoma. Clinico-pathologic observations, *Cancer* 8:437, 1955.

17. Allen MS, Hertig AT: Carcinoma of the ovary, *Am J Obstet Gynecol* 58:640, 1949.

18. Schwartz PE: Ovarian masses: serologic markers, *Clin Obstet Gynecol* 423-432, 1991.

19. Bergman F: Carcinoma of the ovary, *Acta Obstet Gynecol Scand* 45:211-231, 1966.

20. Ozols RF, Young RC: Ovarian cancer: where to next? *Semin Oncol* 18:307-310, 1991.

21. Young RC, Fuks Z, Hoskins WJ: *Cancer of the ovary.* In DeVita VT Jr, Hellman S, Rosenberg SA, editors: *Cancer: principles and practice of oncology,* vol 1, ed 3, Philadelphia, 1989, JB Lippincott, pp 1162-1196.

22. Hoskins W: The influence of cytoreductive surgery on progression-free interval and survival in epithelial cancer, *Clin Obstet Gynecol* 3:59, 1989.

23. Deppe G, Malviya VK: Ovarian cancer advances in management, *Surg Clin North Am* 5:1023-1039, 1991.

24. Potter ME, Hatch KD, Soong SJ, et al: Second look laparotomy and salvage therapy: a research modality only? *Gynecol Oncol* 44:3-9, 1992.

25. Chambers SK, Chambers JT, Kohorn EI, et al: Evaluation of the role of second look surgery in ovarian cancer, *Obstet Gynecol* 72:404-408, 1988.

26. McClay EF, Howell SB: A review: intraperitoneal cisplatin in the management of patients with ovarian cancer, *Gynecol Oncol* 36:1, 1990.

27. Benacerraf BR, Finkler NJ, Wojciechowski C, Knapp RC: Sonographic accuracy in the diagnosis of ovarian masses, *J Reprod Med* 35:491-495, 1990.

28. Granberg S, Norstrom A, Wikland M: Comparison of endovaginal ultrasound and cytological evaluation of cystic ovarian tumors, *J Ultrasound Med* 10:9-14, 1991.

29. Herrmann UJ Jr, Locher GW, Goldhirsch A: Sonographic patterns of ovarian tumors: prediction of malignancy, *Obstet Gynecol* 69:777-781, 1987.

30. Meiere HB, Farrant P, Guha T: Distinction of benign from malignant ovarian cysts of ultrasound, *Br J Obstet Gynecol* 85:893-899, 1978.

31. Moyle JW, Rochester D, Sider L, et al: Sonography of ovarian tumors: predictability of tumor type, *AJR* 141:985-991, 1983.

32. Sassone AM, Timor-Tritsch IE, Artner A, et al: Transvaginal sonographic characterization of ovarian disease: evaluation of a new scoring system to predict malignancy, *Obstet Gynecol* 78:70-76, 1991.

33. Fleischer AC, McKee MS, Gordon AN, et al: Transvaginal sonography of postmenopausal ovaries with pathologic correlation, *J Ultrasound Med* 9:637-644, 1990.

34. Rodriquez MH, Platt LD, Medearis AL et al: The use of transvaginal sonography for evaluation of postmenopausdal ovarian size and morphology, *Am J Obstet Gynecol* 159:810-814, 1988.

35. Di Santis DJ, Scataridge JC, Kemp C, et al: A prospective evaluation of transvaginal sonaography for detection of ovarian disease, *AJR* 161:91-99, 1993.

36. Fleischer AC, Daniell JF, Rodier J, et al: Sonographic monitoring of follicular development, *J Clin Ultrasound* 9:275-280, 1981.

37. Filly RA: *Ovarian masses—what to look for—what to do.* In Wilson SR, Charboneau JW, Leopold GR, editors: *Ultrasound Categorical Course Syllabus,* San Francisco, 1993, American Roentgen Ray Society, pp 11-19.

38. Campbell S, Geossens L, Goswamy R, Whitehead M: Real-time ultrasonography for determination of ovarian morphology and volume, *Lancet* 1:425-426, 1982.

39. Goldstein SR, Subramanyam B, Snyder JR, et al: The postmenopausal cystic adnexal mass: the potential role of ultrasound in conservative management, *Obstet Gynecol* 73:8-10, 1989.

40. Levine D, Gosink BB, Wolf SI, et al: Simple adnexal cysts: the natural history in postmenopausal women, *Radiology* 184:653-659, 1992.

41. Wolf SI, Gosink BB, Feldesman MR, et al: Prevalence of signal adnexal cysts in postmenopausal women, *Radiology* 180:65-71, 1991.

42. Rulin MC, Preston AL: Adnexal masses in postmenopausal women, *Obstet Gynecol* 70:578-581, 1987.

43. Luxman D, Bergman A, Sagi J, David MP: The postmenopausal adnexal mass: correlation between ultrasonic and pathologic findings, *Obstet Gynecol* 77:726-728, 1991.

44. Hall DA, McCarthy KA: The significance of the postmenopausal simple adnexal cyst, *J Ultrasound Med* 5:503-505, 1986.

45. Andolf E, Jorgensen C: Simple adnexal cysts diagnosed by ultrasound in postmenopausal women, *J Clin Ultrasound* 16:301-303, 1988.

46. Baltarowich OH, Kurtz AB, Pasto ME, et al: The spectrum of sonographic findings in hemorrhagic ovarian cysts, *AJR* 148:901-905, 1987.

47. Quinn SF, Erickson S, Black WC: Cystic ovarian teratomas: the sonographic appearance of the dermoid plug, *Radiology* 155:477-478, 1985.

48. Tessler FN, Perrella RR, Fleischer AC, Grant EG: Endovaginal sonographic diagnosis of dilated fallopian tubes, *AJR* 153:523-525, 1989.

49. Osathanondh R, Berkowitz RS, de Cholnoky C, et al: Hormonal measurements in patients with theca lutein cysts and gestational trophoblastic disease, *J Reprod Med* 31:179-183, 1986.

50. Lawrence PH, Lyons EA, Levi CS: Hyperreactio luteinalis, *J Ultrasound Med* 2:375-376, 1983.

51. Rankin RN, Hutton LC: Ultrasound in the ovarian hyperstimulation syndrome, *J Clin Ultrasound* 9:473-476, 1981.

52. Gammill SL, Shipkey FH, Himmelfarb EH, et al: Roentgenology-pathology correlative study of neovascularity, *AJR* 126:376-385, 1976.

53. Fleischer AC, Rodgers WH, Rao BK, et al: Assessment of ovarian tumor vascularity with transvaginal color Doppler sonography, *J Ultrasound Med* 10:563-568, 1991.

54. Fleischer AC, Rodgers WH, Kepple DM, et al: Color Doppler sonography of ovarian masses: a multiparameter analysis, *J Ultrasound Med* 12:41-48, 1993.

55. Bourne T, Campbell S, Steer C, et al: Transvaginal colour flow imaging: a possible new screening technique for ovarian cancer, *Br Med J* 299:1367-1370, 1989.

56. Weiner Z, Thaler I, Beck D, et al: Differentiating malignant from benign ovarian tumors with transvaginal color flow imaging, *Obstet Gynecol* 79:159-162, 1992.

57. Kawai M, Kano T, Kikkawa F, et al: Transvaginal Doppler ultrasound with color flow imaging in the diagnosis of ovarian cancer, *Obstet Gynecol* 79:163-167, 1992.

58. Kurjak A, Zalud I, Alfirevic Z: Evaluation of adnexal masses with transvaginal color ultrasound, *J Ultrasound Med* 10:295-297, 1991.

59. Tekay A, Jouppila P: Validity of pulsatility and resistance indices in classification of adnexal tumors with transvaginal color Doppler ultrasound, *Ultrasound Obstet Gynecol* 2:338-344, 1992.

60. Timor-Tritsch IE, Lerner JP, Monteagudo A, Santos R: Transvaginal ultrasonographic characterization of ovarian masses by means of color flow–directed Doppler measurements and a morphologic scoring system, *Am J Obstet Gynecol* 168:909-913, 1993.

61. Brown DL, Frates MC, Laing FC, et al: Ovarian masses: can benign and malignant lesions be differentiated by color and pulsed Doppler ultrasound? *Radiology* 190:333-336, 1994.

62. Hamper UM, Sheth S, Abbas FM, et al: Transvaginal color Doppler sonography of adnexal masses: differentiation in blood flow impedence in benign and malignant lesions, *AJR* 160:1225-1228, 1993.

63. Brown DL, Muto MG, Cramer DW: *Brigham and Women's Hospital Program.* In Fleischer AC, Jones HW, editors: *Early detection of ovarian carcinoma with transvaginal sonography,* New York, 1993, Raven Press, pp 183-191.

64. Hata K, Hata T, Manabe A, et al: A critical evaluation of transvaginal Doppler studies, transvaginal sonography, magnetic resonance imaging, and CA-125 in detecting ovarian cancer, *Obstet Gynecol* 80:922-926, 1992.

65. Kurjak A, Shalan H, Zalud I: Evaluation of adnexal masses with transvaginal color ultrasonography (letter), *J Ultrasound Med* 11:332, 1992.

66. Kurjak A, Predanic M: New scoring system for prediction of ovarian malignancy based on transvaginal color Doppler sonography, *J Ultrasound Med* 11:631-638, 1992.

67. Fukuda T, Ikeuchi M, Hasimoto H, et al: Computed tomography of ovarian masses, *J Comput Assist Tomogr* 10:990-996, 1986.

68. Sawyer RW, Vick CW, Walsh JW, McClure PH: Computed tomography of benign ovarian masses, *J Comput Assist Tomogr* 5:179-186, 1981.

69. Friedman AC, Pyatt Rs, Hartman DS, et al: CT of benign cystic teratomas, *AJR* 138:659-665, 1982.

70. Muramatsu Y, Moriyama N, Takayasu K, et al: CT and MR imaging of cystic ovarian teratoma and intracystic fat balls, *J Comput Assist Tomogr* 15:528-529, 1991.

71. Skaane P, Heubner KH: Computed tomography of cystic ovarian teratomas with gravity-dependent layering, *J Comput Assist Tomogr* 7:837-841, 1983.

72. Quinn SF, Erickson SE, Black WL: Cystic ovarian teratomas: the sonographic appearance of the dermoid plug, *Radiology* 155:477-478, 1985.

73. Matsumoto F, Yoshioka H, Hamada T, et al: Struma ovarii: CT and MR findings, *J Comput Assist Tomogr* 14:310-312, 1990.

74. Fishman EK, Scatarige JC, Saksouk FA, et al: Computed tomography of endometriosis, *J Comput Assist Tomogr* 7:257-264, 1983.

75. Lewis E: The use and abuse of imaging in gynecology cancer, *Cancer* 60:1993-2009, 1987.

76. Megibow AJ, Hulnick DH, Bosniak MA, Balthazar EJ: Ovarian metastases: computed tomographic appearances, *Radiology* 156:161-164, 1985.

77. Cho KC, Gold BM: Computed tomography of Krukenberg tumors, *AJR* 145:285-288, 1985.

78. Walsh JN, Rosenfield AT, Jaffe CC, et al: Prospective comparison of ultrasound and computed tomography in the evaluation of gynecologic pelvic masses, *AJR* 131:955-960, 1978.

79. Sanders RC, McNeil BJ, Finberg HJ, et al: A prospective study of computed tomography and ultrasound in the detection and staging of pelvic masses, *Radiology* 146:439-442, 1983.

80. Ghossain MA, Buy J, Ligneres C, et al: Epithelial tumors of the ovary: comparison of MR and CT findings, *Radiology* 181:863-870, 1991.

81. Cohen DJ, Kucera PR: Percutaneous biopsy of pelvic masses, *Semin Interven Radiol* 9:138-151, 1992.

82. Eriksson O, Hagmar B, Ryd W: Effects of fine-needle aspiration and other biopsy procedures on tumor dissemination in mice, *Cancer* 54:73-78, 1984.

83. Leahy AL, Stephens RB, Daly PA: Pseudomyxoma peritonei complicating biopsy of an ovarian cyst, *Ir J Med Sci* 154:476, 1985.

84. Bret PM, Atri M, Guibaud L, et al: Ovarian cysts in postmenopausal women: preliminary results with transvaginal alcohol sclerosis. Work in progress, *Radiology* 184:661, 1992.

85. Feigen M, Crocker EF, Reid J, et al: The value of lymphoscintigraphy, lymphangiography and computer tomography scanning in the preoperative assessment of lymph nodes involved by pelvic malignant conditions, *Surg Gynecol Obstet* 165:107-110, 1987.

86. Buy J, Moss AA, Ghossain MA, et al: Peritoneal implants from ovarian tumors: CT findings, *Radiology* 169:691-694, 1988.

87. Bergman F: Carcinoma of the ovary, *Acta Obstet Gynecol Scand* 45:211-231, 1966.

88. Walkey MM, Friedman AC, Sohotra P, Radecki PD: CT manifestations of peritoneal carcinomatosis, *AJR* 150:1035-1041, 1988.

89. Mitchell DG, Hill MC, Hill S, Zaloudek C: Serous carcinoma of the ovary: CT identification of metastatic calcified implants, *Radiology* 158:649-652, 1986.

90. Stern J, Buscema J, Rosenchien N, Siegelman SS: Can computed tomography substitute for second-look operation in ovarian carcinoma? *Gynecol Oncol* 11:82-88, 1981.

91. Goldhirsch A, Triller JK, Griener R, et al: Computed tomography prior to second-look operation in advanced ovarian cancer, *Obstet Gynecol* 62:630-634, 1983.

92. Clarke-Pearson DC, Brandy LC, Dudzinski M, et al: Computed tomography in evaluation of patients with ovarian carcinoma in complete clinical remission, *JAMA* 255:627-630, 1986.

93. Giunta S, Tipaldi L, Diotelleri F, et al: CT demonstration of peritoneal metastases after intraperitoneal injection of contrast media, *Clin Imaging* 14:31-34, 1990.

94. Halvorsen RA, Panushka C, Oakley GJ, et al: Intraperitoneal contrast material improves the CT detection of peritoneal metastases, *AJR* 157:37-40, 1991.

95. Nelson RC, Chezmar JL, Hoel MJ, et al: Peritoneal carcinomatosis: preoperative CT with intraperitoneal contrast material, *Radiology* 182:133-138, 1992.

96. Weinreb JC, Barkoff ND, Megibow A, et al: Value of MR imaging in distinguishing leiomyomas from other solid pelvic masses when sonography is indeterminate, *AJR* 154:295, 1990.

97. Togashi K, Nishimura K, Kimura I, et al: Endometrial cysts: diagnosis with MR imaging, *Radiology* 180:73-78, 1991.

98. Kier R, Smith RC, McCarthy SM: Value of lipid- and water-suppression MR images in distinguishing between blood and lipid within ovarian masses, *AJR* 158:321-325, 1992.

99. Mitchell DG, Gefter WB, Spritzer CE, et al: Polycystic ovaries: MR imaging, *Radiology* 160:425-429, 1986.

100. Stevens SK, Hricak H, Stern JL: Ovarian lesions: detection and characterization with gadolinium-enhanced MR imaging at 1.5T, *Radiology* 181:481-488, 1991.

101. Thurhner S, Hodler J, Baer S, et al: Gadolinium-DOTA enhanced MR imaging of adnexal tumors, *Comput Assist Tonogr* 14:939-949, 1990.

102. Perkins Ac, Powell MC, Wastie ML, et al: A prospective evaluation of OC 125 and magnetic resonance imaging in patients with ovarian cancer, *Eur J Nucl Med* 16:311-316, 1990.

103. Smith FW, Cherryman GR, Bayliss AP, et al: A comparative study of the accuracy of ultrasound imaging, x-ray computerized tomography and low field MRI diagnosis of ovarian malignancy, *Magn Reson Imaging* 6:225-227, 1988.

104. Rahmouni A, Tempany C, Jones R, et al: Monitoring of lymphoma by magnetic resonance imaging, *Radiology* 188:445-451, 1993.

10 MRI in Pregnancy

Karen M. Horton and Clare M.C. Tempany

Since the development of nuclear magnetic resonance (NMR) imaging techniques and their extension into whole body imaging, investigators continue to discover new and exciting clinical applications. One such use of magnetic resonance imaging (MRI) is for maternal, fetal, and placental imaging during pregnancy. Although ultrasonography continues to be the primary imaging modality during pregnancy, some conditions such as very large or complex masses, obesity, overlying bony structures, or gas-filled organs interfere with ultrasound images. MRI, which, like ultrasonography, lacks ionizing radiation, is capable of supplying important clinical information in these circumstances and has the ability to produce multiplanar images with excellent tissue contrast. This chapter reviews the safety issues of MRI in pregnancy and discusses its current applications for maternal, fetal, and placental imaging. As with any new diagnostic imaging tool for use during pregnancy, it is important to investigate any potentially adverse biologic effects of MRI.

SAFETY CONSIDERATIONS

Although MRI does not involve ionizing radiation, several other potential health hazards have been identified and investigated. In 1979, Budinger[1] reviewed the importance of such MRI features as the static magnetic field, radiofrequency power, and time-dependent magnetic fields. He concluded that, as employed in MRI experiments at that time, these parameters posed no substantial biologic hazards. Bacteria, human lymphocytes, and Chinese hamster ovaries have all been exposed to conditions similar to those encountered during clinical MRI without any reports of lethal, mutagenic, or adverse chromosomal effects.[2-4] Prasad et al[5] studied the effects of 0.15T MR imaging on murine splenocytes and discovered that the low-strength magnetic field had no effect on the natural killer cell cytotoxicity. Later, Prasad et al[6] conducted a similar study but this time investigated the potential effects of MRI exposure with 2.35T magnetic field strength on the natural killer cell cytotoxicity of human peripheral blood mononuclear cells. Once again, they concluded that natural killer cell cytotoxicity is not adversely affected by MRI.

These studies helped support MRI as a safe imaging tool. However, as applications of MRI expanded and magnetic strengths increased, worries about the potential hazards have multiplied. There were concerns about the possible effects of repeated or long-term exposures to strong magnetic fields. Also, many feared that the use of MRI during pregnancy, particularly during organogenesis, might have disastrous consequences. Over the past several years, many studies have been conducted to help investigate these concerns.

In 1985, Withers et al studied the cytotoxic effects of MRI on spermatogenesis in mice and found that 66 hours of continuous exposure to a 3T magnetic imaging device failed to produce any significant cytotoxicity.[7] Next, McRobbie and Foster investigated the effect of exposure to pulsed magnetic fields on the pregnancy of mice and on the postnatal development of their litter.[8] No adverse effect on the pregnancy was detected, and there was no significant difference between litter number or growth rates of the experimental group compared with controls. In a similar 1988 study by Heinrichs et al, pregnant BALB/c mice were exposed to MRI conditions. No overt embryotoxicity (resorptions, stillbirths) or teratogenicity (homeotic shifts) was revealed.[9] However, a slight but significant reduction in fetal crown rump length was detected in the group of MRI-exposed fetusus compared with controls. In 1990, Prasad et al, prompted by recent concerns over increased magnetic field strengths, studied the effects of low and

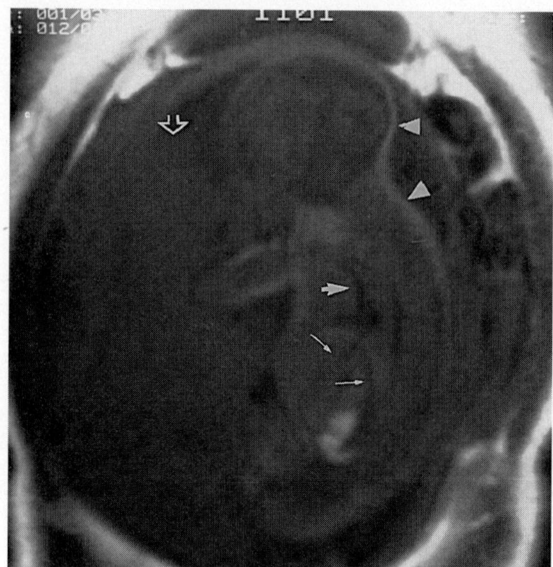

Fig. 10-1 Coronal T1-weighted image (TR 600, TE 20) of the mother (inverted to show the fetal anatomy), showing a 29-week fetus in the parasagittal plane. The subcutaneous fat outlines the skull and upper body of the fetus *(white arrowheads)*. The right side of the heart is seen with the superior vena cava *(white arrow)* draining into the right atrium. The diaphragm is seen with the inferior vena cava and hepatic veins in the liver inferiorly *(long white arrows)*. The placenta lies on the left lateral aspect of the uterus *(open white arrow)*.

high magnetic field strengths on frog sperm or fertilized eggs and found that MRI did not affect the developmental pattern of the frog embryos.[10]

Although these studies using amphibians and mammals repeatedly concluded that MRI posed no significant biologic hazards to subjects or their offspring, investigators were reluctant to study pregnant women. The first reports of MRI in women during early pregnancy studied those who had decided to terminate the pregnancy.[11,12] Investigators were amazed at the quality of images, which clearly showed the size of the pregnant uterus and its relationship to other pelvic structures. The placenta and its relationship to the uterus and to the cervix could also be visualized easily. During MR studies, no changes in fetal heart rate or in umbilical artery flow have been detected.[12] Investigators were very optimistic that MRI would find a role in fetal imaging, especially in later pregnancy when the fetus is known to move less and thus create less motion artifact.

In the last several years, the applications of MRI during pregnancy have multiplied. Although ultrasonography remains the primary obstetric imaging tool, MRI has been shown to have several advantages. It allows excellent maternal-fetal and placental soft tissue definition (Fig. 10-1), visualization of the cervix and uterus, and good visualization of the extrauterine regions, including the ovaries.

FETAL IMAGING

Extensive scientific investigation has failed to reveal any adverse biologic effects of MRI, which consequently may prove a useful, noninvasive imaging tool for examination of the fetus to complement obstetric sonography, and for use in situations in which ultrasonography has known limitations, such as maternal obesity and oligohydramnios. However, the application of MRI to fetal imaging has been limited by several important factors. These are problems relating to fetal motion and altered positions.

In 1985, Weinreb et al imaged 26 fetuses with MRI after ultrasound examination.[13] The fetal anatomy was reviewed and many normal structures were identified in the first, second, and third trimesters. This group of investigators noted that many fetal structures were not delineated, even during the third trimester, despite their obtaining multiple planar views. Because of the relatively long imaging time required in this study, fetal movement was a concern, especially early in pregnancy, as this movement degrades image quality. Since fetal movement is random, it cannot be overcome with gating techniques such as those used for respiratory and cardiac imaging. To lessen the problem of image degradation due to fetal motion, some investigators have used sedation, either intravenous sedation of the mother with benzodiazepines or, as reported by Lenke et al,[14] fetal intramuscular injections of pancuronium bromide. These drugs temporarily decrease fetal activity and therefore result in superior image quality. However, the use of these substances introduces additional and sometimes unacceptable risks. To decrease the impact of fetal movement on image quality, Garden et al[15] used a fast scan imaging technique and produced clearer fetal images. This and other fast spin echo (FSE) sequences are superior to the conventional spin echo techniques, which are limited by long imaging times. Currently, the most significant difficulty with the use of MRI in fetal imaging continues to be image degradation by fetal movement. Other authors have had fewer problems in the third trimester, as most of the motion is now only from the limbs.[16]

Fetal position is another limiting factor for visualization of fetal structures, as noted by Weinreb et al.[13] Since the fetus is often not aligned in one of the standard imaging planes, fetal structures are often imaged in unusual planes, which can make their identification difficult. Also, many fe-

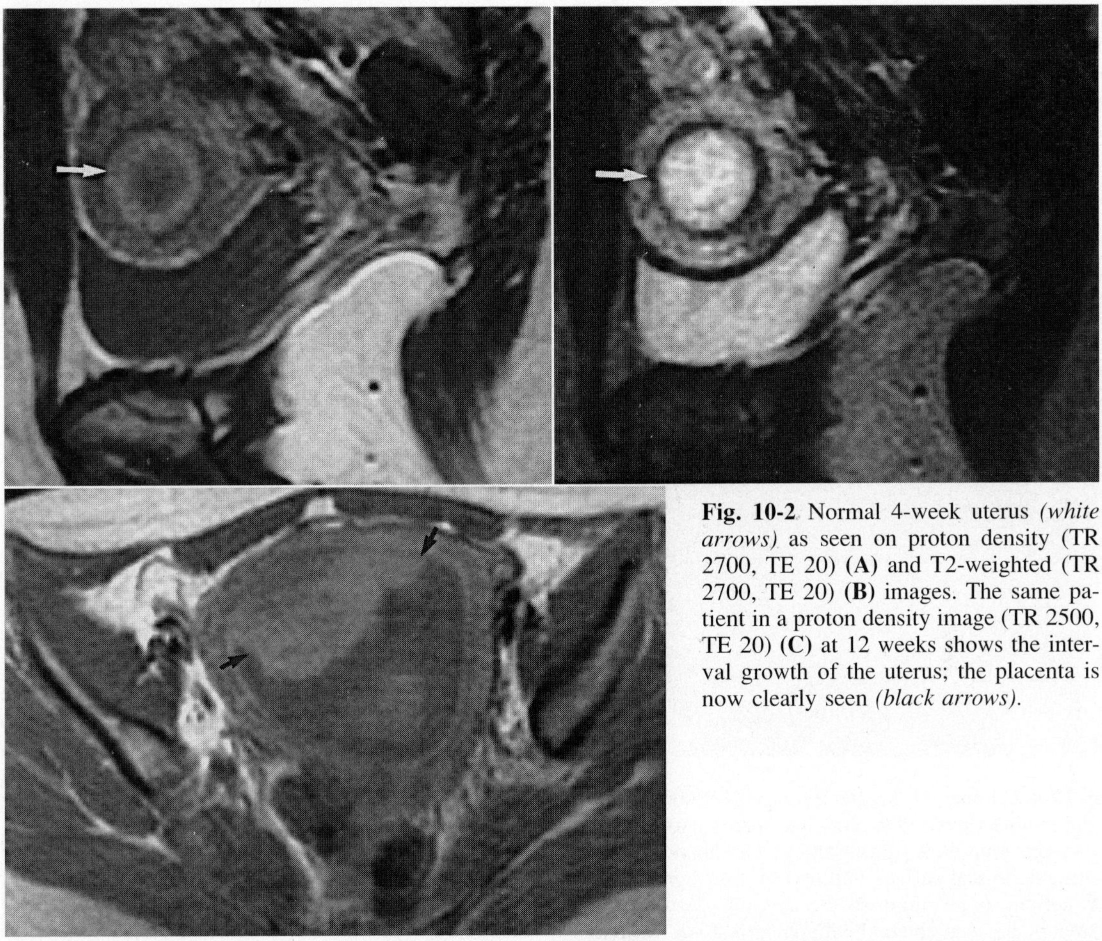

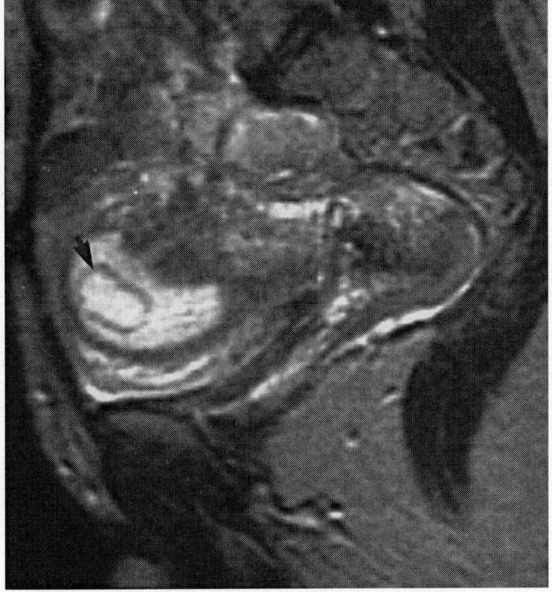

Fig. 10-2 Normal 4-week uterus *(white arrows)* as seen on proton density (TR 2700, TE 20) **(A)** and T2-weighted (TR 2700, TE 20) **(B)** images. The same patient in a proton density image (TR 2500, TE 20) **(C)** at 12 weeks shows the interval growth of the uterus; the placenta is now clearly seen *(black arrows)*.

tal structures may simply be too small to be clearly imaged with MR or may be missed if much space is programmed between image slices. Last, Weinreb et al noted that decreased fat deposits around fetal organs, as compared with adults, leads to less contrast between tissues and thus affects the imaging and identification of fetal structures.[13] However, we have found that fetal subcutaneous fat can aid in identifying the normal fetal parts such as the limbs, abdominal wall, and skull on T1-weighted images ((Fig. 10-1). Early pregnancies can be visualized by MRI as on ultrasonography, with the distended endometrial cavity and gestational sac visible (Figs. 10-2 and 10-3).

Despite these many problems associated with the use of MRI of the fetus, current MR units and applications are consistently successful in obtaining useful images of the fetal heart (see Figs. 10-1 and 10-4), brain (Figs. 10-4 and 10-5), and liver (see Fig. 10-1). Identification of the kidneys, stomach, and bowel (see Fig. 10-4) is often inconsistent and dependent on other factors. Identification

Fig. 10-3 Normal 4-week gestational sac *(black arrow)* on this sagittal T2-weighted image (TR 2700, TE 80).

of bowel, for example, often depends on the presence of meconium or fluid.

On MRI the fetal heart is visible as early as 15 weeks of gestation, but it is not routinely imaged successfully until week 25 (see Figs. 10-1, 10-4, and 10-5). A case report by McCarthy et al in 1984 suggested that, unlike diagnostic imaging of the adult heart, imaging of the fetal heart does not require electrocardiographic gating.[17] This was attributed to very small excursion of the cardiac walls during the normal fetal rapid heart rate. Therefore, the heart can sometimes be resolved into right and left chambers (see Fig. 10-4), and occasionally all four chambers can be identified. The ventricles appear devoid of signal and are separated by signal from the interventricular septum. The right ventricle is larger than the left owing to its dominant role during fetal development. The major vessels appear as tubular structures devoid of flow, but are often difficult to visualize because of their small size. Fetal motion and unpredictable fetal position sometimes prevent useful visualization of intracardiac structure.

The fetal liver is usually easily identified since it occupies most of the fetal upper abdomen and since the liver diaphragmatic interface can be defined. (Figs. 10-1, 10-4, 10-5, and 10-7). The liver appears as homogeneously high signal intensity on T1-weighted images (see Figs. 10-1 and 10-5), although there is a signal texture change in the third trimester thought to reflect changes in the chemical composition of the liver as well as in glycogen stores.[16]

The fetal brain, since it lacks myelination, appears featureless, without differentiation between white and gray matter (see Figs. 10-4 and 10-6). The spin echo technique with long TR demonstrates fetal brain anatomy better by highlighting T2 differences between tissues.[16] Also, as with an

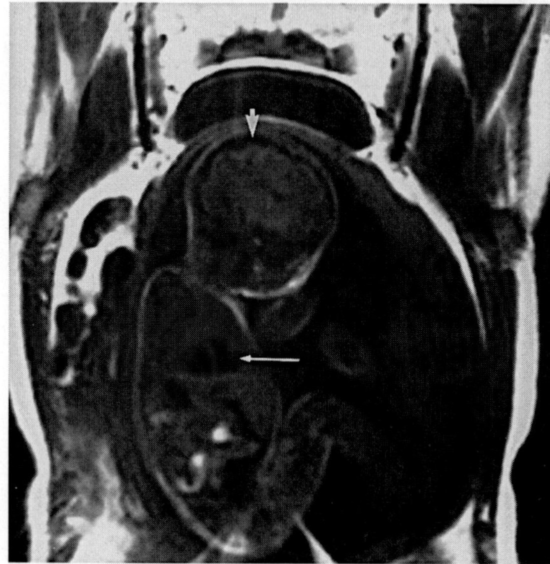

Fig. 10-4 Coronal T1-weighted image (TR 600, TE 20) of the mother (inverted to show the fetal anatomy) with a 29-week fetus in a parasagittal plane shows the fetal brain and cortical surface outlined by low signal intensity cerebrospinal fluid *(white arrow)*. Two cardiac chambers are seen above the diaphragm *(long white arrow)*, and several fat-filled (high T1-weighted signal) bowel loops *(black arrow)* are seen in the abdomen.

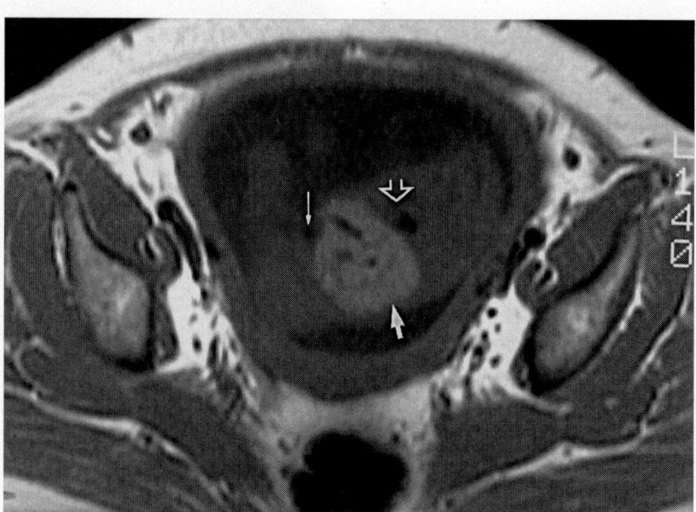

Fig. 10-5 Axial T1-weighted image (TR 500, TE 11) shows a 19-week fetus; the liver is seen with a high T1-weighted signal *(white arrow)*. The hepatic vessels are seen in the parenchyma. The umbilical vein can also be seen as it approaches the liver in the falciform ligament *(small white arrow)*. The fetal heart is seen above the diaphragm *(open white arrow)*.

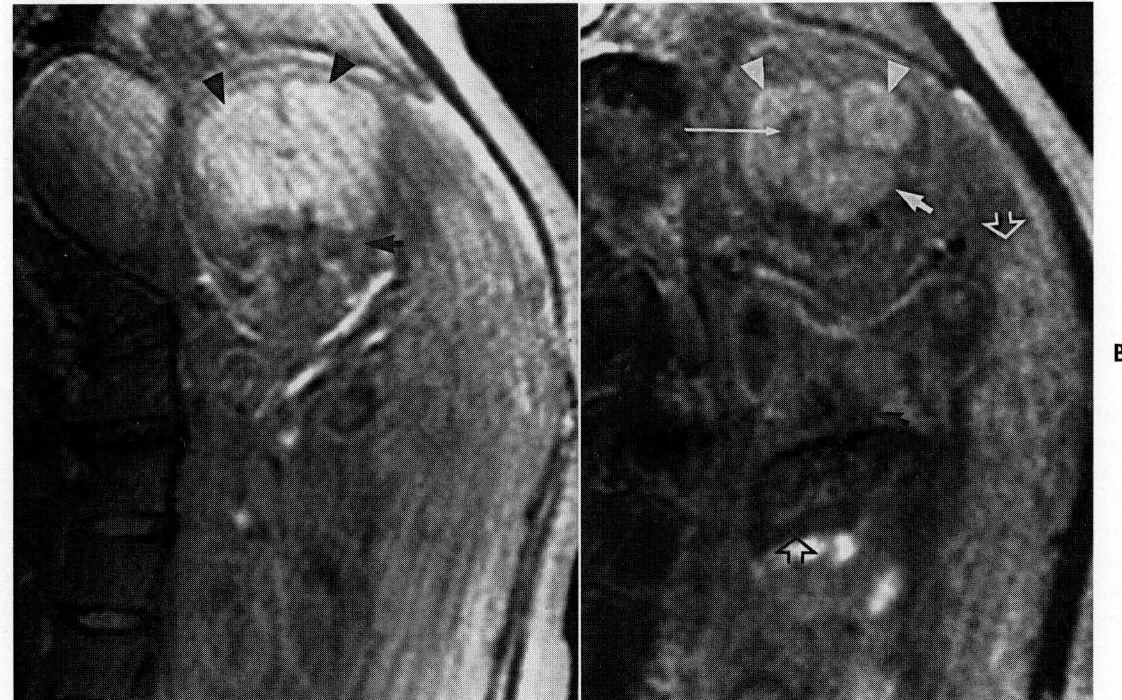

Fig. 10-6 A, Sagittal proton density image of the mother shows a 29-week fetus in the coronal plane anteriorly. The cerebral hemispheres *(black arrowheads)* are identified with the orbits inferiorly *(black arrow)*. **B,** Sagittal proton density image shows posteriorly the cerebellum *(white arrow)* and the posterior aspect of the occipital lobes *(white arrowheads)*. The occipital horn of the right lateral ventricle is seen *(long white arrow)*. Note the cardiac chambers *(black arrow)*, liver *(open black arrow)*, and placenta *(open white arrow)* anteriorly.

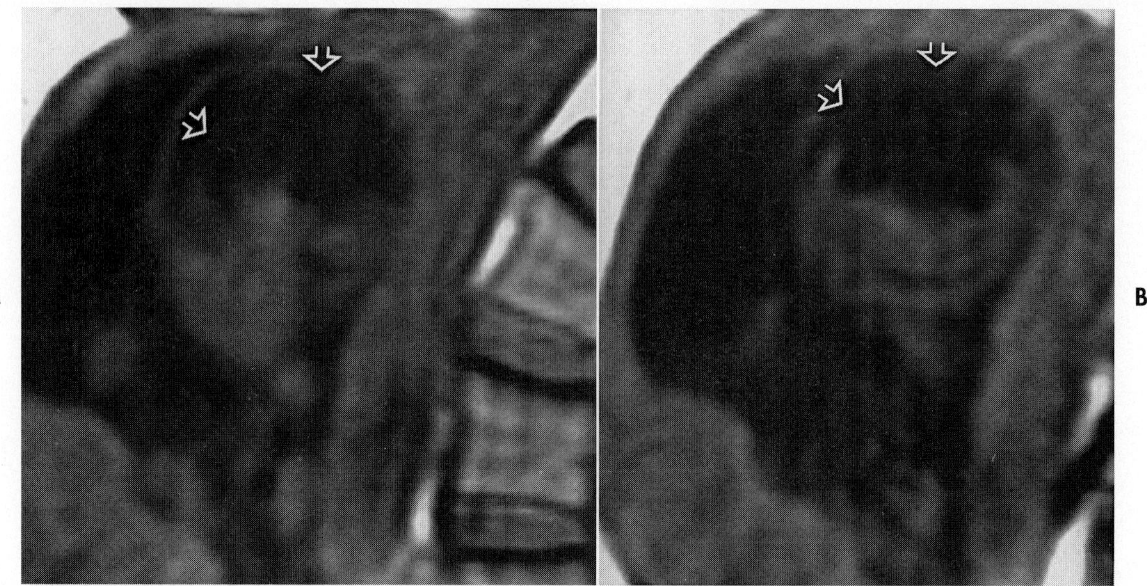

Fig. 10-7 Holoprosencephaly. **A** and **B,** Sagittal T1-weighted images of the mother show the coronal images of the fetal brain, demonstrating the extensive replacement of the cerebrum with a large cystic ventricle *(white open arrows)* in this fetus with alobar holoprosencephaly. (Courtesy Harold Posniak, MD, Maywood, IL.)

adult, the cerebrospinal fluid (CSF) intensity is low and increases with longer TR or TE because of its long T1 and T2.[17] Abnormal structures containing CSF can be identified and distinguished from the surrounding parenchyma. Arachnoid and porencephalic cysts have been identified, as well as holoprosencephaly (Fig. 10-7) and Dandy-Walker malformations.[18] Images of posterior fossa–cerebellum, tentorium, and craniocervical junction have also been reported but are not imaged consistently.[16] The spine can also be seen, but it is usually difficult to seen its entire length (Fig. 10-8).

Another exciting application of MRI is for use in detection of intrauterine growth retardation (IUGR). Some of the normal fetal measurements can be obtained from the T1-weighted images (Fig. 10-9). Currently, the diagnosis of IUGR is often inadequate and not made until the time of delivery, when there is evidence of soft tissue wasting.[19] Ultrasonography is routinely used to measure the head, abdomen, and extremities in an attempt to identify IUGR, but it is unable to image soft tissue stores; it therefore is often inaccurate because it cannot always distinguish between an IUGR fetus and a normal fetus that is simply small.[20]

The ability of MRI to image soft tissues and delineate fetal subcutaneous fat stores has been studied as a possible technique to complement ultrasound diagnosis of IUGR. Results have been promising. Because it is able to clearly image fat

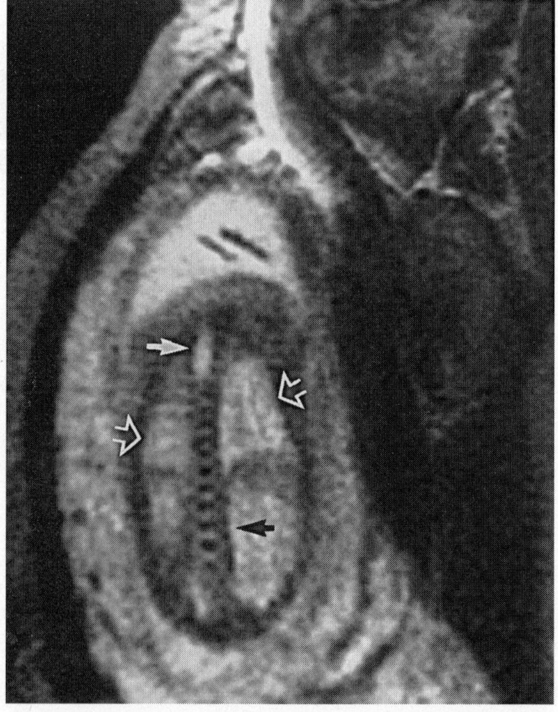

Fig. 10-8 Parasagittal T2-weighted image of the mother (inverted to show the fetal anatomy) shows the 29-week fetus in the coronal plane, revealing the fetal lungs *(open white arrows)* posteriorly and the thoracic and lumbar spine *(black arrow)*. The upper aspect of the cervical cord is seen centrally in the spine *(white arrow)*.

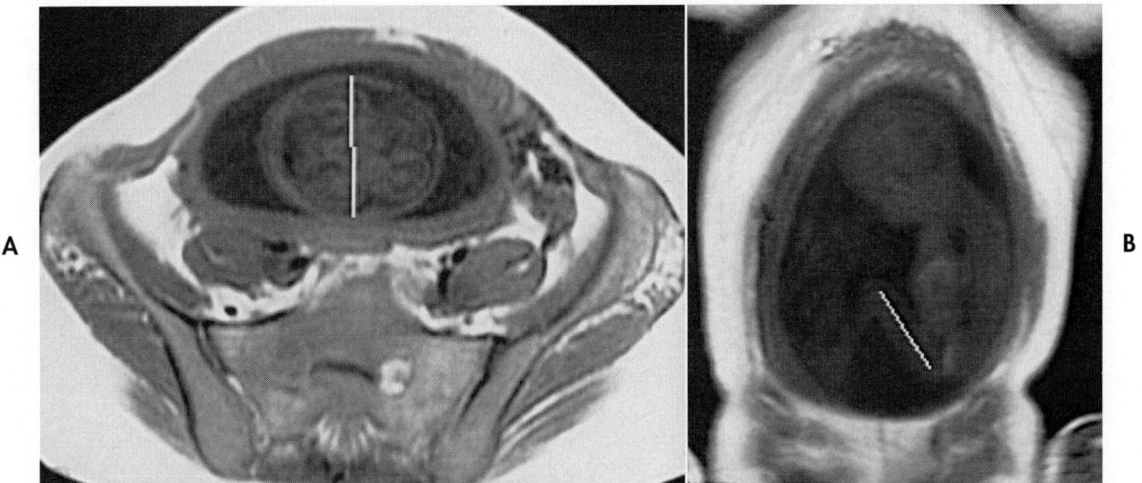

Fig. 10-9 Fetal measurements can be obtained, as shown in this 22-week fetus with the axial T1-weighted image showing the biparietal diameter **(A)** and the coronal T1-weighted image showing the femur length **(B).**

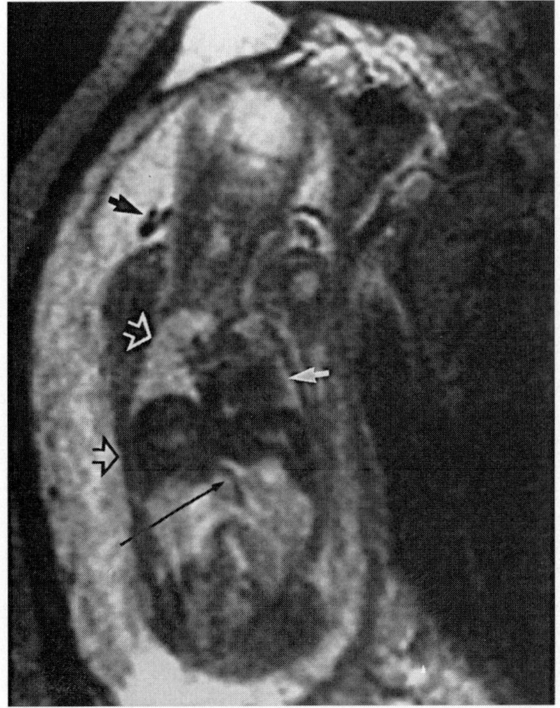

Fig. 10-10 Coronal T2-weighted image of a 29-week fetus shows the normal third trimester appearance of the fluid-filled lungs with high T2-weighted signal *(open white arrow).* The mediastinum and vascular structures are seen centrally *(white arrow).* The right and left diaphragms are seen clearly in normal position. Below the diaphragm, the umbilical vein *(long black arrow)* is seen surrounded by bowel loops, entering the liver. The cord is seen above the right shoulder *(short black arrow).*

stores, MRI has been shown to greatly aid in distinguishing the well-nourished small fetus from the malnourished fetus.[21] However, MRI's exact role in prenatal diagnosis of IUGR has not yet been determined.

Another area of investigation has been in the assessment of fetal lung maturity. A study by Wax et al has shown the normal appearance of the lung in the third trimester (Figs. 10-8 and 10-10).[22] The goal is to find a noninvasive method to assess lung maturity. This is currently done using the lecithin-sphingomyelin (L:S) ratio from amniotic fluid. Further studies comparing the appearance of the lung tissue with the L:S ratios are ongoing.

Therefore, although the potential uses of MRI for fetal brain, heart, and liver imaging, as well as for determination of fetal fat stores and lung maturity, are exciting fields of investigation, MRI often results in unsatisfactory imaging of many other fetal structures, particularly early in pregnancy. Already, through the introduction of FSE sequences, the imaging times have been reduced significantly. However, until investigators can overcome such difficulties as fetal movement and position and decreased tissue contrast due to decreased fat deposit, the utility of MRI for fetal imaging may be limited.

PLACENTAL IMAGING

For many years, ultrasonography has been the imaging modality of choice for placental localization and characterization, and it remains so. In fact, the diagnostic accuracy of ultrasound examination for

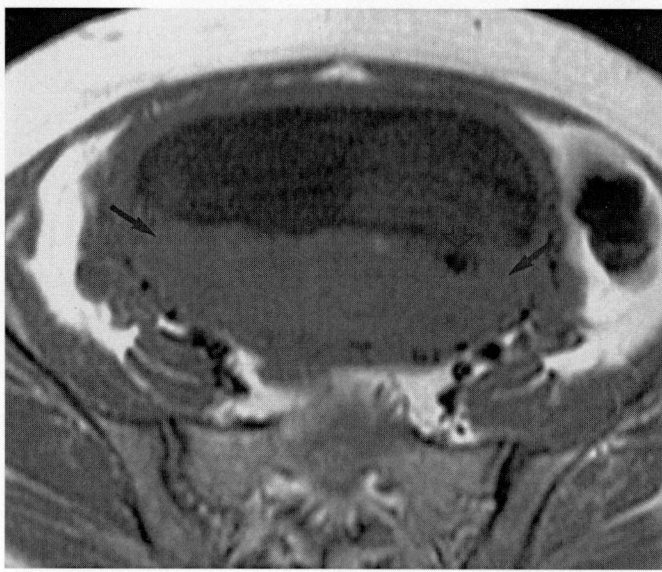

Fig. 10-11 Normal placenta. T1-weighted image (TR 500, TE 11) at 19 weeks shows the placenta isointense to the myometrium *(black arrows),* and one of the cord vessels is seen on the left.

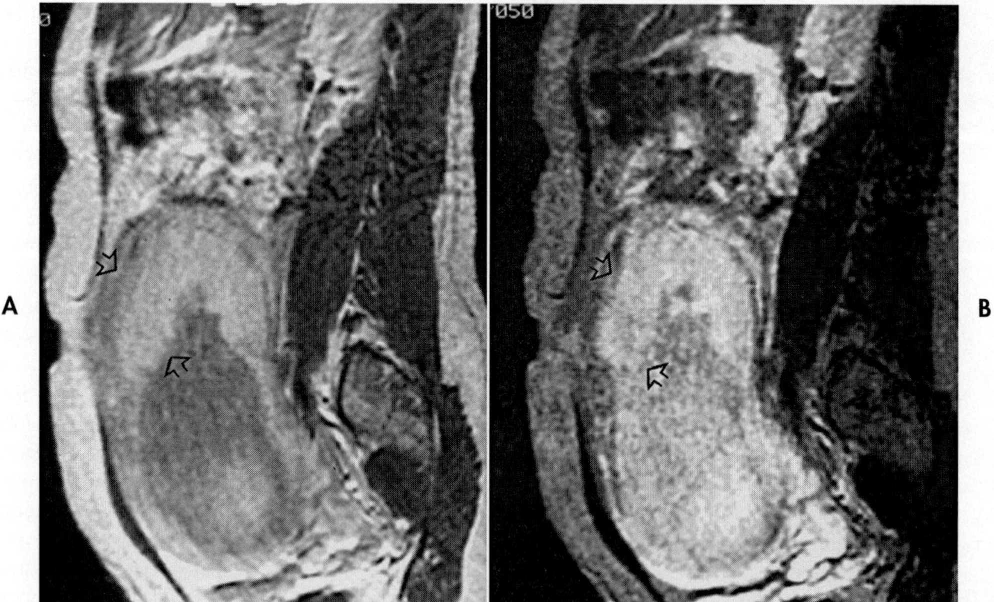

Fig. 10-12 A, Proton density image (TR 2500, TE 30) shows this 22-week fundal placenta *(open black arrows).* **B,** T2-weighted image (TR 2500, TE 80) shows the placenta again; it is now slightly less distinct owing to the increased signal of the amniotic fluid. The demarcation of the placenta and underlying myometrium and the edge of the placenta against the myometrium are seen on both images.

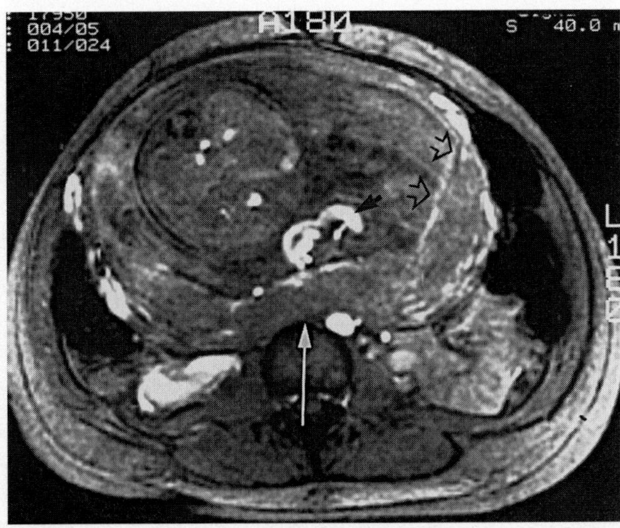

Fig. 10-13 Axial GRASS (gradient recalled acquisition in the steady state) image, acquired with the patient supine, shows obliteration of the maternal inferior vena cava due to compression *(long white arrow)*. The three-vessel cord *(black arrow)* is seen between the fetus and the placenta; several placental vessels are seen on its surface *(open black arrows)*.

placenta previa has been reported to be as high as 93%.[23] However, the supplemental role of MRI in obstetrics is currently attracting much interest in the field of placental imaging. Its ability to produce images with excellent soft tissue contrast allows accurate visualization of placental position (Figs. 10-11 to 10-13) and of the relationship of the placenta to the internal cervical os. The placental size, location, and umbilical cord insertion (see Fig. 10-11) were seen clearly in all patients in McCarthy et al's study.[16] MRI's ability to image blood is also an important advantage. Accurate placental imaging and detection of bleeding is extremely important in the management of third trimester bleeding and such conditions as placenta previa and placental abruption.

Placental tissue has relatively long T1 and T2 relaxation rates and therefore can be readily identified with a T1-weighted sequence, since the surrounding amniotic fluid has low signal intensity with this sequence (Fig. 10-11). It can also be seen on T2-weighted images but may be isointense to the myometrium (Fig. 10-12). It is usually possible on T2 and proton density images together to define the borders of the placenta. The cervix has its characteristic low signal intensity and easily recognizable trilaminar appearance. With the use of both sagittal and axial imaging, the placental position can be determined, and its lower margin and its relationship to the cervical os identified. Gradient echo images will show the normal placental

blood flow and help localize the cord (Fig. 10-13). The number of vessels can be counted in the cord on these and T1-weighted images (see Figs. 10-6, C and 10-13).

In a study of 25 patients with an ultrasound diagnosis of placenta previa in the third trimester, MRI proved equal to ultrasound in localization of the placenta. In addition, it was found to be more accurate than ultrasound in precise determination of the degree of placenta previa.[24] In fact, in this series, ultrasound diagnosis had overestimated the degree of previa in seven of the 25 cases. One reason for this overestimation is that ultrasonography sometimes has difficulty distinguishing a low-lying placenta from a marginal one or placenta previa, especially if the placenta is posteriorly located. MRI, with its superior images in many planes, was able to illustrate the degree of previa accurately in all the cases (Fig. 10-14).[24]

In addition to its use in placental localization, MRI's ability to distinguish blood collections from other fluids makes it potentially useful in the diagnosis of placental abruption. This would be an important application, since the diagnostic accuracy of ultrasonography for abruptions is reported to be less than 50%,[25] and because of the high maternal and fetal morbidity and mortality associated with the condition. In a study of the use of MRI in third trimester bleeding, the three cases of placental abruption were associated with identified abnormalities on the images.[26] This is an exciting

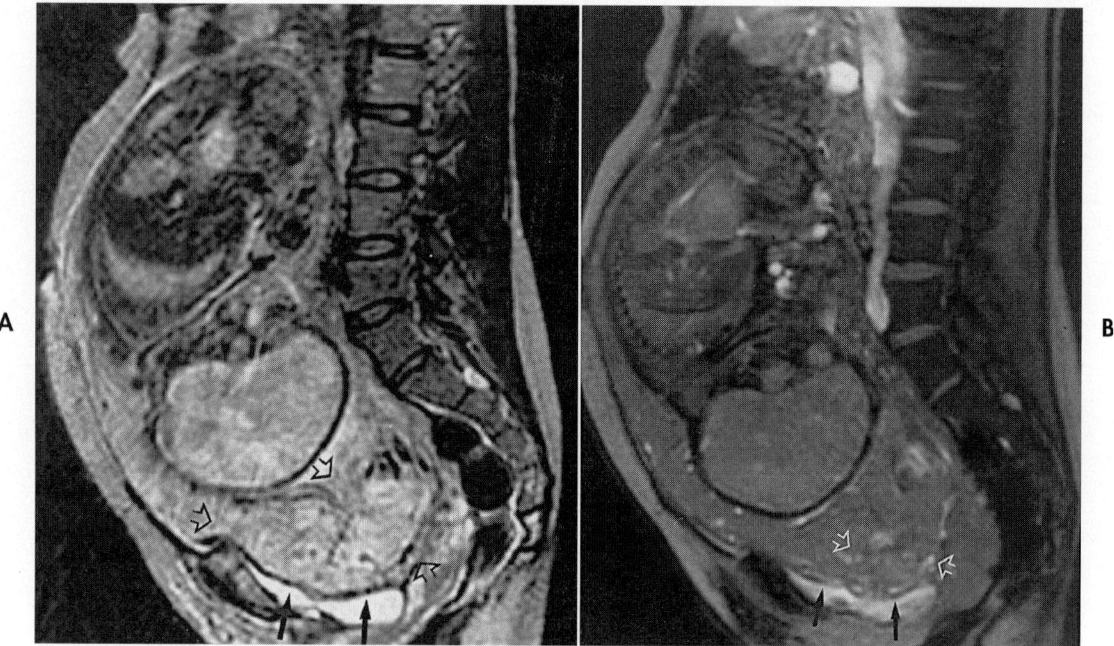

Fig. 10-14 This 36-year-old woman presented with a known placenta previa and possible increta. **A,** Sagittal fast spin echo (FSE) image (TR 4000, TE 102) shows the vertex-presenting fetus, the complete previa *(open black arrows)*. There was no evidence of placenta percreta invading the bladder *(black arrows)*. **B,** Sagittal GRASS image (TR 33, TE 12, flip angle 30) shows the abnormally increased vascular pattern in the placenta, suggestive of an increta *(open white arrows)*, and again no invasion of the bladder is seen *(black arrows)*.

future application of MRI techniques that needs further investigation to define its ultimate role.

Placenta accreta

Another current use of MRI is to evaluate the placenta for possible placenta accreta, a rare condition that may follow a previous cesarean section or uterine instrumentation. The placenta grows deep into the myometrium and occurs more commonly with placenta previa. The placental tissue grows through the myometrium to varying depths. A superficial invasion is known as placenta accreta, deeper invasion is placenta increta (Fig. 10-14), and invasion through the wall of the myometrium is placenta percreta. This last-named condition is the most serious because it can invade adjacent organs such as the bladder.[27] MRI can be helpful to diagnose this rare entity and also to estimate the depth of invasion into the myometrium. These women are delivered by cesarean section followed by a hysterectomy (Fig. 10-15). These forms of invasion can be difficult to differentiate, the most difficult being the increta type. The increta can be detected by thinning of the normal myometrial wall. An unusual case of percreta presenting 3 months postpartum dramatically demon-

strates the aggressive invasive nature of the trophoblastic tissue (Fig. 10-16). In this case the differential diagnosis included a form of gestational trophoblastic disease, a rare placental site trophoblastic tumor, and a placenta percreta.

Ectopic pregnancy

Abnormal sites of implantation can be assessed by MRI. The diagnosis of an ectopic pregnancy is made upon finding an extrauterine embryo and an empty uterus. MRI can define both of these and is used as a problem-solving tool after the ultrasound examination. Difficult cases such as advanced second or third trimester ectopics can be difficult to define on ultrasonography and require careful and full evaluation, especially of the placental implantation site (Fig. 10-17).[28-30] The case seen in Fig. 10-17 showed extensive extrauterine abdominal extension, which was difficult to define completely on ultrasonography. Low cervical canal ectopic pregnancy can also occur, especially after attempted in vitro fertilization, and can also be identified on MRI (Fig. 10-18), allowing for depiction of the level of the internal os.

In summary, MRI may prove a valuable imaging tool for the evaluation of third trimester bleed-

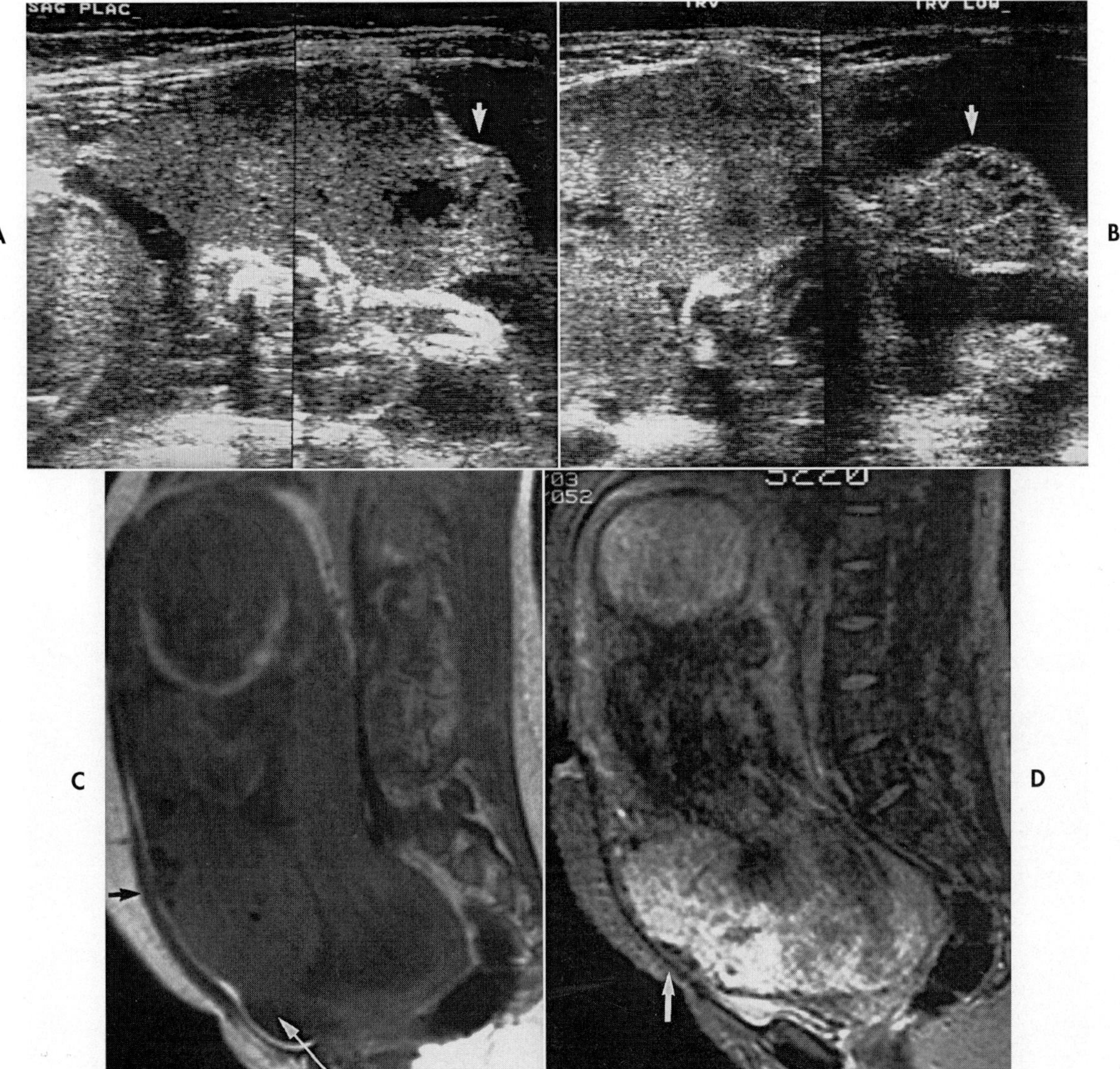

Fig. 10-15 Placenta increta. A 24-year-old woman P2G1, with a history of a previous cesarean section. Ultrasound examination, sagittal (**A**) and transvaginal (**B**), noted the placenta to be anterior with prominent vessels *(white arrows)*, and raised the possibility of placenta accreta. **C**, Sagittal T1-weighted MRI at 30 weeks of gestation showed the anterior placenta with abnormal vessels close to the serosal surface of the myometrium *(black arrow)*. There was also some suggestion that the placenta might cover portions of the cervical os (placenta previa). **D**, T2-weighted images show the thin myometrium anteriorly and cannot be followed completely on the anterior margin *(white arrow)*. The patient underwent an elective classic cesarean section at 39 weeks' gestation. A 2999 g male was delivered with an ApGAR score of 7/8. The placenta was located just under the bladder flap and bled profusely. The patient required 18 units of blood. A hysterectomy was performed and then a repair of the cystotomy. Gross pathologic examination revealed a myometrium with intervening placental tissue, giving a marble-like appearance throughout. Microscopic examination identified placenta increta.

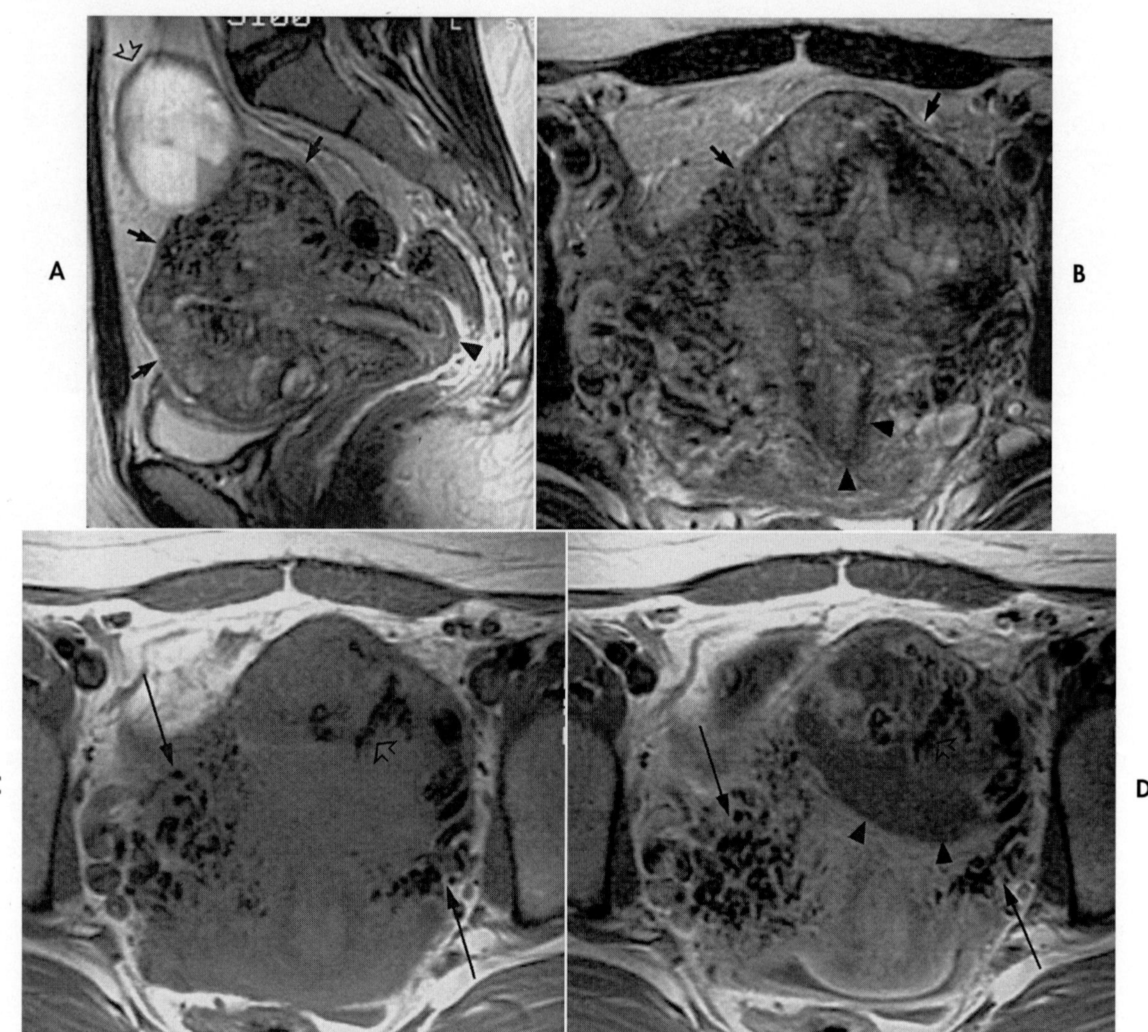

Fig. 10-16 Placenta percreta. This 30-year-old woman presented with vaginal bleeding 3 months postpartum and had a normal-to-low human chorionic gonadotropin (hCG) level. Sagittal **(A)** and axial **(B)** FSE images (TR 4000, TE 95) show the markedly abnormal myometrium *(black arrows)* with multiple foci of low signal throughout the wall. The cervix and endocervical canal are normal *(black arrowheads)*. There is an adnexal cyst noted superior to the uterine fundus on the sagittal image **(A)** *(open black arrow)*. Axial T1-weighted images before **(C)** and after **(D)** administration show the markedly increased vascularity of the parametrium and uterus *(long black arrows)*. The post-gadolinium image shows the central necrotic (nonenhancing) portion *(black arrowheads)* with large vessels coursing through this area *(open black arrows)*.

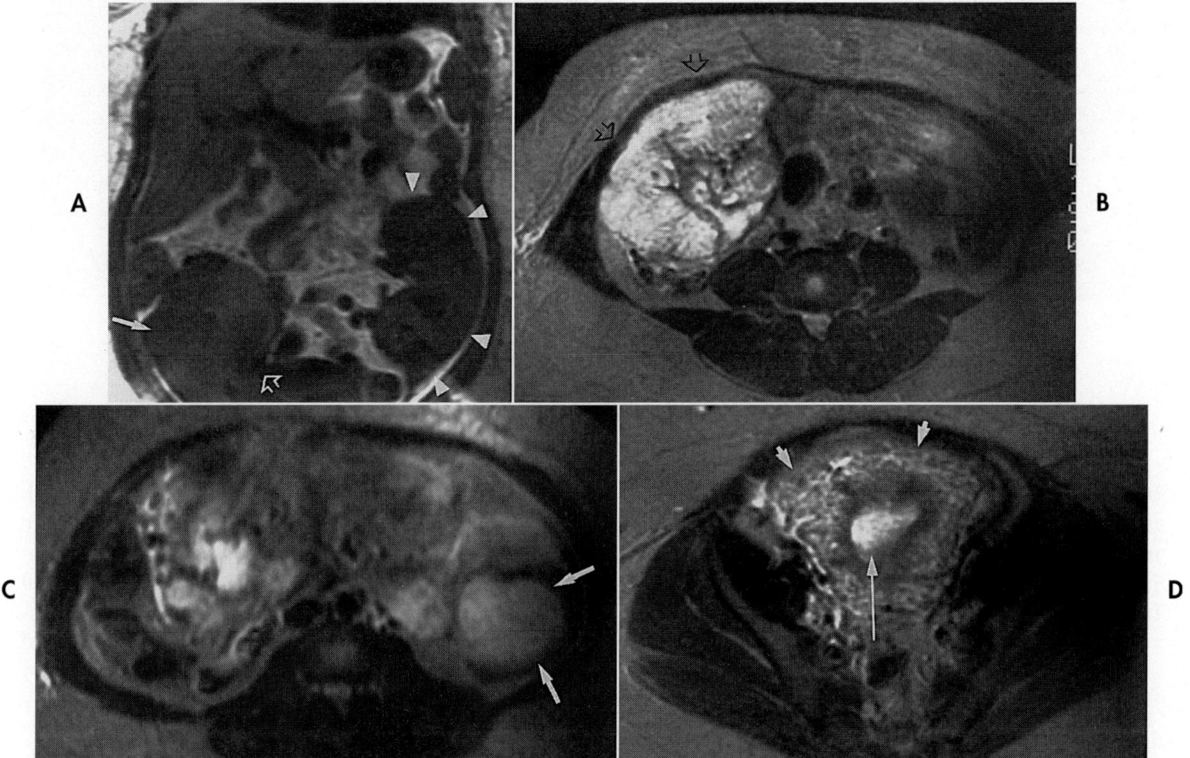

Fig. 10-17 Abdominal ectopic pregnancy. This 35-year-old P3003 underwent a tubal ligation in 1980 and presented to her physician complaining of abdominal pain of 2 months' duration. She reported her last menstrual period to have been 6 weeks before presentation. Ultrasound examination demonstrated an extrauterine pregnancy in the left lower quadrant. The fetus was noted to be breech. **A,** Coronal T1-weighted MRI demonstrated an intra-abdominal pregnancy *(white arrowheads)* with umbilical vein and artery crossing the midline. The placenta was located in the right lower quadrant *(white arrow)*, implanting on the serosal surface of the bladder *(open white arrow)*. **B,** Axial T2-weighted image shows the placenta in the right lower quadrant *(open black arrows)*. **C,** Axial T2-weighted image more superiorly shows the fetal brain in cross-section *(white arrows)*. **D,** Axial T2-weighted image through the pelvis shows the empty uterine cavity *(long white arrow)* with prominent vascular engorgement of the myometrium *(white arrows)*. At surgery, a fetus weighing 850 g was removed from the left lower quadrant. The cord was found to traverse the abdomen and attach to the placenta, which was encroaching on the broad ligament and bladder side wall. The placenta was not removed. (Courtesy Andrew Yang, MD, Baltimore, MD.)

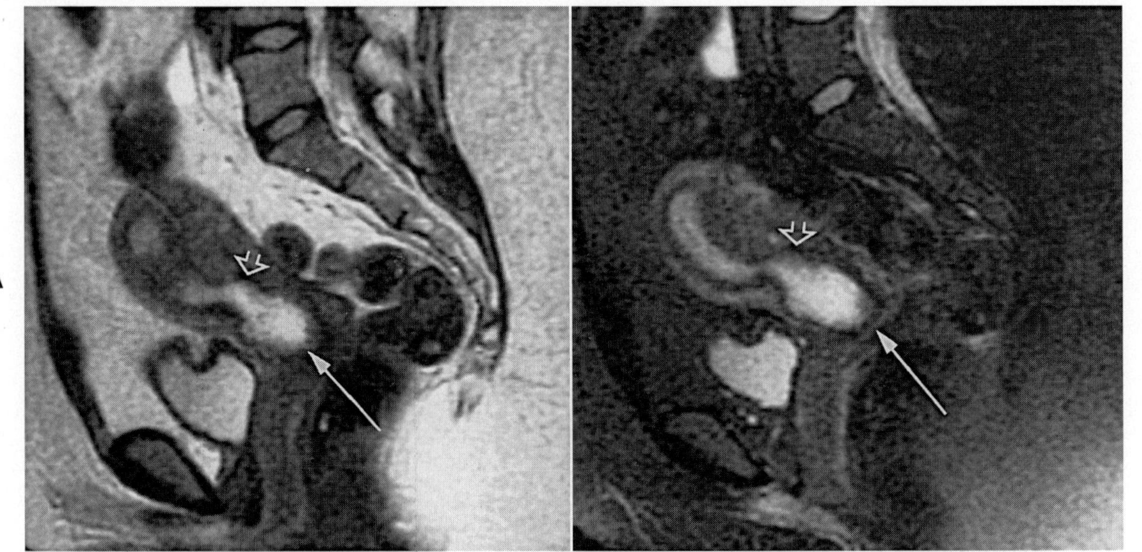

Fig. 10-18 Cervical ectopic pregnancy after in vitro fertilization. Sagittal T-2 weighted image **(A)** and sagittal T2-weighted image with fat suppression **(B)** show the abnormal implantation in the endocervical canal *(long white arrows)* below the level of the internal os *(open white arrows)*.

ing. Its ability to clearly identify anatomic structures, to highlight tissue contrast, and to identify intrauterine blood collections may be a useful adjunct to negative or equivocal ultrasound examinations for the diagnosis of placenta previa and abruption.

MATERNAL IMAGING

Although ultrasonography continues to be the main obstetric imaging modality, MRI with its recent advancements is gaining acceptance as a useful tool for imaging maternal anatomy and pathology during pregnancy. Ultrasound examination of pelvic masses during pregnancy is often limited by physical constraints due to either displacement by the gravid uterus, the size of the mass, poor tissue characterization, or reliance on operator skill. In addition, overlying bowel gas can interfere with image quality. However, precise characterization of the mass, while avoiding ionizing radiation, is essential for planning the delivery of the baby and possible surgical management. Thus, the potential role of MRI in the diagnosis of pelvis masses during pregnancy has attracted much interest over the last several years.

Adnexal masses

MRI has proved superior to other modalities in the identification and diagnosis of pelvic masses.[31,32] Several studies have been carried out to compare the roles of MRI and ultrasound examination in the diagnosis of pelvic masses during pregnancy. Kier

et al conducted a study of 17 pregnant patients with sonograms that suggested a pelvic mass who were subsequently imaged with MRI.[33] The latter improved characterization in 47% of the cases (eight out of 17) and was found to supply additional information to supplement both transabdominal and transvaginal ultrasound examinations. This study also determined the origin of the pelvic mass successfully in all of the cases, compared with ultrasound's 71% accuracy for determining mass origin. A similar study by Weinreb et al also concluded that MRI provided additional important information to ultrasound examination in 44% of pregnant patients (seven out of 16) who presented with a pelvic mass.[34]

Many pelvic masses have easily identifiable characteristics on MRI. In the first trimester the most common pelvic mass is the corpus luteal cyst, which has been described on MRI as a round or oval structure with thin walls and a homogeneous low signal intensity on T1-weighted and high signal intensity on T2-weighted images.[34] Since most corpus luteum cysts spontaneously regress by the end of the second trimester,[35] MR evaluation of a woman early in pregnancy with a mass resembling a corpus luteum cyst on ultrasonography should be delayed and performed only if the mass persists. Mature cystic teratomas also have unique appearances on MRI. These masses typically tend to exhibit signal intensity consistent with fat and may display chemical shift artifacts at higher field strength.[36] They may, however, persist into later pregnancy (Fig. 10-19), and although their detection is not usually difficult, they need to be accurately localized to plan delivery. If the mass is in the pelvis, the pressure exerted by it may be such that the lower uterine segment fails to develop normally. It may thus be small and preclude a vaginal delivery.

If the mass appears complex, the possibility of cystadenoma or cystadenocarcinoma should be considered. Ovarian cystadenocarcinomas, however, exhibit a variety of appearances, such as a complex, multiseptated mass and thick walls, with internal nodules or wall vegetations. Thus, it may be difficult to distinguish them from cystadenomas (Figs. 10-20 and 10-21). Gadolinium is not recommended for routine use in pregnancy as it would normally be used for characterization of a pelvic mass.

Other pelvic masses such as neurogenic tumors may present for the first time in pregnancy. The multiplanar capability of MRI allows for the origins of these masses to be clearly defined (Fig. 10-23). This is particularly important in pregnancy, as

Text continued on p. 254.

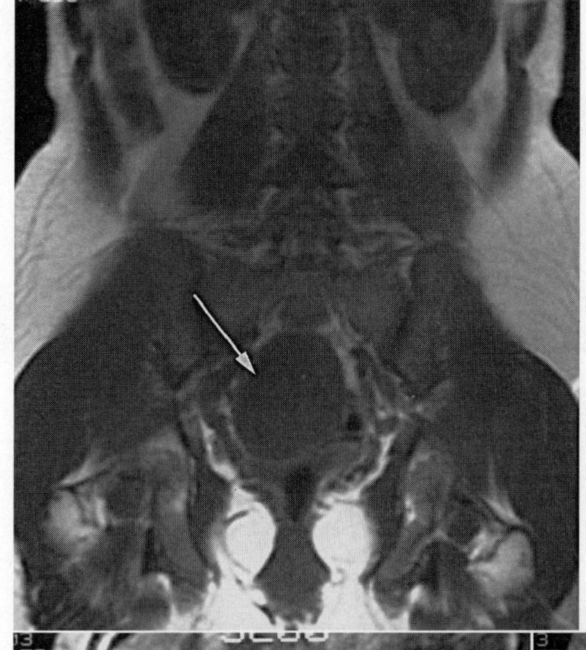

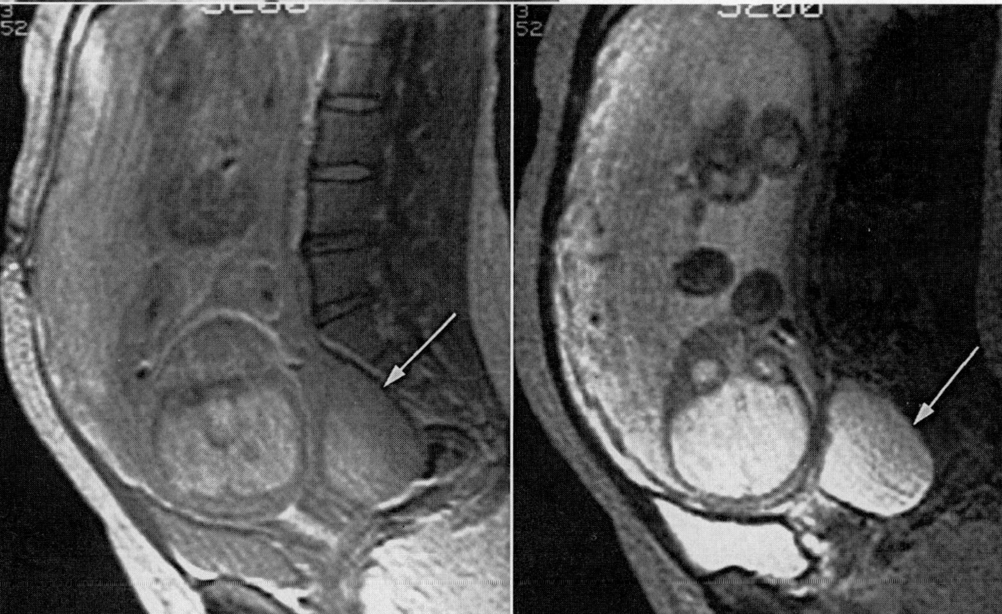

Fig. 10-19 Corpus luteal cyst. In this patient, an 18-year-old woman imaged at 29 weeks, ultrasound examination had shown a 7.3 × 5.5 cm cystic mass in the cul-de-sac with a septation and a probable small rind of ovarian tissue. The differential diagnosis, according to the ultrasound appearance, included endometrioma, cystadenoma, and cystic dermoid. **A,** Coronal T1-weighted images show the low signal mass *(long white arrow)* deep in the pelvis. Sagittal proton density **(B)** and T2-weighted images **(C)** show this to be a typical simple cyst *(long white arrows)* with high T2 signal. It is close to the cervical canal but separate from the uterus.

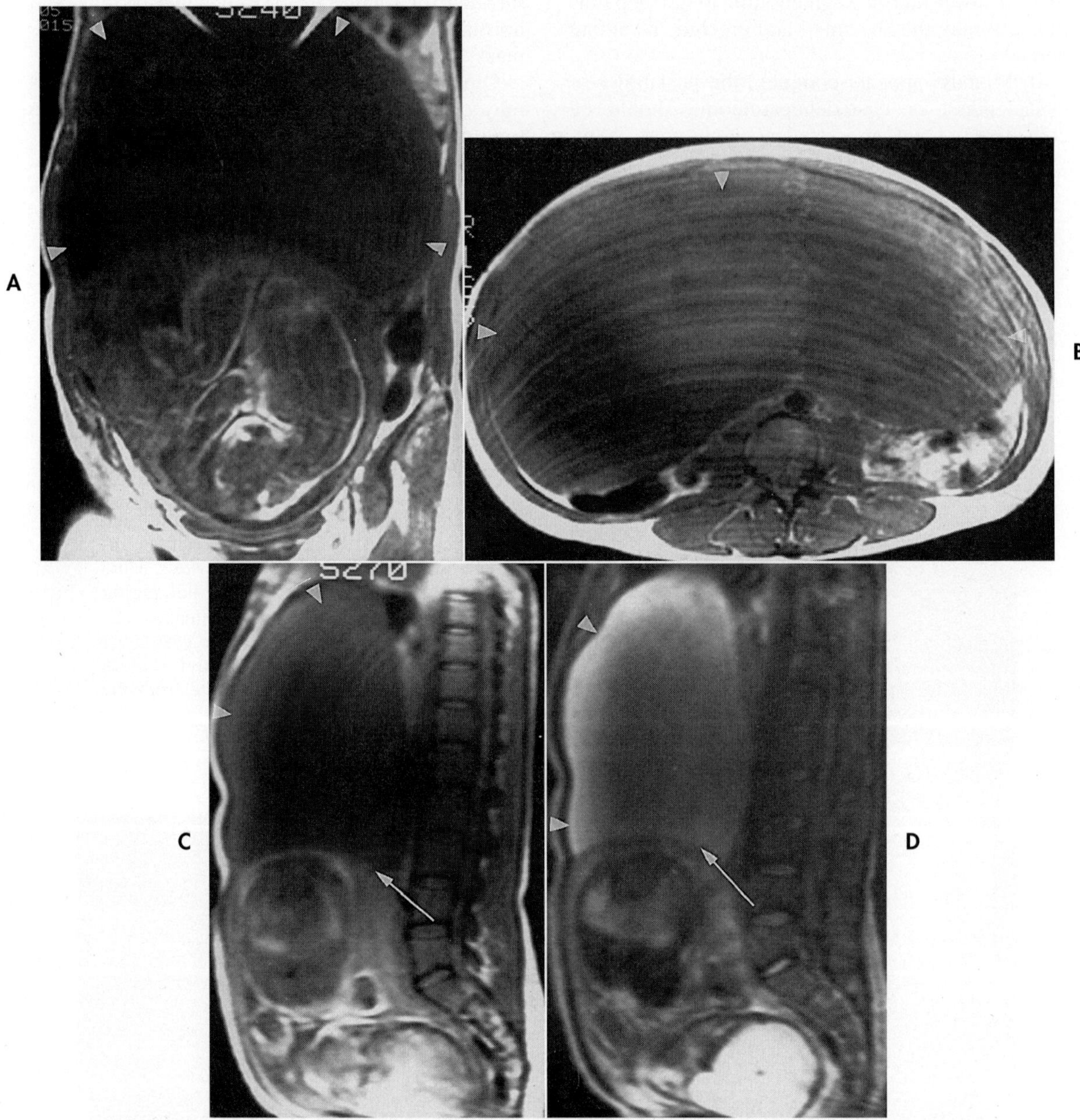

Fig. 10-20 Benign cystadenoma of the ovary. This 23-year-old woman in her late third trimester, presented for evaluation of an abdominal mass. **A** and **B,** Coronal and axial T1-weighted images (TR 600, TE 20) show a large low signal intensity mass superior to the uterus occupying the upper abdomen *(white arrowheads).* **C** and **D,** Sagittal proton density and T2-weighted images (TR 2500, TE 20/80) show this mass to be a large fluid-filled cyst that is simple and unilocular *(white arrowheads).* It is clearly separate from the uterus *(long white arrow).*

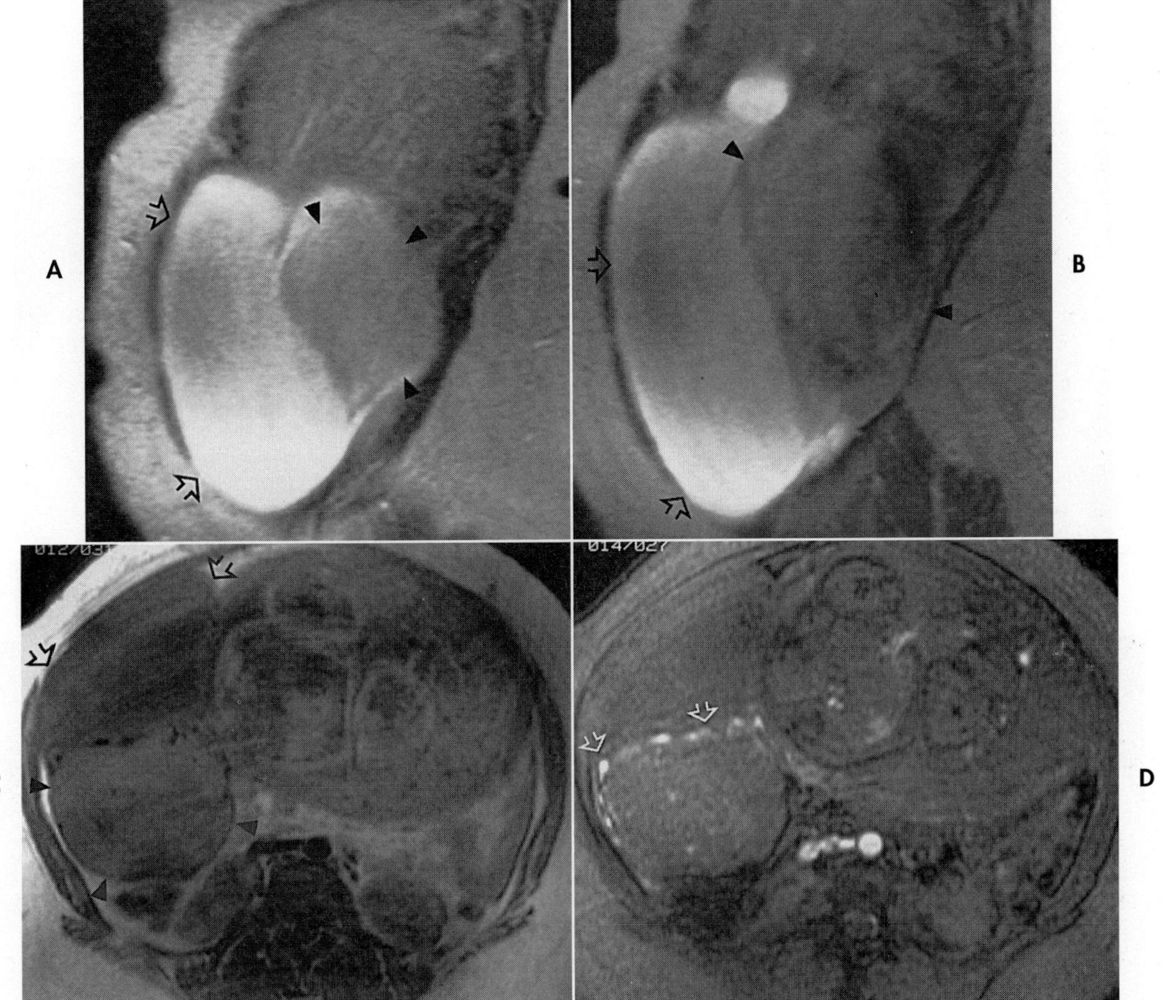

Fig. 10-21 Benign sclerosing stromal cell tumor of the ovary. In this 17-year-old P1G0 woman at 36 weeks' gestation, a routine ultrasound examination demonstrated a large mass in the right abdomen with both solid and cystic components. Areas of calcification and shadowing were also identified. The mass was thought to be extrauterine, and Doppler studies identified feeding vessels extending from the myometrium to the mass. The mass was thought to be consistent with teratoma or dermoid, although malignant degeneration could not be excluded. **A** and **B,** Sagittal T2-weighted images (TR 3000, TE 80) show a large mass in the right flank extending from the subhepatic space to the right lower quadrant. The posterior component is of low to intermediate signal intensity *(black arrowheads)* compatible with solid tissue, and the anterior component is of uniform high signal intensity compatible with fluid *(open black arrows).* **C,** Axial T1-weighted image (TR 800, TE 20) shows the complex mass in the right flank, containing solid tissue posteriorly *(black arrowheads)* and fluid anteriorly *(open black arrows).* The gravid uterus is seen separate and to the left of midline. **D,** Axial GRASS image shows the neovascular flow *(open white arrows)* to the solid component of this mass and the avascular cystic component anteriorly. After delivery of a healthy baby by cesarean section, a 20 × 20 cm solid and cystic mass was removed. Pathologic examination revealed a benign sclerosing stromal cell tumor with a simple cyst anteriorly.

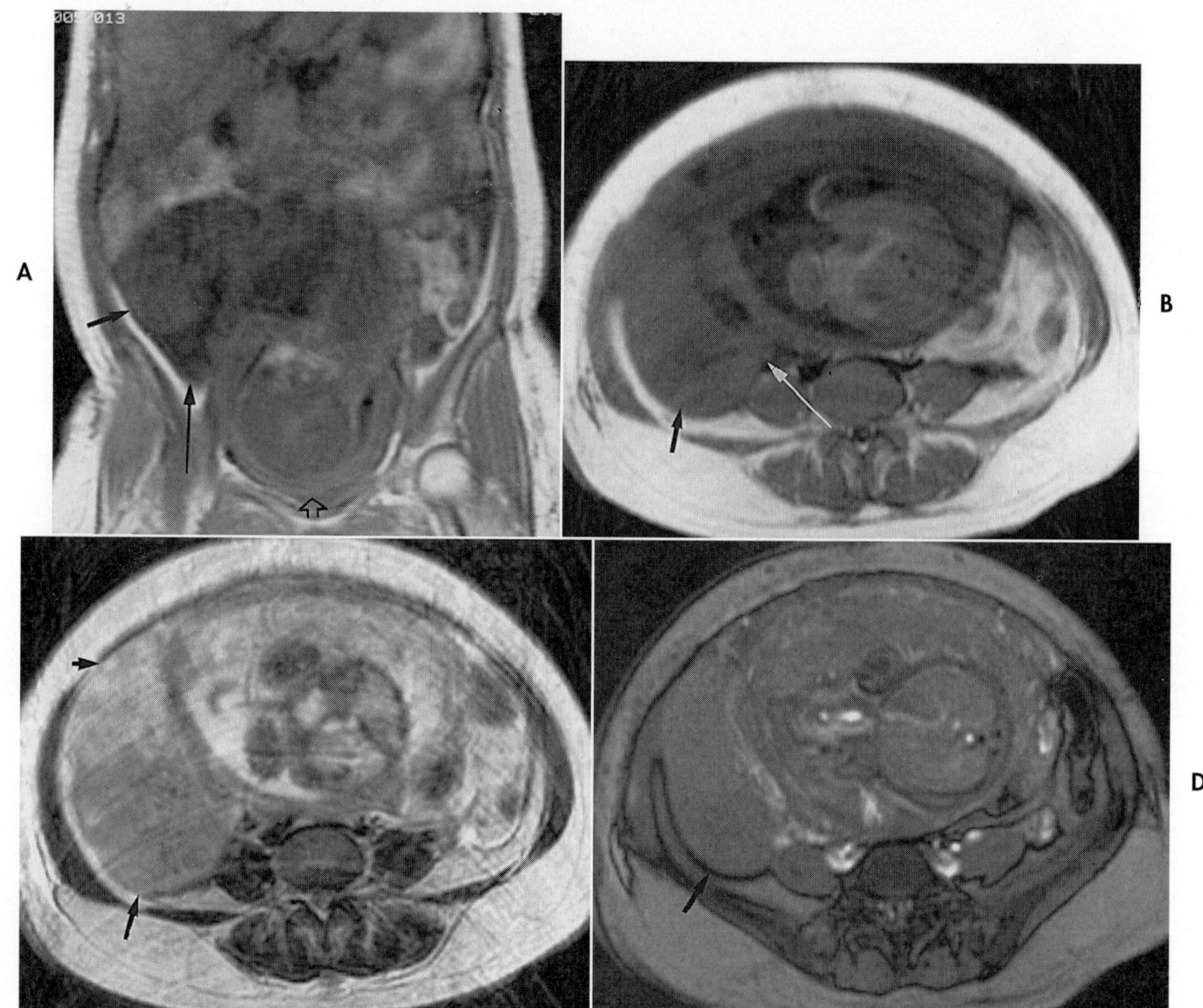

Fig. 10-22 Krukenberg tumor of the right ovary. This 29-year-old woman presented at 29 weeks' gestation with a right-sided abdominal mass. **A** and **B,** Coronal and axial T1-weighted images (TR 600, TE 12) show a solid mass *(black arrows)* in the right flank with associated ascites *(long black arrow)*. The mass is separate from the uterus *(white arrow)*. **(C)** Axial FSE T2-weighted image (TR 4000, TE 102) shows the mass *(black arrow)* and a possible peritoneal implant anteriorly *(short black arrow)*. **D,** Axial GRASS image shows the extrauterine tumor to be relatively hypovascular. This patient underwent a cesarean section and removal of the metastatic gastric adenocarcinoma in the right ovary; at surgery, multiple peritoneal implants were found.

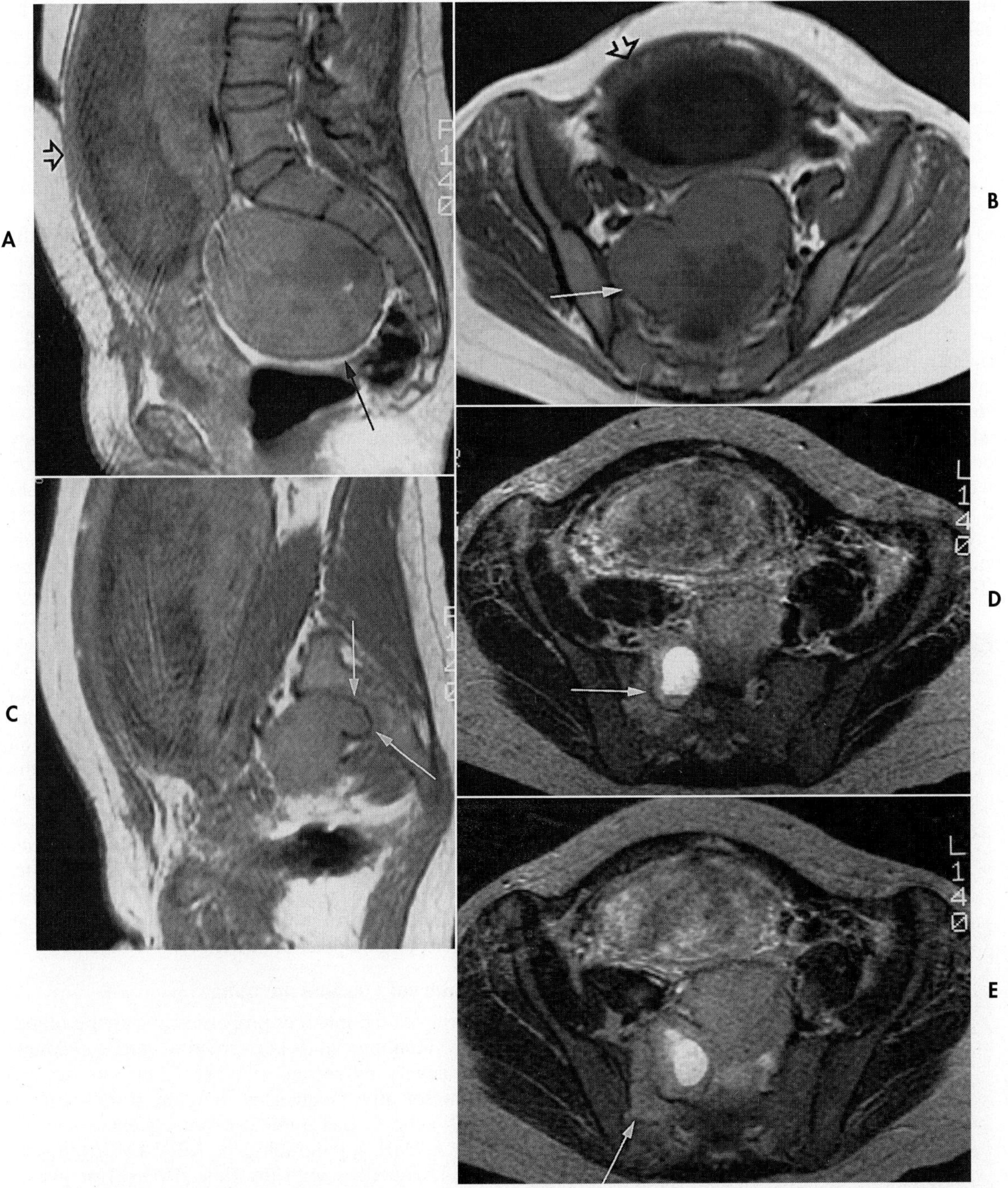

Fig. 10-23 Benign schwannoma of the right sciatic nerve. **A,** Sagittal proton density image shows a large heterogeneous signal intensity mass in the posterior pelvis *(long black arrow)*. **B,** Axial T1-weighted image shows the mass *(white arrow)* posterior to the uterus *(open black arrow)*. **C,** Sagittal proton density image shows the communication between the mass and a sacral neural foramen *(white arrows)*. **D** and **E,** Axial T2-weighted images show the hyperintense signal of the center of the mass, which arises from the right sacral foramen *(white arrow)* and the associated bone invasion to the right of the foramen *(white arrow)*. This signal intensity is compatible with a neurogenic tumor. This patient had a cesarean section that showed the lower uterine segment to be poorly developed, owing to the long-standing pressure from the mass. The mass was subsequently removed by the neurosurgery.

the spinal origin of these tumors requires neuro-surgical intervention.

MR imaging of leiomyomas in pregnancy, as in all women, is characterized by the typical appearance of these lesions and their clear definition. They present specific problems in pregnancy, i.e., obstruction to implantation, obstruction of the birth canal, and difficult-to-define masses on ultrasonography. Another important MRI application is in situations in which the ultrasound examination is unable to distinguish confidently between a subserosal or pedunculated leiomyoma and an ovarian lesion. MRI, with its excellent tissue characterization, can distinguish these lesions with confidence because of the characteristic MR appearance of leiomyomas as homogeneous low intensity structures on both T1- and T2-weighted images, which consist mostly of smooth muscle along with occasionally areas of either high T1W or T2-weighted signal intensity that represent degeneration.[37,38] MRI can be very helpful in imaging the pregnant woman with leiomyomas; if present, the size and locations of these can be clearly defined (Fig. 10-24). Leiomyomas are hormonally sensi-

tive will grow and often degenerate during pregnancy. Myometrial bulges may be seen, appearing as areas of hypointensity on T2-weighted images. These can be differentiated from leiomyomas (Fig. 10-25), as they are transient, distorting only the inner contour of the myometrium and not the outer uterine contour.[39]

MRI of the cervix in pregnancy

MRI may also come to play a potentially significant role in cervical imaging during pregnancy, since ultrasound assessment of the cervix during pregnancy is often limited. MRI is uniquely suited for characterization of the internal structure of the cervix, because the walls of the cervix appear as low signal intensity bands with high signal in between on T2 images, representing the mucous plug in the canal. As in nonpregnant women, MRI may be used during pregnancy to stage cervical cancer. It is especially useful when combined with an abdominopelvic scan for full local, nodal, and liver staging. The advantages are that the examination is noninvasive and uses no ionizing radiation, and intravenous contrast material is not needed. Evaluation of the cervix defines the mass's size and location, along with its relationship to the uterus, endocervical canal, vagina, and parametrium (Fig. 10-26). Thus, the delivery and the cancer treatment can be planned together. If the cancer appears confined to the cervix without parametrial invasion (FIGO stage IIa/TNM T2b. See appendix), the baby can be delivered by cesarean section, followed by a hysterectomy and lymphadenectomy. If there is evidence of tumor spread into the parametrium (FIGO stage IIb/TNM T2b), a hys terectomy is not indicated (Fig. 10-26). MRI may also be able to provide useful information in such conditions as cervical incompetence and cervical dystocia.

Maternal vascular imaging

Owing to the inherent properties of moving blood, flow imaging can be performed with ease and noninvasively by means of MRI. There are several flow-sensitive sequences, ranging from standard spin echo to the gradient echo sequences and the MRA (MR angiography) or MRV (MR venography) sequences with the time of flight or phases contrast techniques. These can all be used in pregnancy to assess both the arterial and venous systems.

When imaging the venous system in pregnancy, it is important to remember to image the woman in both the supine and decubitus positions or in the decubitus position alone. This is because, as pregnancy progresses, so does the amount of pressure exerted by the gravid uterus on the inferior vena cava (IVC) in the supine position. The amount of

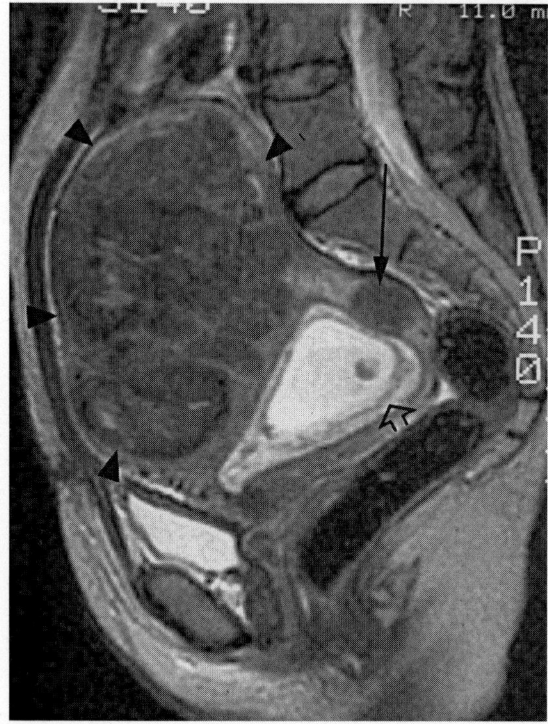

Fig. 10-24 Uterine leiomyomas. Sagittal T2-weighted FSE image (TR 4000, TE 102) shows an early intrauterine pregnancy (gestational age 9 weeks) *(open black arrow)*. The uterus is markedly enlarged and contains multiple intramural leiomyomas *(black arrowheads);* a small submucosal one is seen just above the endometrial cavity *(long black arrow).*

pressure is enough to cause the IVC to appear occluded in the supine position (Fig. 10-27). Thus, to ensure detection of normal flow in the IVC, the patient should be imaged in the decubitus position. In fact, this is often a more comfortable position for the patient, especially in the third trimester.

MRI can be useful in the diagnosis of gestational trophoblastic disease and can be used to monitor tumor response to chemotherapy. A study by Hricak et al of nine women with gestational trophoblastic disease demonstrated that the tumor distorted the MR appearance of uterine zonal structures, and showed hypervascular masses of heterogeneous signal intensity with indistinct boundaries between tumor and myometrium.[40] The study also demonstrated a regression of the abnormalities and return to normal uterine MR appearance, which correlated with chemotherapy and decreasing serum β-subunit human chorionic gonadotropin (hCG) concentration.[40] In a 1993 review, MRI was shown to detect abnormalities in two thirds of patients with hCG levels greater than 500 MIU/ml.[41] The MR findings consisted of abnormalities in the myometrium itself or evidence of extrauterine disease.

Postpartum complications

MRI can be used to evaluate women with postpartum complications such as ovarian or pelvic vein thrombosis (Fig. 10-28). Computed tomography can also be used to detect and assess the extent of venous thrombosis; this must be done with a bolus of intravenous contrast (Fig. 10-29). The sensitivity of MRI in detecting thrombosis in a noninvasive manner makes this a useful technique. Other uses are for detection of complications of abortions, such as retained products or clot (Fig. 10-30), and for detection of infections such as endometritis and abdominopelvic abcesses. Incomplete abortions have been shown as endometrial masses or abnormal distention of the endometrial cavity.[41,42]

In summary, although ultrasonography will continue to be the primary imaging modality in obstetric diagnosis because of its low cost, lack of radiation, and widespread availability, MRI is

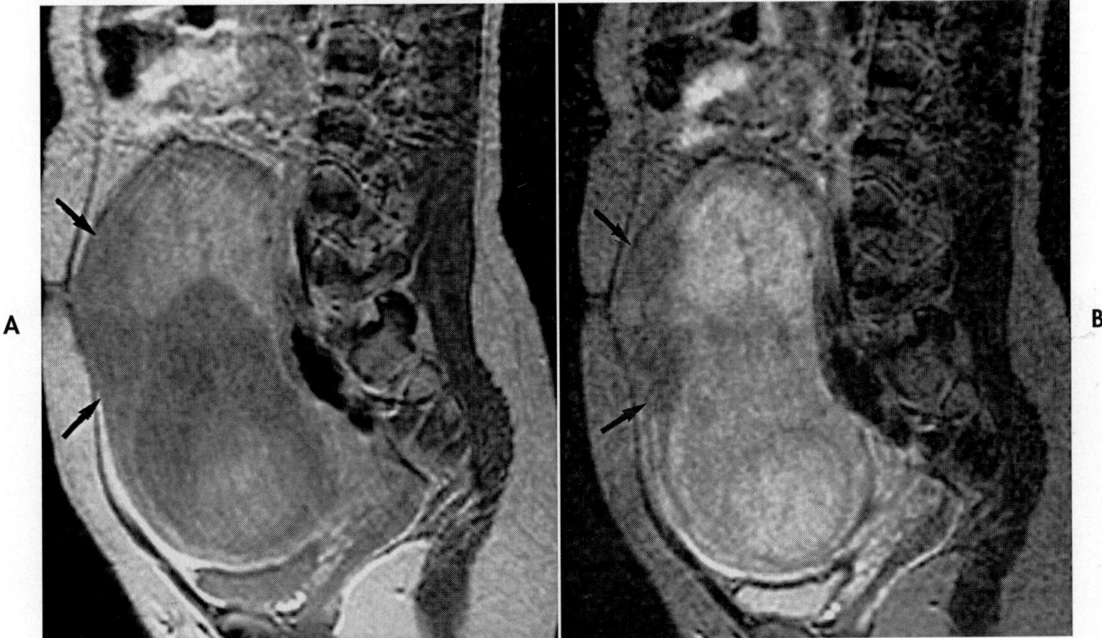

Fig. 10-25 In this 28-year-old woman, a routine ultrasound examination at 21 weeks' gestation revealed a solid mass at the left border of the uterus that measured 5.4 × 3.8 cm. In order to better characterize the mass, the patient underwent MRI. **A** and **B,** Sagittal proton density and T2-weighted images demonstrate the pregnant uterus with a single fetus in the cephalic position. The placenta is clearly identified superior and fundal in location and extending across the midline. There is mild thickening of the anterior wall of the myometrium, which has a diffusely low signal intensity *(black arrows)*. This did not change appearance on subsequent images and sequences, and was thus compatible with a mural leiomyoma. The patient went on to deliver a 3110-g baby girl with an ApGAR score of 9/9 by spontaneous delivery.

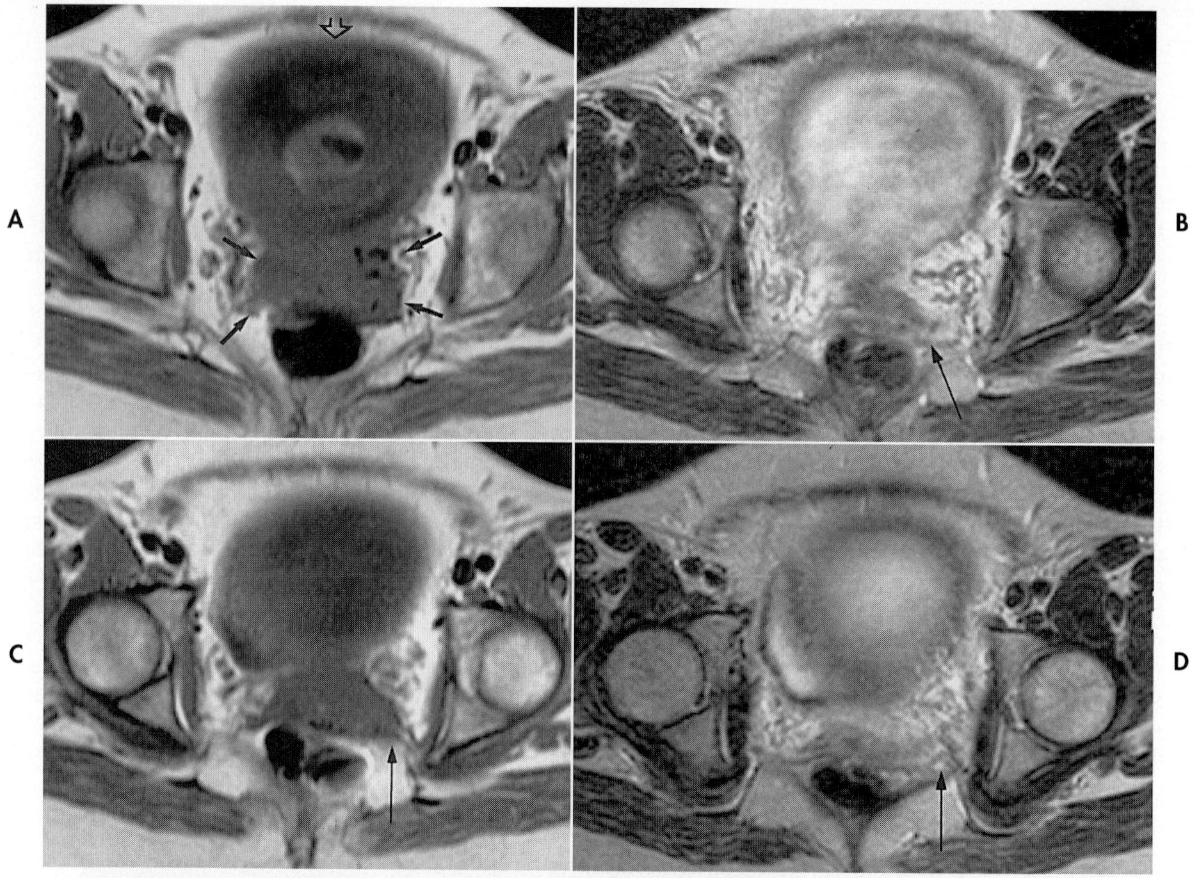

Fig. 10-26 Squamous cell carcinoma of the cervix. This 40-year-old woman presented at 19 weeks' gestation with biopsy-proven cervical carcinoma. **A** and **B,** Axial T1- and T2-weighted images at the same level show a mass in the cervix *(black arrows);* the gravid uterus is seen anteriorly *(open black arrow).* The T2-weighted image **B** shows the normal cervix to be replaced by high signal intensity tumor *(long black arrow).* **C** and **D,** Axial T1- and T2-weighted images at the same level (below the level in **A** and **B)** show extension of the mass into the parametrium on the left side *(long black arrows).* This patient had a normal vaginal delivery at term, followed by radiation therapy to the cervix.

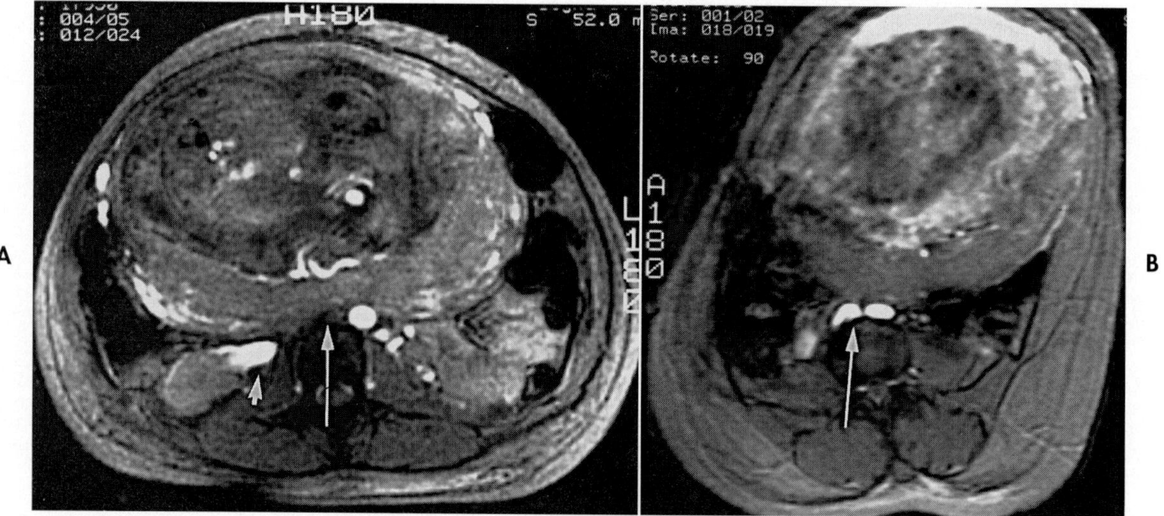

Fig. 10-27 Axial GRASS images of the maternal inferior vena cava (IVC). **A,** The patient is supine, showing complete compression of the IVC *(long white arrow);* note the right-sided hydronephrosis of pregnancy *(short white arrow).* **B,** The patient is turned on her side, and normal flow is seen in the IVC *(long white arrow).*

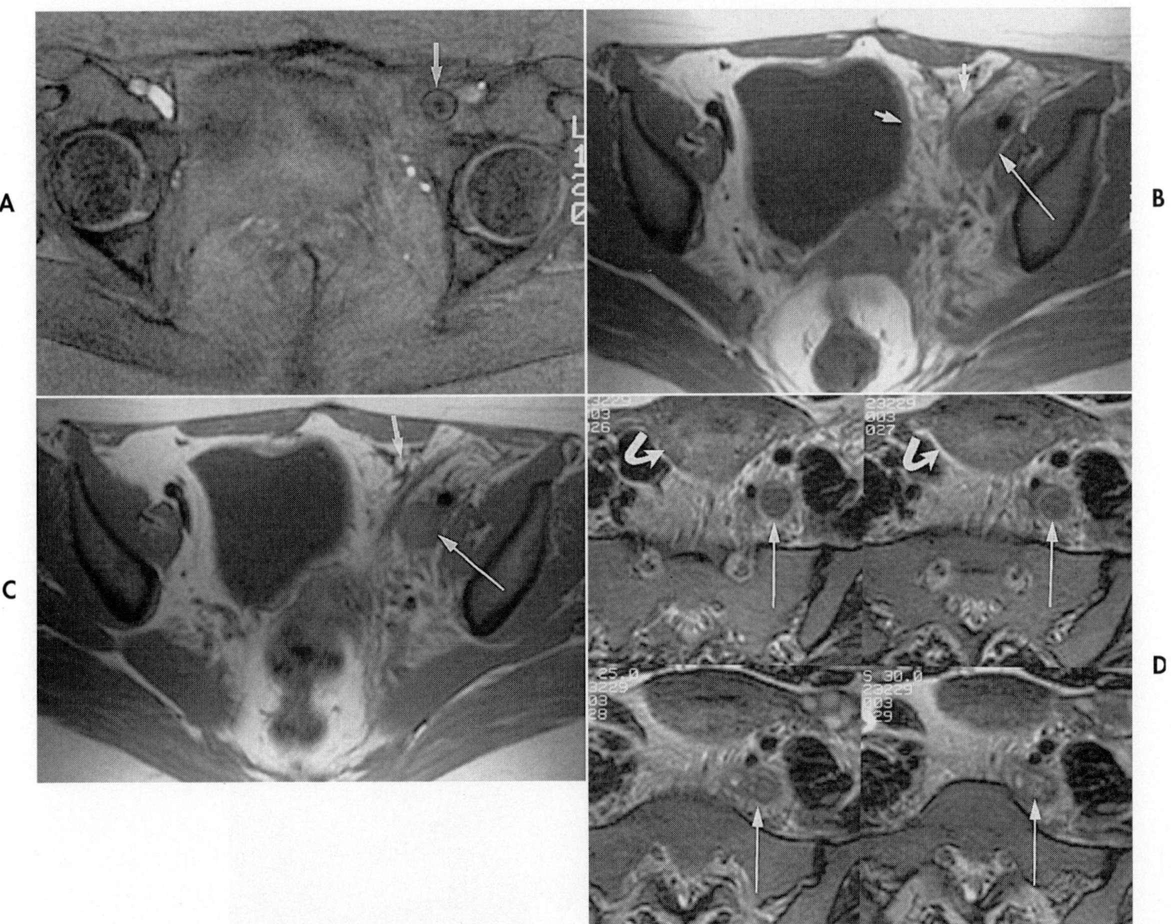

Fig. 10-28 Postpartum septic thrombophlebitis. This patient presented 7 weeks after an uncomplicated vaginal delivery with left leg swelling, fever, and elevated white blood cell count. **A,** Axial GRASS image at the groin shows complete occlusion of the left common femoral vein, which is distended with clot *(white arrow).* **B** and **C,** Axial T1-weighted images show the enlarged left external iliac vein *(long white arrow)* with extensive infiltration of the adjacent fat *(short white arrows),* compatible with inflammation. **D,** Axial FSE images progressing cephalad show the thrombus extending up into the common iliac vein *(long white arrows).* The postpartum uterus is seen *(curved white arrows)* anteriorly. The zonal architecture has not yet been restored.

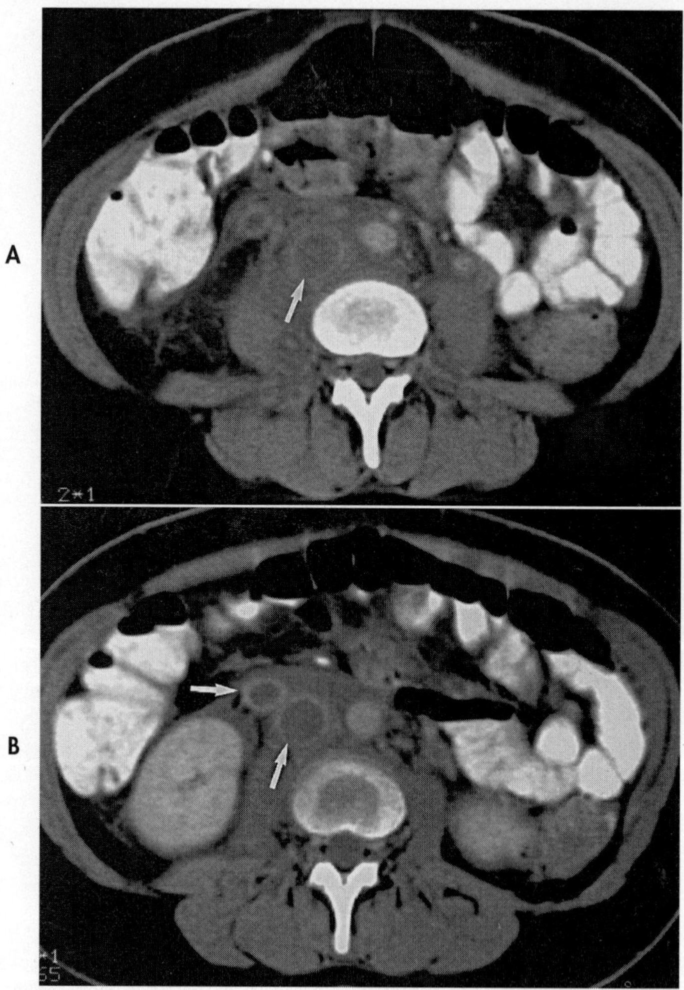

Fig. 10-29 Ovarian vein thrombosis. Axial computed tomographic images of the mid-abdomen show a large, low attenuation filling defect *(white arrows)* expanding the IVC and right gonadal vein in this woman 2 weeks postpartum.

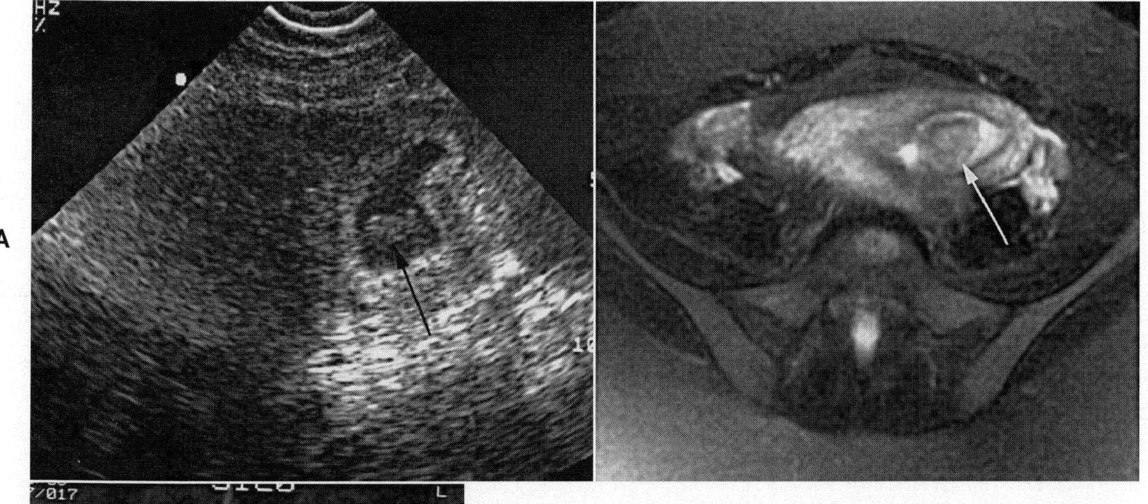

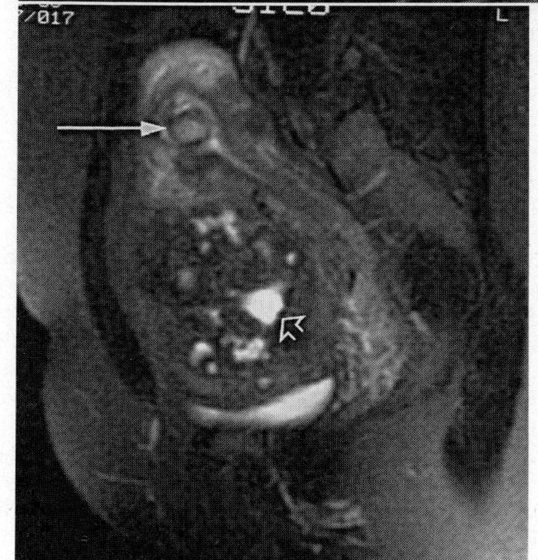

Fig. 10-30 Retained products of conception and a large leiomyoma. This 30-year-old woman presented 2 days after a miscarriage with persistent bleeding. **A,** Transvaginal ultrasound examination shows distention of the endometrial cavity, which contains echogenic material *(long black arrow)* compatible with clot or retained products. **B,** Axial fat-suppressed FSE image (TR 4000, TE 102) shows the same findings as the ultrasound examination; the cavity is distended with low signal intensity material *(long white arrow)*. **C,** Sagittal fat-suppressed FSE image shows the low signal material *(long white arrow)* to be in the fundus of the uterus, and the large anterior submucosal and intramural degenerating leiomyoma. The multiple foci of high signal *(open white arrow)* in the center of the leiomyoma are areas of cystic degeneration and necrosis.

gaining wide acceptance as an effective and safe imaging tool that supplies valuable information about maternal anatomy and pathology during pregnancy.

REFERENCES

1. Budinger TF: Thresholds for physiological effects due to RF and magnetic fields used in NMR imaging, *IEEE Trans Nucl Sci* NS-26:2821-2825, 1979.
2. Wolff S, Crooks LE, Brown P, et al: Tests for DNA and chromosomal damage induced by nuclear magnetic resonance imaging, *Radiology* 136:707-710, 1980.
3. Thomas A, Morris PG: The effects of NMR exposure on living organisms. I. A microbial assay, *Br J Radiol* 54:615-621, 1981.
4. Cooke P, Moris PG: The effects of NMR exposure on living organisms. II. A genetic study of human lymphocytes, *Br J Radiol* 54:622-625, 1981.
5. Prasad N, Lotzova E, Thornby JI, et al: Effects of MR imaging on murine natural killer cell cytotoxicity, *Am J Radiol* 148:415-417, 1987.
6. Prasad N, Lotzova E, Thornby JI, Taber KH: The effects of 2.35-T MR imaging on natural killer cell cytotoxicity with and without interleukin-2, *Radiology* 175:261-263, 1990.
7. Withers HR, Mason KA, Davis CA: MR effect on murine spermatogenesis, *Radiology* 156:741-742, 1985.
8. McRobbie D, Foster MA: Pulsed magnetic field exposure during pregnancy and implications for NMR foetal imaging: a study with mice, *Magn Reson Imaging* 3:231-234, 1985.
9. Heinrichs WL, Fong P, Flannery M, et al: Midgestational exposure of pregnant BALB/c mice to magnetic resonance imaging conditions, *Magn Reson Imaging* 6:305-313, 1988.
10. Prasad N, Wright DA, Ford JJ, Thornby JI: Safety of 4-T MR imaging: study of effects on developing frog embryos, *Radiology* 174:251-253, 1990.
11. Smith FW, Adams A, Phillips WP: NMR imaging in pregnancy, *Lancet* 1:61, 1983.
12. Johnson IR, Symonds EM, Kean DM, et al: Imaging the pregnant human uterus with nuclear magnetic resonance, *Am J Obstet Gynecol* 148:1136-1139, 1984.
13. Weinreb JC, Lowe T, Cohen JM, Kutler M: Human fetal anatomy: MR imaging, *Radiology* 157:715-720, 1985.
14. Lenke RR, Persutte WH, Nemes JM: Use of pancuronium bromide to inhibit fetal movement during magnetic resonance imaging, *J Reprod Med* 34:315-317, 1989.
15. Garden AS, Griffiths MD, Weindling AM, Martin PA: Fast-scan magnetic resonance imaging in fetal visualization, *Am J Obstet Gynecol* 164:1190-1196, 1991.
16. McCarthy SM, Filly RA, Stark DD, et al: Obstetrical magnetic resonance imaging: fetal anatomy, *Radiology* 154:427-432, 1985.

17. McCarthy S, Stark DD, Higgins CB: Demonstration of the fetal cardiovascular system by MR imaging, *J Comput Assist Tomogr* 8:1168-1169, 1984.
18. Lowe TW, Weinreb JR, Santos-Ramos R, et al: Magnetic resonance imaging in human pregnancy, *Obstet Gynecol* 66:629-633, 1985.
19. Creasy RK, Resnik R: *Intrauterine growth retardation.* In Creasy RK, Resnik R, *Maternal-fetal medicine,* Philadelphia, 1984, WB Saunders, pp 491-510.
20. Deter RL, Hadlock FP, Harrist RB: *Evaluation of normal fetal growth and the detection of intrauterine growth retardation.* In Callen PW, editor: *Ultrasonography in obstetrical gynecology,* Philadelphia, 1982, WB Saunders, pp 113-140.
21. Stark DD, McCarthy SM, Filly RA, et al: Intrauterine growth retardation: evaluation of magnetic resonance, *Radiology* 155:425-427, 1985.
22. Wax JR, Kuhlman JE, Callan NA, et al: Magnetic resonance imaging of the third trimester lung, *J Maternal-Fetal Invest* 1994;4:73-75.
23. Bowie JD, Rochester D, Cadkin AB, et al: Accuracy of placental localization by ultrasound, *Radiology* 128:177-180, 1978.
24. Powell MC, Buckley J, Price H, et al: Magnetic resonance imaging and placenta previa, *Am J Obstet Gynecol* 154:565-569, 1986.
25. Jaffe MH, Schoen WC, Silver TM, et al: Sonography of abruptio placentae, *AJR* 137:1049-1054, 1981.
26. Kay HH, Spritzer CE: Preliminary experience with magnetic resonance imaging in patients with third trimester bleeding, *Obstet Gynecol* 78:424-429, 1991.
27. Thorp JM, Councell RB, Sandridge DA, Wiest HH: Antepartum diagnosis of placenta previa percreta by magnetic resonance imaging, *Obstet Gynecol* 80:506-508, 1992.
28. Spanta R, Roffman LE, Grissom TJ, et al: Abdominal pregnancy: magnetic resonance identification with ultrasonographic follow-up of placental involution, *Am J Obstet Gynecol* 157:887-889, 1987.
29. Cohen JM, Weinweb JC, Lowe TW, Brown CB: MR imaging of a viable full term abdominal pregnancy, *AJR* 145:407-408, 1985.
30. Harris Gj, Al-Jurf AS, Tuh W, Abu-Tousef MM: Intrahepatic pregnancy: a unique opportunity for evaluation with sonography, computed tomography, and magnetic resonance imaging, *JAMA* 261:902-904, 1989.
31. Crooks LE, Sheldon PE: Magnetic resonance imaging of the female pelvis—initial experience, *AJR* 141:1119-1128, 1983.
32. Powell MC, Worthington BS, Symonds EM: The application of magnetic resonance imaging to gynaecology, *Br J Hosp Med* 35:393-403, 1986.
33. Kier R, McCarthy SM, Scoutt LM, et al: Pelvic masses in pregnancy: MR imaging, *Radiology* 17:709-713, 1990.
34. Weinreb JC, Brown CE, Lowe TW, et al: Pelvic masses in pregnant patients: MR and ultrasound imaging. *Radiology* 159:717-724, 1986.
35. Lavery JP, Koontz WL, Layman L, et al: Sonographic evaluation of the adnexa during early pregnancy, *Surg Gynecol Obstet* 163:319-323, 1986.
36. Togashi K, Nishimura K, Itoh K, et al: Ovarian cystic teratomas: MR imaging, *Radiology* 162:669-673, 1987.
37. Hricak H, Lacey C, Shriock E, et al: Gynecologic masses: value of magnetic resonance imaging, *Am J Obstet Gynecol* 153:31-37, 1985.
38. Hamlin CJ, Petterson H, Fitzsimmons J, Morgan LS: MR imaging of uterine leiomyomas and their complications, *J Comput Assist Tomogr* 9:902-907, 1985.
39. Togashi K, Kawakami S, Kimura I, et al: Sustained uterine contractions: a cause of hypointense myometrial bulging, *Radiology* 187:707-710, 1993.
40. Hricak H, Demas BE, Braga CA, et al: Gestational trophoblastic neoplasm of the uterus: MR assessment, *Radiology* 161:11-16, 1986.
41. Barton JW, McCarthy SM, Kohorn EI, et al: Pelvic MR imaging findings in gestational trophoblastic disease, incomplete abortion and ectopic pregnancy: are they specific?, *Radiology* 186:163-168, 1993.
42. Brown JJ, Thurnher S, Hricak H: MR imaging of the uterus: low signal intensity abnormalities of the endometrium and endometrial cavity, *Magn Reson Imaging* 8:309-313, 1990.

Appendix: TNM/pTNM Classification of Malignant Tumors

The cervix uteri, corpus uteri, and ovary are discussed in Tables A-1 to A-3 and illustrated in Figures A-1 to A-14.

Table 1 Cervix uteri: TN clinical classification

TNM categories	FIGO stages	
TX		Primary tumor cannot be assessed
T0		No evidence of primary tumor
Tis	0	Carcinoma in situ
T1	I	Cervical carcinoma confined to uterus (extension to corpus should be disregarded)
T1a	IA	Preclinical invasive carcinoma, diagnosed by microscopy only
T1a1	IA1	Minimal microscopic stromal invasion
T1a2	IA2	Tumor with invasive component 5 mm or less in depth, taken from base of epithelium, *and* 7 mm or less in horizontal spread
T1b	IB	Tumor larger than T1a2
T2	II	Cervical carcinoma invades beyond uterus but not to pelvic wall or to lower third of vagina (Fig. A-1)
T2a	IIA	Without parametrial invasion
T2b	IIB	With parametrial invasion
T3	III	Cervical carcinoma extends to pelvic wall and/or involves lower third of vagina and/or causes hydronephrosis or nonfunctioning kidney (Fig. A-2)
T3a	IIIA	Tumor involves lower third of vagina, no extension to pelvic wall
T3b	IIIB	Tumor extends to pelvic wall and/or causes hydronephrosis or nonfunctioning kidney
T4	IVA	Tumor invades *mucosa* of bladder or rectum and/or extends beyond true pelvis (Fig. A-3) *Note:* The presence of bullous edema is not sufficient evidence to classify a tumor as T4
M1	IVB	Distant metastasis

T, Primary tumor.
From Spiessl B, et al, eds: TNM atlas: illustrated guide to the TNM/pTNM classification of malignant tumors, ed 3, 2nd revision, New York, 1992, Springer-Verlag.

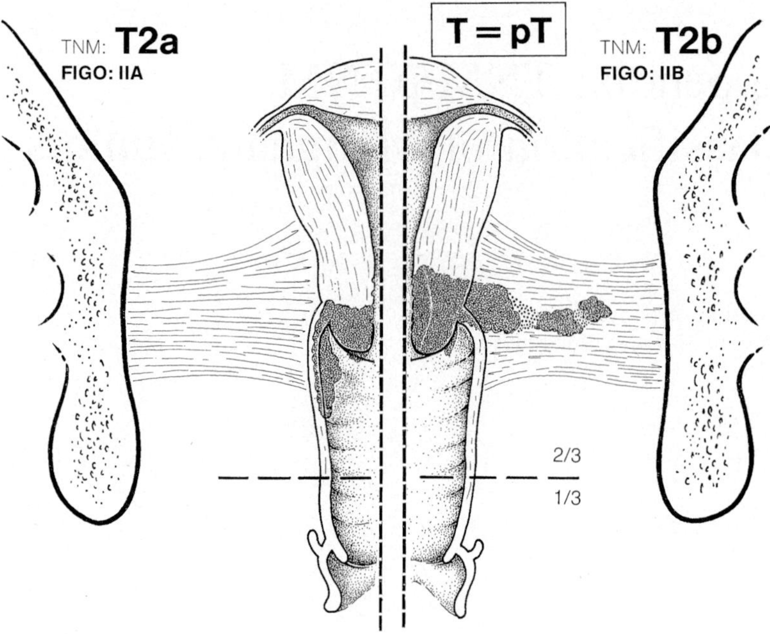

Fig. A-1 (From Spiessl B, et al, eds: TNM atlas: illustrated guide to the TNM/pTNM classification of malignant tumors, ed 3, 2nd revision, New York, 1992, Springer-Verlag.)

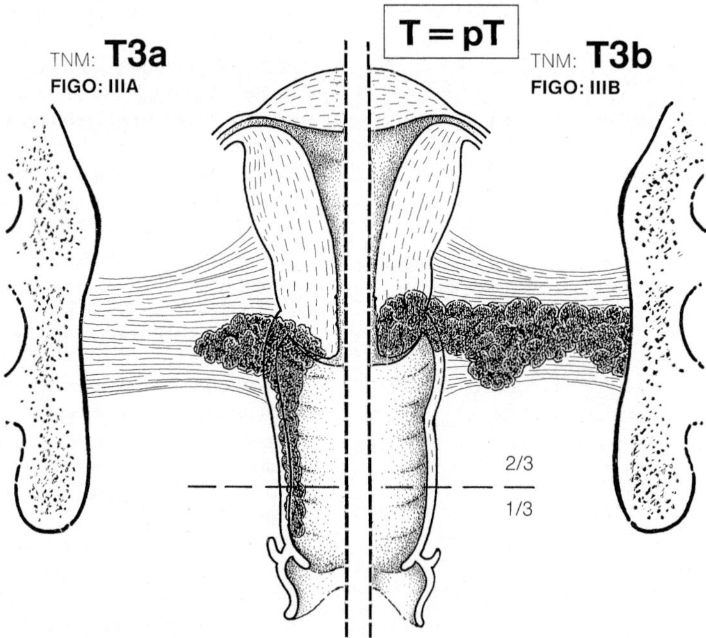

Fig. A-2 (From Spiessl B, et al, eds: TNM atlas: illustrated guide to the TNM/pTNM classification of malignant tumors, ed 3, 2nd revision, New York, 1992, Springer-Verlag.)

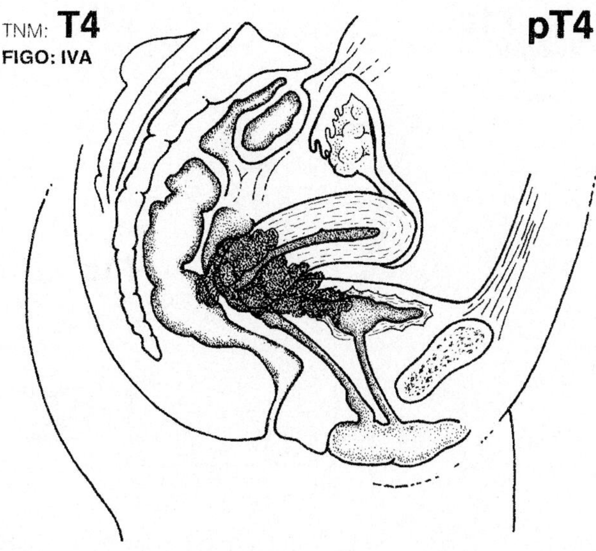

Fig. A-3 (From Spiessl B, et al, eds: TNM atlas: illustrated guide to the TNM/pTNM classification of malignant tumors, ed 3, 2nd revision, New York, 1992, Springer-Verlag.)

Table 2 Corpus uteri: TN clinical classification

TNM categories	FIGO stages	
TX		Primary tumor cannot be assessed
T0		No evidence of primary tumor
Tis	0	Carcinoma in situ
T1	I	Tumor confined to corpus (Fig. A-4)
T1a	IA	Tumor limited to endometrium
T1b	IB	Tumor invades up to or less than one-half of myometrium
T1c	IC	Tumor invades to more than one-half of myometrium
T2	II	Tumor invades cervix but does not extend beyond uterus (Fig. A-5)
T2a	IIA	Endocervical glandular involvement only
T2b	IIB	Cervical stromal invasion
T3 and/or N1	III	Local and/or regional spread as specified in T3a, b, N1 and FIGO IIIA, B, C below
T3a	IIIA	Tumor involves serosa and/or adnexa (direct extension or metastasis) and/or cancer cells in ascites or peritoneal washings (Fig. A-6)
T3b	IIIB	Vaginal involvement (Fig. A-6) (direct extension or metastasis)
N1	IIIC	Metastasis to pelvic and/or para-aortic lymph nodes (Fig. A-8)
T4	IVA	Tumor invades bladder *mucosa* and/or bowel *mucosa* (Fig. A-7)
M1	IVB	Distant metastasis (*excluding* metastasis to vagina, pelvic serosa, or adnexa, *including* metastasis to intra-abdominal lymph nodes other than para-aortic and/or inguinal lymph nodes)

T, Primary tumor.
Note: The presence of bullous edema is not sufficient evidence to classify a tumor as T4.
From Spiessl B, et al, eds: TNM atlas: illustrated guide to the TNM/pTNM classification of malignant tumors, ed 3, 2nd revision, New York, 1992, Springer-Verlag.

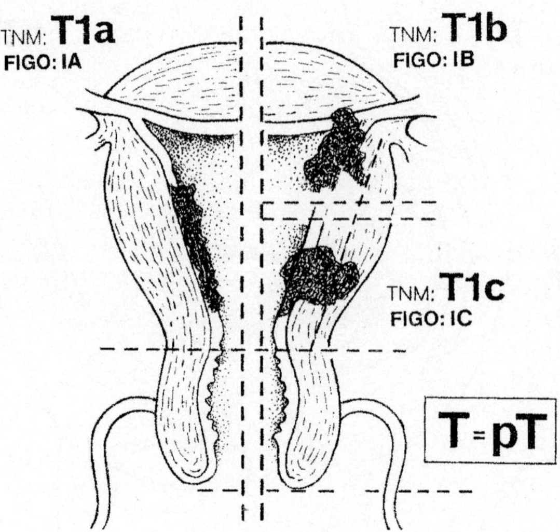

Fig. A-4 (From Spiessl B, et al, eds: TNM atlas: illustrated guide to the TNM/pTNM classification of malignant tumors, ed 3, 2nd revision, New York, 1992, Springer-Verlag.)

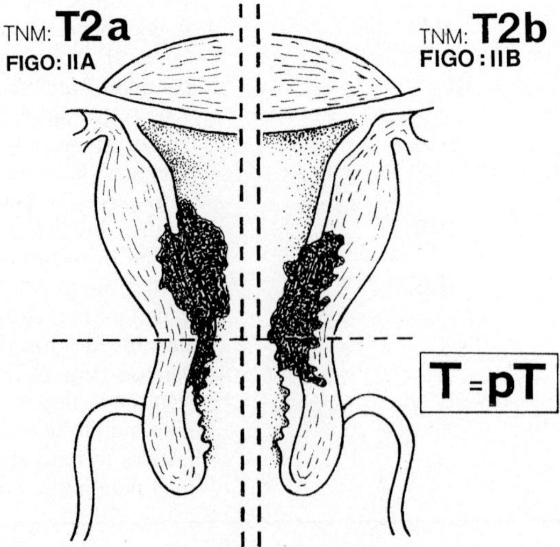

Fig. A-5 (From Spiessl B, et al, eds: TNM atlas: illustrated guide to the TNM/pTNM classification of malignant tumors, ed 3, 2nd revision, New York, 1992, Springer-Verlag.)

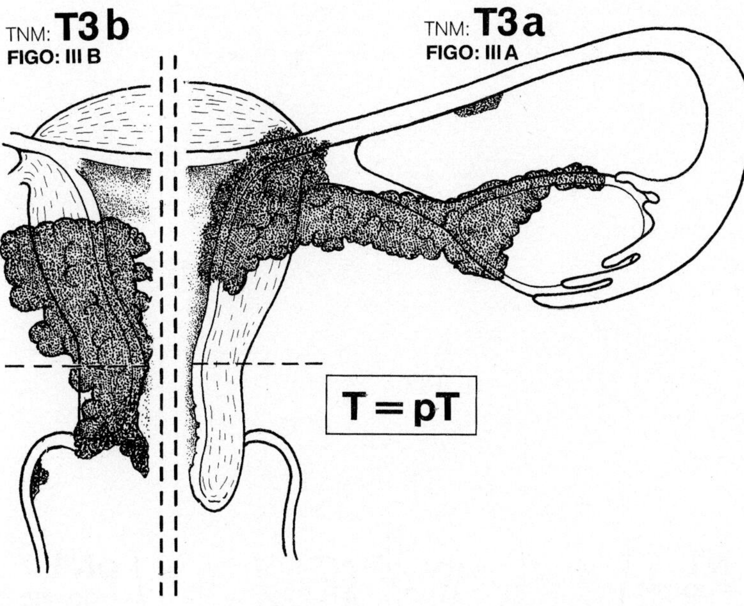

Fig. A-6 (From Spiessl B, et al, eds: TNM atlas: illustrated guide to the TNM/pTNM classification of malignant tumors, ed 3, 2nd revision, New York, 1992, Springer-Verlag.)

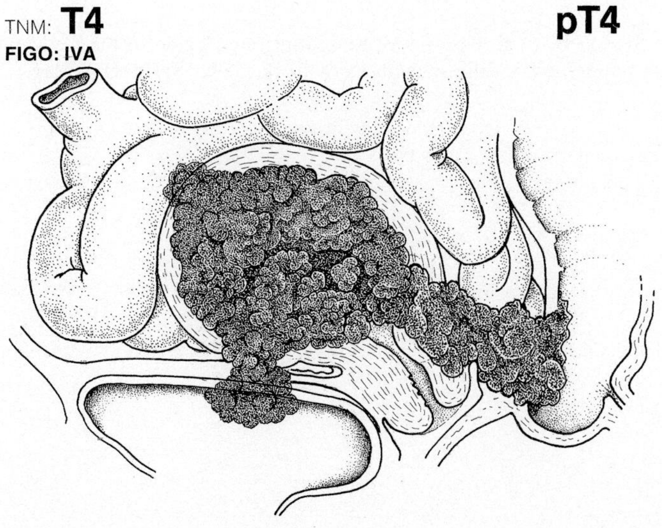

Fig. A-7 (From Spiessl B, et al, eds: TNM atlas: illustrated guide to the TNM/pTNM classification of malignant tumors, ed 3, 2nd revision, New York, 1992, Springer-Verlag.)

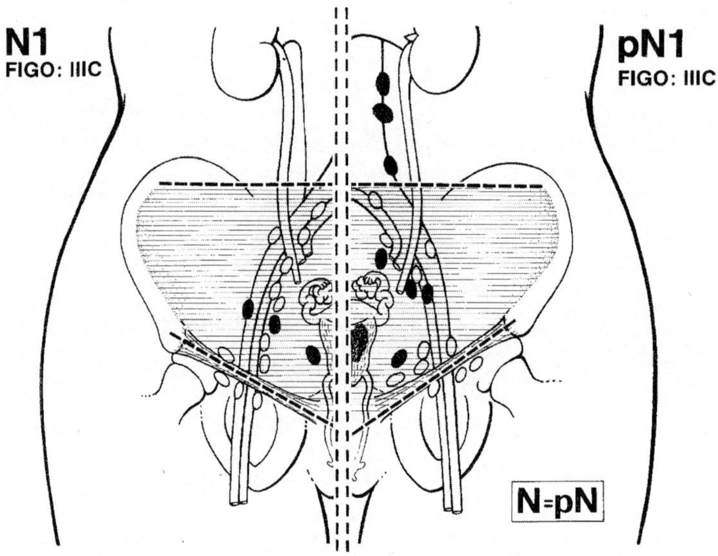

Fig. A-8 (From Spiessl B, et al, eds: TNM atlas: illustrated guide to the TNM/pTNM classification of malignant tumors, ed 3, 2nd revision, New York, 1992, Springer-Verlag.)

Table 3 Ovary: TNM clinical classification

TNM categories	FIGO stages	
TX		Primary tumor cannot be assessed
T0		No evidence of primary tumor
T1	I	Tumor limited to ovaries
T1a	IA	Tumor limited to one ovary; capsule intact, no tumor on ovarian surface; no malignant cells in ascites or peritoneal washings (Fig. A-9)
T1b	IB	Tumor limited to both ovaries; capsules intact, no tumor on ovarian surface: no malignant cells in ascites or peritoneal washings (Fig. A-10)
T1c	IC	Tumor limited to one or both ovaries with any of the following: capsule ruptured, tumor on ovarian surface, malignant cells in ascites or peritoneal washings (Fig. A-11)
T2	II	Tumor involves one or both ovaries with pelvic extension
T2a	IIA	Extension and/or implants on uterus and/or tube(s); no malignant cells in ascites or peritoneal washings (Fig. A-12)
T2b	IIB	Extension to other pelvic tissues; no malignant cells in ascites or peritoneal washings (Fig. A-13)
T2c	IIC	Pelvic extension (2a or 2b) with malignant cells in ascites or peritoneal washings (Fig. A-14)
T3 and/or N1	III	Tumor involves one or both ovaries with microscopically confirmed peritoneal metastasis outside pelvis and/or regional lymph node metastasis
T3a	IIIA	Microscopic peritoneal metastasis beyond pelvis
T3b	IIIB	Macroscopic peritoneal metastasis beyond pelvis 2 cm or less in greatest dimension
T3c and/or N1	IIIC	Peritoneal metastasis beyond pelvis more than 2 cm in greatest dimension and/or regional lymph node metastasis
M1	IV	Distant metastasis (excludes peritoneal metastasis)

T, Primary tumor.

Note: Liver capsule metastasis is T3/stage III, liver parenchymal metastasis M1/stage IV. Pleural effusion must have positive cytology for M1/stage IV.

From Spiessl B, et al, eds: TNM atlas: illustrated guide to the TNM/pTNM classification of malignant tumors, ed 3, 2nd revision, New York, 1992, Springer-Verlag.

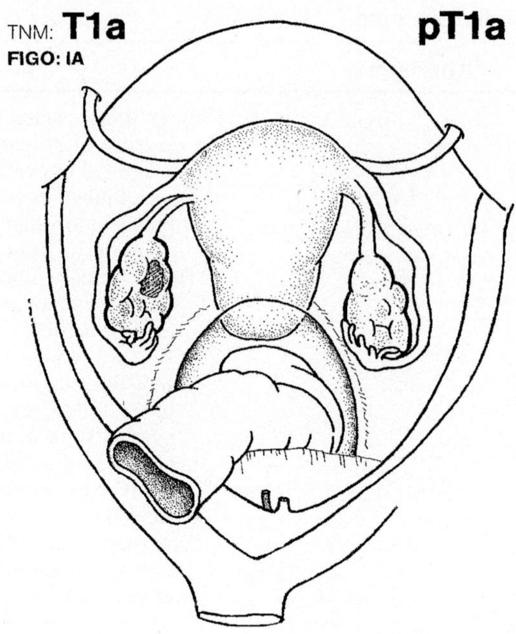

Fig. A-9 (From Spiessl B, et al, eds: TNM atlas: illustrated guide to the TNM/pTNM classification of malignant tumors, ed 3, 2nd revision, New York, 1992, Springer-Verlag.)

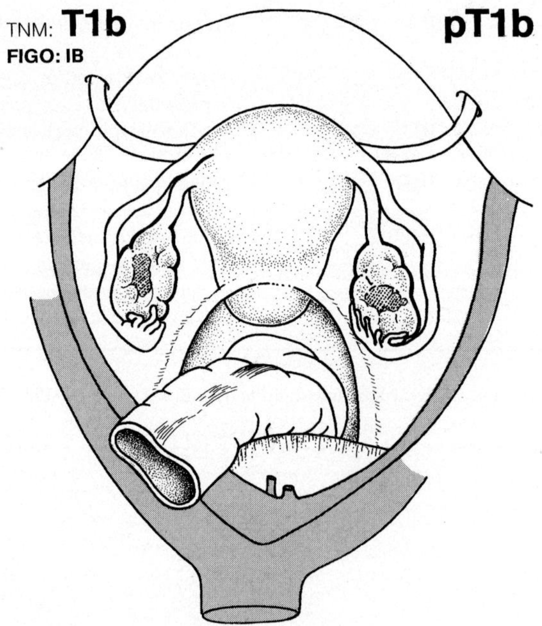

Fig. A-10 (From Spiessl B, et al, eds: TNM atlas: illustrated guide to the TNM/pTNM classification of malignant tumors, ed 3, 2nd revision, New York, 1992, Springer-Verlag.)

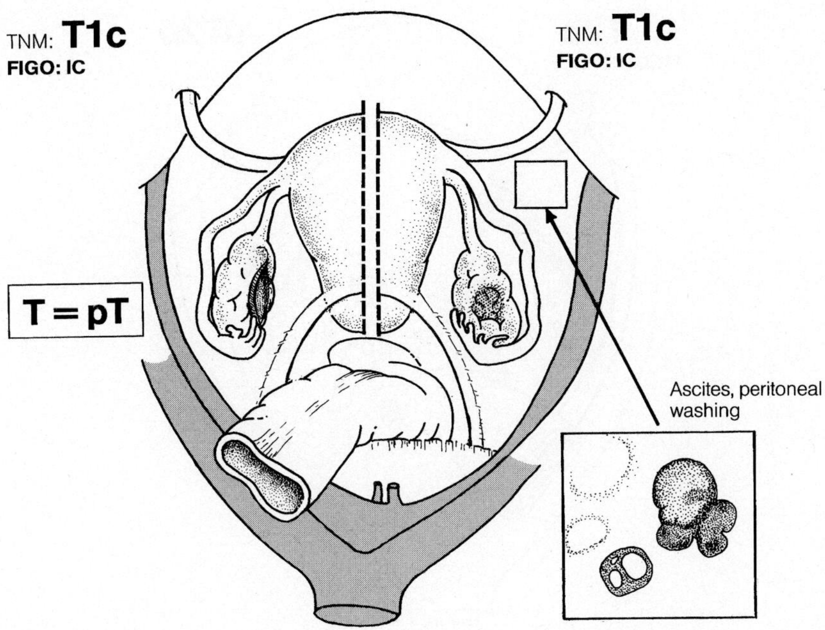

Fig. A-11 (From Spiessl B, et al, eds: TNM atlas: illustrated guide to the TNM/pTNM classification of malignant tumors, ed 3, 2nd revision, New York, 1992, Springer-Verlag.)

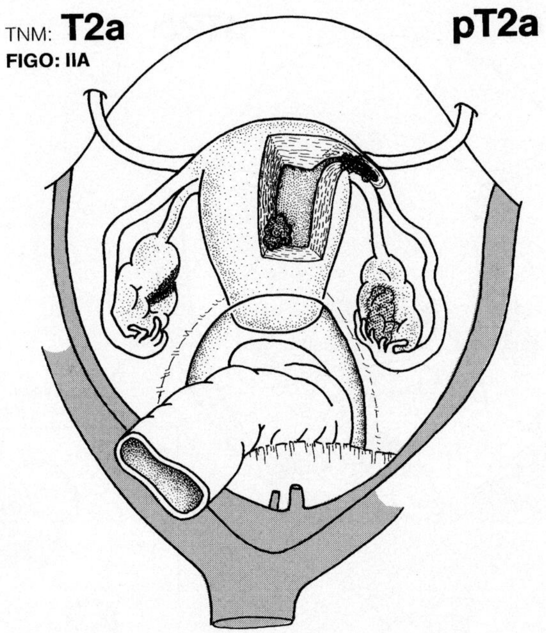

Fig. A-12 (From Spiessl B, et al, eds: TNM atlas: illustrated guide to the TNM/pTNM classification of malignant tumors, ed 3, 2nd revision, New York, 1992, Springer-Verlag.)

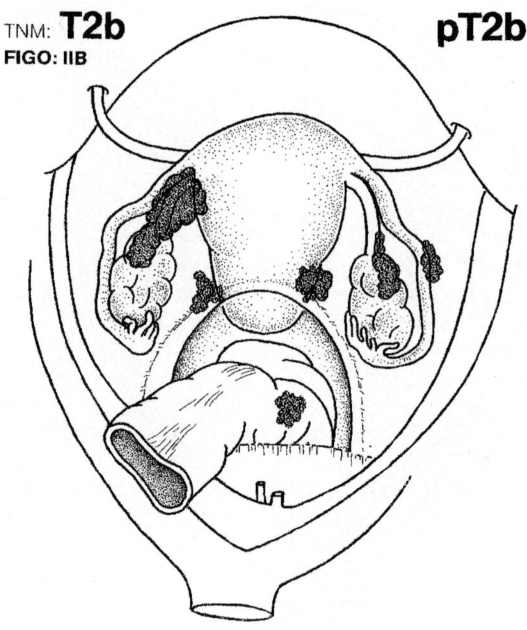

Fig. A-13 (From Spiessl B, et al, eds: TNM atlas: illustrated guide to the TNM/pTNM classification of malignant tumors, ed 3, 2nd revision, New York, 1992, Springer-Verlag.)

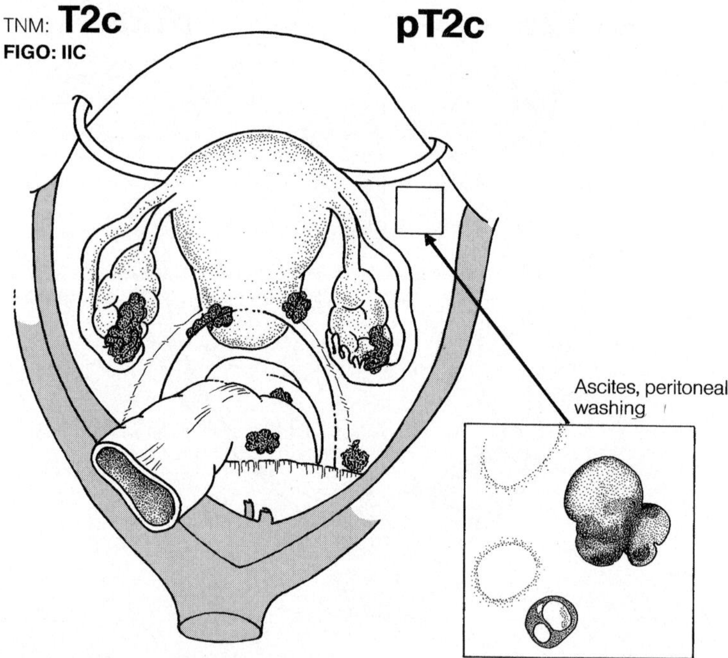

Fig. A-14 (From Spiessl B, et al, eds: TNM atlas: illustrated guide to the TNM/pTNM classification of malignant tumors, ed 3, 2nd revision, New York, 1992, Springer-Verlag.)

Index

A

Abdominal wall motion reduction, 62
Abdominopelvic abscesses, postpartum, 255
Abortion, spontaneous, 78, 86-88
Acquisition time, 32
Adenocarcinoma
    ovarian, 217
    poorly differentiated, 225f
    sigmoid, 221f
    uterine, 183
Adenomyoma, uterine, 151f
Adenomyosis, 149
    clinical presentation of, 149
    diagnostic techniques for, 149-153
    endometrial, 133f
    epidemiology of, 149
    multiple leiomyomas and, 153f
    pathology of, 149
Adnexal mass
    benign, 196-198, 199f
    computed tomography for, 200-205
    cystic, 200-201
    diagnosis of, 190-231
    Doppler ultrasonography for, 194-200
    GRASS image of, 230f
    high signal intensity, 212f
    with high vascular resistance, 197f
    hyperchoic, 201, 202f
    large, right, 224f
    with low vascular resistance, 196f
    malignant, 195-196
    MRI assessment of, 187-188
    during pregnancy, 248-254
    ultrasonography of, 185-186
    vascularity of, 198
Aging, patterns in bone marrow, 50-52
Air-stool interfaces, 50
Amenorrhea
    with Asherman's syndrome, 137
    with müllerian abnormalities, 86
American Fertility Society, müllerian abnormality
        classification of, 83, 84-85
Amniotic fluid, 242f
Anorectal anomalies, 100
Anorectal stenosis, 100
Antinuclear antibodies (ANA), 78
Anus
    ectopic, 100
    imperforate, 100, 101f
Arachnoid sleeve, 53
Artifact(s)
    phase encoding or ghost, 62
    techniques for reduction of, 62-70
    water/fat chemical shift, 27-28
Ascites
    detection of, 223
    in peritoneal carcinomatosis, 205
Asherman's syndrome
    diagnosis of, 137-138
    pathology of, 137
Avascular necrosis, 50
Axial plane T2-weighted images, cervical, 41

B

Barium
    enema catheter, 105
    oral and rectal, 59

Bicornuate uterus, 84, 86, 88, 94
    class IV, 77f, 89f, 93f
Biomagnetic effect, 30
Bladder, 46-48
    continence of, 53
    exstrophy of, 94, 97-99
    full, 49f
    pheochromocytoma, 217, 222f
    transitional cell carcinoma of, 106
Body coil, 59-60, 119f
    for cervical imaging, 116, 126-127f
    parameters for, 73
Bone marrow, 50
    assessment of, 50-52
    T1-weighted images of, 66
    tissue contrast in, 50-52
Bone metastasis, 174f
Bowel
    contrast agents in, 57-59
    lumen of, 48-50
    malrotation, shortening, and duplication of in cloacal
            exstrophy, 100
    peristalsis, blurring from, 62
    small, 48-50
Brain, fetal, 237-238
Breech birth, 88

C

Calcification
    of metastatic ovarian cancer, 208-209
    myometrial, 141-142
    ovarian, 217
Calcium-125, 189, 190
Cancer, ovarian, 189. *See also* Carcinoma, ovarian
    management of, 189-190
Carcinoma
    cervical, 118-120
        MRI of, 120-129
        recurrent, 129
    endometrial, 156-175
    ovarian
        CT staging of, 205-209
        MRI for, 188
        MRI in staging of, 223-231
    transitional cell, bladder, 106
Carcinomatosis, peritoneal, 226f
Cerclage, 94
Cerebrospinal fluid, 53
    intensity of in fetus, 239-240
Cervical carcinoma, 118-129
    bulky stage IIa, 124f
    exophytic, 122-123f
    extension of into parametria, 120-125
    extent of, 120
    FIGO staging criteria of, 120
    FIGO staging of, 254
    invading rectum and bladder, 125
    with invasion through cervical stromal ring, 125f
    metastatic, 68f
    pelvic side wall invasion of, 125
    squamous cell, 256f
Cervix, 35
    anatomy of, 116
    axial FSE T2-weighted images of, 44f
    axial image of, 118, 119f
    benign conditions of, 129
    endometrial tumor extension into, 165
    enlargement of, 64f